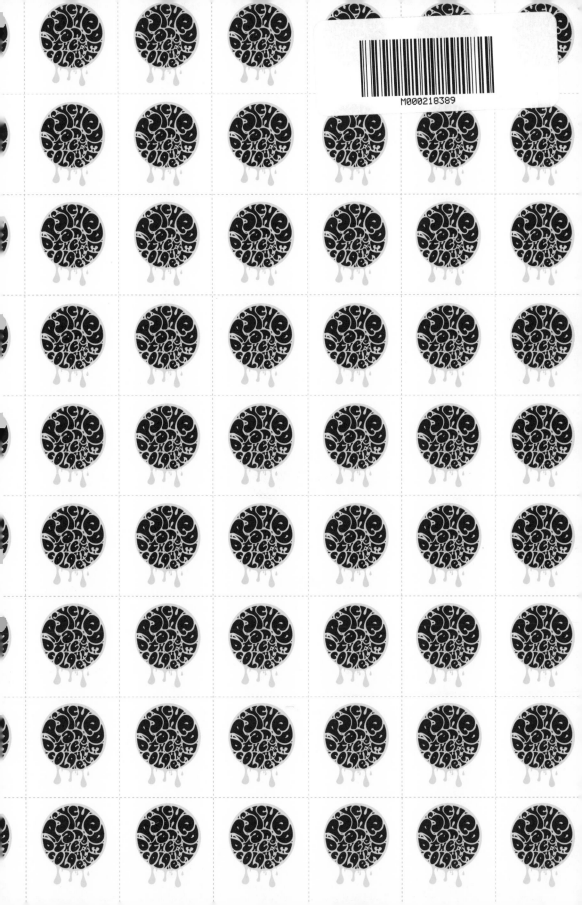

Psychedelia and Other Colours

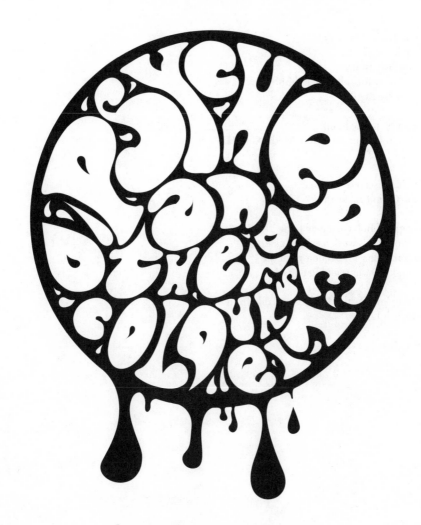

by ROB CHAPMAN

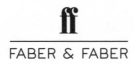

FABER & FABER

First published in 2015 by
Faber & Faber Ltd
Bloomsbury House
74–77 Great Russell Street
London WC1B 3DA

Typeset by Ian Bahrami
Printed in Germany by GGP Media GmbH,
Pößneck

A CIP record for this book is available from
the British Library

ISBN 978–0–571–28200–5

10 9 8 7 6 5 4 3 2 1

For Alice

CONTENTS

FOREWORD

by Andrew Weatherall

You're either on the bus or off it.
KEN KESEY

I owe my psychedelic nativity to Sarah 'Reb' McSweeney, the rockabilly queen of the Old Dean estate, and my pathetic, bravado-reeking attempts to woo her. 'Of course I've done acid before' – the answer to her question, 'Have you ever done acid before?'

I'd never done acid before.

I'll give you the full details of what ensued when next we meet, but it started with a rainbow piss and ended up with me recumbent on a bed (*sans* Ms McSweeney), a transistor radio pressed tightly to one ear, listening to the static between stations. Little did I know at the time that I was creating my own version of Terry Riley's 'Mescalin Mix', where 'everything seems to slow to a subsonic white noise that drifts in and out of audibility'. The bedspread was a universe in and of itself – sonic cathedrals and every molecule a majesty. The merest of triggers, like the merest of collisions that brought the universe into being, brought my psychedelic world into existence. And from day one I had no need for fractal orthodoxy. I was wearing Aldous Huxley's mythical grey flannel trousers. I was on the bus.

I got off the bus, after a decade's lysergic adventuring, at Silbury Hill in Wiltshire, where it dawned on me that the journey was over. This is the conclusion I came to when I found myself standing atop said structure, where, as Adam Thorpe writes in *On Silbury Hill*, 'a progress up the hill would enact the deepest movements of nature, a shape found in the double helix of DNA and in the structure of galaxies'. I was clad in monks' robes and clutching a gnarled staff which, in my mind, was instrumental in creating thunder and lightning. I eventually made it home and put myself to bed after very nearly jumping from a third-floor balcony into an imaginary swimming pool and then being moved to tears while watching the visual extravaganza accompanying 'It's All Too Much', courtesy of the Beatles' *Yellow Submarine*. Thankfully, I realised that were I to continue any further on my journey, my return ticket might expire and the next stop could well be a secure institution.

Sadly, this is a realisation that many don't get blessed with – a realisation that LSD is a key which, as Rob Chapman puts it, 'apportions its insights and discoveries in bright, spectacular starbursts, but the rest, my friend, is up to you'. A realisation that, in the words of the Zombies' Rod Argent, LSD 'always seemed quite a crude way to expand your mind'. What's also sad is that sometimes we imbue with superior magic the work of those artists who have incurred psychic injury having banged their heads on their way through the doors of perception. Somebody else's darkness brings light to our own. It's a price to be paid for art's vicarious thrills. It's why Kevin Ayers

is as underrated as Syd Barrett is overrated. It's pure conjecture, but Ayers's realisation could well have led him to write the line 'Beautiful people are queuing to drown' in 'Song for Insane Times'. I also think he knew that, rather than providing answers, LSD just threw up even more complex questions. Questions that would eventually gnaw at the guy ropes of sanity. Spend too much time focusing on definitive answers and you eventually forget the original question. Meanwhile, the real answers go sailing past in the midst of simply being and living. The answer, as Ayers pointed out in 'Whatevershebringswesing', is 'right there in front of your nose . . . so let's drink some wine and have a good time'.

I'm not saying don't get on the bus, because if you do there's every possibility of entering a world in which you are simultaneously both a central nucleus and a tiny atom in a universe of kaleidoscopic synapses. Strangely enough, a world just like the one described in *Psychedelia and Other Colours*: a world comprised of a central truth surrounded by a breathtaking network of mind-expanding connections.

Large works of historical synthesis based on secondary reading and the observation of contemporary history can only be written in maturity.

ERIC HOBSBAWM, April 2012[1]

Writing is in fact never anything but the poor and skimpy remains of the wonderful things each person has inside himself. What ends up as writing are erratic little clumps of ruins when compared to a complicated and splendid ensemble.

ROLAND BARTHES, April 1979[2]

ALL DRESSED UP AND LAUGHING LOUD

An Introduction

All of those present become comically iridescent. At the same time one is pervaded by their aura.
WALTER BENJAMIN[3]

I think the only remotely interesting drug was acid. I had a slightly peculiar attitude towards it I think. Just about everything about hippydom I hated. I liked the 60s up to about '65 or '66. I liked the mod clothes, I liked the look . . . I only did it three times myself and found it very interesting . . . I remember being very taken by very obvious things like sunsets and the silhouettes of buildings. But beyond that I wasn't very interested in the drug culture. I could see that the drug culture did not need to be like that. It could have been sharp suits and LSD.
JONATHAN MEADES[4]

We're taking the scenic route. I hope you're OK with that. The world really doesn't need another book about the psychedelic sixties, not one that tells the same story about the same bunch of people from the same tired old perspectives at any rate. Very early on in proceedings, when I was still undecided about whether or not to try and solicit new information from those who were there at the time, I was watching the DVD extras for *Magic Trip*, the 2011 documentary about Ken Kesey's fabled bus ride across America. Co-director Alex Gibney mentioned that he had originally intended to include new interviews with the surviving Merry Pranksters, but when he came to synch up the memories to the footage, he found them, as he put it, 'too rehearsed'. It's that over-rehearsed version of the story that I want to avoid

here. And besides, there's another tale that needs to be told. Several others, in fact.

The book's subtitle – 'And Other Colours' – gives me carte blanche to go the scenic route. It's my creative licence, my get-out-of-jail-free card (or at least on bail), but it's also an acknowledgement that psychedelia didn't just appear out of nowhere or exist in a vacuum. Part of my reluctance to go the well-trod route stems from my dissatisfaction with the increasingly crass way in which pop history is presented in the media. Pop documentaries on TV and radio (and most interviews in what is left of the quality music press) seem to have settled on an agreed history of the past. Guided by market-driven editorial edicts regarding who the significant artists are, who the permissible cult figures are and what the important events are, they present a non-negotiable narrative of epochs, icons and myths which becomes as self-fulfilling as it is tiresomely repetitious. This book is about many things but it's not about creating or consolidating orthodoxies. As grandiose and fanciful as it's going to look in print, I'm more interested in how this stuff might play out a century or two after we're all gone, when reputation and cultural baggage count for nothing and all that's left for future historiographers to haggle over is our memory essence and the residue of vibrating air. I'm also interested in what led up to all this – the first two hundred years of psychedelia, if you will. My 1960s might therefore be a little more elongated and expansive than the one you're used to. You might also find certain reputations inverted and others inflated beyond what you've previously encountered, but please remember there are no in-groups and out-groups here. Everyone is in.

I'm not one for regurgitating endless biographical details about band line-ups and the record labels they were on. You can find that kind of information in any number of well-researched (and sometimes not-so-well-researched) sources, if cataloguing is your thing. I'm fascinated by genealogy, but it's the genealogy of ideas that interests me here.

Similarly, if you weigh a book simply by its absences I can save you a lot of time right now. Countless groups – from Blue Cheer to Blues Magoos, from the Misunderstood to Skip Bifferty – don't get the attention that you might think they deserve in a book of some quarter of a million words. Leaving them out agonised me as much as it will you. My first draft contained half as many words again, and the stuff I sketched out or thought about, or envisaged including but didn't, is unquantifiable. In the process of writing *Psychedelia and Other Colours* I listened to thousands of hours of music, and hundreds of worthy endeavours didn't make the final cut. So if you get to the end of the concluding chapter and find yourself thinking, 'Hasn't he heard "Lazerander Filchy" by 49th Parallel or "Cover Me Babe" by the Sunshine Trolley?', well, yes, I have, and countless others like them. In fact, I listened to so much music that in the end it all became pleasingly, almost perversely generic. I began to appreciate psychedelia for its similarities as much as its differences. My listening aesthetic was rarely guided by records that were outstanding or exceptional, although many of them clearly are. As often as not I have mentioned them because they were typical – typical of the commercial tendencies of their time, typical of the marketing strategies that promoted them, typical of the mainstream they all swam in. In such transcendent moments music became codified patterns of noise, free of all extraneous detail. The moment I realised I was probably in too deep with this approach came early one Saturday morning as I was driving to the shops. 'Heroes and Villains' came on the radio and in my half-awake state I initially failed to recognise a record I'd heard a thousand times before. Instead, in those thirty seconds or so before cognition kicked in, I heard the extraordinary sound of a barbershop quartet on acid, much like Brian Wilson must have heard it on that first morning of creation. So, before you castigate me for not mentioning your favourite track off *Minnesota Garage Punk Rarities Volume 23*, please bear all this in mind.

For most publishers, including this one, the house style for indicating ellipses is three dots (. . .). I'd like you to imagine three dots on virtually every other page of this book as I stripped my 'grand ensemble' to its essence and left several themes unattended. At the outset I naively thought that there would be an opportunity to venture far beyond the Anglo-American model and to look at psychedelia's various global manifestations. When he was researching *The Right Stuff*, Tom Wolfe originally envisaged that the book would end with the moon landing. When he was a thousand pages into his draft and had only reached John Glenn's 1962 orbiting of the Earth, his wife commented, 'They're not going to the moon, honey. Not in this book anyway.' Getting to the moon in this book proved relatively easy, given the subject matter. Getting to Turkey, Brazil, Japan and Nigeria, on the other hand, proved to be impossible. Another book. Another lifetime.

On the subject of psychedelic music my subjectivity will be clear. On the subject of psychedelic drugs my philosophy might best be summarised as 'Neither a proselyte nor a prohibitionist be.' This is neither a book for drug bores nor drug banishers (he says hopefully). Much of what Jonathan Meades says above resonates with me; it didn't need to be like *that* is pretty much my watchword too. I was never much inclined towards the Cheech & Chong and Furry Freak Brothers end of things or the uniform (and uniformity) that went with all *that*. But either way, please try and keep an open mind. As the late lamented Trish Keenan of Broadcast once sang, 'It's not for everyone.' And if you don't agree with the categories I have constructed in order to make sense of the landscape, then create your own and may they serve you well. Better they serve you than the other way round. Ultimately, music is, I believe, a forum for our imaginations, not for fixed readings or what Alan Watts calls 'keenly callipered minds'. It ceases to belong to the artists the minute they present it to the world.

I had more to tell you but a person from Porlock called upon some urgent business an hour or so ago and the rest, I discover, is now just a blur.

Spending Some Time with Paradise People: Thanks and Acknowledgements

To Lee Brackstone and Dave Watkins, my editorial overlords at Faber, for keeping me off the straight and narrow. To my agent Sarah Such for helping bring all this to fruition. To Ian Bahrami for meticulous copy-editing. To Rob Young and Audun Vinger Johanssen for allowing me to dress-rehearse some of these thoughts at the By:Larm festival in Oslo in 2014. Likewise Deborah Carmichael at Michigan State University for the invitation to appear at the PCA/ACA annual conference in Boston in 2012, when this book was still just a kaleidoscopic gleam in my eye and a folder full of scribble.

Figuring that anecdotage and reminiscence wasn't really the way to go I carried out very few new interviews for this book, but I did incorporate and expand upon material from articles I have previously written on the Soft Machine, Kevin Ayers, Robert Wyatt, Marc Bolan, the Zombies, Procol Harum, Brian Jones, the Beach Boys, the Blossom Toes and Syd Barrett. Anyone who feels short-changed by the brief chapter on Pink Floyd is directed to my 2010 Syd Barrett biography A Very Irregular Head. Offcuts and an altogether better class of afterthought from the material gathered for that book also found a place here, for which I thank Peter Baker, Barry Miles, Pete Brown, Sebastian Boyle, Libby Gausden, Andrew Rawlinson, Anthony Stern, Nigel Lesmoir-Gordon and the irascible, cussed spirit of the late and very much missed Storm Thorgerson. Thanks also to Stan Shaff for additional information on Audium and Peter Coyote for his thoughts on the Diggers.

For additional research material I would like to thank the BBC Written Archive at Caversham, the British Library, JSTOR for access to all journals cited in the bibliography, Barney Hoskyns and the team at rocksbackpages.com for access to all pop press articles that weren't already in my attic archive, Ace Records, William McGregor and Jim Irvin, Janet Greenwood at the University of Huddersfield's library, Isabel Turner and Derek Ham at the BBC in Salford, Professor Rohan McWilliam at Anglia Ruskin University, and Cindy Keefer at the Center for Visual Music in Los Angeles.

Closer to home and to where the heart is: to Pete Upcraft and Neil Dell, with whom I've spent the best (and worst) part of forty years discussing, arguing, ridiculing and revering this stuff. To Gavin Brownrigg, Colin and Kate Lyall and all my fellow Salonistas at Lyall's bookshop in Todmorden. And finally to my wife Caroline, the ultimate cook of cakes and kindness, and to my daughter Alice, to whom this book is dedicated. It's dedicated to all the Alices, in fact, whether by name or by nature.

Rob Chapman, Todmorden,
autumn equinox, 2014

1

TO MAKE THIS TRIVIAL WORLD SUBLIME

The man who comes back through the Door in the Wall will never be quite the same as the man who went out. He will be wiser but less cocksure, happier but less self-satisfied, humbler in acknowledging his ignorance, yet better equipped to understand the relationship of words to things, of systematic reasoning to the unfathomable Mystery which it tries, forever vainly to comprehend.

ALDOUS HUXLEY, *The Doors of Perception*[1]

I am about to embark upon a hazardous and technically unexplainable journey into the outer stratosphere.

THE WIZARD OF OZ

'It Must Be to Do with Orange. Not Only with Orange'

'So far, are these visual things the only effects you've had?' asks the inquisitor, in his soft Scottish brogue.

'No,' says the dark-haired, wild-eyed girl from the planet Freecloud. As she speaks she rolls an orange in her hands like it's warm Play-Doh.

'What other effects?' the inquisitor persists.

'It's all to do with colour. It's all to do with round, with shapes,' she says in a hushed, childlike voice.

She inhales and lets out an exasperated gasp.

'Ah, everything's coloured,' she says, making a sudden dismissive hand gesture as if she's warding off some approaching cosmic storm.

'Ah, it must be to do with orange. Not only with orange,' she says, comically admonishing herself as she comes out with the qualifier. She opens her eyes wide when she speaks the second sentence, as if startled by her own sudden discovery about the nature of orange. She makes another delicate theatrical hand gesture and lets out another little gasp. Her thoughts continue to spill thick and fast.

'I haven't seen colour. I live in a monochromatic world,' she says, fixing her inquisitor with a witchy stare. All the time she continues to grasp the orange tightly, occasionally rolling it from palm to palm, as if letting go would break the spell.

'I can't use colour,' she says, and shakes her head sadly at this realisation.

She pauses again for a millisecond, or possibly several lifetimes. A look of infinite contentment plays across her face. She opens her palms as if to release the orange, like it's an exotic bird.

'I can do everything,' she says.

Later our softly spoken Scottish inquisitor talks to another well-elocuted young woman with shining saucer eyes. It's another sunny day in the long hot summer of 1966 and she's sitting on the grass outside. The hum of nearby traffic can be heard as she wriggles and fidgets.

'You've had a drug. Has it done anything to you yet?' the inquisitor enquires.

'Oh yes, yes, it's affected me,' she replies with commendable understatement. She leans forward, eager to help her inquisitor with his enquiries.

'In what ways?' he persists.

'Um, colours have become quite a lot brighter,' she says. 'It's like paisley effects in the sky.' She cups her chin in the dish of her hand and glances shyly skywards, avoiding her inquisitor's gaze. There is a suppressed giggle in her voice as she pronounces the vowel sounds of the word 'paisley' in a long-drawn-out posh-girl drawl.

'What do you mean by that?' asks the inquisitor sternly.

'Um, all the boxes are falling paisley patterns,' she says, making a trickle

pattern with her fingers and dissolving into cosmic merriment.

'If you haven't heard of LSD, you will,' the BBC presenter Fyfe Robertson warned viewers as he introduced a special edition of the magazine programme *24 Hours* on 27 July 1966, from which the above other-worldly encounters are taken. And he was right. Just three months after the programme was aired LSD was made illegal both in Britain and America. Despite the impending threat of legislation, the BBC's investigation into LSD use was remarkably fair, even-handed and non-sensationalist. Two separate groups of young people were filmed while high on the drug, one in London, the other in Brighton. The participants ran the gamut of psychedelic volunteers, from earnest scholarly explorers to giggly socialites. Subjects were captured in various stages of contemplation, befuddlement and bliss, but overall everyone seemed to be bearing up well despite the sensory onslaught and Fyfe Robertson's looming presence and cautionary tone. Essentially it is a meeting of two worlds. Watch what happens when planets collide, planet normal and planet otherworld. The orange girl and the paisley-patterns girl in particular look like they might have been pleasingly captivating company in which to while away an interstellar hour or two. Both are clearly airborne and mid-voyage by the time they submit themselves to the unfathomable how, why, what, where and when of their inquisitor's questions.

To the uninitiated – in other words, almost everyone – their responses would have seemed facile and empty-headed, verging on the imbecilic. 'They all struck me as being terribly pathetic and certainly didn't appear to be enjoying themselves,' was one response from an internal BBC panel viewer.[2] Another was equally disapproving: 'The film is quite frightening enough to put one off . . . if we came out like the girl with the orange it would be even more chilling.'

Viewing-panel participants were asked the question, 'If you found an easy source for obtaining LSD-25 and you knew it to be pure, would you take it?' Some answered the question directly; others took it as an opportunity to comment more expansively on the programme. 'NO,' said one participant. 'The look on the London group's faces put me off. Especially those awful girls!' 'I agree with it being used for medical research,' said another. 'But it is obviously too unknown a substance to be taken just for kicks.' Of those who answered yes, most stressed 'under medical supervision'. One or two made

it very clear that they might be amenable to kicks and were clearly intrigued enough by the film to want to experience the drug. 'Is the film meant to deter anyone?' asked another. 'I don't think that the type who would take it would be put off.' 'To the sensation seeker this film would be a sort of commercial,' agreed another. 'For this reason I don't think it should be shown.' 'It needs a warning . . . before the film and a sombre summing up afterwards,' said another. 'I don't think Robbie's present ending will do. It calls for something admonitory, but not too Calvinistic.'

The most astute respondent of all acknowledged that it might be too late for admonishments, Calvinistic or otherwise, and that the cat was already out of the bag. 'Although I would expect many marginal groups of young people to make an immediate effort to get hold of LSD-25 I would not expect this film to cause a large and permanent increase in the use of this drug. I think the real importance of the film is that it would be simply one of many factors making a probably minute contribution to the change of traditional values. This kind of change is intrinsically disturbing and some would say undesirable. But I think it is inevitable and anyway it's in mid swing.' And indeed it was. In the event the airing of the programme caused little fuss. There were no letters of complaint. The BBC's audience research for that night's transmission focused on the long-running antiques programme *Going for a Song* and the *Herb Alpert and His Tijuana Brass* show.

'The Most Extraordinary Gradations of Mauve'

Ten years prior to these jolly japes a more sedate, although no less revelatory, meeting took place. On Friday 2 December 1955, in the drawing room of his Surrey home and with television cameras present, the Labour MP and broadcaster Christopher Mayhew took 400 mg of mescaline under the medical supervision of his old school friend, Dr Humphrey Osmond, the man who just happened to have launched Aldous Huxley on his own maiden voyage. Stating that he was 'as sane as I ever am', Mayhew took the drug at midday. At ten past one the camera captured him sitting slightly slouched in his armchair, glazed and relaxed and grinning a Cheshire Cat grin that never left his face for the duration of the filming. At this point in proceedings he was particularly taken with a reddish curtain behind the cameraman.

'It's the colour of . . . damn, Humphrey,

I warned you that on colours my vocabulary is bad.'

Pressed to continue Mayhew was only able to confirm that 'it has the most extraordinary gradations of mauve'.

His interviewer conceded that he could only see a dullish red and wondered aloud whose judgement we should believe. 'Ah, now you're asking me the $64 question,' said Mayhew. 'Whether I'm seeing the curtain normally . . . or whether I'm intoxicated and seeing pink elephants.' He continued to gaze at the curtains, laughed, stared intensely, pondered some more and conceded defeat. 'Well, all I can say is it's still the $64 question,' he shrugged, with the distant air of a man who looked like he could ponder the $64 question all day long. Given the circumstances it seemed a cheap price to pay for his insight, genial company and urbane good manners. 'I'm looking very hard now, beyond the camera,' he continued. And indeed he was, off into distant galaxies and undiscovered solar systems, the location of which appeared to be somewhere among those mauve gradations of curtain, just below the pelmet.

A little later Humphrey Osmond informed the viewer that 'the time's now just on 14.00, and in the last half hour or so Christopher has been preoccupied to a very great extent with time, and we've had numerous discussions on this'. Issues of space and time exercised Mayhew greatly during the interview and he later described his mescaline experience as 'a state of euphoria that went on for months'. During the filming, though, he described it like this:

> *It's now eighteen minutes to three but I know now that my time and space changes, and that soon I shall go into a different time and a different space, which will seem instantaneous to you, I know, and therefore it will be as though I'm talking gibberish, as though I'd been here all the time . . . I quite see that, from your point of view, that'll look nonsense, but I do try and assure you that, from my point of view, between the time that I, perhaps, begin this sentence and the time that I end it, I shall have gone . . . a long time has elapsed, Humphrey.*

Mayhew drifts away several times during the afternoon. At one point Osmond tries to engage him in discussion about his altered notion of the 'here and now'. 'Could you tell us in what way that has altered?' he asks. 'You've told us there's another time which you're

experiencing, but I don't think you've said very much about what it means to you.' Mayhew responds with the same charm and civility he would have expressed had he just accidentally taken another man's brolly from the umbrella stand at his gentlemen's club. 'I'm sorry, you've just asked that question as I was going off, Humphrey,' he says distractedly. 'When I say "going off" . . . I didn't mean I was going to sleep . . . I mean that I was leaving your space, and your time . . . and going to this other space and time. And now I'm back again!'

At the peak of his mescaline trip Mayhew informs Osmond that 'I am moving, at this moment, from one time into another time . . . and back again. I'm not so conscious, Humphrey, of moving myself in space, but I am extremely conscious . . . of moving in time, of things having no succession and of there being no absolute time, no absolute space. It is simply what we impose on the outside world . . . and the more closely I feel this, the more relaxed I feel . . . the less I feel inclined to talk. Now I'm becoming of your level again, back again, Humphrey, and I know that you'll be smiling at that, probably.'

Director's voice (*off*): 'Cut!'

'About a name for these drugs – what a problem!' Aldous Huxley pondered in a letter to Osmond in 1956.[3] 'Psyche-delic' was the term everyone eventually settled for, but if Huxley had got his way the phonetically cumbersome 'phanerothymes' might have become the accepted synonym for the medicine chest of hallucinogens that was beginning to fascinate military minds, mystics, clinical researchers and intellectuals alike. Not that Huxley himself found it cumbersome. 'Euphonious and easy to pronounce,' he maintained. Huxley's original rhyming couplet read:

> *To make this trivial world sublime*
> *Take half a gramme of phanero-*
> *thyme.*

Osmond, dear sweet Humphrey Fortescue Osmond, a man with a kindly butter-wouldn't-melt face, countered with the phrase that launched a trillion trips:

> *To fathom hell or soar angelic*
> *Just take a pinch of psychedelic.*

'I have looked into Liddell and Scott and found that there is a verb phaneroein, "to make visible or manifest", and an adjective phaneros meaning "manifest, open to sight, evident",' said Huxley. 'Or what about phanerothyme? Thumos means soul . . . and is

equivalent of the Latin animus.' Humphrey's 'psychedelic' also derives from Greek: *'psihi'* (psyche) and *'diloun'* (manifest), which literally translates as psyche- or soul-manifesting, to make the soul visible. As we now know, Osmond won the terminology game – and it was a game. It's intriguing to note that the future language of Western consciousness expansion was settled by the playful exchange of rhyming couplets by two eminent men of letters, but while Osmond may have won the semantic battle, Huxley won the dialectic war, and his original suggestion retained more resonance. On the surface there is not a great deal of difference between manifesting the spirit and making the soul visible, but there is a world of difference in the assumptions behind each couplet. Osmond's version emphasised the demonic and the divine and gave rise to the enduring notion that LSD triggers mind-altering visitations that are either heavenly or hellish, with little in between. It was Huxley who wrote a book called *Heaven and Hell* and claimed that hallucinogenic drugs might allow us, briefly at least, to commune with saints and sages and see what Adam might have seen on the morning of his creation, but on his first mescaline trip Huxley also said that he marvelled at the folds in his grey flannel trousers. This mention of his drab apparel has always been held up as one of the ultimate symbols of the staid and starchy philosopher being transformed by his visions of beauty. In fact, the story is a myth. He was wearing blue jeans that day and his wife Maria made him change it in the manuscript, insisting that he ought to be better dressed for his readers. 'Oh, what a disservice she did there to Aldous,' said Huxley's biographer, Sybille Bedford. 'Blue cotton, blue linen, light-washed, sun-rinsed – who has not seen these transfigured in impressionist and post-impressionist paintings; postman's trousers, French railway porters' tunics, are magical almost by definition. How much more tolerable, more comprehensible, Aldous's raptures might have appeared had he only been allowed to admit to his blue jeans.'[4]

Indeed, those folds in his trousers ('a labyrinth of endlessly significant complexity!') led Huxley into a rapturous and slightly dotty digression on the role of drapery in the arts. He mused on the 'inexhaustible theme of crumpled wool and linen' in representations of the Madonna or the Apostles, El Greco's 'disquietingly visceral skirts and mantles' and Watteau's 'silken wilderness of countless tiny pleats and wrinkles', and seemed every bit as exercised by the infinite shimmering possibilities of the colour spectrum as Mayhew had been with his extraordinary gradations of mauve. Significantly, though, when Huxley was asked to close his eyes and contemplate the inner world, the results were 'curiously unrewarding', as he put it. Compared with his intensified visual impressions his inscape was altogether less marvellous. 'Brightly coloured, constantly changing structures that seemed to be made of plastic or enamelled tin,' as he wrote. '"Cheap", I commented. "Trivial. Like things in a Five and Ten."'[5] This 'suffocating interior' of dime-store trinkets and trivia, Huxley decided, was his own inner self reflecting back at him with a surprising degree of mundanity and self-loathing. 'I felt the lesson to be salutary,' he said, 'but was sorry none the less that it had to be administered at this moment and in this form.'[6]

In contrast to Osmond's heavenly highs and hellish lows, Huxley surmised that in order to reach the sublime a fair amount of trivia might have to be filtered out first. Everyone understands the commonplace and the mundane. We deal with it on a daily basis. The Romantic poets elevated it to a guiding principle. Keats called it the 'material sublime'. Concepts like heaven and hell are more intangible and abstract. One person's diabolic visitations might be another's pretty patterns. It was Huxley who told us that hallucinogens would allow us a glimpse into the world as Blake saw it, but he also made it clear that it was the everyday world that had to be transcended in order to get there. He warned that the euphoric effects were temporary – 'The Revelation dawned and was gone again within a fraction of a second,' he says at one point in *The Doors of Perception*[7] – and that the trivial would still be there when the drug wore off. 'We were back at home, and I had returned to that reassuring but profoundly unsatisfactory state known as "being in one's right mind",' he said with discernible regret at the end of his first mescaline experience.[8]

Nirvana by Numbers

Ever since Albert Hofmann first synthesised the chemical compound that is lysergic acid diethylamide-25 in the Sandoz pharmaceutical laboratory in Basle, Switzerland, in 1943, the history of LSD has never been anything less than contentious. 'The man who comes back through the Door in the Wall will never be quite the same as the man who went out,' said Huxley in *The Doors of Perception*. On that everyone was pretty much agreed. They agreed about little else. The only thing that remained indisputable was that once Albert Hofmann's colourless, odourless dream genie was out of the bottle, there was no getting it back in again.

LSD's powerful psychoactive properties eluded many of the existing criteria that mighty normally be applied to pharmaceutical analysis. The dosage is measurable not in milligrams, thousandths of a gram, but micrograms, millionths of a gram, and its effects are notoriously unpredictable. Two people given the same dosage in the same circumstances might yield wildly differing results. 'The variety is bewilderingly complex,' said G. Ray Jordan of LSD's multitude of effects, 'extending from schizophrenic-like delusion to enhanced perception of visual relationships; from paranoiac withdrawal to expansive recognition of the living interrelatedness of all beings in everyday life; from chaotic anxieties to a liberating experience of "union with God", which carries over into the commonplace.'[9] Neither a stimulant nor a depressant in the conventional sense, it is impossible to overdose on LSD. It is not physically addictive and has no biological side effects. Any damage that can be caused through misuse is almost entirely psychological.

From 1953 the CIA began to secretly fund LSD research and the US military tried to find a use for its psychoactive properties. LSD was tested as a truth serum, as an interrogative tool, as an agent of biological warfare and as an enabling and destabilising component in military operations. Although covert military experiments continued in both Britain and America throughout the 1950s and 1960s, it was conceded that the drug's volatile nature counted against it. It was hard to assess the reliability of an enemy's confession if at the same time he was telling you that he was at one with the moon, the stars and the sun.

The Christopher Mayhew footage, originally intended for use in an edition of *Panorama* called 'The Mescaline Experiment', was not shown at the time. A nervous BBC decided that a committee of psychiatrists, philosophers and theologians should assess whether the programme was suitable for broadcast. One of the main critics of the programme, Canon Besson of Cambridge University, decreed that Mayhew's mescaline-inspired insights were 'mystical adventures achieved on the cheap'. The Corporation eventually decided not to air the programme on moral and ethical grounds. No records of it remain in the BBC Written Archive

and the footage of Mayhew and Humphrey Osmond shot at the former's Surrey home did not resurface for many years. Watching it again thirty years later for a BBC2 *Everyman* special, broadcast in November 1986, Mayhew was unrepentant. 'It was the most interesting thing I had ever done,' he maintained, describing his mescaline experience as 'profoundly interesting and thought-provoking'. He accepted the psychologist's judgement made at the time that his space–time perceptions were impaired by the drug and that little time had in fact elapsed at all. 'But at the same time *they* didn't have the experience,' he remarked. Mayhew summarised that experience as 'not so many minutes in my drawing room interrupted by these strange excursions in time but years and years of heavenly bliss. I had these experiences and they were real,' he insisted, 'and they took place outside of time.' He strongly rejected the criticisms made by Canon Besson about the validity of his experience. 'You can dismiss it as a dreamlike hallucination which lasted a fraction of a second, owing to the disintegration of my ego and so on, or you can say it was a real experience that happened outside time. I would say that on that occasion *I did visit by a short cut* the world known to mystics and to some mentally sick people [emphasis mine].'

This 'short cut' aspect of the hallucinogenic experience – the idea that people were getting enlightenment on the cheap – was particularly problematic to theologians, but they were not alone in their concern. Prominent intellectuals and academics resented the application of what they perceived as pseudoscience to something as complex as human consciousness. Huxley controversially indicated that hallucinogens might allow temporary access to the world as the prophets and poets saw it, but this claim had come with caveats. He compared his mescaline experiences with 'what Catholic theologians call "a gratuitous grace," not necessary to salvation but potentially helpful and to be accepted thankfully, if made available'.[10] In their rush to condemn Huxley most of his critics chose to ignore the caveats. Louis Lasagna, academic dean of the School of Medicine at Tufts University, considered *Doors of Perception* 'the result of unusual . . . romantic proclivities',[11] while the scientist Ronald Fisher remarked that 'the book contained 99 per cent Aldous Huxley and only one half gram mescaline'.[12] R. C. Zaehner, in his book *Mysticism, Sacred and Profane*, had no truck with Huxley's view of the trivial made sublime and experienced only the trivial when he took the drug. 'In Huxley's terminology "self-transcendence" of a sort did take place,' he admitted, 'but transcendence into a world of farcical meaninglessness. All things were one in the sense that they were all, at the height of my manic state, equally funny.'[13] 'Not everyone who took one or another of the psychedelic substances understood the experience alike,' said R. A. Durr, in a far more conciliatory tone. 'Some understood it not at all – their visions were meaningless marvels – and some understood simply that their minds and senses were temporarily abnormal.'[14] This rationalist riposte was favoured by many of Huxley's critics, who declared that his visionary impulses were fraudulent and those romantic proclivities of his were not to be trusted.

Arthur Koestler also criticised Huxley in his essay 'Return Trip to Nirvana', evoking the Austrian mountains he had climbed in his schooldays, when it used to take five to six hours to scale a 7,000ft peak. 'Today, many of them can be reached in a few minutes by Cable-Car, or ski-lift, or even by motorcar,' he noted. 'Yet you still see thousands of schoolboys, middle-aged couples and elderly men puffing and panting up the steep path, groaning under the load of their knapsacks.' Koestler clearly favoured the individual who climbs the mountain over the one who takes the easier route. 'My point is not the virtue of sweat and toil,' he said. 'My point is that, although the view is the same, their vision is different from those who arrive by motorcar.'[15]

Philosopher and religious teacher Alan Watts encountered no such problems when he took the cable-car ride to the summit. Well acquainted with Chinese, Japanese and Hindi sacred texts, with Zen Buddhism and the rigorous teachings of yogis, Watts thoroughly enjoyed what he called his 'eight-hour exploration courtesy of the Sandoz Company'. 'For me the journey was hilariously beautiful. I and all my perceptions had been transformed into a marvellous arabesque or multidimensional maze in which everything became transparent, translucent and reverberant with double or triple meaning. Every detail of perception became vivid and important, even ums and ers and throat clearing when someone read poetry, and time slowed down in such a way that people going about their business outside seemed demented in failing to see that the destination of life is this eternal moment.'[16]

Koestler's judgement was coloured in no small part by his own less than favourable experience as a volunteer patient, when he clearly experienced more of Osmond's heaven and hell than Huxley's trivial made sublime. 'At the University of Michigan there was an awfully nice English psychiatrist. It was because he was so nice that I first took the psilocybin mushroom,' he told the *Paris Review* in 1984. 'It was extremely frightening. When I was under, I noticed that the nice English psychiatrist had a scar on his neck – from a mastoid operation perhaps. His face went green and the scar started gaping as a wound and for some reason I thought, "Now at last the Gestapo have got me." Or was it the KGB? It was one of the two. The psychiatrist had a standard lamp and the base of it suddenly developed bird's claws. Then I flipped for a moment into normality and told myself, "You are hallucinating, that's all – if you touch the claws they'll go away." So I touched them. But they didn't go away. Not only a visual but also a tactile hallucination . . . when I came back from this experience of induced schizophrenia, the after effects lasted for several months . . . I came to the opposite view to Huxley's. These things have no particular spiritual value but they might have clinical value.'

The psychiatric community agreed and initially utilised LSD as a psychotomimetic in order to replicate the conditions of psychosis and other delusional mental conditions so that they might further understand those same schizophrenic episodes that Koestler had endured. Many eminent medical practitioners, including Humphrey Osmond in Canada, Sidney Cohen in the US and Ronald Sanderson in Britain, tested the drug on themselves to gain insight into what it did to others. Cohen, who had first observed how the drug caused 'a transient psychosis in all subjects',[17] was one of the first to foresee its potential use in understanding the biochemical factors behind mental illness. When he took the drug in October 1955, he was pleasantly surprised by the results. Instead of being catapulted into madness he found that 'the problems and strivings, the worries and frustrations of everyday life vanished; in their place was a majestic, sunlit, heavenly inner quietude'.[18]

In 1957 Cohen and his assistant Betty Eisner began administering LSD to volunteer psychotherapy patients. This strategy represented a radical shift in the psychiatric use of LSD, away from the psychotomimetic model towards rehabilitation of the patient. Eisner was at the time a doctoral student at UCLA and had been Cohen's first LSD test volunteer in 1955. She had a less clinically objective approach towards the drug's uses, which would

eventually lead to a falling out with Cohen, but while they worked together their results were impressive. Cohen, though, began to distance himself from Eisner's more empathetic approach. 'It does not seem to me that Betty is the ideal therapist for an investigation of this sort,' he wrote in March 1958. 'Her personal investment in the success of LSD therapy tends to reduce the validity of her results.'[19]

Paradoxically, those same kick-start methods that theologians and philosophers objected to would come to play a crucial role in the therapeutic application of LSD. Using LSD as a 'booster mechanism' became a central tenet of psychotherapy in the 1950s. The drug's capabilities were seen as beneficial to releasing early-life trauma and other issues that might be buried deep in the unconscious. Outlining 'the advantages of LSD therapy as compared to conventional therapy', Eisner stated: 'LSD makes available, from the very first session, other levels of consciousness which might require months or years of conventional therapy to effect. Rapport is greatly enhanced, transference is speeded, and material from the past is far more accessible.'[20] Some distrusted this approach for the very same reasons they dismissed the spiritual benefits of the drug, and they cast doubt on the revelatory dimension of LSD use. Disparaging the drug's use in treating alcoholics, William Vernon Caldwell stated: 'Can we believe that in one session, a maximum of four to six hours of therapy, fifteen years of bad childhood conditioning, traumatic experiences, and a lifetime of lopsided neurotic adjustment can be erased?'[21]

Humphrey Osmond was similarly wary of some of the more tenuous claims made on behalf of Freudian analysis. 'It is all very well trotting out the old oceanic uterine womb life stuff,' he said, 'but far from explaining anything that only makes it all the more odder.'[22] Osmond was equally sceptical about past-life regressions. 'Deeply interested in the previous existences business,' he wrote to Betty Eisner, 'but the great danger is that it may become just a fad.'[23]

Bears Not Squirrels

What clearly emerged from the early days of LSD research was that everyone was getting the results they wanted. Those who adopted the psychotomimetic model found the psychosis they were looking for. Psychoanalysts expressed their findings in psychoanalytical terms, physiologists described them in physiological terms.

Freudians found evidence of their Freudian theories, Jungians validated their Jungian archetypes. Behavioural therapists identified appropriate behaviour traits. Prohibitionists described LSD in morally problematic terms, proselytes described it in evangelical and utopian ones. Others who trod a more neutral path doubted if LSD had any value at all, and treated it as one of those periodic medicinal aberrations to be filed away next to phrenology, trepanning and bloodletting.

LSD was also put to uses that were ethically dubious to say the least. In the 1950s it was frequently used in conjunction with ECT on vulnerable psychiatric patients. In the US treatment often involved a cocktail of LSD and methylphenidate (i.e. Ritalin). It was also administered to children as young as five and to pregnant women. Equally contentiously LSD was used to treat marital problems, female frigidity, male impotence, homosexuality and perversion. All of these were grouped together for the most dubious of classificatory purposes. Treating frigidity with LSD involved little more than making sexually unresponsive women compliant to the desires of their undesirable husbands. The methods used (and the coercive psychobabble that often went with it) seemed expressly designed to turn a generation of recalcitrant proto-feminists into Stepford Wives. If those dubious strategies seemed guaranteed to singlehandedly politicise a generation of women, the use of LSD in the 'treatment' of homosexuality came from the Dark Ages and was often used in conjunction with the then fashionable technique of aversion therapy, in which the patient was shown a photo of an attractive male and simultaneously given an electric shock. These treatments formed part of a wider strategy of using LSD to reintegrate undesirable and antisocial elements back into normal society. Such usage was clearly ideological and the fact that these barbaric methods were given legitimacy (and funding) speaks volumes about the priorities of clinical psychology back then. Even though some of these social-conditioning techniques were no different to those developed by the CIA, they raised very little apprehension among the psychiatric community at the time. It was far more worried that its more liberal practitioners might be taking fraternisation too far and indulging in LSD free-for-alls with their patients.

Hovering over all this, of course, is the spectre of Timothy Leary and his colleagues, whose unconventional research methods got them kicked out of Harvard in 1963. But the arguments in favour of criminalisation had begun long before Leary appeared on the scene. The received wisdom is that prohibitive laws were passed in response to Leary's irresponsible behaviour and his increasingly messianic role in promoting the drug. Such a viewpoint readily assumes that people were not already taking LSD recreationally. In 1959 film star Cary Grant told a Hollywood gossip columnist that he had taken it over sixty times in therapy, remarking that since he took the drug, 'young women have never before been so attracted to me'.[24] When Timothy Leary later made similar claims for LSD's libidinous properties in a *Playboy* magazine interview, these salacious details were readily seized upon by the sin- and sensation-seekers of the popular press. But the truth is that several years before the free-love generation began preaching its sexual politics, LSD was being used freely at swingers parties, among Hollywood and New York socialites, and by the Hugh Hefner *Playboy* crowd, as hosts began to spice up their gatherings with a little lysergic aphrodisiac. As well as being fashionable LSD therapy was lucrative too. 'What frightful people there are in your profession,' wrote Aldous Huxley to Humphrey Osmond. 'We met two

Beverly Hills psychiatrists the other day, who specialized in LSD therapy at $100 a shot – To think of people made vulnerable by LSD being exposed to such people is profoundly disturbing.'[25] Others claimed that therapists were charging up to $500 for a session, even though Sandoz Pharmaceuticals provided the drug without charge. A lot of therapists got rich quick off this kind of exploitation, and their unethical activities did much to remove LSD from the realm of the mystics and the medics and into the opportunist hands of the alternative snake-oil salesmen. In this respect Timothy Leary's unconventional research methods at Harvard were simply part of a well-established lineage of medicine-show hucksterism.

In 1957 Sidney Cohen acted as technical consultant on a US TV special about LSD called *The Lonely World*. The following year he was an advisor on an eight-part series called *Focus on Sanity*. In the latter he is seen interviewing a young housewife who describes her LSD experience in awe-struck detail. The footage is readily accessible on the Internet and shows a pretty, petite, dark-haired American housewife undergoing a similarly transformative experience to that enjoyed by Fyfe Robertson's subjects in the BBC *24 Hours* documentary. 'Everything is in colour and I can feel the air. I can see it, I can see all the molecules – I'm part of it. Can't you see it?' she says an hour after taking LSD at the Veteran's Administration Hospital in Los Angeles. Dr Cohen asks her how she feels inside. 'Inside?' she replies. 'I don't have any inside.' She remains poised throughout her experience, her expression frozen in permanent childlike wonder, as if planets are whizzing by at a million miles an hour right in front of her face. 'I am one. You have nothing to do with it,' she says softly and without a trace of rancour. 'The dimensions and all the prisms and the rays. I've never seen such infinite beauty in my life.' She talks slowly, deliberately, as if measuring the value of every word. 'It's too beautiful. Can't you feel it? Can't you see it?' she implores. 'What should I see?' asks Cohen. There is a lengthy pause. 'I wish I could talk in Technicolor,' she says. 'Such a pity that America squandered its greatest natural resource,' says one of the comments on YouTube: '1950s housewives.'

Long before American housewives started appearing on prime-time TV to share their LSD experiences it had become abundantly clear that there was a lack of adequate terminology with which to describe the drug's euphoric effects. Conventional vocabulary was found wanting when it came to articulating the sheer otherness of the voyage, and even the most distinguished practitioners fell back on the familiar romantic tropes of the infinitesimal when it came to illustrating the drug's sensory parameters. Early LSD pioneer Al Hubbard called the drug 'my god of the galaxies'. Sidney Cohen called a book *The Beyond Within*. Alan Watts called one of his *A Joyous Cosmology*. Stanislav Grof's pioneering study was entitled *LSD: Doorway to the Numinous*. From their titles alone these works acknowledged that although heaven might be glimpsed in a grain of sand or from a cable-car ride to a mountain top, the insights gained were not readily expressible in common everyday parlance. For many participants the profundity of the experience could only be conveyed by a string of inadequate superlatives as everything was reduced to a universal 'wow'.

Even more problematic was the research environment itself. Psychiatrists favoured controlled experiments in a closely monitored clinical setting, while psychotherapists preferred more informal and relaxed encounters involving group interaction. To advocates of the latter the problem with the former was the very notion of a controlled environment. Betty Eisner called it 'putting parameters around infinity' and recalled without fondness the test conditions of her own maiden voyage. 'All I could remember of that first LSD experience was that I was constantly being interrupted in order to take tests,' she remarked.[26]

When Alice is undergoing her rapid changes in size in Wonderland she attempts numerous strategies in order to cling to clarity and reason. First she attempts her multiplication tables: 'Let me see: four times five is twelve, and four times six is thirteen, and four times seven is – oh dear! I shall never get to twenty at that rate.' Next she tries her hand at geography: 'London is the capital of Paris, and Paris is the capital of Rome . . .' She also tries to recite 'How Doth the Little Busy Bee' but, as she later explains to the caterpillar, 'it all came out different'.[27] Christopher Mayhew was required to put parameters around infinity too as he embarked upon his mescaline journey, and like Alice he found words and logic inadequate tools for the task. This being the scientifically rational 1950s rather than Carroll's scientifically rational 1850s Mayhew was also required to undergo his own version of the 'How Doth the Little Busy Bee' test. At different stages during the afternoon

Humphrey Osmond gets him to repeat the adage 'To be rich and prosperous a nation must have a safe, secure supply of wood.' When he attempts the sentence at 1.10 p.m., seventy minutes into his trip, Mayhew misses out the words 'safe' and 'secure'. When he attempts it again at 2.00 p.m., he repeats it faultlessly. 'I got the two,' he exclaims with schoolboyish glee, so pleased is he at having negotiated the alliteration hurdle. 'Well done,' says Osmond politely. Mayhew was also required to undertake a subtraction test, taking seven from a hundred in successive stages, 'until there's nothing left', as Osmond puts it, a statement that might have messed considerably with a less finely tuned mind. Subtraction proves a little harder than memorising a mantra about the nation's dependence on a safe supply of wood. Mayhew does OK until he gets down to twenty-three, at which point he departs from the task, offering a cheery 'Now I'm off again, Humphrey' by way of explanation. 'In my period of time, I'm off again for long periods,' he adds. 'But you won't notice, probably, that I've gone away at all.'

Psychologist Arthur Kleps defined the limits of Eisner's infinity parameters best when he stated: 'If I were to give you an IQ test and during the administration one of the walls of the room opened up, giving you a vision of the blazing glories of the central galactic suns, and at the same time your childhood began to unreel before your inner eye like a three-dimensional colour movie, you too would not do well on an intelligence test.'[28]

Problems of a similar kind were noted in P. G. Stafford and B. H. Golightly's 1967 anthology *LSD – The Problem-Solving Psychedelic*. One patient explained the difficulties he had when trying to take a simple Rorschach test. 'I tried very hard to find something to say, but there was just very little there to be said. Only Card VIII was definitely something. I wanted to say "Squirrels," and I tried a long time but I couldn't get the word out. Finally, I gave up and decided to try "Animals." Before I had worked on that word very long, I figured out vaguely that "Animals" wouldn't do because then the psychologist would ask me what kind, and I would have to say "Squirrels," and I just couldn't. So I said "Bears." They didn't look like bears but it was better to say "Bears" than not say "Squirrels."'[29] Clearly (or even fuzzily), if the whole cosmic paradigm could be reduced to a conundrum about bears and squirrels, then standard procedures and methodologies were to be found wanting in more ways than one.

Keenly Callipered Minds

When Alan Watts's *The Joyous Cosmology* was published in 1962, it brought him into closer contact with the psychiatric profession. Watts, in his own words, was 'astonished at what seemed to be their actual terror of unusual states of consciousness'. Perusing their research he found 'only maps of the soul as primitive as ancient maps of the world. There were vaguely outlined emptinesses called Schizophrenia, Hysteria, and Catatonia, accompanied with little more solid information than "Here be dragons".'[30] When Watts met an eminent analyst at a New York party, 'his personality became surgically professional' as soon as Watts admitted he had taken LSD. 'He donned his mask and rubber gloves and addressed me as a specimen, wanting to know all the surface details of perceptual and kinesthetic alterations, which I could see him fitting into place, zip, pop and clunk, with his keenly callipered mind.'[31]

Those same keenly callipered minds were not so keen when it came to the liberalisation of LSD use that was spreading among their own fraternity. Betty Eisner was one of those whose reputation was called into question when she and some of her colleagues began having group sessions. Eisner and her circle held weekly or biweekly LSD parties, usually on Friday evenings after dinner. These were casual, informal and utterly anathema to the respectable medical community. Eisner herself documented one occasion when twenty-two people took the drug at one of these social gatherings. 'Those who were present at that wild Halloween session remember the actress who refused to come out from under the piano, and the patient who talked in voices and had to put her hands in pans of water to disengage from the witch inside or whatever it was,' she recalled.[32] But, empathetic as she was, even Eisner expressed concern at the activities of Timothy Leary and his associates. 'There seems to be quite a movement developing around Tim and Dick [Richard Alpert] for personal research in expanding of consciousness,' she wrote in a letter to Humphrey Osmond in December 1962. 'You probably have heard about their place they rent in Mexico in the summers. There was something that bothered me about the whole thing – some sort of separateness or rather a special sort of language, which seems to be developing. I wonder why so much of the drug work has led to fractionation rather than fusion.'[33]

Alan Watts also distrusted the course that Leary and Alpert were taking. 'To his own circle of friends and students he had become a charismatic religious leader who, well trained as he was in psychology, knew very little about religion and mysticism and their pitfalls,' he said.[34] Citing 'the messianic megalomania that comes from misunderstanding the experience of union with God', he noted that 'as time went on I was dismayed to see Timothy converting himself into a popular store-front messiah with his name in lights'. Watts was equally dismayed at the divisiveness that opened up in the LSD debate, as positions hardened and all sense of rationale went out of the window. He found himself taking part in a televised debate on David Susskind's *Open End* show between proselytes and prohibitionists. 'In the ensuing uproar and confusion of passions I found myself flung into the position of moderator,' he said, 'telling both sides that they had no basis in evidence for their respective fanaticisms.'[35] Aldous Huxley also found that TV appearances only encouraged fundamentalism and did little to encourage informed debate. 'One gets plenty of lunatic fringe forever after,' he said. 'I had a letter a few days ago from Mauritius, from a gentleman who went out there twenty years ago to achieve enlightenment and has now written the most extraordinary book on the world's history and would I please write an introduction . . . and I say nothing of the gentleman in Chicago who has discovered the Absolute Truth and sends letters and telegrams about it to President Eisenhower and Bertrand Russell . . . nor the young man from Yorkshire who ate a peyote button and for three days heard all music one tone higher than it should have been.'[36]

Huxley's advice was that everyone in the psychedelic research community should keep a low profile and discuss matters 'in the relative privacy of learned journals, the decent obscurity of moderately highbrow books and articles'. But keeping a low profile wasn't Leary's style. Sidney Cohen had written to his sponsors as early as 1960, stating, 'I deplore some of the fringy goings on with this group of drugs.'[37] It is also worth noting that the first bust for the illegal manufacture of LSD occurred during that same year in Los Angeles, well before the moral panic set in. By 1963 many in the medical community were actively disassociating themselves from what they called the 'kicks and cults' activities of Timothy Leary and the Millbrook set. 'I spent an evening here with him a few weeks ago – and he talked such nonsense that

I became quite concerned,' Aldous Huxley wrote to Humphrey Osmond in December 1962. 'Not about his sanity – because he is perfectly sane – but about his prospects in the world; for all this nonsense talking is just another way of annoying people in authority, flouting convention, cocking snooks at the academic world; it is the reaction of a mischievous Irish boy to the headmaster of his school . . . I am very fond of Tim but why oh why does he have to be such an ass.'[38] Osmond, like Huxley and Betty Eisner, also continued to voice serious misgivings about Leary. 'Am concerned about Tim, but have found it hard to maintain contact with him,' he wrote to Eisner in May 1963. 'He has acted as if these powerful chemicals, many of whose actions are still obscure, were harmless toys. They aren't.' Osmond's view was that Leary was mistaking the apparent inertia of the US legislature for indifference. 'One of these days the headmaster will lose patience,' Huxley warned prophetically, and so it would prove. Osmond noted how both Huxley and Al Hubbard strongly disagreed with Leary's strategy. 'They both believed for quite different reasons that working inconspicuously but determinedly within the system could transform it in the long run. Timothy believed that it could be taken by storm.' Working inconspicuously was not, of course, Leary's style. Taking America by storm was. 'Tim had too much show biz in his nature to allow him to pursue such a reasonable and gradual approach,' said Eisner. Some blamed Leary outright for the curtailment of legitimate research; others blamed liberal practitioners like Eisner. In the end it was all academic anyway, or rather not academic enough.

Another crucial factor that helped accelerate the prohibition of LSD was thalidomide. Thalidomide didn't merely cast doubt on the idea that lysergic acid could be an effective panacea for a range of ailments, it introduced sheer apocalyptic horror into the debate itself. It is interesting to compare the way in which thalidomide and LSD were treated in the early 1960s. Both were the subject of inefficient trial periods and uncertainty about their long-term effects, but only one of these substances wreaked global havoc. However, it was the more benign chemical that was banned. In the late 1950s and early 1960s an estimated 10–20,000 children worldwide were born with serious physical malformations due to thalidomide being prescribed to pregnant women during their first trimester, despite not having been properly tested for its effect on the foetus. In

Germany, where it was first manufactured, thalidomide was even available over the counter as a non-prescription drug. Despite the resulting scandal and campaign for compensation that ensued, thalidomide was only ever withdrawn temporarily from the market, and in many countries was never subject to a formal ban. It was only withdrawn in Canada in March 1962, one of the last Western countries to do so, but it was that country's subsequent actions that sealed LSD's fate. A new classificatory system was introduced in Canada called Schedule H, which contained drugs that could be neither sold nor distributed. The first drugs placed on that list were thalidomide and LSD. As a result of this and subsequent initiatives by the Food and Drug Administration in the US, LSD and thalidomide became inextricably linked with misuse and malformation. LSD was damned by association and scare stories soon began to trickle down from the medical community via the media to the public. Similar warnings about birth defects and irreparable chromosome damage were disseminated and the first moral panics and urban myths began to develop: 'LSD – the drug that will give you deformed babies.'

The effects of prohibition were soon felt by everyone in the psychiatric community. In November 1962 the Sandoz laboratory stated that it would continue to provide LSD 'for animal work only'. In June 1963 new legislation came into effect that gave the FDA control over all new investigational drugs. Ostensibly aimed at amphetamine abuse, it did nothing to quell the supply of legal 'mother's little helpers' available over the counter. What it did do was initiate an embargo on all legitimate LSD research. So thorough and rapid was the subsequent clampdown that by autumn 1963 FDA agents were raiding accredited research establishments in an attempt to impound any remaining LSD supplies. In June 1966 California and Nevada became the first two US states to legislate against LSD; by October it was illegal in the entire country. In the same month similar legislation was passed in Great Britain.

The cessation of the legal manufacture and distribution of LSD and the formal withdrawal of permits and grants in the early 1960s brought to an end a decade of fruitful medical research. This curtailment occurred precisely at a time when black-market manufacture and self-experimentation were flourishing. As Stanislav Grof noted, 'LSD research was reduced to a minimum and, paradoxically, very little new scientific information was being generated at a time when it was most needed.'[39] Alan Watts was dismayed at the turn of events and saw only disaster and misinformation arising from LSD's suppression. 'I was seriously alarmed at the psychedelic equivalents of bathtub gin, and the prospect of these chemicals, uncontrolled in dosage and content, being bootlegged for use in inappropriate settings without any competent supervision whatsoever,' he said. 'But the state and federal governments were as stupid as I had feared, and by passing unenforceable laws against LSD not only drove it underground, but prevented proper research.'[40]

'At present I am strongly inclined to feel that its major use may turn out to be only secondarily as a therapeutic and primarily as an instrumental aid to the creative artist, thinker, or scientist,' Watts had written prophetically in 1958,[41] and so it would prove, but no one at the time quite envisaged that it would eventually be the pop musicians of the 1960s who would best express what Aldous Huxley referred to as those 'partial nirvanas of beauty'.[42] With battle lines being drawn so rigidly around the three Ms – the military, the mystical and the medical – no one really paid much attention to the fourth – music, the one that would soon choreograph an entire culture. 'Would a naturally

gifted musician *hear* the revelations which, for me, had been exclusively visual?' Huxley asked tantalisingly in *The Doors of Perception*. 'It would be interesting to make the experiment.'[43] But until the mid-1960s nobody did. Certainly not Timothy Leary, which is remarkable to consider given the prominent role he would play in the 1960s counter-culture. Articles about the relationship between music and creativity were almost entirely absent from the pages of the *Psychedelic Review*, the hallucinogenic house journal which he, Richard Alpert and Ralph Metzner ran between 1963 and 1971. When the writer Anaïs Nin met the Millbrook crowd she was unimpressed with their lack of aesthetic insight. 'Leary discussed a statement he had made, that there was no language, no way to describe the LSD experience. I did not agree. I mentioned the poets. I mentioned Michaux. I mentioned the surrealists. All unknown to them. They were scientists, not poets . . . They were making links with ancient religions, but not with literature, I felt.'[44] The contents of the *Psychedelic Review* confirm Nin's misgivings. There was a preponderance of articles about spirituality and mysticism but very little about the creative realm. The journal did, though, run an extremely thoughtful overview of Aldous Huxley's life in its special tribute issue of 1964. 'Huxley's regard for mysticism was well known,' wrote Huston Smith. 'What some overlooked was his equal interest in the workaday world . . . To those who greedy for transcendence deprecated the mundane, he counselled, "We must make the best of both worlds."'[45]

Dismissed, disregarded or prematurely abandoned before their full potential had been realised, psychedelic drugs continued to be used widely and would provide the catalyst and inspiration for some of the most creative popular music of the 1960s. In the end it was neither the military, the medical establishment nor indeed the mystical establishment who would offer that cable-car ride to the mountain top. It was left to the creatives and the hedonists to take up the challenge. Needless to say, some were far from happy with this state of affairs. Stanislav Grof contrasted 'responsible clinical or spiritual use' with what he called 'the naïve and careless mass self-experimentation of the young generation, or deliberately destructive experiments of the Army or the CIA'.[46] He appeared to be suggesting that there was little to choose between the two. But that 'naïve and careless mass self-experimentation' he so readily dismissed gave us 'Tomorrow

Never Knows', 'God Only Knows', 'Good Vibrations', 'White Rabbit', 'Penny Lane', 'Strawberry Fields Forever', 'See Emily Play' and, lest we forget, 'The Reality of Air Fried Borsk' by the Driving Stupid and 'Like a Dribbling Fram' by Race Marbles. Those blazing insights and euphoric visions which were so distrusted in the worlds of psychiatry and military interrogation lent themselves perfectly to the partial nirvanas and fragmentary insights of the pop world. And so began the greatest pharmaceutical field experiment in the history of Western civilisation, as thousands and then hundreds of thousands and eventually millions of willing participants swallowed hard, soared angelic and went about their psychedelic business.

'Our culture has always revered the power of imaginative insight and must in reason value any agency, chemical or otherwise, capable of releasing such powers in large numbers of people,' wrote R. A. Durr in the introduction to his sober and scholarly study *Poetic Vision and the Psychedelic Experience*. 'No creative advance has been made without some usually considerable risk,' he pointed out. 'In respect of their immense power and the great wide-ranging service they give promise of rendering, the psychedelic drugs appear to be astonishingly benign.'[47] Durr's caveat was a familiar one: LSD was 'trustworthy under controlled conditions, when set and setting are supportive'. To hedonists and truth-seekers alike, though, the only pertinent issue was who controlled those conditions. As psychologia gave way to psychedelica, 'set and setting' became increasingly determined by the users, not the dispensers. And if recreational drug use was to become one huge social experiment, then the new laboratory would be the users' own social environment – the streets, parks and playgrounds, the recording studios, the discotheques and dance halls.

Nobody tried to make the trivial more sublime than the pop musicians who took acid during the psychedelic era. Those who found themselves negotiating Huxley's 'best of both worlds' were dipping into a rich legacy. 'Not peculiar, extravagant, but universal and close at hand,' said Durr as he appraised the attempts of the Romantic poets to awaken the power of imagination. 'For in so far as the other-worldly visions are revelations of the "collective" as distinct from the "personal" unconscious – are universal, recurrent or archetypal – they are expressive of mankind.'[48] He could just as easily have been referring to the wealth of great music that was about to be unleashed upon the world. The molecular structure of the universe remained unshaken but for a brief moment in the 1960s the particles would be rearranged by those who embraced the pharmacological muse sufficiently for everyone to notice.

And so in the end it all comes back to that terminological parlour game played out by Humphrey Osmond and Aldous Huxley, as they batted their skittish correspondence back and forth in 1956. You can hang an entire philosophical debate on the battle between Huxley's '*thumos*', the rational, and Osmond's '*psyche*', the transcendent. It's a debate that originates with the ancient Greeks and echoes down the centuries, through dark ages and enlightened ages alike, through Blake's freshly cleaned doors, through De Quincey's confessional, through George Crabbe, Wilkie Collins and all those other opiated acolytes, on through the sacred pleasure domes of Coleridge and the material sublime of Keats. On it goes, hurtling past the dimmed lights of the Parisian Club des Hashischins and the slumped silhouettes of Rimbaud, Verlaine, Baudelaire and all the other systematic disorganisers of the senses, on past the *fin de siècle* decadents and *flâneurs*, on through Walter Benjamin's Protocols, through Jean Cocteau's stupor and sacrament, through André Breton's surrealist beauty that would be convulsive or not at all, via Burroughs and the Beats and all the part-time fakirs and full-time illusionists who followed in their wake, until the moon's a pretty balloon and the clouds are all made of paisley and the sun topples from the sky, turns into an orange and rolls into a wood-panelled English drawing room in 1966, where the cameras are rolling and a wild-eyed girl child is being interviewed by Fyfe Robertson for a BBC documentary about LSD. The girl picks up the spherical object and exclaims, 'Ah, it must be to do with orange. Not only with orange.' And, of course, she was right. It was all 'to do with orange. Not only with orange.' But, in order to explain just how right the orange girl was, we have to go back to the beginning. Not only the beginning. Before the beginning.

PSYCHEDELIA USA

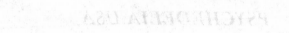

2

PAINTING WITH LIGHT

My! People come and go so quickly here.
DOROTHY, *The Wizard of Oz*

'San Francisco Rock Bands'. That's all it says on the handbill designed by Rick Griffin for the Human Be-In, the legendary gathering of the tribes that took place in Golden Gate Park on Saturday 14 January 1967. No other detail than that. The only people who get a namecheck are the North Beach laureates of beat culture and the star turns and alternative medicine men of the emerging psychedelic underground: Timothy Leary, Richard Alpert, Gary Snyder, Allen Ginsberg, Jerry Rubin, Dick Gregory, Lawrence Ferlinghetti, Michael McClure. Buddha gets a mention too. Not the deity, but a well-known local ex-Marine drill instructor who occasionally got up on stage with Big Brother and the Holding Company and encouraged everybody to do their thing. But no mention of bands. Another poster for the event, created by Stanley Mouse and Michael Bowen, states something similar. 'All SF Rock Groups', it says on that one. Again there's a namecheck for Leary, Ginsberg, Snyder et al., but no further info about the music. In fact, all but one of the five handbills and posters that were designed for the Be-In just offer a simple variant on 'San Francisco Rock Bands'.

On one level the absence of group names can be read as a hip and knowing nod to the Bay Area cognoscenti – the tight-knit community of heads and freaks who would have been going to the Be-In anyway and, in all probability, knew who was likely to play. But it's also an acknowledgement of something more telling, a touching reminder that January 1967 still seemed an age away from a time when record companies, managers and promoters would be prepared to pull all kinds of stunts to make sure their band got top dollar and prominent publicity. Five months after the Be-In came the Monterey Pop Festival. At that event groups were asked to sign a release form granting world-wide rights for use of their performance footage. The Grateful Dead refused, so they weren't filmed. Two members of Country Joe and the Fish were ripped to the gills on the powerful hallucinogen STP and refused too. They were filmed anyway. Big Brother and the Holding Company also refused, so their opening-day performance wasn't captured on camera either. However, their singer, Janis Joplin, was persuaded by Albert Grossman, her soon-to-be manager, that it might be in her interest to sign, forcing the organisers to hastily reschedule a second Big Brother performance on the festival's closing night. The official reason given at the time was 'popular demand' due to the phenomenal success of the band's Friday-night appearance, but those on the inside knew otherwise.[1] When the Monterey movie was released, the other members of Big Brother couldn't help noticing that the close-ups were all of Janis.

There are, though, more significant absentees from those Be-In handbills, and their omission downplays the importance of a whole range of other cultural initiatives. The flowering of west-coast psychedelia was never just about the music, and before we can even begin to talk about the Grateful Dead, Jefferson Airplane, Big Brother and the Holding Company, Country Joe and the Fish et al. we have to bring on a whole cast of miscellaneous characters, bit-part players and illuminating extras who gave the great passing pageant its colour and its context.

Music arrived on the scene relatively late in the day and a whole range of earlier innovations helped shape psychedelia's landscape. In the spring of 1964, when Ken Kesey's Merry Pranksters painted up their dayglo bus and went off in search of 'Furthur', the Grateful Dead was still a jug band, Joe McDonald was a Berkeley folk musician, Janis Joplin was still in Texas taking speed, and pretty much everybody else, from the Byrds to the Lovin' Spoonful, was still in thrall to the four loveable moptops from Liverpool they'd seen on *The Ed Sullivan Show*. In *Noise: The Political Economy of Music* Jacques Attali stated that 'Music is prophecy: its styles and economic organisation are ahead of the rest of society because it explores, much faster than material reality can, the entire range of possibilities in a given code. It makes audible the new world that will gradually become visible.'[2] Not in the case of psychedelia it didn't. If we're talking about exploring 'much faster than material reality can, the entire range of possibilities in a given code', then we first have to examine psychedelia's prehistory, all those inchoate impulses that anticipated not just what the future might sound like but what it would look like too. If we're talking prophecy and new worlds that 'will gradually become visible', we have to begin our journey by observing basic principles. Light travels faster than sound.

'Vision in Motion'

'Painting with light is an old chapter of human activity,' wrote Bauhaus co-founder Lázló Moholy-Nagy in 1939, in an essay entitled 'Light: A New Medium of Expression'.[3] The merging of art, light and music has a long and illustrious history and Moholy-Nagy evoked a rich legacy of illumination and shadow play as evidence: theatre performances under canvas, lit by pitch oil and back projections; colourful displays that used tinted glass chips and rudimentary prisms; Isaac Newton's experiments with filtered light; the magic lantern; the *trompe l'oeil* lighting effects of the baroque opera; the nineteenth-century invention of

limelight; the creation of 'colour organs' and other contraptions designed to play what was then called 'light music'. All of these played their part in shaping the terrain that would make psychedelia possible.

Moholy-Nagy rewrote 'Light: A New Medium of Expression' for his book *Vision in Motion*, a work which was completed just months before he died in 1946. In his valedictory masterpiece he made one small but significant amendment to his original statement: 'Painting with light is an old chapter of human activity' now read 'Painting with light is an old chapter in artistic Utopias.'[4] Having been forced to flee Nazi Germany, Moholy-Nagy and his Bauhaus colleagues had ample time to reflect on both human activity and artistic utopias, having seen what tyrannical regimes could do to either. The Italian Futurists, for all their revolutionary rhetoric about machine music, were ultimately undone by their masturbatory relationship with fascism. The grand schemes of the Russian Constructivists and Suprematists were derailed by the merciless orthodoxy of Soviet socialist realism. The twentieth century is peppered with accounts of noble projects in art, architecture, music and theatre that were never realised. 'Like their Italian

Futurist contemporaries none of the more extreme kinetic fantasies of the Russian architectural avant-garde were ever built,' noted Chris Salter.[5] In his plans for an 'Electromechanical Peep Show' El Lissitzky envisaged 'beams of light refracted through prisms and mirrors, following the movement of bodies',[6] just one of many precursors to the immersive environments that lay forty years ahead in the unenvisaged psychedelic future. El Lissitzky's proposals for a multi-perspective performance space were intended to merge the most advanced forms of art, science and technology into a radical new totality of creative space. Unfortunately for him, totality ran up against totalitarianism, not in the form of the purge, the midnight knock, the show trial or the banishment to the salt mines – all that came later – but in the shape of something far more mundane: the procedures of petty officialdom. The grand plans that Bauhaus founder Walter Gropius had for his Total Theatre in the creative fervour of 1920s Germany were similarly undone by their sheer financial impracticality.[7]

'Machines of Loving Grace'

'It is fake, ersatz. Instant mysticism,' Arthur Koestler told Timothy Leary the day after his unhappy psilocybin trip to magic-mushroom land. 'There's no wisdom there. I solved the secret of the universe last night, but this morning I forgot what it was.'[8] This exchange is usually taken as prima facie evidence of the limitations of the hallucinogenic experience, but it also suggests that what we really need to do is construct an appropriate aesthetic to go with the experience, an aesthetic that fully embraces temporality and the ephemeral. 'The Hacienda must be built,' wrote Ivan Chtcheglov in his 1953 call to arms 'Formulary for a New Urbanism', but the overwhelming evidence suggests that the haciendas never are built except in our dreams. Chtcheglov's architectural utopia was doomed to join all the others that dazzle with their bold ambition but remain locked in the sanctuary of our imaginings. The psychological residue that these dream worlds accumulate is modernism's great unsung legacy. What we are documenting as much as anything else here is a history of impermanence, a history which at some point in the mid-1960s witnesses a kaleidoscopic collision between mind-expanding drugs and mind-bending music performed, initially at any rate, under mind-warping environmental circumstances. Ultimately, that's how the history of painting with light and all the other precursors to psychedelia can be read: as a series of anticipatory forces that offered brief tantalising glimpses of utopia. These initiatives envisioned a time yet to come, a future just out of reach, a hacienda that resolutely refused to yield up the secrets of its architectural blueprint.

At a certain point midway through the twentieth century LSD imposes itself upon this narrative and reinvigorates the aesthetics of impermanence. Psychedelic drugs in context can be read as a fresh attempt to address a seemingly irresolvable paradox: how to give substance to abstraction. New cultural spaces would be needed in order to accommodate these previously unclassifiable ideas, these 'machines of loving grace', as poet Richard Brautigan put it, and new ways of thinking too. To paraphrase André Breton, the new performance environment had to be transformative and multisensory or not at all. 'Our imaginations, haunted by the old archetypes, have remained far behind the sophistication of the machines,' wrote Chtcheglov. 'The various attempts to integrate modern science into new myths remain inadequate.'[9]

The colour organ that Moholy-Nagy refers to in *Vision in Motion* was devised in 1734 by the French Jesuit mathematician Louis Bertrand Castel. Castel envisaged a 'harpsichord for the eyes' and designed the *clavecin oculaire*, a light organ that was intended to produce simultaneous sound and colour. It was just the first of many such devices. In 1789 Erasmus Darwin (grandfather of Charles) proposed that the newly invented Argand oil lamp could be used to produce 'visible music' via light projection through coloured glass. In his 1844 pamphlet 'Colour Music', D. D. Jameson prophetically imagined a darkened room containing walls lined with reflective tin plates. Glass containers enclosed within these walls ('the bottles seen in the windows of druggist shops can be used for this purpose') would be filled with coloured liquids which would act as filters for back projections that would bathe the room in light.

Various modifications of the colour organ were devised during the nineteenth century, including Frédéric Kastner's pyrophone, a gas-driven device that could replicate the human voice; when domestic electricity became available, it was adapted to incorporate illuminated crystal tubes. In 1877 the American inventor Bainbridge Bishop patented an electromechanical device designed to provide what he called 'painting music'. The attachment was placed on top of an organ and projected sunlight via a system of levers and shutters while music was being played. In 1893 Alexander Wallace Rimington, a professor of fine arts at Queen's College London, patented his own colour organ, a ten-foot-high instrument which used arc lamps and filters, with organ stop settings to control hue, luminosity and colour purity.[10]

In 1915 Alexander Scriabin became the first composer to write a piece specifically scored for projected light. His so-called 'colour symphony' *Prometheus, the Poem of Fire* premiered in Moscow in 1911, but on that occasion the light machinery failed to operate. When it was performed in 1915 at Carnegie Hall, critics dismissed it as a 'pretty poppy show'. Later that same year, shortly before his death, Scriabin began to devise a performance piece called *The Mysterium*, which would embrace all the senses, utilising music, dance, theatre, perfume and coloured light. He envisaged *The Mysterium* as his musical and cosmological masterpiece. It is the Brian Wilson *Smile/ Dumb Angel* of the late classical era and all that remained of it after Scriabin's death were thirty pages of notes, fifty-three pages of score (mostly

unrelated fragments that sketched out themes and harmonies) and the poetic text for the 'Prefatory Action', a grand orchestral piece in itself, but one which was merely intended to serve as the prelude to the masterwork. Scriabin's instruction for the 'Prefatory Action' was that it should be performed in a semi-circular hall, with spiralling tiers of seats rising from the centre. He insisted that there should be no separation between spectators and performers. The performance arena would be bathed in waves of shadow and light, accompanied by flashes of flame and other pyrotechnic delights. The actual *Mysterium* required an even grander setting. Scriabin specified that his magnum opus would commence with bells suspended from clouds over the Himalayas and would end after seven days with the enlightenment of mankind. The impracticalities of a conventional auditorium accommodating such ideas were perhaps obvious.

The Mysterium stands as the ultimate unrealisable project of the twentieth century. It offers a tantalising glimpse into the mind of a musical Icarus who, in his delusory rapture, flew too close to the sun, not in order to test the durability of his wax wings but to size up the celestial orb as a stage set. But Scriabin was not alone in his utopian dreams; he was merely the latest in a long line of idealists who wished to embrace the possibilities (and impossibilities) of the polysensory environment. Illogic and disproportion was what did for Scriabin. Subsequent dreamers scaled down their modi operandi but were no less utopian in their intent.

During the 1920s Moholy-Nagy experimented with a series of kinetic light-display machines, using transparent frames, perforated metal discs and light bulbs to create variously patterned motion areas with coloured and colourless spotlights. The idea for the Light Space Modulator, as he called it, came from a 1922 sketch entitled 'Design for a Light Machine for Total Theatre', which utilised revolving rays of projected and filtered light. Later versions used the latest developments in thermoplastics, such as Plexiglas, to create light refractions. Fellow Bauhaus artist Ludwig Hirschfeld-Mack also experimented with reflected colour displays and in 1926 developed the *'Farblichtmusiken'* ('coloured-light music'), a light and colour modulator that provided a visual translation of music. Hirschfeld-Mack saw great potential for these experiments in light and sound and envisaged 'the powerful physical and psychical effect of . . . direct coloured beams

combining with rhythmic accompanying music to evolve into a new artistic genre'.[11] Moholy-Nagy was equally prophetic twenty years later. 'We are heading towards a kinetic, time-spatial existence,' he wrote in 1946. 'Towards an awareness of the forces plus their relationships which define all life *and of which we had no previous knowledge and for which we have as yet no exact terminology* [emphasis mine]. The affirmation of all these space–time forces involves a reorientation of all our faculties.'[12]

In 1922 the Danish-born theosophist Thomas Wilfred sought to create what he called an 'eighth fine art', which would combine music and light. He coined the term 'Lumia' to describe this synthesis of forms. Wilfred's 'Lumia' compositions were performed ('displayed' might be more accurate) on the Clavilux, a contraption similar to a pipe organ that incorporated up to six light projectors controlled by a keyboard. The beams from the projectors varied in intensity and strength and were directed through a complex array of prisms, coloured gels and rotating slides. Wilfred premiered the Clavilux in New York in 1922 and wrote keyboard notations for his light compositions, which lasted between five and ten minutes. The pieces, although meant to be experienced in contemplative silence, were given musical titles like 'Triangular Etude' ('single central forms with diaphanous accompaniment') and 'Study in Rising Form' ('forms ascending in space and unfolding in colour over a restless angular accompaniment'). The stunning effect of these slow-moving visual abstractions resembled the swirling multi-coloured display of the aurora borealis. During the 1920s Wilfred gave well-received concert tours of his Lumia 'compositions' throughout North America and Europe. Presented as if they were musical recitals, they were scored with Wilfred's specially devised form of notation. He had originally trained as a lute player and initially described the technical and aesthetic potential of his invention purely in musical terms. Between 1929 and 1931 Wilfred began to devise automated self-playing versions of the Clavilux, prompting him to shift focus. Influenced by Kandinsky's theories of geometric design and by the critic Willard Huntingdon Wright, who in 1923 had prophesised 'the medium of the new art will be light: colour in its purest, most intense form', he began to distance himself from musical terminology and made a calculated attempt to align his eighth fine art more closely to current developments in abstract painting. Wilfred now envisaged his work being 'hung' statically on gallery walls, and adapted his sense of perspective and proportion accordingly. He scaled down his Lumia projections to the size of a conventional four-foot-by-three-foot canvas and as a result was courted briefly by fine-art patrons and collectors in New York. This strategy received its ultimate validation when Wilfred was included in MOMA's groundbreaking 15 Americans exhibition, which ran from April to July 1952 and introduced the works of Jackson Pollock, Willem de Kooning, Clyfford Still and Mark Rothko to a wider audience. But while Pollock, Rothko and the other abstract expressionists went on to achieve fame, notoriety and critical acclaim, the 15 Americans exhibition represents the sole occasion when Wilfred was deemed worthy of such esteemed company. As Stephen Eskilson noted, 'While Pollock, Still and Rothko secured their place within MOMA's master narrative on the second floor, Lumia and Wilfred were shunted the other way, out of the realm of triumphant modernism and into a basement gallery.'[13]

Wilfred paid a heavy price for not fitting into any of the accepted aesthetic categories of his time. He courted the musical establishment and then the fine-art world, but failed to establish any lasting rapport with either. He had little success in making his colour music part of the symphonic repertoire and, in sacrificing illusionist depth for the requirements of the two-dimensional flat screen – at the very moment when Pollock, Rothko and others were exploring the large-scale possibilities of the abstract canvas – he similarly failed to impress contemporary art critics. Wilfred's proposal for a cross-disciplinary eighth fine art was decades ahead of its time and remained unfulfilled for many years. Those swirling replications of the aurora borealis, which once seemed so wondrous and other-worldly, are now commonplace images on computer screen savers.

In 1952, at around the time that Thomas Wilfred's Lumia was being banished to the MOMA basement, Professor Seymour Locks was invited to inaugurate a new Creative Arts building at San Francisco State College. He chose to pay homage to the Futurists and the Bauhaus theatre presentations of the 1920s and '30s, and did so by filling slides with liquid and running them via overhead projectors, while a jazz group improvised to the visual display. Locks's State College show, and the studio-art course he ran called 'Light and Art', have been widely credited with heralding the birth of the modern-day psychedelic light show. In fact, experiments with liquid and refracted light were as old as Isaac Newton, but by adopting the new and appropriating the obsolete in the way he did Locks was signposting the future. His light-show experiments were made possible by two contrasting tendencies: 'The expansion of materials for the visual artist manufactured by postwar industry, such as Day-Glo and synthetic paints, soluble acrylics, colourful aniline dyes and gelatin, and the salvageable instruments and lighting equipment found in military surplus.'[14] Locks utilised the very latest developments in the petrochemical industry (which also gave us vinyl records and nylon shirts) and adapted outmoded materials – army-surplus viewing screens, education-system cast-offs like slide carousels and overhead projectors – giving them new purpose. Only ten years previously those canvas backdrops were being used to give GIs health education on how to avoid VD. His overhead projectors would normally have been used to instruct graduate students on how to build a good career by going to work for Xerox or IBM. In the hands of Seymour Locks they were transformed into avant-garde sensors.

Several of Locks's students and followers – among them Tony Martin, Elias Romero, Glenn McKay and Bill Ham – trained as abstract expressionist artists. In Gene Anthony's book *The Summer of Love*, McKay talked about experimenting with methods of plugging his painting into the wall, but Anthony doesn't really take the theme and run with it. Poet Michael McClure's introduction to that same book cites Pollock and Rothko, but does so solely in the context of the abstract expressionists' romantic spirit rather than where the really tangible linkage is to be found – in technique, in assemblage, in breaking down artistic barriers, in exposing the limitations of form. Again, there was nothing particularly new about this. In 1917 the painter Robert Delaunay proposed that light could be used to animate abstract paintings. And Moholy-Nagy predicted in 1946 that 'the progressive painter who is struggling with his traditional element, pigment, feels that very soon a transition will come, a transition from pigment to light'.[15] He didn't say that light painting would replace pigment painting, merely that what John Cage archly referred to as 'permanent pigment' would no longer monopolise ideas about what constituted a painting, or indeed visual displays in general.

Moholy-Nagy died in 1947, before his prophecies could be fulfilled, but in the post-war years a new generation of sound and light painters emerged who were intent on living out his vision.

'An Infinite Variety of Emotional Metaphors'

By the simple expediency of laying the canvas flat on the ground for his 'action paintings', Jackson Pollock liberated art from the conventions of the easel. In doing so he echoed wider artistic, musical, cinematic, theatrical and literary instincts that sought to break away from the 'closed flat rectangle' in all its forms. Artists of every experimental persuasion were in flight from the enclosed boundaries of the canvas, the score, the screen, the stage, the page. Non-figurative painting, non-representational forms of dance and street theatre, 'expanded' cinema, free verse and concrete poetry, the found sounds and prepared instruments of those who inhabited the avant-garde fringes of the music scene, they all shared the same impulse. It's no coincidence that Terry Riley compared his earliest improvisations with 'musical abstract expressionism rather than jazz'. When Riley's *In C*, a landmark in the development of minimalism, premiered in November 1964 at the San Francisco Tape Music Center, an accompanying 'light event' was provided by Tony Martin, the Music Center's 'visual composer'. Martin disliked the term 'light show' and claimed that few of his contemporaries ever used the phrase. Echoing Moholy-Nagy he talked of 'light composition', 'non-illustrational abstract light in motion' and 'abstract form in motion'. Martin shared the abstract expressionists' desire to liberate art from the shackles of convention and technique. 'When I got there,' he said of his arrival in the Bay Area in 1962, 'it seemed natural to go beyond the canvas, to pick up things that were different, to think about assemblage, to put things together in different kinds of ways.'[16] Martin had seen Thomas Wilfred's Lumia but thought they lacked emotional resonance. Favouring chance procedures over the merely decorative he claimed to be more inspired by the infinite variety of sunlight beams that filtered through the geranium-vined windows of his San Francisco apartment than by any painting. Adamant that the role of 'non-illustrational abstract light in motion' was not simply to provide decorative colouration, he spoke of a desire to enlarge 'the visual experience beyond the performer/instrument'.

Like Seymour Locks, he customised his materials, using, as he put it, 'the film projector as a kind of instrument'. Unlike Locks, Martin shunned liquid projections in his early experiments. Instead he utilised 'found' or recycled film stock, clear and reflective glass, slides, flashlights and prisms. This gave his light compositions a very different look to the more amorphous and fluid motifs of those who favoured gelatine and heated oils.

In the 1950s another of Seymour Locks's collaborators, trumpet player Stanley Shaff, began formulating ideas for what would eventually become known as 'Audium'. 'I met Seymour around 1958,' says Shaff. 'We collaborated on weekly improvisational sessions of light and sound, with Seymour exploring the use of overhead projections and with me playing trumpet, coupled with a range of found sounds and other acoustic instruments.' Shaff's initial ideas for a new type of auditorium emerged out of these informal jam sessions with Locks and his wider circle of collaborators. 'Seymour was an influence for many local artists of the time. He was an instructor of sculpture at San Francisco State College and brought into his home many local artists for an afternoon or evening of discussions on art and ideas. I met painters like Richard Wiley, Bruce Conner, Roy De Forest, the sculptor Stephen De Staebler, photographer Jack Wellpot and the dancer Anna Halprin. They expounded on the aesthetics of the day, abstract expressionism, surrealism, the new environmental possibilities like the potential of "Happenings". It helped clarify our own self-examination and creative directions.'

Where Tony Martin spoke of using the projector as an instrument, Shaff and his Audium collaborator, jazz pianist and equipment designer Doug McEachern, began to think in terms of utilising the entire venue as a compositional tool. 'In an immersive environment sound can become an infinite variety of emotional metaphors,' Shaff says. Unlike his contemporaries, who were chiefly influenced by abstract expressionism, Shaff was inspired by surrealism, in particular the idea of dream states. 'Seymour, as a sculptor, had a deep interest in the surreal as it applied to the eye. In our developing dialogue, I was drawn to the idea of a connection between sound and our inner memories. In our dream state any sound can morph into any other sound. Any sound can become evocative. The more I worked with recordings, a new world of audio possibilities opened up.'

While many of their peers were experimenting with mixed media and the multi-layering of visual stimuli, Shaff and McEachern sought to achieve sensory transformation in a pitch-black room; not even dim light, they stressed, but no light at all. By emphasising deprivation rather than overload Shaff and McEachern's experiments stand apart from those multiple-projection environments, where the overriding objective was sensory onslaught. Audium's total darkness encouraged Cageian silence. 'People are sometimes very negative, sometimes ecstatic,' observes Shaff. 'There's very little in the middle save for those who are simply puzzled. But the one thing that seems to be common is the impact of the darkness. There's a primordial feeling about that going back even to the womb. I've always been very intrigued with the ideas and feelings we carry about sound. We carry many sound histories with us, some arising even before birth, which conjure all kinds of subtle emotional responses from us.'

Although the Audium approach had echoes of the psychotherapeutic work with LSD that was going on at the time, Shaff saw little connection between his methodology for unlocking the unconscious and that of the medical community, or the wider drug experimentation that followed. 'My interest comes from an aesthetic focus in expressing oneself in sound,' he says. 'The culture's interest in psychedelic events, and the use of drugs to explore the inner landscape, was not of interest to me. It was simply coincidental that my discoveries of the impact of a specialised sound environment on our perceptual life happened to coincide with the era's search for new, inner worlds.'

The creation of radical new performance environments was not confined to the east and west coasts. In 1957 sculptor Milton Cohen devised his 'Space Theater' in a loft in Ann Arbor, Michigan. The loft was converted into a multimedia performance space by architect Harold Borkin, who created a dome effect by covering the ceiling corners with white reflective tiles and incorporating specially designed units to contain Cohen's projectors and mirrors. In his book *Expanded Cinema* Gene Youngblood describes Cohen's Space Theater as 'a rotating assembly of mirrors and prisms adjustably mounted on a flywheel around which is arranged a battery of light, film and slide projectors. Sight and sound move in complex trajectories throughout a maze of shifting, revolving, faceted surfaces. The movement of the mirror/prism flywheel assembly determines image trajectories as the projections are scattered

throughout the performance environment.'[17] Live electronic music for the Space Theater was provided by fellow Ann Arbor residents Robert Ashley and Gordon Mumma, who, inspired by these collaborations, went on to create their own Co-Operative Studio for Electronic Music in 1958. Ashley and Mumma built much of their own equipment and audio-processing circuitry, and gave twice-weekly performances at the Space Theater on their home-made instruments. Adopting the same strategy as Seymour Locks, the vast majority of the components for their self-constructed equipment was acquired from second-hand and military-surplus stores.

The Space Theater ran for seven years between 1957 and 1964, initially to invited audiences and then to the public. A small gathering of around forty people sat on the floor or sprawled on cushions as projected images swirled around them. Pre-recorded music tapes were combined with live improvised electronics during the performances, which usually lasted between an hour and ninety minutes. John Cage and David Tudor were frequent visitors when they were in town, and the Spanish composer Roberto Gerhard later told Ashley that he had never missed a single Space Theater performance during his time as composer-in-residence in Ann Arbor.[18]

The largest-scale light-and-sound events to be set in a domed auditorium were Jordan Belson and Henry Jacobs's Vortex Concerts, a series of 'live performance' programmes that ran from May 1957 to January 1959 at the Morrison Planetarium in San Francisco. Experimental film-maker Belson described Vortex as 'a new form of theater based on the combination of electronics, optics, and architecture. Its purpose is to reach an audience as a pure theater appealing directly to the senses . . . In Vortex there is no separation of audience and stage or screen. The entire domed area becomes a living theater of sound and light.'[19] Electronic music curated by radio engineer and musique concrète composer Henry Jacobs was projected from a playback system consisting of thirty-eight speakers hidden in the planetarium's sixty-five-foot dome. The soundtrack included Jacobs's own compositions as well as music by Karlheinz Stockhausen, Toshiro Mayuzumi and Vladimir Ussachevsky, plus selections of Balinese gamelan and Afro-Cuban rhythms. Belson showed brief manipulated fragments of his own experimental films as well as work by Hy Hirsh and James Whitney. His projection equipment included specially customised devices to produce flicker effects and spirals, along with zooms, prisms, strobes, star projectors, kaleidoscopes, an irising projector (which made areas of light expand and contract), a rotational sky projector and four special dome projectors for interference patterns. Belson and Jacobs made full use of the planetarium's dome facility 'so that things would come pouring down from the center sliding along the walls', as Belson put it. They also took advantage of the hushed acoustics to create an all-enveloping surround sound. Like Shaff and McEachern's Audium events, they also made full use of darkness. 'We could tint the space any color we wanted to,' said Belson. 'We could get it down to jet black and then take it down another 25 degrees lower than that so you really got that sinking-in feeling.'[20]

Around thirty-five performances of the Vortex shows were given, including one at Expo 58, the Brussels World's Fair. Belson was utopian about what he was trying to achieve and described 'being in that dome as a holy experience. The entire theater was like an exquisite instrument.' Nonetheless, he was modest about the outcome. Film, he said, 'was simply a transitional form between conventional theater and whatever theater will be in the future'. He thought of Vortex as 'the most advanced form of theater yet developed' but acknowledged that the Morrison showings were just blueprints, 'just demonstrations that it can be done'.[21]

Many of the techniques Belson demonstrated at Vortex also featured in his 1961 film *Allures*, which he described as 'a combination of molecular structures and astronomical events mixed with subconscious and subjective phenomena – all happening simultaneously . . . a trip backward along the senses from matter to spirit'.[22] Within five or six years an entire musical subculture would be tracing those same psychic footprints. Belson candidly acknowledged the correlation between his light projections and the visual effects experienced under the influence of LSD – this at a time when LSD research had not yet ventured out of the clinical establishment and Leary had yet to take magic mushrooms. Belson had taken peyote and LSD in the mid-1950s but claimed that 'in many ways my films are ahead of my own [drug] experience'.[23] He was also heavily influenced by Jungian psychology, Mahayana Buddhism and a rigorous yoga regime. As Gene Youngblood noted in *Expanded Cinema*, 'by bringing together Eastern theology, Western science and consciousness-expanding drug experiences, Belson predates the

front ranks of avant-garde art today in which the three elements converge'.[24]

Another important group who brought together Eastern theology, Western science and consciousness-expanding drug experiences was USCO (short for Us Company or Company of Us), a multimedia collective founded by Gerd Stern, Steve Durkee and Michael Callahan in 1964. Stern was a Jewish refugee who had fled Nazi Germany, arriving in America in 1936, aged eight. He lived much of his early life in Washington Heights, then known as 'Frankfurt on the Hudson' for its high number of German émigrés. Educated in New York, he moved to California in the 1940s. During 1949/50 he spent time at the Columbia Psychiatric Institute with Allen Ginsberg and Carl Solomon. By 1953 he was publishing his own poetry. Frustrated by the limitations of the written word, he began making word collages and developed a style that can best be described as audio-visual concrète. He discovered in around 1961 that, in his own words, his poems 'started running off the paper and into collage and lights and sound'.[25]

Steve Durkee was ten years younger than Stern. Hailing from New York he initially trained as a painter, and in 1957 moved into a Fulton Street studio that had previously belonged to

Robert Rauschenberg and Cy Twombly. Durkee quickly established himself as part of the same downtown scene that included Rauschenberg, James Rosenquist and Robert Indiana. He was mentioned alongside Rosenquist, Indiana, Roy Lichtenstein, Andy Warhol and Jim Dine in Gene Swenson's original survey of the burgeoning pop art movement, which was published in *Art News* in September 1962. This was the first time pop art had been reviewed favourably by an art critic, although Swenson eschewed the term and called the article 'The New American Sign Painters', in homage to Robert Indiana's description of his own work. Durkee and Indiana shared a love for billboards and advertising signage; both were nostalgic for the way America had looked in the 1940s and 1950s. Coenties Slip, where Indiana had his studio in the early 1960s, was at that time an area of abandoned wharves and warehouses, and still bore physical reminders of the old coffee and banana storage facilities of the nineteenth-century docks. Durkee and Indiana both trawled the East River and the streets around the Slip collecting junk, mast timber from old nineteenth-century sailing ships and discarded hoardings with antique stencilling, all of which they incorporated as 'found material' in their work.

Although he shared Indiana's love of roadscapes and retrieved iconography, Durkee had less time for the hard-edged school of pop art, with its emphasis on automated and mass-produced imagery. By 1963 he found that his frustrations with the limitations of painting mirrored Gerd Stern's frustrations as a poet. 'The important thing is not to get stopped by categorization at any point,' he told Richard Kostelanetz. 'I got included but that wasn't what I was into at all,' he said, alluding to Swenson's *Art News* article. 'I saw pop as a very limited type of art and I'm not tremendously appreciative of the culture we live in. What it celebrated was something I didn't care to celebrate. I saw it not as a sensitizer but as a de-sensitizer.'[26]

Born in 1944, Michael Callahan was the archetypal teenage techno-nerd. 'When we should have been out chasing girls we were out chasing surplus oscilloscopes,' he says. While in high school, Callahan designed a rudimentary ring modulator utilising the automatic cruise-control system of a car. He began speculating on what would happen if you reversed the system so that the car went faster downhill rather than slower. 'That was the [conceptual] leap,' he said. 'Rather than designing the systems to be linear and well-behaved, what happens if we change the sense so that it gets chaotic?'[27]

Callahan was introduced to Gerd Stern in 1963, when the latter approached the San Francisco Tape Music Center for a sound tape to be used as part of *Contact Is the Only Love*, a kinetic sculpture piece he was building for an exhibition at the San Francisco Museum of Art. By this time Callahan had become the Tape Center's technical director. *Contact Is the Only Love* was a seven-foot-by-seven-foot octagonal-shaped, three-dimensional 'mechanical poem' mounted on a pole, with a cement-filled airplane tyre as a base. Painted bright yellow, it had a circle of blue lights running in anticlockwise patterns, while an outer circle of white neon lights flashed clockwise. At the centre, signs read 'Go', 'On', 'Yield', 'Merge', 'Do Not Cross Line' and 'Enter with Caution'. The piece was heavily influenced by the sign-painting and numerology motifs of Robert Indiana, whom Stern had been introduced to by Durkee, and directly references Indiana's *Yield Brother #2* and the multipartite *The Demuth American Dream #5*, which contained cruciform panels and a circular mantra reading 'Die', 'Eat', 'Hug', 'Err'.

Again taking their cue from the work of Indiana, Callahan and Stern began to incorporate old pinball-machine and arcade-game parts into their sculptures. Callahan's contribution to these pieces utilised the same techniques of plunder and retrieval that had inspired everyone from Seymour Locks to the pop artists. Callahan began purchasing discarded IBM mainframes from a store called P&D Surplus in Kingston, New York, which he then customised into kinetic art parts. 'In 1964 IBM had just brought out the 360 series,' he remembered, 'so they were able to call in all their old vacuum tube and early computers and basically get people to upgrade to 360's.'[28]

These three – recalcitrant poet Stern, disillusioned painter Durkee and maverick switch doctor Callahan – along with Stern's wife, photographer and weaver Judi Stern, and Durkee's wife, sculptor and photographer Barbara Durkee, comprised the core of the original USCO and in 1964 set up operations in an old church in Garnerville, New York State. They were later joined by a variety of collaborators, most notably experimental film-makers Jud Yalkut and Stan Vanderbeek, and photographer and future *Whole Earth Catalog* founder Stewart Brand. In 1964 Vanderbeek designed and constructed a purpose-built multiple-projection environment called the Movie-Drome in Stony Point, upstate New York. The Movie-Drome was Vanderbeek's own attempt to break out of the closed flat rectangle of conventional cinema architecture by having films multi-projected from a variety of perspectives onto the Drome's curved walls. It was a project driven, like so many others, by utopian aims. 'Unconsciously we're developing memory storage and transfer systems that deal with millions of thoughts simultaneously,' Vanderbeek said. 'Sooner than we think we'll be communicating on very high psychic levels of neurological referencing . . . This business of being an artist in residence at some corporation is only part of the story; what we really want to be is artist in residence of the world, but we don't know where to apply.'[29]

Heavily influenced by Marshall McLuhan, Buckminster Fuller, Ananda Coomaraswamy and Meher Baba, USCO created a range of multimedia events between 1963 and 1966 that combined science, technology, art and mysticism. These purpose-built theatrical environments incorporated light shows, found sounds and tape loops, kinetic art, sculpture and poetry. Like Tony Martin, USCO eschewed liquid light projections, referring to them as 'wet shows'. Early installations like *Verbal American Landscape* were

Indiana-esque slide-show montages of billboards and road signs. For *Who RU and What's Happening?*, staged at the San Francisco Museum of Art in November 1963, they began multi-layering the slides and added street noise and other audio ambience. Allison Becker, the eleven-year-old daughter of sociologist Howard Becker, handed out programmes for the event dressed as a stop–go traffic light. The arts and music critic of the *San Francisco Chronicle*, Alfred Frankenstein, wrote a dismissive review under the heading 'Landmark of a Flop'. While admitting that the slide show of photographs by Ivan Madjrakoff was quite beautiful, he was scathing about the rest of the event. 'It is announced, God save us, to be done again, tomorrow night at the same place,' he noted portentously. On the second night Gerd Stern dropped acid before the performance.

In June 1965 USCO collaborated with Timothy Leary's Castalia Foundation to co-present a show called *Psychedelic Explorations* at the New Theatre on New York's East 54th Street. The show also featured artists Jackie Cassen, Don Snyder and Richard Aldcroft. The presentation would, it was promised, expound upon 'the theoretical background necessary for an understanding of the new techniques of audio-olfactory visual alteration of consciousness'.[30] The evening's schedule was billed as:

> *7.15 to 8.00 Psychedelic*
> *   Improvisations*
> *8.15 to 9.45 Lecture-Discussion*
> *9.45 to 10.30 Psychedelic Theatre*
> *10.30 to 11.00 Informal Question*
> *   and Answer Period*

USCO remained mistrustful of a show where 'psychedelic improvisation' could be contained within a forty-five-minute time slot (or any linear slot at all) and where, according to the programme, 'methods of expanding consciousness ancient and modern will be discussed and where feasible demonstrated', as if LSD was a party trick akin to some fraudulent old medium extracting fake ectoplasm in front of the gullible and the needy. To show their displeasure USCO sabotaged the academic pretensions of the event by playing a tape of Antonin Artaud in full screaming theatre-of-cruelty mode at piercing volume while Leary was speaking.

By November 1965 an increasing sense of religiosity had begun to inform USCO events. When they performed the multi-sensory *We R All One*, with live dancers and music, the piece climaxed with a ten-minute drone chant of 'Om' from the speakers that was designed to bring the participants down gently. Images of Meher Baba's smiling visage were projected onto a screen and Baba instructions such as 'I have come not to teach but to awaken' were shown next to USCO's own flashing messages. The collective also began to sell posters of Baba at their shows, and his image began to appear on the masthead of their stationery. Baba responded to this endorsement by telling Gerd Stern and Steve Durkee that hallucinogenic drugs were destructive and they should stop using them.

The Limits of the Marvellous

Another of Seymour Locks's descendants was San Francisco painter Bill Ham. Ham would play a crucial role in the development of psychedelia and provides a vital link between the post-war light-show activists at State College and the full-blown drug-fuelled experimentation that would explode into life in the mid-1960s. Although he cites a familiar ancestry of light painting and colour music that includes Castel's ocular harpsichord, Kastner's pyrophone and Scriabin's *Poem of Fire*, Ham, by his own admission, came late to such experimentation. 'In 1965, unaware of any of the previous work mentioned above, while working with brushes, pigment and other conventional materials, in the general style called action painting or gestural abstraction, I made my own discovery of the electric wall plug via the transparent overhead projector and began working with light (projected imagery) and music. This was for me a natural extension of the techniques and purpose of action painting including a direct spontaneous method of working.'[31] Inspired by Locks's use of overhead projectors, Ham, like several of his contemporaries, saw the possibilities of plugging his paintings directly into the wall and began experimenting with light and sound at his Pine Street studio. It was the improvisational potential of the light show, its seemingly infinite capacity to generate spontaneous and transient images, that excited him. 'This light art, like music, unless recorded, is totally impermanent,' he stated. He referred to the new possibilities as 'Action painting that ceases with the action. Painting that exists only during the time of its creation . . . These qualities of momentariness, impermanence and free scale required a new painter–viewer relationship. This is an art form in which the artist and viewer share an immediate experience, where

composition, execution and presentation occur simultaneously.'[32]

Forty years after László Moholy-Nagy anticipated the new sensibility and Thomas Wilfred proposed an eighth fine art, the light-show artists and immersive environmentalists of the 1960s were articulating the aesthetics of impermanence with fresh impetus. 'A transience that was yet eternal life,' as Aldous Huxley put it, 'a perpetual perishing that was at the same time pure being, a bundle of minute, unique particulars in which, by some unspeakable and yet self-evident paradox, was to be seen the divine source of all existence.'[33] In the summer of 1965 Bill Ham and a couple of dozen other Pine Street émigrés decamped from San Francisco to the unlikely locale of Virginia City, Nevada. Here they converted a vacant property into an Old West-style bar that they decked out in period furnishings and velvet drapes and renamed the Red Dog Saloon. Virginia City was an old silver-rush town south of Reno, high up in the Sierra Nevada hills. With its glory days long gone its population had dwindled to a few hundred. Ham had shown up in Virginia City with a prototype four-foot-by-six-foot light mural, which was promptly installed in the Red Dog Saloon. Programmed to operate indefinitely, it soon began to pulsate to the sounds of the saloon's resident band, the Charlatans.

The Charlatans were the brainchild of George Hunter, a pretty-boy mod fop who played a bit of autoharp but was best known around San Francisco State College for his dress sense. Eschewing beatnik drab and Ivy League orthodoxy, Hunter decked himself out in a range of early-twentieth-century finery. He envisaged the Charlatans as more a pop-art project than a musical entity and recruited a bunch of like-minded conceptualists to the cause, dressing them in desperado drag and regatta chic and taking hundreds of publicity shots for a group that existed only in theory. In the spring of 1964 one of Hunter's recruits, piano player Byron Ferguson, had opened what is widely credited as San Francisco's first head shop a few doors up from the Tape Music Center on Divisadero Street. Called the Magic Theatre for Madmen Only, in honour of a scene in Herman Hesse's *Steppenwolf* ('price of admittance your mind'), the boutique stocked a range of Victorian and Edwardian period clothing, much of which found its way down to Virginia City the following year.

If significance and prestige are to be measured in record sales alone, then the Charlatans were a glorious failure. They were the right band in the right sort of place at exactly the right time and yet they still managed to blow it. Despite being courted by a succession of record companies, Autumn and Kama Sutra among them, their recording sessions were generally as untogether as they were. They never settled on a convincing lead vocalist, or indeed a convincing musical style, and by the time they did record a proper album the moment had passed. True to Hunter's original philosophy, they made far more sense as a conceptual art installation than as a rock group. Their name, a carefully selected ruse to get their retaliation in first, should have provided sufficient clue as to their intent. Their music, initially an adjunct to their fashion sense, never really caught up with their acid-wracked sense of *esprit de corps*. What did eventually emerge on record – too little, too undistinguished and way too late – pales into insignificance compared with what the Charlatans represented. And what they represented, as Dorothy Parker once said of Tallulah Bankhead, was the proverbial good time that was had by all.

It's somehow appropriate that the Charlatans should have fetched up in an old mining town way off the beaten track. They were psychedelic prospectors, venturing ahead of the pack in order to stake out the viability of the territory and the riches it might yield. For the entire summer of 1965 the band and their entourage tripped their heads off, fooled around with firearms, promenaded in bordello chic and resolutely failed to hone their stagecraft or their chops. Instead, like the rest of the Red Dog regulars, they treated Virginia City as one big dilapidated sound stage full of authentic scenery and beat-up props, a mythological playground for their Old West mind games and their acid masquerades. The handbill for the opening night of the Red Dog on 29 June – a pen-and-ink drawing designed by Hunter and Ferguson – paid homage to the great vaudevillian showman Joseph Hollingsworth, aka Victorina, aka Kar-Mi, a man who plied his trade throughout the US in the early twentieth century as an illusionist, sword swallower and sharpshooter. One of his most famous posters, designed to promote the Great Kar-Mi Troupe, promised 'Originators and Presenters of the Most Marvelous Sword Swallowing Act on Earth – Shoots a Gun Barrel While It Is Down His Throat – Swallows an Electric Light – The $10,000.00 Novelty Act – The Limit of the Marvelous.' Hunter and Ferguson took the last of those phrases and immortalised it on a handbill. And for the entire summer of

1965 that's what the saloon's clientele did: they pursued the limits of the marvellous, especially on Monday nights, when the bar was closed and everyone 'dined electric' behind locked doors.

Naturally, it couldn't last. As a portent of what was to come, the influx of fellow revellers, drawn by word of mouth, alerted the authorities to what was going on in their not-so-sleepy town. Following an inevitable drug bust, the whole operation swiftly shut down and everyone high-tailed it back to San Francisco, but not before they had created the circumstances favourable for the creation of an entire subculture: drug life, fancy dress code, limits of the marvellous and all.

The New Electric Drama

It appears to me that artists and audience are at a threshold of a most exciting period. James Broughton, a poet friend of mine who has known my work for the past ten years, said to me after the recent happening at the Golden Gate, 'They've caught up with you. Now how do you define your task?'
ANNA HALPRIN, 1967[34]

When you look at any of the footage of Bay Area bands, whether they are playing in the open air or under the swirling lights of the Fillmore or the Avalon Ballroom, you will see people dancing. Crazy, wigged-out, weirdly bearded freaks and beautiful young Californian girls with golden flowing locks and gaily painted faces are expressing themselves in the way they know best: not in passive contemplation of the beyond within but by frenziedly shaking their funky stuff. It is an endearing reminder that there is another less cerebral and less celebrated line of development that informs the cultural narrative of the 1960s. It finds form and fruition in the joy of physicality, performance and visible display. Marshall McLuhan used the phrase 'the electric drama' to describe the new circumstances; there has perhaps been too much emphasis on the electric and not enough on the drama.

Anna Halprin's Dancers' Workshop shared its workspace with the San Francisco Tape Music Center in a three-storey Victorian building at 321 Divisadero Street. The two organisations shared an ethos too, and frequently collaborated on group productions. Tony Martin in particular recognised Halprin's seminal role in the development of multimedia performance in the early 1960s. 'I had instincts for a kind of polysensory art

form from the beginning,' he said. 'Ann for me was a catalyst for that.'[35] Stan Shaff also credits Halprin for her pioneering role in shaping the new sensibility. 'She was interested in developing a more encompassing total theatre and recognising music and sound as a stronger force in dance rather than just as a decorative quality.'

'I wanted to explore in a particular way, breaking down any preconceived notions I had about what dance was, or what movement was,' Halprin told Yvonne Rainer in 1965. 'Everything was done for quite a few years with improvisation. *The purpose of the improvisation was not self-expression* [emphasis mine]. I was trying to get at subconscious areas, so things would happen in an unpredictable way. I was trying to eliminate stereotyped ways of reacting.'[36] This emphasis on the instinctual anticipated the way in which a whole generation was learning to feel and think. Halprin expressed her modus operandi in terms of the visceral and the vicarious, stressing the pursuit of spontaneous sensation over the interpretive and the intellectual. Out in the wider cultural landscape a growing number of adherents were beginning to hang a whole philosophy on such principles. 'Inherent in this personal experience was the possibility of discovering in chance relationships some new ways of releasing the mind from preconceived ideas and the body from conditioned or habitual responses,' said Halprin.[37]

Several other dance and theatre companies played their part in the development of this experimental approach to performance in the early 1960s. By far the most important of these was the San Francisco Mime Troupe. Founded in 1959 by Ronnie Davis of the Actors' Workshop, the troupe was a mobile company that performed mainly in parks and other public spaces. It drew upon an eclectic range of techniques adapted from minstrelsy, puppetry, vaudeville, carnival sideshows and the burlesque, but mostly it drew upon the grotesque and parodic mask play of sixteenth-century *commedia dell'arte*.

Exponents of the popular Italian theatrical form travelled in troupes throughout Europe during the Renaissance, performing on impromptu stages in city streets and other public spaces. 'Reviving this comedic form was a stroke of genius on Davis's part. It recuperated the carnivalesque . . . and transposed it to a modern American setting,' said Michael William Doyle.[38] 'Our interest in this 16th century form is not antiquarian,' stated a Mime Troupe programme. 'We use it because it is popular, free, engaging and adaptable.' As LSD began to make its presence felt on the gestural politics of a generation, these centuries-old notions of masque and myth play gained fresh contemporary relevance. John W. Cuncliffe described the sixteenth-century Jacobean masque in terms that anticipated the carnivalesque quality of psychedelia's own theatrical environments. He defined the masque as 'an evening entertainment in which the chief performers were masked courtiers, accompanied by torchbearers, all in costumes appropriate to the device presented; *the elements of song and dialogue were developed later* [emphasis mine]'.[39] As with the psychedelic underground, the masque's musical accompaniment was an afterthought. Initially it was secondary to games, dances, mimicry, role play and all those other aspects of procession and pageantry that informed the new dramatis personae.

By 1963 the Mime Troupe was collaborating extensively with the Tape Music Center, and in March of that year participated in an ambitious city-wide Happening called *City Scale*, written and devised by Ken Dewey, Tony Martin and Ramon Sender. With *City Scale* the Tape Music Center moved completely beyond the traditional fixed performance venue. San

Francisco itself was now the stage. The audience was driven around town in two rented trucks. Highlights included a car 'ballet' in North Beach, with vehicles moving through the streets with coloured gels on their headlights; a woman sitting in the window of a piano tuner's workshop in a bathrobe singing Debussy while a formally dressed pianist accompanied her; a book-returning ceremony at City Lights bookshop in which stolen books were handed back; and a staged argument between two of Anna Halprin's dancers, John Graham and Lynne Palmer, with Graham pretending to be teaching Palmer to drive. At one point Elias Romero's light projections were cast on the walls of the Wells Fargo building in North Beach. The 'performance' ran for six hours until two in the morning. As it was drawing to a close the two truckloads of participants ran into the beginnings of a fight between two street gangs. The conflict came to a complete halt as the rival gangs stood transfixed by the street theatre unfolding before them. 'What was wonderful was the mix of reality and staging. You never knew if what you were experiencing was actually in the piece or not,' said Ramon Sender.[40]

Mime Troupe member Peter Berg coined the terms 'guerrilla theater' and 'life actors' to describe the troupe's working methods. He defined theatre's ability to destroy the demarcation between audiences and artists as 'breaking the glass'. 'If you broke the glass people would stream through to the other side of the stage and become life actors,' he said. Wherever you looked in San Francisco in the early 1960s everyone seemed to be finding novel ways of shattering that glass. In a three-month period during 1963, between Martin Luther King's epochal 'I Have a Dream' speech and John F. Kennedy's assassination, you could see the San Francisco Mime Troupe performing at Capp Street studios, with music by Steve Reich, and the members of the Tape Music Center performing as part of the San Francisco Arts Festival; Tony Martin had a solo exhibition of his work at the Batman Gallery on Fillmore Street; and Audium was being presented in total darkness at the Museum of Art. In the same building Gerd Stern and Michael Callahan were presenting their multimedia event *Who RU and What's Happening?*

'Somewhere there should be a place where the fragmented elements of our musical life could be melted together and recast through the reestablishment of the artist's dialogue with his community in a new and vital way,' stated Ramon Sender in a Tape Music Center mission statement in 1964. 'A place where a new music would find a dynamic and vital expression for our own era . . . There is growing awareness on the part of young composers all over the country that they are not going to find the answers they are looking for in the analysis and composition seminars of the academies.'[41]

It was no coincidence that the Mime Troupe, like their *commedia dell'arte* forebears, took their productions to the parks and other public places. *City Scale* wasn't just a temporary Happening; it was a blueprint for a new state of mind. Standard artistic practices were being challenged in every quarter. In music, theatre, literature, painting and sculpture, art installations and free cinema people were beginning to question what constituted an art form, a performance, a performance environment, even an audience. Wherever you looked the 'closed flat rectangle' was being eroded. Poems were running off the page. The San Francisco Mime Troupe and the Dancers' Workshop were turning a city into a stage. Peter Berg was saying we are all actors and life is the script. Light-show pioneers were making moveable abstract expressionism. Everyone seemed to be in flight from existing artistic forms and

the restrictions of categorisation, from the academy, from the gallery system, from the theatrical, literary and cinematic establishment. Anna Halprin articulated this new spirit of openness and collaboration better than anyone: 'There were no boundaries,' she said. 'There was so much interaction between what was going on . . . What was popular art, what was fine art, what was experimental art all got kind of moved together.'[42]

A questing spirit was abroad. All it needed now was for someone to take the show on the road.

Caution – Weird Load

It was quite a scene. People were bursting into flames everywhere you looked.
HUNTER S. THOMPSON[43]

Ken Kesey called it the 'Neon Renaissance', that loose amalgam of creative tendencies and indefinable life forces that shared a common desire to break free of convention. 'I think a lot of people are working in a lot of different ways to locate this reality,' Kesey said in 1963, citing Ornette Coleman in jazz, Anna Halprin in dance, Lenny Bruce in comedy, the new wave in the movies and a range of authors including

William Burroughs, Joseph Heller and Günter Grass. Equally significant was Kesey's addendum: 'And those thousands of others whose names would be meaningless, either because they haven't made IT yet, or aren't working in a medium that has at its end an IT to make.'[44]

Fittingly it was Kesey himself who would provide both catalyst and launch pad for many of those embryonic impulses. By 1963 he had one successful novel to his name, *One Flew Over the Cuckoo's Nest*, and another, *Sometimes a Great Notion*, on the way, but he was already in flight from what he regarded as a cumbersome literary reputation. He was also uncertain about whether he wanted to carry on writing novels, or indeed whether he wanted to carry on writing at all. In 1964 he found the solution to his creative impasse in the form of a beat-up old school bus which he bought for $1,250 from a sales engineer who had fitted it out with bunk beds, a bathroom and a kitchen with the intention of taking his eleven kids on vacation.

At his La Honda ranch home in the Santa Cruz mountains south of San Francisco, Kesey and his colleagues from the Stanford Creative Writing Program rigged up the bus with a sound system and a generator and put a platform on the rear for extra storage space and a fenced-in turret on top for filming and observation. Then they action-painted the vehicle in splashy random daubs and drips. Artist Roy Sebern added the famously misspelled 'Furthur' to the destination plate, someone else painted 'Caution Weird Load' on the front and back bumpers, and on 14 June 1964 the Weird Load set off for New York. The intention was to attend the launch party for *Sometimes a Great Notion* and then drop in on the New York World's Fair. Along the way they planned to make a movie.

Ken Kesey is frequently cited as the prime mover in liberating LSD from the locked medicine cabinets of the psychiatric community and unleashing it upon America. In fact, he was just one of many who surreptitiously sneaked supplies out of medical establishments – in Kesey's case the Menlo Park Veterans Hospital, where he had been an LSD volunteer in 1959 – but it was undoubtedly his enterprising methods of dispensation that gave the Neon Renaissance its extra-dimensional palette of colours. Kesey embodied a pragmatic, backwoods, muscular kind of bohemianism. Like Jack Kerouac, who had been a promising track athlete and football player in his youth, Kesey was a keen sportsman who had trialled for the US wrestling team for the 1960 Rome Olympics. At college the jocks wondered why he hung around with writers and the writers wondered why he hung around with jocks. In later years, when asked what he considered his greatest work, Kesey always responded with the same reply: 'the bus'. He knew, more instinctively than Marshall McLuhan ever did, that the medium was the message. The bus was simultaneously Kesey's unwritten third novel, a touring art installation, a mobile Happening and a micro-theatre. Kesey's role in the whole cosmic escapade was that of impresario and galvaniser. The narrative of *One Flew Over the Cuckoo's Nest* had been driven by Randle Patrick McMurphy and Chief Bromden, and on the Merry Pranksters' bus Kesey continued to act out the dualism of his protagonists. He was one part McMurphy, manipulator of circumstances, subtle co-ordinator of the psycho-drama going on around him – 'Let's go here and do this and see what happens' – and one part Bromden, passively observing the machinations of the Combine through a medicated dream haze. There is testimony from several fellow bus mates and former writing-group buddies that Kesey, with his beat-era tastes in poetry and jazz, wasn't particularly clued in to the contemporary avant-garde or to electronic music. But that wasn't the point. In bringing together those who were with those who, as he had put it, weren't 'working in a medium that has at its ends an IT to make', Kesey ensured that the bus trip and the Acid Tests that followed jump-started the psychedelic era.

As they time-warped their way across America from west to east and back again ('the unsettlers of 1964 going backwards across the Great Plains', as Kesey described it), the Merry Pranksters spent $70,000 of his money (mostly future book advances and movie-rights money for *Cuckoo's Nest*) and shot forty-five miles of disjointed, unsynched 16-millimetre film and audio tape. By August they were back in La Honda trying to edit all that footage down to something manageable, not yet comprehending that in the process of attempting to make a movie they had in fact become both the process and the movie. Occasionally they showed snippets and rough cuts at Kesey's house or at fellow Prankster Ken Babbs's place in Santa Cruz, an old chicken ranch known as the Spread. These informal gatherings took place between April and November 1965 and were the first unofficial Acid Test parties. There would be a further sixteen

Acid Test events between November 1965 and the so-called 'Acid Test graduation' on 31 October 1966, which took place just weeks after LSD was made illegal in the US. During those twelve months the counter-culture would go from being a loose coalition of kindred spirits to a fully fledged subcultural force with its own socio-economic structure and conflicting ideologies, as well as its own regular gig venues, house bands, alternative newspapers, radio stations and hip entrepreneurs. When the Acid Tests shifted from being small, informal word-of-mouth parties to advertised public events, they unleashed a multi-sensory, drug-fuelled Happening upon the west coast of America. Taking their cue from the psycho-acoustic pioneers of the Vortex and USCO events, the Pranksters rigged up Acid Test venues with light and film projections, strategically placed speakers, sound mixers and concealed microphones. Everything was designed to blow minds and scramble senses. Audio concrète snippets of audience conversation or shrieks of laughter would be picked up by the concealed mics, then filtered, treated and panned around the room. Kesey would later credit USCO's Gerd Stern as being one of the main inspirations behind the Acid Tests, and there was certainly something of the sensory overload of USCO events like *Who RU and What's Happening?* in the Acid Test set-up.

By 1965 Ron Boise and his Thunder Sculptures already had semi-permanent residence as yard art among the abandoned autos and rusting machinery that littered Ken Babbs's old chicken ranch. Now they became a central feature of the Acid Tests. Boise was to die of porphyria at the age of thirty-five before his innovations could be truly appreciated, but his tuned-metal artworks, welded together from the wrecks of old cars, then wired with contact mics, sensor pads and amplified strings for that essential Harry Partch-like tonality, pioneered the kind of kinetic installation pieces that are now commonplace at music festivals and multimedia art events.

Another key participant was Don Buchla, who at the time was in the process of road-testing his 100 Series Modular Electronic Music System, a prototype voltage-controlled synthesizer which, unlike Robert Moog's model, was designed for use in live performance and not just as a studio tool. It also differed from the Moog in that it deployed touch-sensitive plates rather than a keyboard to trigger manually programmed sounds and loops, making it the first commercially produced synthesizer to incorporate a sequencer. The 'Buchla Box', as it came to be known, had originally been commissioned by Morton Subotnick and Ramon Sender at the San Francisco Tape Music Center in 1964. Subotnick would go on to use it on his Nonesuch LPs *Silver Apples of the Moon* (1967) and *The Wild Bull* (1968), but when Buchla brought it to the Acid Tests it was still a work in progress. Buchla happily entered into the spirit of things at the Acid Tests, dropping LSD, making experimental recordings with the Hell's Angels who regularly showed up at the events, and spraying the audience with the random voltage fluctuations that he would later incorporate into another synthesizer system he was working on called the Source of Uncertainty Module. The Acid Tests also featured the light shows of Roy Seburn (billed as 'Roy's Audioptrics') and Glenn McKay (billed as 'the altered statesman of light shows'). 'My first psychedelic experience when I went to the Acid Test was the thing that really formed me as an artist,' says McKay. 'I was painting abstractly then, and I thought I knew what abstract was. But a good load of acid made me realize, wait a minute, this is abstract.'[45]

Those same amorphous abstractions gave birth to the Grateful Dead.

The Dead's evolution from old-timey jug band to R&B covers outfit to free-form psychedelic rock collective is interwoven into the fabric of the Acid Tests. The core of the original line-up – twenty-one-year-old Jerry Garcia on guitar, banjo and kazoo, sixteen-year-old Bob Weir on washtub bass and jug, and eighteen-year-old Ron 'Pigpen' McKernan on harmonica and guitar – had begun life as half of Mother McCree's Uptown Jug Champions in 1964, playing songs from the original jug-band era of the 1920s and '30s, plus a smattering of folk and blues covers. At the end of 1964 they went electric and changed their name to the Warlocks. They continued to play revivalist material, black American music of the 1950s and early 1960s now rather than that of the 1920s and '30s, although a few jug-band originals remained in the set. Initially the Warlocks' music was driven by Garcia and Pigpen's love of the blues, although there was a little of the proto-garage band in there too. They also began to stretch out their forty-five-minute version of Wilson Pickett's 'In the Midnight Hour' with even lengthier solos and tonal experimentation. The style that emerged out of this – not quite rock, not quite jazz, not quite blues – would evolve throughout the period of the Acid Tests into what bass player Phil Lesh called 'some kinda genre-busting rainbow polka-dot hybrid mutation'.[46] Originally a classically trained trumpet player, Lesh brought an avant-garde sensibility to the still-evolving unit. At Mills College he had been a composition classmate of minimalist composer Steve Reich, where the pair studied under Luciano Berio. At the time Reich was also musical director of the San Francisco Mime Troupe, and he collaborated with Lesh on providing musical accompaniment for Troupe productions at their theatre space on Capp Street. In February 1964 the two men provided the sound for the Mime Troupe's *Event III (Coffee Break)*, which also featured visual projections by Elias Romero and choreography by Ronnie Davis and the Mime Troupe. Lesh participated in Reich's 'Music Now Koncerts' in May 1964, playing his own orchestral compositions and contributing to ensemble improvisations with Reich, future Grateful Dead keyboard player Tom Constanten and saxophonist-composer Jon Gibson. He also collaborated with Reich on several of his early tape-recorder experiments, which went on to form the basis of pieces such as *It's Gonna Rain* (1965) and *Come Out* (1966). In his autobiography Lesh is modest about his role in these ventures,

describing how during *Event III* he was required to rise up out of the stage trapdoor playing 'Twinkle Twinkle Little Star' on the trumpet. He described his contribution to the Music Now Koncert 6 & 7/8 for Bernardo Moreno as 'a piece of pretentious crap consonant with all the current avant-garde clichés'. He was, though, astute enough to recognise *Event III* as 'the prototype for what became the Acid Test – at that time lacking of course the main ingredient'.[47] While they waited for the main ingredient to show up, everyone made do with some very potent alternatives. 'One day in 1964 Steve Reich came over to my house with a bag full of these odd-looking little green dried-up buttons,' said Ramon Sender of the Tape Music Center, recalling the day Reich turned him on to peyote. 'We each downed sixteen. I went through a little bit of the nausea thing, but then I was having a great time noodling around at the piano, but finally he said he thought it was time for him to go home. I said, "You're going to go home? But why? We're having a wonderful time." He left and I lay down and began having an absolutely Jungian, back-to-the-womb recap of my life.'[48]

When Jerry Garcia and Phil Lesh attended the inaugural public Acid Test at the Spread on 27 November

1965, they were still performing as the Warlocks. But at some point soon after that Garcia plucked 'Grateful Dead' from Phil Lesh's wife Ruth's Funk and Wagnalls dictionary, and sometime between the third Acid Test at Muir Beach on 11 December 1965 and the fifth Acid Test, the first large-scale event at the Fillmore on 6 January 1966, the Warlocks became the Grateful Dead. During the Acid Tests the group's extemporisation grew ever more abstract. In jazz parlance, they were traddies who became modernists overnight. 'The Acid Test was the prototype for our whole basic trip,' Jerry Garcia told *Rolling Stone* magazine in 1972. 'We were lucky to have a little moment in history when LSD was still legal and we could experiment with drugs like we were experimenting with music. When LSD entered the scene the whole world went kablooey!'[49] The Dead played the majority of the Acid Tests, sometimes performing lengthy sets, sometimes rendered incapable by lysergic circumstances.

'There was no pressure on us,' said Garcia. 'People didn't come to see the Grateful Dead, they came for the Acid Test. Therefore we weren't in the spotlight, so when we did play we played with a certain kind of freedom you rarely get as a musician.'[50]

The most combustible ingredient in the Acid Test laboratory was the audience itself. Participation was compulsory; how could it be otherwise when hidden microphones might pick up your every stoned utterance, amplify them, stereo-pan them and send them booming around the room? Either that or some tape-delay device might mess with your head by replaying something you'd said five minutes (five months? Five centuries?) earlier. Hours after that it might resurface again and be incorporated into one of Neal Cassady's raps. LSD turned everyone into a walking/talking/gibbering *objet d'art*. It was impossible to opt out. You couldn't really be a wallflower or shrinking violet – unless, of course, the acid was convincing you that you were an actual wallflower or shrinking violet. People painted their faces, sewed mirror patches into their clothing and walked around as human reflectors and kinetic receptors, instinctively choreographing their actions to the ultraviolet glow and the light-show bombardiers. At the Acid Tests the event itself was the art form; the participants were their own 'ready made', their own found environment.

At the first Fillmore Acid Test in January 1966, a member of the audience wore a white mechanic's suit with a black cross on the front and a sign on the back saying, 'Please don't believe in magic,' a riposte to the Lovin' Spoonful's recent hit 'Do You Believe in Magic'. When the San Francisco police force brought the Fillmore event to a premature close, they too were coerced into participation, ascribed the role of 'cops' by the Acid Test participants. Their opening line – 'Who's in charge here?' – was the cue for all manner of philosophical discourse and improvised action. Kesey, in his element as high priest and provocateur, hung from the rigging, revelling in the mayhem. 'Be in your own movie,' he shouted, as pandemonium erupted below. 'Be in your own movie.' And for a short while everyone was.

Peter Berg had introduced the concept of life-acting into the Mime Troupe's lexicon. The radical theatre groups and dance workshops were fully exploring the possibilities of masque and myth play. The Acid Tests took these ideas to a whole new level. In his 1970 essay 'Reflections on Happenings', Darko Suvin stated: 'Happenings have some curious and instructive analogies with a number of other non-dramatic scenic genres.'[51] He made explicit comparisons between these avant-garde events and the English masque. Masques were often one-off or two-off events. They took place in the open air or in splendorous surroundings, and were performed and watched by a small social group with shared values and assumptions and an implicit understanding of the symbolism and gestural language on display. 'Most important perhaps,' contended Suvin, 'the Masque also attempted to allegorize the audience, and its appeal, as that of any coterie "myth play," was a curious mixture of the popular and the esoteric; it is popular for its immediate audience but those outside its circle have to make a conscious effort to appreciate it.'[52] The parallels with the Acid Tests, Be-Ins and Love-Ins were obvious. Suvin concluded that the masque 'even at its best was an attempt rather than an achievement, but although it never gained in intrinsic and permanent value, it had a deep, fruitful, and lasting influence [on poetry and theatre] which enriched itself by incorporating many of its elements and ways of using space, music and actors.'[53] Take out the comma between 'space' and 'music' and watch philosophical and artistic boundaries separated by three centuries evaporate into thin air.

At the sixth Acid Test, held in Portland, Oregon, on 15 January 1966, Kesey saw a besuited, umbrella-wielding businessman walk in off the street, take his hit of acid and dance away his nine-to-five blues. As the spotlight hit him he froze momentarily and then announced, 'The king walks!' as he began to choreograph his own Acid Test, shadow-dancing with his twirling umbrella. The Grateful Dead noticed this and began to accompany his movements, synching the music to them.

The Acid Tests peaked with the three-day Trips Festival held at San Francisco's Longshoreman's Hall on the weekend of 21–23 January. The event was organised by photographer and USCO collaborator Stewart Brand and Ramon Sender from the Tape Music Center. As well as regulars like Don Buchla and Ron Boise, the Trips Festival featured Tony Martin's light show, films by Bruce Conner, Bruce Baillie and other members of the Canyon Cinema collective, and Ben and Rain Jacopetti from the Open Theater, whose *Revelations* was set to feature a light show projected onto nude figures. Rock music was provided by the Grateful Dead, the Loading Zone and a pre-Janis Big Brother and the Holding Company. 'The bus' got its own billing, as did 'hell's angels, many noted outlaws & the unexpectable'.

A number of 'Side Trips' were also announced (as if the main event wasn't Off-Off Broadway enough). In one of them dancer Chloe Scott appeared at the Tape Music Center in a performance with composer Lou Harrison. Scott had been part of the original Perry Lane group who had 'dined electric' at Ken Kesey's place in the early 1960s. She had performed with Anna Halprin and ridden the Pranksters' bus as far as San Jose in 1964. She also arranged the apartment in New York where the Pranksters met up with a drunken and disillusioned Jack Kerouac. In another Side Trips event Tape Center resident composer Pauline Oliveros performed the hour-long *A Theater Piece* at the Encore Theatre, a collaborative effort with choreographer Elizabeth Harris and set designer Ronnie Chase. It also featured Tony Martin's slides and Tape Center collaborator Bill Maginnis's 'light instruments'. San Francisco Mime Troupe founder Ronnie Davis made an unforgettable cameo appearance, playing violin in the nude.

The sheer breadth and variety of the Trips Festival billing read like a roll call for the Neon Renaissance, a celebratory coming together of all the separate in-groups and out-groups. 'It was pretty astounding to come to this festival and see how many people were doing related psychedelic stuff,' said Prankster Lee Quarnstrom of the Longshoreman's Hall event. 'Like getting to the North Pole and seeing three or four groups of explorers coming from the other direction.'[54] With a knowing nod to the legendary Vortex concerts of the late 1950s, among those billed to appear on Saturday 22 January was Henry Jacobs with his 'air dome projections'. In the festival programme he was billed as the man 'who first carried out the fantasy of turning on an air dome'. Jacobs was something of a legend in the Bay Area, having broadcast extensively on KPFA in Berkeley since the early 1950s. His show *Music and Folklore* is widely credited as being one of the first to feature what would later be called world music – although, proto-prankster that he was, Jacobs was not averse to announcing completely fictitious biographical information about the artists he played. He invented 'Sholem Stein', a Hebrew musicologist who among other claims to fame had traced the previously undocumented Jewish roots of calypso music. Jacobs was also responsible for a series of Folkways albums that featured his own sound experiments and musique concrète. Shortly before his Vortex collaboration with Jordan Belson he released an album of offbeat humour called *The Wide Weird World of Shorty Petterstein*, on which he played straight man to his actor friend Woodrow Leafer's hipster jazz man.

The LP featured titles like 'Drums in the Typewriter' and 'Chess' (the new three-dimensional variety). In 1963 Jacobs released *The Laughing String* LP, a completely out-there conceptual work featuring a string that, when tied around its victim, caused uncontrollable laughter.

As the Acid Tests gathered momentum an array of wayward spirits entered the Pranksters' orbit, all drawn to the creative possibilities of the grand goof. Hugh Romney (aka Wavy Gravy) is now probably best known for his starring role at the 1969 Woodstock Festival, when he famously announced, 'What we have in mind is breakfast in bed for 400,000 people,' as he and his Hog Farm communards did their loaves and fishes bit with granola for the hungry hordes. Romney, like Jacobs, was a beat survivor. He had been poetry director at the Gaslight Cafe on MacDougal Street in Greenwich Village during the early 1960s and shared a room with Bob Dylan, who wrote 'A Hard Rain Is Gonna Fall' on his typewriter. Lenny Bruce managed him for a while, and as a 'traveling monologist' he MC'd shows for John Coltrane and Thelonious Monk. In 1962 he recorded a live album, *Third Stream Humour*, while opening for Monk, and the following year he joined the San Franciscan improvisational theatre company the Committee. With Tiny Tim and Moondog he performed under the name of the Phantom Cabaret, so named because after their first performance in Greenwich Village the club had been closed down and potential bookers and promoters couldn't get hold of them. By 1964 Romney was financing what he called his 'free-floating lifestyle' by selling marijuana packaged in decorator bags to local and visiting musicians; his calling card read, 'Goon King Brothers Dimensional Kreemo'. Later that year Romney moved into a house with singer-songwriter Tim Hardin. One night Ken Babbs and some friends came calling, wanting somewhere to show their film footage.

If anyone was destined to meet Kesey and the gang, it was Wavy Gravy. During that breakfast-in-bed morning call at the Woodstock Festival he namechecks the Pranksters as co-community workers. As an Acid Test volunteer he was a perfect foil for Neal Cassady, and the pair began riffing in tandem, adding their beat sensibilities to the ever-expanding repertoire of madness and chaos. Del Close, Romney's sometime partner in the Committee theatre group, also joined up with the Pranksters around the time of the first LA Acid Test in February 1966. Anyone

who has listened to the out-takes from the Beach Boys' *Pet Sounds* recording sessions will be familiar with the moment when, just as they are about to commence working on 'Let's Go Away for Awhile', Brian Wilson interrupts his instructions to the Wrecking Crew to ask if anyone has ever heard an album called *How to Speak Hip* by Del Close and John Brent. The album, released on Mercury in 1959, features Close playing straight man to fellow beat John Brent's hipster 'Geets Romo'. Its opening track promised 'a new departure in language instruction for English speaking people who want to talk to and be understood by jazz musicians, hipsters, beatniks, juvenile delinquents and the criminal fringe', and the album offered advice on, among other things, 'Basic Hip', 'Vocabulary Building', 'The Riff' and 'Uncool'.

Like Romney, Close's Prankster credentials were impeccable. He'd signed up for official LSD tests in Brooklyn in the late 1950s as part of the air force's preparation for the Mercury space programme (when he pulled out, he claimed the authorities wrote to him saying, 'Dear Mr Close. You still owe us one dream'), and he'd performed at Hubert's Museum, the freak-show emporium immortalised by Lenny Bruce, alongside Larry Love the

Human Canary, who was later known as Tiny Tim.[55] As a jobbing actor he appeared in the surreal sitcom *My Mother the Car*, starring Jerry Van Dyke as a man whose deceased mother Gladys had been reincarnated as a 1928 automobile, and he also featured in Mel Brooks and Buck Henry's *Man from U.N.C.L.E.* spoof *Get Smart*. And at the same time as he was trying to establish himself in the straight acting world Close put on *Lysergic A Go-Go*, a show that spoofed Timothy Leary's touring lecture events. *Lysergic A Go-Go* was staged in November 1965, and featured Close playing characters such as Dwight David Genuine and Azrad the Incombustible. The audience received capsules filled with Safeway hamburgers as they entered the incense-filled auditorium and were then treated to an hour of satire, a light show and dancers cavorting to a live band called Summer's Children while Close sprayed mist from pressurised cans. Close was listed in the programme as being responsible for the visual effects, which featured 'a battery of transparency projectors, UV lamps, a Lissajous wave-pattern generator, and for the "Retinal Circus" a linear polariscope, and a plane interferometer of his own design'. Close also claimed fallaciously that this was the first time a light show had been used

in conjunction with a live rock-and-roll band, which would have set antennae and trigger fingers twitching among the former clientele of Virginia City's Red Dog Saloon.

The Acid Tests probably ran for about as long as they needed to, and many felt that the Acid Graduation Ceremony on 31 October 1966 came at just the right time. By then Kesey's assembling of the neon tribes had served its purpose and events on the wider horizon were taking on their own momentum. And amid the pandemonium one simple statistic hadn't gone unnoticed: the Trips Festival grossed $12,500 profit. The music business could quantify that in a way that it couldn't quantify the more outlandish exploits of the avant-garde. It couldn't put a price on city-wide art Happenings; it couldn't comprehend three-dimensional mechanical poems, space theatres, expanding cinemas, sensory overload and immersive darkness; it was not equipped to deal with McLuhanesque non-linear discontinuity or Halprinesque experiences of perceptual awakening. But $12,500 it understood only too well. $12,500 made the more astute elements of the music industry sit up and take notice. It certainly made promoter Bill Graham take notice when Stewart Brand and Ramon Sender generously handed him

half the profits for his help in organis-
ing the event. Two weeks later Graham
began to put on regular rock concerts
at the Fillmore, and by the early summer of 1966 San Francisco was host-
ing several regular rock concerts every
week. Bill Graham alone was putting
on Friday, Saturday and Sunday shows
at the Fillmore.

Stewart Brand cites the event he
co-organised as the beginning of the
end of rock music's brief engagement
with multimedia experimentalism.
'The Trips Festival was like a changing of the guard in the Bay Area,' he
said. 'It was the beginning of the Grateful Dead and the end of everybody
else.'[56] Gene Sculatti and Davin Seay
put it more bluntly in their book *San
Francisco Nights*: 'It was a question
ultimately of simplifying. Avantish happenings, droning poetry mantras and
non-scheduled free-form freak-outs
were becoming less daring and shocking than plain boring.'[57]

In a deliberate dig at the more
passé aspects of the Happenings, the
programme for the Trips Festival had
noted:

*the general tone of things has
moved on from the self-conscious
happening to a more JUBILANT
occasion where the audience*

*PARTICIPATES because it's more
fun to do so than not. maybe this
is the ROCK REVOLUTION.
audience dancing is an assumed
part of all the shows, & the
audience is invited to wear
ECSTATIC DRESS & bring their
own GADGETS (a.c. outlets will be
provided).*

Tom Wolfe made a similar point
about the participatory aspect of the
events in *The Electric Kool Aid Acid
Test*, stating that 'suddenly there was
no longer any separation between the
entertainers and the entertained at all,
none of that well-look-at-you-startled-
squares condescension of the ordinary
happening'.[58] Signs that a changing of
the guard was taking place were apparent even during the festival itself, and
Ben and Rain Jacopetti of the Open
Theater experienced the backlash first
hand. It is the Open Theater that is
seen enacting the desert orgy scene
in Antonioni's 1970 movie *Zabriskie
Point*, but the Trips Festival audience
were having none of it. Invited to
appear at the event by Ramon Sender,
they found that when they went to perform their nude *Revelations* show, the
crowd made it clear that they wanted
rock and roll instead. 'The Open Theater part of it was an absolute, total

bomb because it had been conceived as cabaret theater,' remembered Ben Jacopetti. 'All of a sudden there were 5000 freaks that wanted The Grateful Dead! What could I do with 5000 freaks that wanted it up the ass?'[59] In the event Bill Graham sent on a local Berkeley rock group called the Loading Zone to placate an audience who had evidently come for rock music and not 'avantish happenings'.

3

THE GRETA GARBO HOME FOR WAYWARD BOYS AND GIRLS

Exploited and divided as it was, the Haight bustled with life for those in tune with it. The street itself was the real scene, a down and dirty, do your own thing public stage running between Stanyan and Masonic Streets. You could sing, beg, get high, cruise for sex partners, plot the overthrow of the government, sleep, be mad, or do what you would there. It was liberated turf.

PETER COYOTE[1]

FORGET the war in Vietnam. Flowers are lovely. FORGET America's 3300 military bases. Make music. FORGET Mime Troupe, Lenny Bruce, The Beard. Strobe lights are groovy.

DIGGERS PAMPHLET[2]

Although San Francisco had no shortage of suitable venues, rock concerts in the city from the spring of 1966 onwards were largely synonymous with Bill Graham's shows at the Fillmore and Chet Helms's events at the Avalon Ballroom. Helms, notionally at least, attempted a continuation of the 'anything goes' attitude of the Acid Tests and the Red Dog Saloon. In contrast, Bill Graham brought hard-nosed New York business ethics to the west coast. He knew how to put on a show, make it run on time, keep the authorities sweet and the fire exits clear. No freeloaders. No coming and going at will ('No inzy-outzy,' as his infamous door sign read). Graham knew how to hustle, but he introduced an element of old-fashioned paternalism too: balloons, sweets and apples for the punters; stuff on the walls to read for shy people who weren't part of the hip crowd and who might be intimidated wandering in on their own for the first time. This was the complete antithesis of the Acid Test philosophy. Indeed, Graham was appalled at the sheer wanton irresponsibility of the Kool-Aid approach to acid ingestion. He was street-smart enough to know that punters and artists alike were going to do drugs; he just wasn't going to have it get too messy on his watch. Graham shrewdly envisaged how rock concerts would run in the future: streamlined, rationalised, punctual-ish, with the emphasis on the music, not the culture it had sprung from. No 'avantish happenings, droning poetry mantras and non-scheduled free-form freak-outs', as Sculatti and Seay put it. Well, far fewer anyway.

The pragmatic, business-orientated Graham rarely advertised the light

83

shows for his Fillmore events. He wanted clear visuals on the posters, even asking for an out-of-town group's hit single to be highlighted in starbursts and quotes, just like they were on mainstream pop posters. When the Velvet Underground played the Fillmore, Nico was billed as the 'Pop Girl of '66'. When the Grateful Dead were in transition from the Warlocks to the Dead, Graham insisted that their billing read, 'The Grateful Dead (formerly The Warlocks)'. It was this quaint mix of old-school showbiz techniques and sensitivity to the core values of the culture that made Graham such a complex and compelling impresario. Bands both loved and hated him for it. A watershed moment in the evolution of rock stagecraft occurred one night after Jefferson Airplane had played a three-hour set to an ecstatic Fillmore crowd. Graham asked guitarist Paul Kantner to go out and take a bow. 'Fuck that, that's show business,' Kantner responded. Graham's reply was priceless: 'I turned to him and I said, "Schmuck! What do you think you're in?"'[3]

By the late summer of 1966 the San Francisco scene centred on a dozen or so blocks to the south of Golden Gate Park, intersected by two streets whose very names would become synonymous with the Summer of Love: Haight and Ashbury. At the time the district was in decline. Its spacious but run-down Victorian buildings housed a mix of students from the nearby State University, blue-collar working-class whites, poor blacks from the bordering Fillmore district, displaced Chinese from an overcrowded Chinatown, a smattering of East Bay radicals, and beat migrants from North Beach, who had fled an area now garishly lined with strip clubs.

Among the creative community everyone knew everyone. The Tape Music Center, Anna Halprin's Dancers' Workshop and radical radio station KPFA shared premises at the southern end of Haight. Bill Ham's basement workshop was a drop-in centre for likeminded individuals who watched him finesse his *Light Sound Dimension* show. The property Ham rented out at 1836 Pine Street housed members of the Family Dog commune. At the Charlatans' house on 1090 Pine Street Chet Helms ran 50-cents-a-night jam sessions. 1090 was also where Big Brother and the Holding Company formed and where Helms introduced Janis Joplin to the band. The Great Society and the Jefferson Airplane rehearsed in the San Francisco Mime Troupe's attic. Most of the Grateful Dead lived at 710 Ashbury, and during the heyday of 'Hashbury' a walk of a few blocks would take you past Allen Ginsberg's apartment, the Drugstore Café, the Psychedelic Shop, the Blushing Peony, the House of Richard boutique, Quaser's Ice Cream Store, the Free Clinic, the I-Thou and Blue Unicorn coffee shops, the Print Mint art supplies and posters shop, the Straight Theatre and the Radha Krishna Temple.

This had all come about via a combination of happenstance and cheap rent. In 1966 an apartment in the area could be rented for $90 a month, two floors of an old mansion for $175, and an entire three-storey multiple-occupancy house for as little as $200. The dance halls could be hired cheaply too – the Fillmore for $65 a night or $500 a month. This sense of community would be the defining characteristic of Haight-Ashbury as it blossomed throughout 1966. Musically the scene centred on a handful of bands: the Grateful Dead, the Great Society, Jefferson Airplane, Big Brother and the Holding Company, Quicksilver Messenger Service, Mystery Trend, the Rising Sons and the Charlatans. Once the Fillmore Auditorium and Avalon Ballroom gigs were up and running, you could see at least one of these bands on a weekly basis somewhere in the Bay Area. This sense of community would be the defining characteristic of the San Francisco

rock sound, but it would foster a certain insularity too.

In his book *The Haight-Ashbury*, Charles Perry describes the mounting sense of curiosity and anticipation when Andy Warhol's *Exploding Plastic Inevitable* descended upon the west coast to play three shows at the Fillmore at the end of May 1966. The Velvet Underground Perry found to be 'self-consciously decadent', playing 'mannered high school rock'. The light show was 'nothing but ordinary stage lighting spotlights'. 'So that was what was happening in New York,' he concluded. 'Heroin, perversion, vanity, stasis. Maybe San Francisco wasn't so provincial after all.'[4] In fact, Perry's response, perhaps unwittingly, illustrated precisely how provincial it was. That east coast/west coast legacy line would play out very differently over the next ten or fifteen years, but for now this was the Bay Area in its parochial pomp.

West-coast harmony was pitted against east-coast ego. Pacific bliss was affronted by Atlantic abrasion. Andy Warhol's *Exploding Plastic Inevitable* was perceived as cacophonous, brutalising and cathartic, and by the summer of 1966 the Velvet Underground had come to represent everything that psychedelia was not. The psychedelic bands were acid, mescaline, peyote; the Velvets were opiates and amphetamine rapture. The west coast was lapping waves and beach satori; New York was anomie and alienation. West-coast lights were amorphous, beatific, oceanic; the east coast was hyper-optics, searchlights and strobes. The west coast was multicolour; the east coast was monochrome. California dreamlight versus New York white light (and white heat). Bill Ham's liquid drift versus Tony Conrad's *Flicker* movie. West-coast music was meandering and unmeasured; the Velvets were all motorik repetition and drone. The Avalon Ballroom was a kaleidoscopic blast; Billy Name painted or tinfoiled everything in the Factory silver. 'It must have been the amphetamine, but it was the perfect time to think silver,' Warhol wrote. 'Silver was the future, it was spacey – the astronauts . . . And silver was the past – the Silver screen . . . And maybe more than anything else, silver was narcissism – mirrors were backed with silver.'[5]

Even the most enthusiastic chroniclers of the scene admitted that the appeal of west-coast music might have seemed baffling to outsiders. 'Talent scouts came to the San Francisco dance halls and saw sloppy-looking bands who took forever to tune up and didn't always play on time or in tune,' reported Charles Perry. He defined the San Francisco sound as 'basically folkies learning how to play electric instruments', which meant 'a lot of solemn, chiming chords on the beat'.[6] Ron Nagle of the band Mystery Trend was less diplomatic in his appraisal, referring disparagingly to what he called 'psycho-babble in A Minor'. Sculatti and Seay go so far as to suggest that 'by late '66 the San Francisco sound had, for all practical purposes, been codified . . . For all the lip service played to experimentation and Doing One's Own Thing, the music was adhering to a specific set of criteria,' they claimed. 'Long meandering songs with big spaces for jams and improvisation, obscure and/ or obtuse lyrics and a sense of self-importance directly proportional to the growing status of musicians as quasi-religious warrior/heroes.'[7]

Most San Francisco rock bands were happier playing live than they were in the studio. 'The Beatles are too complex to influence anyone around here. They're a studio sound,' Marty Balin of Jefferson Airplane told Richard Goldstein. An unnamed member of the Airplane expresses similar sentiments about the Beach Boys. 'What Brian Wilson is doing is fine but in person there's no balls. Everything is fabricated like the rest of that town. Bring them into the Fillmore and it just wouldn't work.' *Pet Sounds* and *Revolver* were summarily dismissed because they couldn't be recreated in a live context. This privileging of live performance over studio recording undoubtedly reflected San Francisco's communitarian milieu and its rich legacy of street theatre and spontaneous joy. More worryingly, it manifested itself in a wariness both of technology and of the very modernist tendencies that had informed the Bay Area's cultural activity up to that point. Jazz, Balin told Goldstein, 'started out as dance music and ended up dead as something to listen to'. Gary Duncan of Quicksilver Messenger Service approached recording as an unwelcome chore, a mere by-product of the live show. 'Playing something in a studio means playing for two months,' he said. 'Playing live, a song changes in performance. In a studio you attack things intellectually; onstage it's all emotion.' Elsewhere in Goldstein's piece, an unnamed member of Big Brother puts down the Byrds because 'they had to learn to perform after they recorded'.[8]

This wariness of the recording process and, indeed, of intellect – expressed during the period when the Beatles and the Beach Boys were beginning to fully explore the sonic possibilities of the studio – reveals a residual conservatism in the west-coast ethos. Most Bay Area bands had their roots in folk, blues and country music, and it's perhaps no coincidence that the first song to contain the word 'psychedelic' was a cover version of an old jug-band standard. 'Hesitation Blues', recorded by the Holy Modal Rounders in 1964, amended the original's chorus to: 'Got my psychedelic feet in my psychedelic shoes / I believe, Lordy mama, I got the psychedelic blues.' Apart from that simple change the rest of the song remained faithful to blues lingua franca and country-music phrasing, but it showed how easily the new chemical sensibility could be incorporated into what was up to that point a traditionalist repertoire. This strategy would serve most west-coast bands well throughout the psychedelic era. For all the pharmaceutical intake, there was still an awful lot of 'gonna see/find/ ball/lose my woman down Louisiana way' in the lyrics. Before lyricist Robert Hunter refocused the Grateful Dead's grasp of the metaphysical, their early material was full of blues archetypes and idioms. In fact, what becomes obvious from listening to a lot of the early west-coast rock is that groups who took psychedelics didn't necessarily make overtly psychedelic music.

The Grateful Dead's eponymously titled debut LP, released on Warner Brothers in the spring of 1967, was essentially an attempt to replicate their live set. Recorded in just four days, with the help of a considerable intake of Dexamyl diet pills, the album contained just two group compositions: 'The Golden Road (to Unlimited Devotion)' and the garage-y 'Hey Joe' soundalike 'Cream Puff War'. The rest of the album was made up of cover versions. These included 'Sitting on Top of the World' (also covered by Cream), Bonnie Dobson's 'Morning Dew', Pigpen's Sonny Boy Williamson showcase 'Good Morning Little Schoolgirl' and an extended vamp on the old jug-band tune 'Viola Lee Blues', which had been in the band's repertoire since their earliest jug-band days. Anyone acquainting themselves with this music for the first time and expecting the full-on Kesey Kool-Aid experience will be bemused by the absence of mind-blowing experimentation.

Jefferson Airplane's debut LP *Jefferson Airplane Takes Off* was released in September 1966. Recording commenced just weeks after they signed with RCA in November 1965 and was completed in March 1966. Like the Dead's debut, it was largely a reprise of the band's stage act, although unlike the Dead album it contained mostly group compositions and just three cover versions: Memphis Minnie's 'Chauffeur Blues', John D. Loudermilk's 'Tobacco Road' and Chet Power's west-coast anthem 'Get Together'. The group compositions are characterised by the airy contralto of original vocalist Signe Toly Anderson and Marty Balin's earnest tenor. There are folk harmonies aplenty and a preponderance of 'solemn, chiming chords on the beat', as Charles Perry put it. Anderson modelled her rendition of 'Chauffeur Blues' on Miriam Makeba's version, while Balin took Lou Rawls's version of 'Tobacco Road' as his inspiration. Despite the eclectic source material there was little on the Airplane's debut to justify their manager's crass attempt to label them as 'fojazz', a hybrid of folk and jazz.

The one band that could accurately be called fojazz was the Great Society. Formed by guitarist Darby Slick, his film-student brother Jerry, who played drums, and Jerry's wife Grace, on vocals, the band played regular live dates in San Francisco between October 1965 and October 1966. Just as they were about to sign a record deal with Columbia, Grace Slick accepted an invitation to replace Signe Anderson in the Jefferson Airplane and effectively brought the Great Society to an end.

Slick came from privileged stock. She was the daughter of a wealthy investment banker, hung out with the Palo Alto bohemian set, modelled clothes for a while and was an early adopter of the mod style, wearing her hair in an English fringe. Already in her mid-twenties by the time the Beatles hit the *Ed Sullivan Show*, she was in an open marriage with her husband Jerry, and the lyrics she penned for the Great Society had a maturity to match. 'Didn't Think So' had an 'I Put a Spell on You'/'You Don't Own Me' arrangement and offered worldly-wise advice on how to let someone go without drama or tears. 'Often as I May' was a similarly mature exploration of unshackled love, told from a proto-feminist point of view. Both songs lent a telling counterpoint to the prevailing blues machismo of most west-coast lyrics. 'Father Bruce' was dedicated to Lenny Bruce, and related the tale of how the comedian, much the worse for wear, fell out of a window at the Swiss American Hotel in North Beach in March 1965 and broke his ankle. The band's folk-pop influences came to the fore on an extended version of the spooky, enigmatic girl-group classic 'Sally Goes Round the Roses'. The song had been a Top 10 hit for the Bronx-based outfit the Jaynetts in 1963 and was later covered by

Pentangle and Tim Buckley. The Great Society also covered 'Nature Boy', a chart hit for Nat King Cole in 1948 that was composed by Eden Ahbez, a former drifter and commune dweller who looked and lived like a hippie ten years before most people even knew what a beatnik looked like.

All that survives of the Great Society on record is a handful of sessions produced by Sylvester 'Sly' Stewart at Autumn Records between October and December 1965, and a sixty-seven-minute, seventeen-track compilation of live performances taped at the Matrix Club in the summer of 1966. At the time the Great Society was clearly still a work in progress. Fluctuating between their folk-rock roots and more exploratory influences, the group offered an adventurous hybrid. Their sound was dominated by Darby Slick's tentative raga approximations on the guitar and Grace Slick's strident alto voice. Had they stayed together, who knows what they might have achieved. No doubt had the Grateful Dead split up immediately after the Acid Tests they would have cast an equally enigmatic shadow over the subsequent development of west-coast rock. As it was, Grace went on to fame, fortune and rehab, while Darby devoted himself to the classical music of northern India and went off to study full-time with Ali Akbar Khan for twelve years.

When Grace left to join the Jefferson Airplane, she took two Great Society songs with her: the Darby Slick-penned 'Somebody to Love' (originally entitled 'Someone to Love') and her own composition, 'White Rabbit'. Heard in their original Great Society setting both are revelatory. Darby had written 'Someone to Love' early one morning while coming down off an acid trip, having spent the night waiting in vain for his girlfriend to call. The original is taken at a slower pace than the Airplane version, which allows Slick's vocal to convey the necessary measure of quiet despair. In Jefferson Airplane's hands the stretched-out syllables and emasculated howl of the original are replaced by a rallying cry for free love – sentiments that were more in keeping with the licentious spirit of the times, of course, but they rob the song of its subtlety and fragile tenderness.

If the Airplane's version of 'Somebody to Love' trades acid-comedown anxieties for libido-driven declaration, their overhaul of 'White Rabbit' takes the sprawling, unpolished original and transforms it into one of the Summer of Love's undisputed classics. 'White Rabbit' captures the spirit of Lewis Carroll's time-warped Victoriana as

well as anything produced in England at the time. On the original Great Society version Grace Slick's lyrics are preceded by Darby's lengthy raga meanderings. It's the right idea for the wrong song and Darby hasn't got his Eastern chops sufficiently together for it to work. In response, the vocal delivery is stilted and uncertain; Grace sounds as if she is still trying to work out the best way to sing the song, and awkwardly attempts to adjust the flow of her lyric to the music's irregularity. Jefferson Airplane's pared-down version replaces the raga explorations with a simple folk-rock bolero that allows the lyric to spiral and soar all the way to its jubilant 'Feed your head' climax. Slick emphasises Alice's abandonment of logic and proportion by maintaining logic and proportion in her delivery, and by keeping things rigid and regimented 'White Rabbit' gains what the Airplane's version of 'Somebody to Love' loses – impetus and elegance. It's a cleverly constructed song that aligns Alice's dream world to its wider subcultural context, hookah-smoking caterpillar, pills that make you larger and all. The Alice imagery is used sparingly (and, in the case of the White Knight talking backwards, inaccurately), but calling the song 'White Rabbit' rather than 'Alice' puts the emphasis on the chase rather than the central character. References to Alice herself are saved for an aside. Go ask Alice. She understands. It's a knowing and smart song, and Grace Slick in those early days was a knowing and smart lyricist, certainly smart enough to get an overt drug song past the censors and into the Top 10.

LSD was never particularly the drug of choice for Big Brother and the Holding Company. They favoured alcohol and speed, preferences that endeared them to the bourbon-swigging Janis Joplin when she joined them in June 1966. Critical evaluation of Big Brother's music has been all but eclipsed down the years by the Joplin myth. One part beatnik Bessie Smith, one part lost little ingenue adrift in a man's man's world, Joplin's talents have been eulogised and vilified in equal measure. The excesses she displayed in her voice were symptomatic of the excesses that helped kill her, but when she first made her way up from Port Arthur in Texas to the North Beach hootenannies in the early 1960s she played a bit of autoharp and sang Rose Maddox songs with a pronounced southern lilt. Something of that delivery could be heard in the version of 'Amazing Grace' she performed with Big Brother in their early days. Following her Bessie Smith epiphany (although some say her transformation

owed just as much to an impromptu Odetta impression she did one night at a Port Arthur party) and five years dedicated to seasoning her voice with cigarettes and Southern Comfort, Joplin returned to San Francisco in 1966 with the husky blues holler that became her trademark. Also in her repertoire were a gospel rasp, an Otis Redding impression and a show-tune vamp. Instead of taking acid like most of her peers, Joplin grew maudlin and belligerent on spirits or numbed and stupefied on opiates. In order to cope with fame and notoriety she adopted a succession of creative guises that seemed to ensnare as much as liberate her. 'Perhaps Janis found refuge in this cosmic narcissism that gradually remained more real than whatever remained of herself,' David Dalton noted perceptively. 'These disguises seemed to relieve her of the responsibility of her own existence. Crawling into the lives of others she set at rest momentarily the forces within her and without her, triggered as they often were by her own volition, which constantly seemed to seek out her own destruction.'[9]

Joplin could be a bitter drunk. She snarled and raged and bit the hand that fed her. 'Rolling Stone? Those shits?' she railed to journalist Stanley Booth in January 1969. 'They don't know what's happening, they're out in San Francisco feeling smug because they think they're where it's at. This is where it's at, Memphis!' San Francisco, she suggested, was merely a stopping-off point, a hitching post. Had circumstances been different she might easily have fetched up in Muscle Shoals or Memphis. Had the dice rolled more favourably she could have been Bonnie Bramlett or Bonnie Raitt instead of the love generation's Billie Holiday and all that entailed. Throughout it all she remained avowedly, unrepentantly unpsychedelic. Her wardrobe owed more to Zelda Fitzgerald and the New Orleans bordello than it did to the flowery Tinkerbells who whiff-whaffed their way through the streets of Haight-Ashbury. Her band sounded exactly like what they were – dedicated speed freaks and juicers. Big Brother and the Holding Company were no great shakes as instrumentalists. Their fanciful attempts to replicate the free-jazz flights of Pharoah Sanders and Cecil Taylor were exactly the kind of thing Ron Nagle had in mind when he talked about 'psycho-babble in A Minor'. Their music possessed little of the fluency or prowess of a Jerry Garcia or a Quicksilver Messenger Service, and was always closer in spirit to the raw-edged Detroit sound of the MC5 and the Amboy Dukes. One thing Big

Brother did have in common with other west-coast bands was that they never really captured their live sound in the studio and were best experienced in the flesh. They rapidly disowned their debut album, recorded for the Chicago jazz label Mainstream in just three days in the summer of 1966, and Joplin later thanked critic Ralph J. Gleason in person for being honest about what she called 'our shitty record'. Like most debut efforts by their west-coast contemporaries, it sounds inhibited and reined in and all the other things that Bay Area bands complained about when they suspected their natural inclinations were being compromised by the soul-sapping requirements of the recording process. Vocal duties were shared democratically between the members; there were prettified harmonies and distinct signs that the producer was trying to present Joplin as a sweet-voiced coffee-bar folkie rather than the R&B banshee she was clearly cut out to be. Nothing illustrates this better than the album's polite version of 'Down on Me', which has nothing like the intensity levels of the version that would prove to be one of the highlights of the Monterey Pop Festival. And it sounds like a demo next to the version that appeared on the posthumously released *Joplin in Concert* album, recorded in Detroit – the band's spiritual home perhaps – in February 1968.

Of all the groups who might seem baffling to outsiders Quicksilver Messenger Service is the outfit that most singularly fails to transcend its milieu. What may have sounded great blitzed out of your skull in the Bay Area ballrooms sounds rambling, formless and unfocused to ears unattuned to the Haight-Ashbury zeitgeist. The last of the big San Francisco groups to sign a record contract, Quicksilver made their name with lengthy extemporisations on Bo Diddley's 'Who Do You Love?' and 'Mona'. The former was stretched out over a whole side of their second album, *Happy Trails*, while a version of 'Mona' opened side two. Greil Marcus hailed 'Who Do You Love?' in *Rolling Stone* magazine in May 1969, detecting 'never an iota of sloppiness' in the performance and claiming that 'Quicksilver finds dimensions of that "bump buddy bump bump – bump bump" beat that no one has even suggested before'. Leaving aside the strong possibility that Diddley himself found dimensions in that shuffle beat that no one had suggested before, less elevated sensibilities might have merely detected generic chord sequences that rarely looked like giving Wes Montgomery, Buddy Guy or Albert King a run for their money. They might even detect an iota of sloppiness. Quicksilver Messenger Service were probably the supreme purveyors of a hybrid musical tendency – blues-ish, folk-ish, country-ish, classical-ish, borrowing from all but never really nailing any of them – that has been given disproportionate attention and uncritical approval by chroniclers of the west-coast scene. Fuelled by a complacent and complicit underground press that rarely offered genuine close musical analysis, preferring instead to take as read the standing and status of selected outfits as bona fide counter-cultural heroes, this benign critical orthodoxy flourished well into the early part of the 1970s. To twenty-first-century ears such unqualified approvals must sound as puzzling as the attention formerly meted out to some long-forgotten swing-band leader or a New Orleans Kid Ory copyist.

'I came out to San Francisco in December 1966, a month before the Human Be-In,' said David Rubinson. 'The best band out here then was Moby Grape. Bar none. Moby Grape and then Steve Miller. Big Brother was terrible. The Airplane were terrible. The Warlocks who then became the Grateful Dead were terrible. All these people they were horrible. They couldn't play.

They couldn't tune their guitars. And they were doing what to me was the ultimate injustice. They were doing Elmore James badly.'[10] Rubinson went on to co-manage Moby Grape and produce their second album, so he possibly had a vested interest in making such a statement, but he did undoubtedly hit on one of the chief characteristics of the west-coast sound: its close musical affiliation to the blues. There were blues aficionados in almost every Bay Area band and a lot of them never strayed very far from their roots. Even Rubinson's own Moby Grape regularly reverted to the twelve-bar boogie as a default position. Initially the group was managed and produced by fojazz perpetrator Matthew Katz. Katz and ex-Airplane drummer Skip Spence put the group together in late 1966 and their debut album, *Moby Grape*, was issued in June 1967. For a publicity stunt Columbia issued five singles from the album simultaneously, thus guaranteeing minimum sales and maximum accusations of hype. 'Hey Grandma', the only single to reach the *Billboard* Top 100, was a blues workout with druggy lyrics written by guitarist Jerry Miller and drummer Don Stevenson, even though Skip Spence was the only member of the band to take acid. Spence's 'Omaha', the stand-out cut on

the album, had some of *Safe as Milk*'s mutant gothic blues feel to it, but was sweetened by the kind of chiming, harmonised vocals that characterised much of the Bay Area output. Elsewhere on the album 'Naked If I Want To' was slowed-down, good-timey, jug-band folk, 'Someday' was a contemplative ballad with a distinctly Byrds-like feel to it, 'Lazy Me''s earnest, yearning vocal sounded like Jefferson Airplane, and 'Sitting by the Window' sounded like Jefferson Airplane had David Crosby joined them. The most avant-garde thing they did – indeed, the only avant-garde thing they did – was 'The Lake', which appeared on their second album, *Wow/Grape Jam*, released in April 1968. 'The Lake' combined some distinctly of-its-era verse ('Slip through the green velvet sounds slowly'), submitted by Michael Hayworth, the winner of a writing competition on radio station KFRC, and abstract musical accompaniment performed by the band and treated by David Rubinson during the mixing process. The *Grape Jam* portion of the album was mostly given over to lengthy blues jams, with the regular band line-up augmented by Al Kooper and Mike Bloomfield. Bloomfield had some serious chops as a musician and was also a member of Mike Butterfield's Blues Band, the ultimate musician's musicians combo of the sixties. Their most fruitful deviation from the Delta holy grail was the thirteen-minute title track to their summer of '66 *East–West* album, but even this much-lauded rock–raga hybrid was book-ended by twelve-bar bluesology and only took flight briefly into other musical realms. After showcasing the kind of soloing that would characterise heavy-rock playing for a generation, 'East–West' slips into cruise control at around the eight-and-a-half-minute mark and is safely back at base camp with a good two minutes to go. The Butterfield Blues Band always had other modal options in their locker, but they were just as content paying homage to the down-home Mississippi tradition.

Steve Miller was a Butterfield and Bloomfield devotee. He played electric blues in Chicago before fetching up in San Francisco, where he formed the Steve Miller Blues Band. The group eventually dropped the word 'Blues' from its name and recorded the mildly psychedelic *Children of the Future* album in London early in 1968. The LP opens with a blizzard of atonal noise but soon settles down into mellow and mellifluous song structures, with regular rock-and-roll beats and soulful inflections. The whole thing is rounded off with a couple of blues standards: Buster Brown's 'Fanny Mae' and Big Bill Broonzy's 'Key to the Highway'. As on Moby Grape's *Wow/Grape Jam*, psychedelic impulses are signified by the judicious addition of sound effects and other studio trickery. Stripped of these fripperies the Steve Miller Band sound like a polished rock band with commercial potential.

The one psychedelic-era outfit that did truly transcend its blues roots was Captain Beefheart and His Magic Band. They were also the group who, although lacking the all-important Greil Marcus endorsement, genuinely did take that Bo Diddley beat somewhere else. Their *Safe as Milk* album, released in the autumn of 1967, is the one undeniable space-age Delta masterpiece of the era and it set into motion a series of blues mutations that would lead Beefheart and his ever-evolving Magic Band to the outer reaches of rock's avant-garde. These explorations reached their peak of complexity with the vast, sprawling, free-form canvas of *Trout Mask Replica* in 1969, but the blueprint was laid down on *Safe as Milk*. Recorded in the spring of 1967 at RCA's studios in LA, much of the material reflects that town's hard-edged heritage. LA, though, found the Magic Band way too uncommercial and the group had to be beamed into the Avalon Ballroom before it all made sense. *Safe as Milk*'s songs are characterised by short flurries of notes rather than the expansive noodling of other contemporary outfits. It's a different approach to the blues, a dissonant dislocation rather than assonant affirmation. Harmonies are eerie and gothic. Drum patterns are tribal and rarely in 4/4. Alex St Clair's lead guitar and Ry Cooder's fluid bottleneck lines frequently disintegrate into staccato abrasions. Beefheart's lyrics, several of them co-written with beat poet Herb Bermann and hatched in the parched, searing heat haze of the Mojave desert, are gussied up in a Howlin' Wolf growl. 'There's no dense chromatics going on there; it's just a simple juxtaposition of things that belong in slightly different universes,' said Stephen Walsh as he set about code-breaking Stravinsky's *Rite of Spring* and its 'octaves gone wrong'.[11] Same goes for *Safe as Milk*.

Although Beefheart took plenty of acid around this time, he was reportedly less than pleased when producer Bob Krasnow added phasing and other distortion effects to the Magic Band's second album, *Strictly Personal*, in order to psychedelicise the sound. Despite the apparent furore this caused, the effects were liberally applied and were utterly

in keeping with the other-worldly vibe of the album. But Beefheart was no literalist and figured, quite rightly, that his music was strange enough without the psychedelic window dressing.

The most surreal and psychedelic of the Bay Area bands was also the most politicised and satirical. The two albums that Country Joe and the Fish recorded for Vanguard in 1967, *Electric Music for the Mind and Body* and *I-Feel-Like-I'm-Fixin'-to-Die*, remain the finest examples of the psychedelic sound to emerge from the west coast. Phil Lesh described the Grateful Dead's music as a 'genre-busting rainbow polka-dot hybrid mutation' and boldly told a Family Dog gig promoter that 'what your little séance needs is us', but what the play politics and astral mind games of the Bay Area really needed was Country Joe and the Fish. The band's founder members, singer Joe McDonald and guitarist Barry Melton, were both born of Jewish émigré mothers and card-carrying communist fathers who had been victimised by the FBI during the McCarthy-era witch hunts. McDonald was named after Joseph Stalin, and he named his band in honour of a revolutionary simile attributed to Chairman Mao, who instructed the victorious Red Army to 'swim among the people as fish swim in the sea'. McDonald and Melton met at the Berkeley Folk Festival and initially performed together in jug-band combos at the Jabberwock coffee house in Berkeley. Between November 1964 and November 1965 they were part of the Instant Action Jugband, a loose conglomeration of musicians that eventually evolved into Country Joe and the Fish.

In September 1965 the Instant Action Jugband contributed to a 'talking issue' of local folk-music magazine *Rag Baby*. Another talking issue of the mag followed a few weeks later and the four tracks that featured – 'Superbird', 'Bass Strings', 'I-Feel-Like-I'm-Fixin'-to-Die Rag' and 'Section 43' – would become staples of the Country Joe and the Fish repertoire. To illustrate the rapid development that the band's music underwent between 1965 and 1967 you only have to listen to the two versions of the anti-Lyndon Johnson song 'Superbird' that appeared on the *Rag Baby #1* EP and *Electric Music for the Mind and Body*. On the former McDonald delivers the words talking-blues style over a 'Smokestack Lightning' riff and washboard percussion. He adopts a Woody Guthrie rasp, punctuates the lyric with mannered whoops that betray a Hootenanny apprenticeship, and throws in an acerbic 'Gonna make

him an agricultural worker – part of his own poverty programme,' in reference to Johnson's grand plan for the great society. By the time the group came to re-record the song for their debut LP, 'Superbird' had been transformed into a splenetic polemic which married Marvel-comic imagery with the new cosmic sensibilities. Had the Merry Pranksters formed a band during this period they might have written something like 'Superbird'. Its sardonic tone is closer to the Washington Square Park rabble-rousing of the Fugs than the more beatific and blissed-out atmosphere radiating from Golden Gate Park. Country Joe and the Fish were a product of their environment, most decidedly a Berkeley band rather than a Haight-Ashbury one. Berkeley was a radicalised district famous for its organised protests against the House Un-American Activities Committee when the Committee's members came witch-hunting in May 1960. The FSM (Free Speech Movement) grew out of these protests and forged direct political links between the southern civil-rights movement and northern campaigners for civil liberties – this at a time when the incumbent president, John F. Kennedy, was disinclined to give his public support to the activities of Martin Luther King for fear of alienating the southern Democratic vote. Another Berkeley-based organisation, the SDS (Students for a Democratic Society), attempted to build a broad alliance of radical pacifists, left-of-centre Democrats and non-aligned anti-war groups. It refused to exclude the participation of known communists, and it was as representatives for the SDS that McDonald and Melton recorded their songs for the *Rag Baby* EPs. The organisation also sponsored the duo's short tour of north-western colleges in the autumn of 1965. In reality, this comprised a Greyhound bus ride from Oakland to Portland, Oregon, where McDonald and Melton played a handful of dates, mostly in people's living rooms, and enjoyed their first experience of LSD.

Berkeley had a very different scene to the one across the bay. While San Francisco hosted political street theatre and chanted for peace, campaigners in Berkeley plotted active resistance and troop-train stoppages. In October 1965, when the University of Berkeley campus hosted its second International Day of Protest and Vietnam Day Committee teach-in, Joe McDonald organised the line-up of folk singers who performed at the event. The teach-in culminated in a march of 15,000 people on the draft-board offices of the Oakland Army Induction Center. Among the marchers were Ken Kesey and the Merry Pranksters; music was provided by McDonald, Melton and Bruce Barthol, three-fifths of what was about to become Country Joe and the Fish. The band first formally used the name in November 1965 for a gig at the university campus supporting Allen Ginsberg, Ed Sanders and the Fugs. They were billed as 'folk-rock-mantra'.

Country Joe and the Fish were a combustible unit, full of creative tension and discord, but their music possessed a grace and elegance that transcended their internal feuding. Eschewing the rambling improvisations of other Bay Area bands, they married their blues and folk leanings to tightly crafted songs full of sudden unexpected tempo shifts. They were especially big on waltz time: old-time country waltzes, military waltzes, show-tune waltzes, sometimes combining all three into their psychedelic hoedown. The most distinctive elements of their sound were Barry Melton's piercing shards of lead guitar and the thin, reedy tone of David Cohen's 'crappy little Farfisa organ', as Cohen himself put it. He had joined the band primarily as a guitarist, and rather than attempt to play the keyboard as a lead instrument he transposed his guitar lines for organ.

He also liked to play blocks of sustained chords modulated by the Farfisa's wobbly vibrato. That same Farfisa drone could be heard on a thousand garage-band records, but when the Fish used it, it sounded transcendental. They could also play like a half-decent surf band when the occasion presented itself. On the instrumental 'The Masked Marauder' they sound like a narcoticised Ventures. On 'Section 43', which featured in the Monterey movie, they construct a west-coast tone poem in three parts that, unusually for the times, makes no concession to raga rock or 'psycho-babble in A Minor'. Instead it takes its cues from Buffy Sainte-Marie's E-to-D drone, Holst's *Peer Gynt* and John Fahey's studied guitar miniatures in order to construct an acid spaghetti western full of slow-building tension, eerie harmonica and desert-mirage shimmer. 'Colors for Susan', the slow meditation that concludes their second album, is a similar E-to-D meditation, with melodic deliberations influenced by Eric Satie's *Gymnopédies* and John Fahey's purposefully rambling extemporisations. 'Colors for Susan' doesn't really belong to the west-coast school of instrumental noodling; it comes from some other way of thinking, and lodges itself somewhere between the cool guitar abstractions of Gábor Szabó and Robbie Basho (whom McDonald knew well and had performed with) and the meditative Zen jazz of Paul Horn and Tony Scott.

Joe McDonald's lyrics frequently relayed a barbed sense of humour rarely evident in some of the more earnest outpourings of his west-coast peers. 'Flying High', track one, side one on the debut album, was a true account of the time McDonald tried hitch-hiking on the freeway out to LA airport in November 1965. Originally entitled 'I Went Flying High All the Way', it tells the tale of the longhair whom no one offers a lift to, until two shining knights of the road pick him up, dose him and send him merrily on his way, sky-bound in every sense.

'I-Feel-Like-I'm-Fixin'-to Die', recorded for the *Electric Music for the Mind and Body* album but eventually included on the follow-up to which it gave its title, is one of the most memorable protest songs of the 1960s. To an accompaniment of fairground calliope and catcalls from a derisory kazoo, the song is one long polemic against the futility of war. It nails its targets in four cutting verses and a cheerleader chorus of savage intent. With pinpoint precision the song singles out the bungled foreign policies of Uncle Sam and his hawk-baiting generals, who had been humiliated in Cuba and now had itchy trigger fingers and a taste for revenge. It shames the Wall Street profiteers for whom there is no such thing as a bad war, and most topically of all, in one devastatingly understated line – 'Put down your books, pick up a gun' – it summarises what the draft extension meant for the college campuses of America. 'I-Feel-Like-I'm-Fixin'-to-Die' has all the disdain of a Pete Seeger or Tom Paxton song, but its shocking denouement – 'Be the first one on your block / to have your boy come home in a box' – sets it apart.

When he wasn't writing acerbic anti-war songs, McDonald could spin acid madrigals and elegant courtship gallants with the best of them. 'Not So Sweet Martha Lorraine', 'Porpoise Mouth', 'Grace' and 'Janis' are full of florid imagery and sensibilities that sound closer in spirit to the English baroque than the Midwest dustbowl of his musical roots. 'Janis', set to an old-time country waltz, offered a carefree portrait of Joplin far removed from the bellicose southern belle the singer often presented to the world. McDonald obviously saw another, more gentle side to her during the brief time that they were lovers. 'Grace' reveals an equally sensitive side to the McDonald muse. The singer was awestruck when he first saw Slick performing with the Great Society, comparing her to Yma Sumac. He was less enamoured with her band, however, and thought her material 'was really crap', so he wrote her a song to sing but was then too shy to present it to her. For all the band's eclecticism 'Grace' was the only overtly Eastern-influenced track on their debut LP; Barry Melton picks out delicate koto lines on his guitar, while McDonald offers a mantric recitation to unrequited love. 'Porpoise Mouth' harks back to McDonald's first acid trip. Its rococo lyric skips a light fandango from 3/4 to 6/8 and back again, while alluding to the beauty of nature, marching bands, children skipping rope and some decidedly priapic desires. 'Not So Sweet Martha Lorraine' transforms the traditional blues lingua franca of 'She gone done me wrong' and replaces it with 'She gone done me weird'. According to McDonald, Martha Lorraine was a composite of three separate women, but several people have suggested that it's solely about Pat Sullivan, the former wife of the group's manager, Ed Denson, briefly McDonald's girlfriend and also the subject of John Fahey's 'Raga Called Pat'. The song offers a knowing nod to the kind of beat-chic women who flitted through Bob Dylan's life during his *Blonde on Blonde* period. It speaks of an infuriating, soul-sapping, self-obsessed bookworm who throws the I Ching and drives her men insane. The same woman reappears in less maddening guise as on the second album's 'Pat's Song', where to an understated accompaniment of bells and acoustic guitars McDonald serenades sappily to a love-sharing child of the elements who has a smile that colours the sky. In one of the most moving and elegiac moments the band ever recorded, the lovey-dovey lyric gives way to a requiem waltz, complete with military drum roll to signify love's passing.

There was a palpable old-time showbiz element to McDonald's song arrangements that always managed to stay just the right side of schmaltz. The unreleased orchestral version of 'Janis' offers glimpses of a Randy Newman or Harry Nilsson in the making. In an earlier era McDonald could easily have been a Hoagy Carmichael or a George Gershwin or a Screen Gems house writer with a pad up in the Hollywood Hills – providing he hadn't already been blacklisted, of course.

The Dead Scene Scrolls

In the late summer of 1966 twenty or so members defected from the San Francisco Mime Troupe to take their ideas of guerrilla theatre directly to the streets, parks and panhandles. They included writers Peter Berg, Peter Coyote, Emmett Grogan, Kent Minault, Billy Murcott, James Broughton and Richard Brautigan, and sculptor Robert La Morticella. They called themselves the Diggers in honour of a group of seventeenth-century English dissenters and took confrontational play-politics to a whole new level. If the Merry Pranksters were the supreme court jesters of the counter-culture, the Diggers were its conscience, its provocateurs and its Greek chorus all rolled into one. As Dominick Cavallo put it, they 'provided moral substance to a hippie love ethic that often amounted to little more than self-absorption, hedonism, and solipsistic trances masquerading as "self-exploration"'.[12] The Diggers were responsible for many of the key events that took place in Haight-Ashbury during 1966 and 1967, including free food distribution in Golden Gate Park, the Free Store, the Death of Money Parade and the Death of Hippie Pageant. Participation in Diggers events involved stepping through the ever-present Free Frame of Reference, a thirteen-foot-tall (or twenty-five foot, depending on which version you believe) construction built by Billy Murcott out of two-by-four blocks of wood bolted together and painted gold (or yellow, depending on . . . etc.) by Emmett Grogan. The purpose of the device was to invite the participant to 'change their frame of reference' – this might be their immediate outlook, it might be their entire consciousness. The Frame of Reference was both a physical and symbolic manifestation of the Diggers' activist credo. They recognised that 'effecting changes in objective reality', as Michael William Doyle put it, 'had to be preceded by altering people's perspective on the assumed fixity of the status quo. Renegotiating those under-examined assumptions might well produce new and more imaginative ways of organizing social relations.'[13]

If the Frame of Reference could be read both literally and metaphorically, there was nothing remotely analogous about the distribution of free food. Every afternoon at 4 p.m., from October 1966 onwards, vegetable-and-chicken stew was served in the Fell Street Panhandle of Golden Gate Park. This was no loaves-and-fishes parable – i.e. 'None of us have got very much but most of us have got a little, and if we learn to share it, everything will be groovy.' This was a direct acknowledgement that many of the new arrivals in the Haight had insufficient nutrition.

First in line in the free-food queue, as Emmett Grogan recognised, were 'the casualties of the so-called Love Generation. Kids who were beaten down by the mean streets or the cold, wet, foggy, San Francisco climate.'[14]

The Diggers favoured anonymity and stealth but they came to wider public prominence on 31 October 1966, when they enacted a 'Full Moon Celebration of Halloween' at the intersection of Haight and Ashbury. Hundreds of leaflets were handed out before the event, promising 'PUBLIC NONSENSE NUISANCE PUBLIC ESSENCE NEWSENSE PUBLIC NEWS'. The celebration commenced with the parading of the ubiquitous Frame of Reference and a pair of nine-foot puppets constructed especially for a Mime Troupe presentation by Robert La Mortadella (as Robert La Morticella called himself). The puppets were made to resemble Vietnam correspondent and anti-war activist Robert Scheer and pro-war Berkeley Congressman Jeffery Cohelan. Scheer had recently challenged Cohelan in the local primaries, and with strong support from local activists, civil-rights supporters and the anti-war movement had only been narrowly defeated. A puppet show called 'Any Fool of the Street' was improvised around the recent campaign, while three-inch miniature frames were handed out to the crowd. By 6 p.m. six hundred people had gathered to take part in the activities. When the police arrived, they were incorporated into the action too. This led to a surreal stand-off, with the cops at one point addressing the puppets directly and threatening them with arrest. When their patience ran out, both puppeteers and puppets were bundled into the police wagons. According to Grogan, while the arrested Diggers were at the police station the nine-foot puppets stood propped against a side wall. A procession of duty cops came and went, did startled double takes and commented on their size. Grogan referred to the event as 'a goof, a fun bust, the only time being arrested [had] ever been a fun thing in [my] life'.[15]

There is a famous shot, taken by newspaper photographer Bob Cambell, of five of the Diggers stumbling out of the courtroom on Tuesday 29 November 1966 after the charges against them had been dropped. The photo, which made the front page of the following day's *San Francisco Chronicle*, is one of the most iconic of the era. It is to the counter-culture what Lee Evans and John Carlos's Black Power salute at the Mexico Olympics was to the civil-rights movement. Although

the piece did not specifically mention the Diggers or the Mime Troupe, it was the first time that any of their number had been publicly named and 'unmasqued'. The photo captures the quintet in spontaneous poses of ridicule and contempt. Prominent at the front is Emmett Grogan, bleary-eyed, with a cigarette between his lips. He is wearing a scarf knotted varsity style and an IRA croppy-boy cap. He gives the camera a defiantly un-Churchillian two-finger salute, not so much V for Victory as 'Fuck you'. Grogan later claimed that his well-publicised pose inadvertently gave birth to the hippie peace sign. Behind him to his right sculptor and puppet-maker Robert La Morticella makes devil horns (or the sign of the cuckold) above Grogan's head. Behind him to his left actor Kent Minault, arms outstretched and teeth clenched, aims a playful right boot at Grogan's backside. Crouched beside Minault, Peter Berg, the chief instigator of life acting and guerrilla theatre, pulls a vinegary bah-humbug face and gives an ambiguous thumbs-up. It could be a victory sign or, as Grogan suggests in his autobiography, a stick-this-up-your-ass salute. Next to him Brooks Bucher, described in the photo caption as 'unemployed', tugs on a scarf and sticks out his tongue.

On the same day that the Diggers enacted their Full Moon Celebration they opened the first of their Free Stores at a formerly derelict six-car garage on 1762 Page Street. What had been donated (or stolen) afforded plenty of opportunity for creative role play. 'Fire helmets, riding pants, shower curtains, surgical gowns and World War I army boots are parts for costumes. Nightsticks, sample cases, water pipes, toy guns, and weather balloons are taken for props,' noted the Diggers manifesto, 'Trip Without a Ticket'. 'When materials are free, imagination becomes currency for spirit.' Such provocative tactics ran counter to the way in which most local entrepreneurs were attempting to run their businesses. Several got together to form the Haight Independent Proprietors (HIP), an organisation for which the Diggers reserved some of their greatest animosity. Peter Coyote disdainfully referred to the hippies' 'Hallmark Card philosophies' and, like Emmett Grogan, was sceptical about the motives of those who were attempting to extract a profit from the community. The Diggers, he noted, were 'piqued with the HIP Job Co-Op, which took advantage of the desperation of runaways by offering them sweatshop wages to make the "love" objects sold in local

stores'.[16] Similar contempt for the profit motive was evident in the 'Death and Rebirth of the Haight' parade (aka 'The Death of Money'), which took place on Saturday 17 December 1966. Several of the Diggers' former colleagues in the Mime Troupe took part in the procession, which, in the accustomed manner – and with a time-honoured nod to the 1963 *City Scale* event and the principles of seventeenth-century masques – involved a semi-improvised street ballet. A black coffin carried by pallbearers wearing animal masks was led down Haight Street by a chief mourner swinging a kerosene lamp. Behind it hooded figures bore a silver dollar sign on a pole. Members of the Mime Troupe were kitted out as *commedia dell'arte*-style beggars, cripples and dwarves. To the tune of Chopin's Funeral March everyone sang, 'GET – OUT – MY LIFE – WHY – DON'T – YOU – BABE', a line taken from the Supremes' 'You Keep Me Hanging On'. Mirrors, penny whistles, incense, candles and placards bearing the word 'NOW' were handed out to the crowd.

Aside from knowing how to throw a great disruptive street party, the Diggers were, like their seventeenth-century forebears, committed pamphleteers. Their mimeographed broadsides regularly took a scatter gun to the sacred cows of hippiedom, and the ranting agitprop of their communiqués spared no one. Sometimes it came in the form of scathing, sub-'Howl' parodies of City Lights verse:

Our bowels quake in constipated
   false alarms.
We are often naked and nameless
in boring rooms with tedious
   records
and toy tops that make colored
   sparks
for drug stained eyes.
(from 'Let Me Live in a World
Pure')

Other targets were more strategically chosen:

When will BOB DYLAN quit
   working on Maggie's Farm?
When will RALPH GLEA-
   SON realize he is riding in a
   Hearst?
When will TIMOTHY LEARY
   stand on a streetcorner wait-
   ing for no one?
When will the JEFFERSON
   AIRPLANE and all ROCK-
   GROUPS quit trying to make
   it and LOVE?
(from 'Let Me Live in a World
Pure')

The Diggers' broadsides, as Emmett Grogan reminded everyone, were a reaction against 'the SF *Oracle* underground newspaper and the way it catered for the new, hip, moneyed class by refusing to reveal the overall grime of Haight-Ashbury reality'. Grogan dismissed what he called 'the self-proclaimed, media-fabricated shamans who espoused the tune-in, turn-on, drop-out, jerk-off ideology of Leary and Alpert'.[17] As well as the regular distribution of broadsheets on the streets, Diggers communiqués were also sent to the local underground press. 'We're not foiled anymore by the romantic trappings of the marketers of expanded consciousness. Love isn't a dance concert with a light show at $3 a head,' read one such item, printed in the *Berkeley Barb* on 18 November 1966. In the next edition of the *Barb* a communiqué called 'In Search of a Frame' and signed 'Zapata' laid down the gauntlet more explicitly: 'There has been talk of a psychedelic revolution. It is yet to be seen. Why is it necessary to pay two and a half dollars to go to a dance. What's revolutionary about that?' In a plea that precedes the Bronx hip-hop block parties by more than a decade, it stated: 'Why pay rent on a hall? Why not pressure the city into putting on block dances, parking lot dances,

FREE dances. Would Chet Helms and Bill Graham oppose that? That would be a revolution; something joyous and free in America.' Like Mime Troupe founder Ronnie Davis, who argued that 'the substance of the music is trash . . . absolutely reactionary', the Diggers saw nothing implicitly revolutionary in the activities of the rock groups. 'Where will Jefferson Airplane, Grateful Dead et al. go but up to bigger gigs, better publicity, managers – etc. until they are °°°STARS°°°,' they asked.

Some felt that the Diggers' hostility towards the rock groups was unjustified. The Grateful Dead barely played a paid gig from one week to the next, and although Jefferson Airplane confirmed some people's deeply rooted suspicions by doing a radio ad for Levi's jeans, they too regularly put their beliefs on the line when it came to benefit concerts. A few isolated outlets did escape the Diggers' wrath, notably Ron and Jay Thelin of the Psychedelic Shop, but when the Drugstore Café introduced a fifty-cents minimum purchase between the hours of 6 p.m. and 2 a.m., most people were aware that even the right to sip a groovy coffee came with a price. The Diggers were particularly sceptical about the Golden Gate Park Human Be-In. Grogan saw it as little more than 'the brainstorm of the

Haight Independent Proprietors and their market researchers and consumer consultants'.[18] Timothy Leary and his colleagues came in for considerable enmity too. 'Neither Leary nor Alpert could carry the tune,' Grogan maintained. 'But there they were every time you turned around – on the covers of magazines, on the radio and TV, all over the fucking place – representing them, the young people, the alternative culture. Two creepy, whisky-drinking schoolteachers!'[19]

'The Human Be-In was publicized as a "Gathering of The Tribes",' said Grogan, 'but it was actually more of a gathering of the suburbs with only a sprinkling of nonwhites in the crowd.'[20] What angered Grogan most was the almost universally positive media attention the event received. 'The love shuck was given momentum by all the coverage, and the press even began calling the Love Ghetto of Haight-Ashbury things like "Psychedelphia" and "Hashbury",' he sneered.[21] He was angry about the magnetic effect the coverage was having on the youth of America, 'angry about how their newsmongery was drawing a disproportionate number of kids to the district that was already overcrowded', as he put it, 'thousands of young foolish kids who fell for the Love Hoax and expected to live comfortably poor and take their place in the district's kingdom of love'. In particular, Grogan feared for 'the future of a mob of middle-class kids who were just experimenting with hunger – youngsters who were playing hookie [sic] from suburbia to have an adventure of poverty'.[22]

Bill Graham, who like everybody else stepped through the Diggers' Free Frame of Reference when required to do so, made some astute observations both about Grogan and his own trepidation about the coming Summer of Love. 'Grogan and I got along because underneath it all he knew that he was running another riff,' said Graham. 'He was a scammer but he had good in him . . . he could get down and get high and he had a very strong street sense and he knew a lot. He was a mature street person at a time when there were so many novices. In that era puppies were being born by the truckloads.'[23]

By the summer of 1967 the influx of puppy trucks was at its peak, and Haight-Ashbury was a fully fledged media spectacle. 'Haight cynics joked about bead-wearing *Life* reporters interviewing bead-wearing *Look* reporters,' noted Abe Peck.[24] When the Gray Line San Francisco tour buses started including Haight-Ashbury in their itinerary for $6 a throw, the Diggers handed out mirrors which the locals held up so the tourists could – in the words of 'Happy Freuds' by the Nice – 'see yourself as other people see you'. Richard Brautigan carried his own mirror, which he handed out to likely looking tourists, exclaiming, 'Know thyself!' Peter Coyote reported how 'middle-class people from faraway places began photographing us as if we were exotic natives observed on Safari'. The Diggers' response was to up the ante. 'The tourism diminished when we responded by spray painting the windows of the buses and the camera lenses,' noted Coyote.[25]

In 1968 United Artists released a movie called *You Are What You Eat*. It didn't fit easily into any of the established categories. Neither voyeuristic documentary nor psychsploitation movie, it incorporated cinematic techniques that were far more experimental than would normally be seen in a film ostensibly aimed at a mainstream audience. *You Are What You Eat* featured some of the Haight's most prominent street players, including the Family Dog commune, local bikers and legendary drug supplier Superspade. The film was directed by Barry Feinstein, who had been one of the camera operators on the *Monterey Pop* movie, and was edited by Howard Alk, who also worked with Bob Dylan on *Eat the Document* and *Renaldo and Clara*. The soundtrack featured Peter Yarrow, of Peter, Paul and Mary, who also put up some of the finance; John Simon, who produced the first two Big Brother albums; and, in one of its unforgettable sequences, Tiny Tim performing Sonny and Cher's 'I Got You Babe', with Tim playing the Cher role and Eleanor Barooshian of the all-female band Cake singing Sonny Bono's part, to musical accompaniment by Screamin' Jay Hawkins's backing group the Hawks. It was the last session the Hawks played on before they became the Band. There are many memorable moments in *You Are What You Eat*, but hearing Tiny Tim's piercing falsetto backed by those unmistakably thick swampy textures of Levon Helm, Robbie Robertson et al. arguably beats them all. The movie ends with seven minutes of footage of Frank Zappa and the Mothers performing at the Shrine Auditorium in LA, accompanied by a blitz of a light show and some frantic freaky dancing (although for licensing reasons the music dubbed over the Mothers' performance is by the Electric Flag).

One lengthy sequence was shot at an unrenovated five-floor hotel that stood at the corner of Sutter and Laguna streets. Nicknamed 'the speed palace'

due to its clientele's favoured drug habits, the building was also known as the Greta Garbo House by many locals. According to one former resident, 'The building was overrun with hippies and the lobby was full of runaways just hanging out. Must have been 50 or 60 young kids there. There were two SFPD detectives walking around with a poster board covered with photos asking: "Have you seen any of these people" . . . The floors of the building had been informally divided up by drug of choice, with potheads on the first floor, acidheads on the second and Meth Monsters on the 5th. As you walked the hallway you could see that every door had been kicked in at least once (management? cops? thieves?) and had hasps and padlocks on them.'[26] The former resident also recalls that 'When they were first opened some of the residents found a cache of old but never worn high button shoes in the basement and soon hippie chicks all over the Bay Area were wearing them.'

The movie footage shot at the house is accompanied by the soundtrack's catchiest tune, 'My Name Is Jack' by John Simon. The song's chorus directly references 'the Greta Garbo home for wayward boys and girls', and Simon namechecks several of the hotel's occupants. The 'Carl over there with his funny old hair' was Carl Franzoni, to whom Frank Zappa dedicated 'Hungry Freaks, Daddy' on the Mothers' debut album, and who would play a major part in the Byrds' early set-up. Superspade also gets a mention, and puts in a cameo appearance on the roof of the hotel. There is extensive footage of the interior of the house, with its graffiti-decorated walls, distressed furniture and general drug-den ambience. In a scene without audio young kids are seen motor-mouthing silently to the producer while rolling joints. According to Franzoni, 'It wasn't an acid house, it was a speed house. There's a vignette he [Feinstein] does in the lobby of this hotel and he's talking to some of these kids and they're so loaded they're (munchkin speedfreak blabber), y'know.'[27]

Manfred Mann had a UK Top 10 hit in the summer of 1968 with a cover of 'My Name Is Jack', although they changed the line 'Here comes Superspade, who really gets it on' to the more radio-friendly 'Here comes Superman, who really puts it on'. They also left out the line 'There is Dave with the paints he made from the food the Diggers found', which completely robs the song of its context. But it's that chorus line that really nails it, and ultimately that's what Haight-Ashbury was – the Greta Garbo Home for Wayward Boys and Girls. Speaking of those who flocked to San Francisco full of hope and joy, Peter Coyote made explicit connections between the guerrilla theatrics of the Mime Troupe and the life actors on the streets: 'It was if the participants at a costume ball suddenly found the event too silly and simultaneously dropped their masks. Farm boys from Nebraska were writing poems, preppy girls from Grosse Point were throwing the Tarot and studying herbs. Kids with no idea of what they wanted to become could idle on the teeming streets among people who would not judge them for their confusion.'[28]

The Diggers were hip to the fact that the game was up before most people even knew it had started, before they had perceived that it was a game at all, in fact. They weren't the only group to cast doubt on the 'Love Hoax'. There were plenty of other sceptical voices abroad and their thoughts were aired regularly in the *Oracle* and other outlets. For all its flaws, the counterculture could be ruthlessly self-analytical, but the Diggers were the most vociferous of those who detected that there might be something rotten in the state of hippiedom. 'Don't come to San Francisco,' the more conscientious advocates urged. 'Start up your own Haight-Ashbury where you live.' The Diggers' activities suggest that the issue was more complex than that. 'Inventing a culture from scratch is an exhausting process since everything must be reinvestigated,' said Peter Coyote. 'As edge dwellers, we were proud of being tougher, more experimental, more truthful and less compromised than our peers, most of whom seemed more interested in easy assimilations – dope and long hair at the office or the marketing possibilities of the counter-culture – than in real social alternatives.'[29] Many thought that such incorporation was simply inevitable. Some called it hip capitalism, while Irwin Silber used the phrase 'handicraft capitalism' to indicate the increase in leather workers, sandal-makers, jewellery-makers and all the other tie-dye and embroidery artisans who set up shop in the Haight. Merry Prankster Del Close, who bridged the worlds of the original beats and the hippies, had a more pragmatic response. 'This whole psychedelic thing was co-opted so quick,' he said. 'As soon as people started wearing beads they opened up bead shops.'[30]

4

THE SAVANT-GARDE

Surfadelica, Girl Groups and Garage Land

For the sake of you 'historians' out there I can tell you that some of these bands hailed from here, some from there and the rest from who knows where. They were all rejects from their local boring scenes, they all got booed off stage at the Tiger A-Go-Go clubs where kids were waiting to hear real winners like the Rainy Daze of the Bloos Magoos, they all came in fourth or worse at every Battle of the Bands they ever played and for all these reasons and more these records are now traded for MILLIONS OF DOLLARS by addle brained collectors and fools who love the sound of stoopidiocy as much as I do.

A. SELTZER [sic], Rock Critic at Large, sleeve notes to *Pebbles Volume 2*

As the Bay Area scene was taking shape there was another west-coast agenda going on, one that had little to do with light shows and Merry Pranksters. It pointed to another kind of liquid immersion and another kind of transcendence. It is entirely fitting that the first rock-and-roll record to utilise the term 'LSD' was a surf instrumental, and a surf instrumental B-side at that. 'LSD-25' by the Gamblers was released in 1960 on the flipside of a cut called 'Moon Dawg'. The fact that the title is supposed to have been chosen arbitrarily by a studio engineer is neither here nor there. The significant point is that LSD first entered into the rock-and-roll lexicon because of its logocentric properties rather than its pharmaceutical ones. The Gamblers' random appropriation of the chemical formula for tripping sat well with a musical genre that was gloriously, transcendentally formulaic.

'Moon Dawg'/'LSD-25' was produced by Nick Venet, who would later sign the Beach Boys to Capitol Records and go on to produce their early material. The group featured Derry Weaver on lead guitar, Elliot Ingber on rhythm guitar, Larry Taylor on bass and Bruce Johnston on piano. The A-side was a typical rock-and-roll pounder, driven by Weaver's surf licks and Johnston's piano. 'LSD-25' is a slower, bluesier affair, with Weaver's riffing punctuated by Ingber's echo-laden slide guitar. Ingber subsequently played on Frank Zappa's *Freak Out!* LP and with Little Feat; in the early 1970s he would resurface as Winged Eel Fingerling in Captain Beefheart's Magic Band. The handspan between his snaking reverberated blues glides on 'LSD-25' and his stuttering staccato showcase 'Alice in Blunder-land' on Beefheart's 1972 LP *The Spotlight Kid* encompasses a rhythmic revolution. In the intervening years the beats gestate and mutate and the sonics run increasingly wild and free.

The history of recorded music for most of the twentieth century was a history of coming to terms with extra-neous noise. From the 1930s, when big bands first attempted to harness the wayward and erratic amplification of the electric guitar to the post-war urban blues of Howlin' Wolf, Muddy Waters and Elmore James, over-modu-lation, intentional or otherwise, formed an integral part of the psycho-acoustic fabric. Once studio engineers realised that the trick was to let distortion take its course rather than try to contain it, spillage and side effects came to define the very sound of rock and roll. Echo, initially a consequence of insufficiently soundproofed studios and rudimentary recording techniques, became part of the sonic grain of amplified music. By the time Phil Spector, Jack Nitzsche and Shadow Morton got round to bot-tling the twin genies of leakage and compression in the early 1960s, distor-tion was a working model rather than an aberration.

As aberrations go, 'Rocket 88' by Jackie Brenston and His Delta Cats is as good a place to start this sonic history as any. 'Rocket 88' is post-war popular music's source of the Nile, the R&B record that helped kick-start rock and roll itself. The song was recorded for Chess Records in March 1951 at Sam Phillips's Sun studios in Mem-phis and features Ike Turner and his house band the Kings of Rhythm, with Turner on piano and Willie Kizart on guitar. It was Kizart's distorted guitar that gave the song its distinctive and unusual tone, the distortion supposedly coming about as a result of rain dam-age to Kizart's guitar amp sustained on the way to the session. Phillips liked the muffled sound the soggy amp pro-duced and incorporated it into the tim-bre of the record. The song itself was nothing special: written in homage to the recently introduced V8 Oldsmobile 88, it was just the latest in a series of car-based R&B numbers that rolled off the pressing-plant production line in the post-war years. Neither was Kizart's guitar sound the most arrest-ing feature of 'Rocket 88'. The song is predominantly piano and sax driven and the guitar is embedded low in what might charitably be called 'the mix', but it's Kizart's dirty, atonal drone that has reverberated down the years. Entire careers have subsequently been built around that sound.

In the early 1960s surf music would take 'Rocket 88"s roar of distortion and turn it into a genre. Stripped to its fundaments, like a drag-track chassis or beat-up roadster, 'Rocket 88' reveals the twelve-bar pulse and the I–IV–V chord permutations that fuelled two closely associated activities. Surfing and hot-rod racing were youth culture's most physically active lifestyle movements until hip hop came along. Like hip hop, which spawned a plethora of cultural activities – block parties, turntablism, graffiti art, break-dancing, etc. – the surfing and hot-rod world of the early sixties drew upon a multitude of influences and reference points. The raw adolescent passion and bone-shaking reverberations of early rock and roll were clearly evident in the music, and it's perhaps no coincidence that Gene Vincent had played rhythm guitar in Link Wray's combo Lucky Wray and the Palomino Ranch Hands in the 1950s, for it was Wray, thanks to one fortuitous 1958 instrumental called 'Rumble', who forged the connection between rock and surf. 'Rumble' was actually named in honour of the street-gang fights in *West Side Story* rather than a noise, but its bass-heavy growl fed directly into the instrumental sound of the early 1960s. Equally crucial to the music's early

development was guitarist Dick Dale, who started off picking out Tennessee Williams tunes on the ukulele before developing the heavily percussive technique that would become synonymous with the surf style. Dick Dale and the Del-Tones' 1961 recording 'Let's Go Trippin'' mutates a riff inspired by Chuck Berry (who was actually trying to emulate Charlie Christian, one of the first amplified guitarists) into something more Eastern and exotic. Wray was part Shawnee Indian, while Dale was of Lebanese and Polish descent. Together they brought a unique otherness to rock and roll and weaved an exotic tapestry into its thunderous wall of noise.

Other exotic flavours found their way into the mix too. Surf iconography drew prominently on Polynesian Tiki culture and frequently referenced exotica's holy trinity: Les Baxter, Martin Denny and Arthur Lyman. Socially it attracted a mixed crowd, not just the strutting jocks and blond bronzed Adonis types of Californian legend. Many a City Lights longhair from Venice Beach opted out of the passive contemplation synonymous with the beat lifestyle in favour of a more active form of meditation. For the more robust descendants of beat, surf culture represented a form of physical Zen, living proof that the frontier didn't end at the coast. There was a spiritual undertow to surf culture, one which belies its beach-bum and B-movie stereotypes, and it was best expressed in instrumental form. Surf songs were unashamedly trite celebrations of material wealth and sexual acquisition, full of vainglorious boys boasting about their boards, cars and girls. Had Brian Wilson not retired to his room in 1964 and begun writing melancholic reflections while watching the waves from a distance he would merely be remembered now for a series of songs about spoilt kids having fun fun fun until daddy took the T-Bird away. The best surf songs were laments, the brooding Brian Wilson of 'In My Room', 'Lonely Sea' and 'Please Let Me Wonder' rather than the closet locker-room towel-flicker who wrote 'Surfin' USA' and 'Little Deuce Coupe'. Surf's existential soul is embedded in the Trade Winds' diasporic 'New York's a Lonely Town' ('from Central Park to Pasadena's such a long way'), a tale of a bereft spirit exiled to the east coast, and it can be found in countless other songs that essay distance and angst, and ache with endless summer longing and empty-beach remorse.

Surf instrumentals, on the other hand, were two-and-a-half minute rapid-fire missives that allowed the listener to plant sensory footprints in the sand without having to experience the real thing. Surf was a state of mind, readily adopted by hundreds of bands that lived nowhere near surf-friendly waters, combos who were transported out of their land-locked existence by an echo of something both physical and metaphysical. Bands from Milwaukee with dreams of Waikiki. Bands like the Toads from New Jersey, who semaphored the sound of how they imagined it might be if they had clear blue Pacific waves to ride rather than oil-stained sludge. The Toads made one independently pressed LP in 1964, copies of which now trade for $500 on eBay. Like all surf exotica, it translates its urgency into Morse signals, tone bends and codified modulation. It's the sound of sine waves merging with breaker waves, pick-up clicks syncopated to euphoric heartbeats that rise and fall with the ocean swell. Surf instrumentals painted sound pictures of an imagined negotiation with the wild, untamed, elemental beyond. In the surf world (real or virtual) the participant genuflects to the Earth's gravitational surge and the moon's secret momentum.

Another booster-rocket route to that metaphorical beyond was the space race and the sci-fi future-nostalgia it projected onto lonely satellites and twilight zones. A plethora of surf titles made reference to outer space. That simultaneous yearning and fear about what lay over the endless rolling horizon – as in sea as in space – became an essential component of the surf sound and an integral part of its emotional repertoire. Surf lyrics paddled in shallow waters; surf instrumentals were deep and immersive. And yet for all its elemental passions and rich iconography the role of surf music has been largely written out of most rock histories. Along with the girl groups (whose rise and fall, roughly between 1961 and 1965, it almost exactly replicates) its influence has been vastly underplayed, suffering as it does (again, like the girl groups) from the commonly expressed fallacy that the early 1960s were a barren time for pop music.

Surf music was all speed and glide and had instantly recognisable motifs: thunderous stampeding percussion and an ominous rumbling of toms, drum rolls as relentless as the waves, guitar chords that rippled like the ocean or ricocheted like a gunshot, rhythmic distortions that sounded like rattlesnakes, riffs made entirely out of high-output pick-up clicks and amplified fretwork, all of it underpinned by those low, growling, Wray-gunned bass strings that precede grunge by thirty years.

Tempo was generally fast or frantic, but when tunes were taken at a slower lick they teased out the music's Hawaiian side and its Bikini Atoll impulses. Slo-mo surf transformed the genre into something more eerie, more reflective. Occasionally surf honoured its rock-and-roll roots and included a rasping baritone saxophone or two. Some tracks were even orchestrated: Jack Nitzsche's 'The Lonely Surfer', 'Surf Finger' and 'Baja' were surf music made epic by the simple addition of a surging string arrangement. Sound effects (usually in the form of crashing waves or a hot-rod roar) were often added to the audio concrète, but surf rarely needed to rely on that kind of literalism. Mostly it's just guitar, bass and drums doused in reverb and echo, a torrent of noise that replicated the roar of the ocean, the rise of the waves, the blood rush of the surfer's inner ear. Those cavernous, elemental acoustics were the extra unseen member of the band, augmenting the basic ensemble sound with distortion's distinctive allure. Surf was echo-chamber music.

Surf-band names blur effortlessly into one another. Run together they form a sound poem of staccato concrète; chanted they evoke the surf logos through which all things are made, as divine. Auto-plate names. Street-gang names. Greco-Roman gods' names. Pop-art matrix names. An endless index of the mythological made real and the mortal recast as statuesque hoodlum gods. The Safaris. The Surfaris. The Stingrays. The Ric-A-Shays. The Clee-Shays. The Chantays. The Shan-Tones. The Velvetones. The Vanqueros. The Vibrants. The Vistas. The Valiants. The Vulcaines. The Surf Teens. The Torquays. The Torquettes. The Tempests. The Fugitives. The Phantoms. The Pyramids. The Persuaders. The Scouts. The Squires. The Ramrods. The Reveliers. The Breakers. The Avantis. The Dantes. The Iridescents.

Track titles speak directly of their intent, their ambition, their holy orders and their goal beyond. Strung together they read like metaphysical shorthand. Every one of them an exclamation. A roar. A quest. 'Wipe Out'. 'Kick Out'. 'Turn On'. 'Hot Line'. 'Motivate'. 'Scramble'. 'Ridin' High'. 'Down Shiftin''. 'Side-Swiped'. 'The Switch'. 'Rev Up'. 'Wax 'Em Down'. 'Echo'. 'Vibrations'. 'Nightride'. 'Moon Relay'. 'Moon Race'. 'Moon Child'. 'Moon Shot'. 'Action Plus'. 'Pulsebeat'. 'Pedal Pusher'. 'Cloudburst'. 'Avalanche'. 'Earthquake'. 'Jet Stream'. 'Surf Blast'. 'Swamp Surfer'. 'Shark Attack'. 'Coral Below'. 'Loophole'. 'High Wire'. 'The Breeze and I'.

'Cry of Atlantis'. '8oft Wave'. 'The Rise'. 'Collision Course'. 'Crash'. 'No Return'. 'The Other Side'.

Surf instrumentals proved to be extremely palatable to a wider audience that had never been near a surfboard, and the sound notched up several chart successes in the early sixties. 'Walk Don't Run' by the Ventures (September 1960), 'Pipeline' by the Chantays (April 1963) and 'Wipe Out' by the Surfaris (July 1963) were all Top 10 hits in both the US and the UK. 'Let's Go Trippin'' by Dick Dale and the Del-Tones (September 1961) only made number 60 in the US singles chart but its influence transcended any mere chart placing. Wrecking Crew drummer Sandy Nelson had a string of percussion-heavy hits between November 1959 ('Teen Beat') and June 1962 ('Drumming Up a Storm'). The biggest of these, 'Let There Be Drums', a Top Three record in the UK and a US Top 10 hit in December 1961, is one of the most audaciously minimalist pop singles of the 1960s. Entirely percussion driven, it celebrates rock and roll stripped to its big-beat basics. From that period only Dick and Dee Dee's 'The Mountain's High', scored for vocal duet, drum roll and echo chamber, has a more primal connection with rock and roll's core principles.

For all its aural splendour it is hard to deny surf music's umbilical connection to schlock. It's clearly evident in all those beach-party movies and the two-girls-for-every-boy goofiness and frat-dream fantasies they celebrate. Jan and Dean, in a genre ripe for parody, wrote a masterly paean to auto-uneroticism called 'Schlock Rod', about an olive-green '48 Buick that falls to bits over the duration of the song. Released in 1963, with a melody and delivery borrowed from the Hollywood Argyles' equally parodic 'Alley Oop', the lyrics are delivered in halting medicated-nerd speak replete with spoof hot-rod slang and a clanging, crashing mélange of sound effects. 'Schlock Rod' sits resplendently, delinquently derelict among all the status-symbol tributes to Mustangs and Stingrays. Along with the burning-tarmac roar and the cowabunga shouts, another essential sound source on surf instrumentals was the low-rent horror feature that played at a thousand drive-ins nightly. The frightmare scream, the creaking castle door, the ominous cackle of laughter all celebrate, in cartoon-style homage, the classic era of Bela Lugosi and Boris Karloff. Link Wray's 'The Shadow Knows' commences with the schlock-horror declamation 'Who knows what evil lurks in the hearts of men?' and plays moody chords off against mock evil cries. Even Sun Ra got in on the act with a pseudonymous 1966 album called *The Sensational Guitars of Dan and Dale*, which featured the core of his exotically garbed Arkestra, along with members of Al Kooper's Blues Project. Together they knocked out some splendidly convincing surf pastiche, over classical melodies by Chopin and Tchaikovsky. It's entirely fitting that the B-side of the Kingsmen's 1963 three-chord anthem 'Louie Louie' was a surf instrumental called 'Haunted Castle'. This upbeat organ and guitar duet doesn't sound in the least bit spooky; its stop–start dance rhythms were tailor-made for Annette Funicello or Teri Garr to shimmy and shiver to at Paradise Cove as they filmed in the dead of winter while pretending that life was one long celluloid summer.

Almost anything lent itself to a surf arrangement: rock-and-roll and R&B numbers, Latin American hits, Tamla hits, Christmas novelty records. It didn't matter if it was Bill Dogget's 'Raunchy' or Jimmy Forrest's 'Night Train', 'Temptation' or 'Jezebel', 'Bali Hai' or 'Ali Baba', 'La Bamba' or 'Hava Nagila' – anything could be given a surf workover. The formula worked especially well on all those snappy sixties TV themes that already sounded like surf records anyway: *The Green Hornet*, *Get Smart*, *Batman*, *The Munsters*. Strip *The Monkees'* theme down to its wordless fundamentals and you have a surf tune. Well into the late 1960s, long after the boom was over, the surf sound was being churned out by seasoned sessioneers and contemporary hits were being given the surf treatment in an attempt to cash in on a scene that no longer existed. One band more than any other, the Ventures, made a speciality out of alchemising base musical instincts into surf tones. The Ventures are one of the crucial evolutionary links that connect the surf sound of the early sixties to the garage-band sound that followed. They were using fuzz pedals as early as 1962 and phasing effects and reversed tape by 1963. Their 1963 album *Ventures in Space* (renamed *Out of Limits* for its UK release) features tracks with titles like 'Fear', 'War of the Satellites', 'Solar Race' and 'The Fourth Dimension'. Cuts like 'He Never Came Back' and 'Exploration in Terror' would not have sounded out of place shaking the rafters of the Avalon Ballroom three years later. The standout track, 'The Bat', could have passed itself off as a scary out-take from Zappa's *Freak Out!* or *Lumpy Gravy*. When they weren't anticipating the psychedelic sound, on the album's

more upbeat numbers the Ventures produced moody noirish pieces that depicted outer space as a foreboding and haunted place. And they did all this while looking like the straightest band in rock and roll. Resplendent in the casual wear that they proudly modelled in most of their publicity shots, there was something decidedly subversive about their straightness. Like the surrealist and Dada group photos taken between 1924 and 1933, in which each and every one of them, from Hans Arp to Louis Aragon, looks like a bank manager, salesman or psychiatrist, the Ventures created outer-space surfadelica while assuming body shapes that were strictly squaresville. Like Sun Ra, they probably were from outer space; they just chose to go about their business in a more subtle human disguise than the one chosen by Sonny Blount from Saturn.

There is, of course, a direct link between the surf sound and what came next. By the mid-sixties several surf bands had evolved a tougher, more R&B-based style, adding vocals (often a fake English adenoidal drawl) to their instrumental sound while still retaining something of surf's three-chord thrill. By 1965–6 there were thousands of these groups all over America. They played local battle-of-the-bands competitions, high-school dances, military bases, strip joints, shopping malls, auto fairs, anywhere. Some made one record and faded into obscurity; others made three and began to shape something resembling a career, and then faded into obscurity. Many are remembered for one stand-out cut, one two-and-a-half minute moment of magic when they reached heights never to be scaled again. Few thought that their efforts would endure and one day be revered as the artefacts of a vinyl golden age. Like hot rods and demolition-derby cars, they weren't built to last. The name retrospectively applied to these combos was 'garage bands', based on the notion that many of them rehearsed and sometimes even recorded in the garages of urban and suburban homes up and down the land. But in the same way that most psychedelic pop wasn't labelled as such at the time – it was just pop – and the girl-group era wasn't known as that either – it was also just pop – the term 'garage bands' wasn't used at all when the phenomenon was at its height. 'Garage bands' is something of a misnomer anyway, a quirk of classification that, like so many others, serves mainly to group a whole bunch of loosely associated tendencies under a common rubric. As Richie Unterberger put it, 'The Music Machine, the Remains, and the Chocolate Watch Band – and numerous others – were not simply "garage bands". They were simply very talented bands that didn't get the success that came to the era's biggest groups, due to ill luck, bad management, the uncommercial nature of some of their music and other factors. They were also top-notch musicians and composers, recording in state of the art studios, not in primitive garages.'[1]

In the great cultural ricochet of life the garage bands were the sound of American beat groups imitating English beat groups who had been imitating American R&B groups in the first place. That's not the full story by any means, but if the garage sound can be reduced to one common factor, then the great Anglo-American pursuit of roots on the rebound – a tendency that echoes back and forth across the Atlantic for most of the twentieth century – constitutes a substantial part of its formula. The garage sound takes as its source material a range of English influences: roughly in order of prominence these were the Rolling Stones, the Yardbirds, the Beatles, the Who, Them, the Pretty Things, the Animals, the Kinks, the Dave Clark Five, the Zombies and the Troggs. This list doesn't even begin to explain the full depth and weight of those influences. 'Gloria' and 'Baby Please Don't Go' by Them have a disproportionate influence way beyond the group's brief period of success in America. Along with 'Louie Louie''s A–D–E chord structure, 'Gloria''s central E–D–A riff was the *spiritus sanctus* for hundreds of garage-band records, while Van Morrison's vocal style (borrowed heavily from his own black R&B influences) is as prevalent as Mick Jagger's.

Hundreds of groups took their inspiration from the Rolling Stones. 'Open Up Your Door' by Richard and the Young Lions is just one of countless records that take the Stones' 'Get Off of My Cloud' as its inspiration. The impossibly tall Mr Richard can be seen on a 1966 American TV clip executing Jagger steps and wildly clawing the air as his backing group (actually a front for a group of session musicians) pound their way through this garage classic. The Electric Prunes' 'Get Me to the World on Time' lifts its chorus melody entirely from '19th Nervous Breakdown'. 'Levitation' by the 13th Floor Elevators is '19th Nervous Breakdown' minus the breakdown. Beatles soundalikes came in all shapes and sizes too. 'Lies' by the Knickerbockers was worthy of the moptops themselves. 'I Wonder' by the Gants referenced 'In My Life'. 'I Must

Run' by Phil and the Frantics lays a gorgeous Farfisa drone over a Mersey quiver. 'It's Cold Outside' by the Choir is just one of countless songs that you can imagine having been written the minute the Beatles concluded their performance on the *Ed Sullivan Show*.

Many garage bands recorded cover versions of UK records that had directly influenced them in the first place: the Moving Sidewalks covered the Beatles' 'I Want to Hold Your Hand'; the Standells did 'Paint It Black' and '19th Nervous Breakdown'; the Count Five, who had started off as a Ventures-influenced surf combo, recorded versions of 'My Generation' and 'Out in the Street' by the Who, a band that had its own surf fixation. Countless other garage bands paid homage to the great cultural ricochet: 'Go Away' by the Plague emulates the Kinks' 'All Day and All of the Night', which itself was a rewrite of 'Louie Louie'; 'I Will Not Be Lonely' by the Fanatics is 'Pushin' Too Hard' meets 'You Really Got Me', which is also 'Louie Louie' in Muswell Hill clothing. The San Francisco-based Oxford Circle added further complexity to the cultural rebound by recording the Animals' 'We Gotta Get Out of This Place' – a west-coast take by an American band with an English name on a Newcastle hit written by Barry Mann and Cynthia Weil in New York's Brill Building. The Oxford Circle weren't the only group with an English-sounding name: Anglophilia was also evident in the Beau Brummels, the Liverpool Set, London Phogg, Sopwith Camel, the Squires, the Brigands, the Sir Douglas Quintet and countless others. Before they established their garage-band credentials with 'Can't Seem to Make You Mine' the Seeds were known as the Lords of London.

Running through all of this, and bigger than any other influence, was the tidal flow of surf. Transition markers are there all the way from 'Run Run Run' by the Gestures – a 1964 surf take on Merseybeat that anticipates the Byrds' folk-rock drone – to 'Back Seat 38 Dodge' by Opus 1, a squalling, echo-drenched throb of a song released in 1966 that takes hot-rod testosterone into new, psychologically damaged terrain. The distance from surf to surf-inspired encapsulated in the intro to the Blues Project's 'No Time Like the Right Time' seems to have taken no time at all. Likewise the distance between Dick Dale's 'Lets Go Trippin'' and 'Pushin' Too Hard' by the Seeds. The moment, one minute ten seconds into 'Pushin' Too Hard', when guitarist Jan Savage unleashes eight bars of surf splendour is the moment when old

fuses with new to form a magical surfadelic hybrid. Jan Savage even sounds like a surf name. Three years earlier he would have been fronting a band called Jan Savage and the Vibrants or Jan Savage and the Buicks. Surfadelica is also there in 'Fire Engine' by the 13th Floor Elevators, with its screaming vocal intro (a common surf motif), its siren drone and its manic three-chord flurry. '1523 Blair' by fellow Texan outfit the Outcasts is the moment when Buddy Holly's 'Peggy Sue' and Dick Dale's 'Miserlou' are formally introduced to Love's '7 and 7 Is'. 'Optical Sound' by Human Expression takes the eerie weirdness of surf instrumentals like 'The Birds' by the Motivations or 'Desert Wind' by the Vaqueros and coats them in drug-rush synaesthesia. The Standells' follow-up to 'Dirty Water', 'Sometimes Good Guys Don't Wear White', slows down the Kingsmen's 'Louie Louie' until it sounds like its B-side, 'Haunted Castle'.

The record that did more than any other to retrospectively consolidate the reputation of the garage sound was Lenny Kaye's *Nuggets* compilation. Released in 1972 with the subtitle *Original Artyfacts from the First Psychedelic Era 1965–1968*, *Nuggets* is still regarded by many as the holy grail of garage-band music. It spawned a plethora of imitations whose very titles – *Pebbles, Boulders, Rubble,* etc. – consciously allude to the seminal role played by the twenty-seven tracks contained on the original *Nuggets* album. Lenny Kaye's taste brought a plethora of classic garage cuts to wider public attention, such as 'Night Time' by the Strangeloves, a studio-ensemble record with a guitar solo that was Bo Diddley without the shuffle, the innuendo-drenched 'I Had Too Much to Dream Last Night' by the Electric Prunes, or 'Oh Yeah' by the Shadows of Knight, with its Bo Diddley-via-the-Yardbirds riff and faux-Eastern bridge. 'Don't Look Back' by the Remains had a Mick Jagger vocal over *Safe as Milk*-era Magic Band backing. 'An Invitation to Cry' by the Magicians was a waltz-time soul ballad written by future Turtles songwriters Garry Bonner and Alan Gordon that anticipated how Flo and Eddie might have sounded had they joined Zappa five albums earlier. 'Open My Eyes' by Todd Rundgren's first group Nazz cribs its intro from the Who's 'I Can't Explain'. 'Sit Down, I Think I Love You' by the Mojo Men weaves pop baroque with a delightful Van Dyke Parks arrangement. Anglophilia was also richly represented by versions of John Carter and Ken Lewis's 'My World Fell Down' by Sagittarius

and the Searchers' 'Sugar and Spice' by the Cryan' Shames. The Amboy Duke performed a cover of Them's cover of Big Joe Williams's adaptation of 'Baby Please Don't Go'. 'Tobacco Road' by the Blues Magoo was a US cover of a UK cover of a US track and contained an extended guitar freak-out that had a discernible influence on the Syd Barrett-era Pink Floyd. Four tracks in particular – 'Pushin' Too Hard' by the Seeds, 'Dirty Water' by the Standells, 'You're Gonna Miss Me' by the 13th Floor Elevators and 'Psychotic Reaction' by Count Five – were so influential that even the bands who recorded them felt compelled to rewrite and regurgitate them endlessly.

The first 13th Floor Elevators LP, *The Psychedelic Sound of the 13th Floor Elevators*, and its follow-up *Easter Everywhere* contain some of the most primal yelps of discomfort and joy heard anywhere in rock and roll. The mere existence of the band's 1966 debut, the first album to use the word 'psychedelic' in its title, posits a parallel Earth theory in which the Rolling Stones, by some evolutionary quirk (or quark), never existed, or if they did, they had been described to Roky Erickson and his gang without access to the records, and possibly by an interlocutor who possessed only the most rudimentary grasp of nuance and no understanding whatsoever of who borrowed what from whom or where in the first place. That's just a fanciful pop-journo conceit, of course. What really happened is that they practised, practised, practised to get that good. It's not even a particularly unique noise that they made; plenty of other Texas R&B bands had that rebel yelp and that primeval production. 'Fluctuation' by the Shades of Night, 'Don't Be That Way' by the Reasons Why, 'Torture' by A440 and numerous other tracks contained on those Tex-psych compilations that treat the Lone Star state's voluminous output with all the reverence of Delta-blues curators all share a sound as ubiquitous as Merseybeat. The 13th Floor Elevators simply distilled it to its impure essence, and did it better than anyone else. Their music is clearly of rock and roll but not entirely in it, and their bottom-of-a-well echo and wailing wall of sound couldn't be further removed from the slick, pristine productions coming out of state-of-the-art New York and LA at the time. Echo and reverb equalise everything into a thick primordial gloop from which individual components re-emerge covered in sticky space dust. They even named a track 'Reverberation' just in case the aural manifesto wasn't clear

enough and the message wasn't getting through. Roky Erickson's lyrics are delivered in two modes: a manic high-pitched cackle or a mournful yearning sob. On 'We Sell Soul' he sounds like Van Morrison. On 'Earthquake' the band sound like the Troggs. On 'Fire Engine' and 'Levitation' they build a rustproof mind car that will work for a thousand years.

More than anything, of course, the garage-band sound is the sound of drugs. Amphetamines added a frisson of nail-chewing neurosis to ever-present male anxieties. The brain-mashing onslaught of LSD heaped further chemical layers on top, either soothing the psyche with delusions or debilitating it with nightmare visions of inadequacy. Drugs are the force field that define the territory. '1000 Micrograms of Love' by Satori is a slow blues homage out of Houston, Texas, that sounds like Big Brother and the Holding Company's arrangement of 'Summertime', until the vocalist begins to growl his precisely measured come-on to chemical amour. 'What I feel for you no poet could describe,' he sings, making it clear that only a spaced-out, teeth-grinding grin can really do that. The B-side, 'Time Machine', is set to a Yardbirds-style Eastern wail and an Arthur-Lee's-Love-channelling-the-Rolling-Stones relentless beat. 'I'm gonna show you things that will turn your head around,' he sings, before being sucked into a vortex of phasing and distortion. The whole affair lasts for one minute thirty-seven seconds. Equally mind-expandingly concise at one minute thirty-one is 'Voices Green and Purple' by the Bees, a homage to watching late-night B-movies while your body is slowly devoured by a flesh-eating incubus that looks like Reg Presley. Similarly synaesthetic was 'Colors' by Hunger, the vision-scented sound of Portland, Oregon, from a time when thousand-foot Farfisas and million-eyed echo units stalked the earth. 'Into the Sun' by Pure Jade Green is another pure, shimmering drug puddle of a song made magnificent simply by virtue of the production effects on the vocals, which send the singer's thought dribbles cascading out into the cosmos with the aid of distorted echo and zero-gravity reverb. 'Tripmaker' by the Seeds ('Watch out, watch out, he's coming your way') casts Johnny in the basement mixing up his medicine into a B-movie scenario of fizzing phials and mad scientists. 'Mr Farmer', which can be found on the same Seeds LP, is another undisguised endorsement of better living with chemistry. 'Trippin' Out' by Something Wild ('Listen, girls, and listen, boys / these little things / they ain't no toys') is a more cautionary

warning about the perils of space travel. Set to a 'Tobacco Road' riff, it spreads its two short verses across a mucusy layer of reverberated fuzz before the singer decides, 'My work here is done,' and the whole things fades into drone tones and squalls of feedback. '99th Floor' by the Moving Sidewalks manages to get barely concealed innuendo into both the song title and the band name. Their 1968 album was called *Flash* and its opening track 'Flashback', just in case listeners hadn't got the message. Hamilton Streetcar sang about 'Invisible People', a Lee Hazlewood production ('She's got red eyes and purple lips / she's always on invisible trips') full of fuzz, Farfisas and what-the-fuck-is-he-singing-about imagery. 'Five Years Ahead of My Time' by the Third Bardo has a spooky *Ventures in Space*-style intro and a classy Teddy Randazzo production. 'It may seem like I'm coming on strong,' sings the slightly unhinged vocalist, who is pumped full of New York neurosis ('Society can't play with my mind') and plans to propel you to a new dimension, where he will screw you on his space carpet. Also full of rocket fuel but minus the sexual intent is the joyously deranged cosmic slop of 'Spazz' by the Elastik Band, a record that is gloriously incorrect on so many levels, from the demented way in which the singer pronounces 'spay-azz' and the appropriately mutated cool-jerk rhythm to the sheer incautious, undiscerning celebration of what happens when mind expansion gets several stages beyond messy. Just as unlikely to be mixing the Mixolydian and the Phrygian was 'I Want to Come Back (from the World of LSD)' by the Fe-Fi-Four Plus Two, indisputably the greatest band name in this entire book. It's a too-late-to-turn-back tale ('I wanna get my kicks but this ain't the way') about what happens when you mix schlock-horror-movie imagery, Yardbirds Gregoriana and a cut-price sugar-cube cable-car ride to the summit of your dream-mares. The dire warning that the singer brings back from his excursion into hell – 'My throat's getting dry and the things I see are loud' – should be enough to convince anyone that Coleridge's stately treasure dome doesn't do day passes. As the opium dream that induced Kubla Khan began to wear off and Samuel Taylor Coleridge was interrupted by the (possibly fictitious) person from Porlock, the last words he wrote moments before the euphoria faded were: 'For he on honeydew hath fed, / And drunk the milk of paradise.' The Fe-Fi-Four Plus Two opt for less luscious pastures. 'Laundromat!' the singer screams. 'I gotta find myself! Puppy toys!'

For all its hybrids and synchronicity, that see-saw relationship between British and American music was tinged with arrogance on both sides. It's amusing to hear certain critics playing down the effect that Merseybeat had on the American garage bands, when approximately every third vocalist appeared to have stolen John Lennon's larynx or Mick Jagger's pout. Conversely, the oft-propagated notion that English beat groups reintroduced America to its own black-music heritage is cultural colonialism taken to new delusory heights of condescension. The very foundation stone of the garage-band sound, 'Louie Louie', was written and first performed by African American Richard Berry with his band the Pharaohs in 1957. Garage-band songs are full of soul and R&B influences mainlined directly from the source. One of the best tracks on *Nuggets*, 'Liar, Liar' by the Castaways, a US Top Twenty hit in May 1965, adds a Little Anthony soul shout to surf rhythms. On the same LP 'Love's Gone Bad' by the Michigan-based Underdogs was a blue-eyed take on Chris Clark's original and came out on the same Motown subsidiary, VIP. Ed Cobb, the production svengali behind the Chocolate Watch Band, also wrote 'Tainted Love' for Gloria Jones and 'Every Little Bit Hurts' for Brenda

Holloway. If you listen to 'Heartbeat', the Cobb-penned follow-up to 'Tainted Love', it's basically a garage stomper with gospel-soul vocals. 'The End' by another Michigan-based outfit, the Ruins – with the wonderfully titled 'Take My Love (and Shove It Up Your Heart)' on the flip – has an organ-based soul sound that spread its dragnet all the way from New Jersey to Michigan in the mid-sixties. The east-coast influence of the early Young Rascals hits ('I Ain't Gonna Eat Out My Heart Anymore', 'Good Lovin'', 'You Better Run', 'I've Been Lonely Too Long') permeates the garage-band era. It's an earthy, Italian-American R&B sound that has travelled from doo-wop to psychedelia with its grittiness intact. It can be heard in many psychedelic soul cuts and would reach its peak – or trough, depending on your point of view – with the Vanilla Fudge, who took soul classics like 'You Keep Me Hanging On', 'Shotgun' and 'Take Me for a Little While' and slowed them to a funereal crawl. Many others tried to repeat the trick but none executed it with the same brutal panache.

If pop and soul shared common antecedents, one clear line of delineation that does emerge during the garage era is the great cultural divide between the Chuck Berry and Bo Diddley camps.

It's a territorial demarcation that cuts a swathe through the entire history of rock and roll. The Berry allegiance is reflected in the early Beach Boys, in trad Beatles rather than modernist Beatles, and in the Rolling Stones (who right up until Altamont were performing Berry covers like 'Carol' in their stage act). It's an allegiance that celebrates American iconography by presenting it as a blur of billboards as seen from a speeding car, and in its celebration of affluence and acquisition it has a particular appeal to white audiences. 'You can't give Chuck Berry to a black. We care less about Chuck Berry,' said Ike Turner, as provocative as ever, in the BBC documentary *Dancing in the Street*. Seated at the piano he elaborated on his reputation-shredding discourse. 'Blacks can accept Jimmy Reed. [sings] "You got me running. You got me hiding." We can accept that. But "way down in Louisiana"? Damn Louisiana!'[2] The Bo Diddley route, on the other hand, celebrates a sound rather than an image. It manifests itself in a staccato shuffle that may or may not have come from Africa, and a particular way of sculpting primitive sonics with customised space-age guitars. Far more garage bands endorsed the Bo Diddley method than the Chuck Berry one. It can be heard shuffle-beating its way across the US via the Yardbirds' cover of Diddley's 'I'm a Man' and 'Mystic Eyes' by Them into hundreds of garage cuts. On *Nuggets* the Bo Diddley influence is prominent on 'Psychotic Reaction' by Count Five and 'I Want Candy' by the Strangeloves. And it's ever present, of course, in the primal pulse-beat of the Velvet Underground and the legions of bands that later copied them.

'Primitive' is the word usually used to describe this sound. It's a culturally loaded term which doesn't begin to explain the complexity of what was going on here, and contrary to the 'sound of stoopidiocy' claims often made on the music's behalf, a lot of it clearly wasn't stupid at all. In 'The Boy Looked at Roxy', a hilarious and scabrous sleeve-note polemic spread out over two successive *Pebbles* compilations (volumes 7 and 8, released in 1979), the pseudonymous Greg Shaw, writing under the pen name 'The Rev & Mrs Tommy Parasite', offers a skewed alternative history of rock and roll. He claims that by the mid-sixties rock's rebellious spirit had been led astray by the agents of international communism and that the garage groups acted as a corrective mechanism to this dour and earnest imposition. 'Hundreds of bands turned the sights of their newly liberated consciousness on the real threats

to their freedom,' wrote the Reverend Parasite. And what was this threat? 'Lying girlfriends and a world that doesn't understand.' In a piece called 'Tales from the Drug Attic', published in *NME* in December 1983 and written at a time when a lot of this music was being freshly discovered by a whole new generation, Julian Cope neatly summarised the lyrical content of *Pebbles Volume 5* as: 'Singer meets girl, girl bogs off. Singer loves girl, girl screws singer's arch rival. Singer loves girl, girl is unaware of singer's existence.' The Reverend Parasite and the Arch Drude Cope both hit upon an eternal truth, one that applies equally to many a mod-psych record coming out of the UK during the same period. It's a viewpoint that applies the 'there are only seven stories' principle to rock and roll and finds that to be at least four too many, but there's something else going too, an altogether different kind of distortion. When you make a Xerox of a Xerox of a Xerox of a Xerox, the image blurs and mutates with each successive copy, and that's precisely (and imprecisely) what happened with the garage groups. In that endless rebounding replication back and forth across the Atlantic certain nuances diminished while others were exaggerated; mannerisms grew ever more warped and dislocated from their source until they bore only the faintest resemblance to their original impulse. By 1966 many garage groups were no longer fronted by snarly wild ones trying to sound like English Home Counties, grammar-school-educated blues aficionados, who were in turn trying to build sonic monuments to a blues life cribbed entirely from what they had read on Chess sleeve notes and glimpsed (or thought they had glimpsed) in the faded spectral apparitions of Delta daguerreotypes. An air of hollow braggadocio had prevailed for some time in British mod pop and American R&B, but this was something different. Filtered through the paranoiac prism of acid, this was nothing less than machismo in peril.

And what did it sound like, this swirling vortex of rancour and confusion, this yelp of pain disguised as a death threat? It sounded like Question Mark as he stuttered 'Too many teardrops / for one heart / to be crying' between gulps of resentful breath in '96 Tears'. It sounded like the Seeds' vocalist Sky Saxon growling that his girl was pushing him too hard. This was the sound of lacerated pride and ego emasculation. It's there in the castrato whine of 'Liar, Liar' by the Castaways. It's there in 'Little Girl' by Syndicate of Sound, 'Why Do I Cry' by the Remains,

'Knock, Knock' by the Humane Society ('Whirling / swirling in a world of grief and sin'), 'Action Woman' by the Litter ('You say you own the world / but you don't own my soul') and 'Enough of What I Need' ('Don't you do it with any other guys') by the appropriately named Stoics. These are songs where emptiness, venom and resentment grow ever more neurotic with each surging burst of fear, where every female action or reaction is a threat, where every retaliatory lyric is a suppressed murder ballad, where fronting up completely fails to cover up the boy-crushing hurt and the wounded pride inside.

These anthems to bruised fragility were a central feature of the garage-band sound, but they featured prominently in soul lyrics too and were just as likely to be found in the gothic splendour of Tamla, Stax and Goldwax. The difference between ? and the Mysterians' '96 Tears' and James Carr's 'The Dark End of the Street', or between the Seeds' 'Pushin' Too Hard' and the Four Tops' 'Seven Rooms of Gloom', was one of style rather than substance. Those melodramatic sobs and sighs come from somewhere else too, of course: the girl groups. Where else do you find relationship-wreckers running around all over town, messing their loyal partner around? Who else builds monuments to jealousy, insecurity, betrayed trust, thwarted longings and lonely nights spent all alone? The girl groups and garage groups reflect mirror images of pain and neurosis back at each other over a chasm littered with heartache and regret. Each choreographs its overwrought assumptions to the other's insensitivity and indifference. She's snared him for now but she knows it's not going to last because his heart is still with the motorcycle gang and he really wants to be back with the guys ('Out in the Streets' – Shangri Las). He still sees her out and about, but now she's got a new love, and even though the new guy is out of town, he knows there is no way she'll give him another chance ('Everything's There' – the Hysterics). All these pain-stained diary pages congeal into one long lament. Doomed lovers full of emptiness and regret think identical thoughts about what they're missing and what they lost. 'Last Time Around' by the Del-Vetts, recorded in 1966, is a garage-angst anthem powered by fuzz pedals and a pounding four-to-the-floor rhythm, but it borrows its emotional cut and thrust entirely from the girl-group sound of three years earlier. The bittersweet 'la la' lilt of its chorus is a direct steal from the Shirelles, the Chiffons and the Cookies. The Del-Vetts began

life as a surf band, but they had a girl-group name and expressed girl-group turmoil. The ultra-snotty vocalist on the strangely titled 'Of Old Approximately' by the Bourbons reverses the traditional gender dynamic completely: he's sitting home alone nursing a bottle and a bruised ego, while she goes out with other guys.

The girl groups and the garage bands were pop's great unrequited double act. Neither really makes sense without the other, and it's more than a shame that they couldn't have spent a little more time inhabiting the same time span rather than only briefly overlapping. Instead their stand-off royal, their *pas de deux* of denial is divided by an epoch and a not altogether healthy shift in critical appraisal. The garage-band outbursts of machismo-in-peril find their most honest reflection in the girl-group songs; not the trite cheerleader chorales and eternity-ring serenades to soppiness and sugar-coated conformity, but in the anthems to defiance and identity. Songs like 'Nobody Knows What's Going on (in My Mind but Me)' by the Chiffons, where the listener feels like they're eavesdropping on someone's innermost thoughts, and if she repeats the title-line mantra often enough, she just might convince herself she's right. Or 'Saturday Night

Didn't Happen' by Reparata and the Delrons, where the chorus plays off denial against desire and wishes that the weekend's indiscretions had all been a bad dream. Or Dawn's epic 'I'm Afraid They're All Talking About Me', which takes the 'Will he still respect me if I sleep with him?' dilemma of Goffin and King's 'Will You Love Me Tomorrow' and answers the next day's gossip and taunting with a simple emotional plea: 'Baby, you can help me / by telling me you love me.' It's one of the most affecting moments in pop. The disapproving looks, whispers and small-town approbation are countered with one simple request to her man: 'Stop being so shallow and show a little emotional support here, baby. And you can start by telling me that last night actually meant something.'

Thanks to a series of latter-day compilation albums (notably the *Girls with Guitars* and *Girls from the Garage* anthologies), many a girl-group effort has retrospectively restored the synchronicity that existed between female pain and male angst in the garage sound of the sixties. The Bittersweets' 'The Hurtin' Kind' and Ellaine and the Shardells' 'Tell Me That You Care' stake out the terrain between tenderness and resentment as well as anything on *Nuggets*. Absence is ever present in moody

minor-chord classics like the Chymes' 'He's Not There Anymore' and Lyn and the Invaders' 'Boy Is Gone'.

Girls in garageland were also expert at collapsing the distance between spooky and voracious, and could sound ethereal and on the prowl at the same time. 'Want You' by the Weekends and 'The Rider' by the Pussycats sound like the kind of field recordings Russ Meyer might have made out in the desert scrubland among the wrecked autos and the lost tribes of feral Amazonian women. Charlotte Vinnedge, singer and lead guitarist on the fuzz-toned 'Up Down Sue' by the Luv'd Ones, anticipates the bratty snarl of 'Rip Her to Shreds'-era Debbie Harry with her vocal delivery and Courtney Love's combo Hole with her tuned-down Gibson guitar sound. 'You Don't Love Me' by the Starlets positions itself amid an R&B legacy line that begins with Willie Cobbs's 1961 adaptation and retitling of Bo Diddley's 1955 'She's Fine, She's Mine' and ends with Dawn Penn's 1993 dance-hall makeover of her own 1967 rocksteady version of the same song.

Perhaps the most combative all-female garage band was Ace of Cups, who were regular fixtures on the Haight-Ashbury scene between 1966 and 1968 and played alongside all the top west-coast acts. Ace of Cups featured guitarist and harmonica player Denise Kaufman, who had previously been a member of Ken Kesey's Merry Pranksters, where she was known as Mary Microgram – although Kaufman's experience of acid predated her involvement with Kesey and his crew. During this period she was also part of a band called the Answers, playing Pretty Things-style R&B, and pre-Moby Grape outfit the Frantics. Kaufman was actually the last member to join the Ace of Cups line-up, but she was its galvanising force, well connected and savvy. Her husband at the time, Noel Jewkes, was a member of Bill Ham's Light Sound Dimension, providing musical accompaniment for Ham's live workshop experiments. Like the Great Society, Ace of Cups never really fulfilled their potential. Musically their output ranged from gospel-inflected a cappella to raucous blues jams. They left only a handful of demo and live recordings, which reveal them to be every bit as versatile (and every bit as shambling) as their Bay Area peers.

Several of the Electric Prunes' most distinctive songs – 'I Had Too Much to Dream Last Night', 'Get Me to the World on Time', 'Antique Doll', etc. – were written by the female writing team of Annette Tucker and Nancie Mantz. 'Most of their material sounded like it was written for a female vocalist,' said Prunes singer James Lowe. 'I felt a bit uncomfortable with some of it, but at the time we couldn't write anything as "commercial" so we just did it . . . They were trying to get hits. When you approached songwriting in a professional manner, you did whatever you had to do to get your songs placed. I knew Annette, and she really enjoyed her craft. We always had a laugh at the variety and scope of the images . . . "placing lipstick kisses on the wall". They were lusty bitches!'[3] Despite also writing hits for the Ventures, the Knickerbockers and the American Breed, Tucker and Mantz barely warrant a mention in the boy's-own pantheon of rock and roll.

The best girl-group songs were melodramatic and hyperreal. The archetypes were age-old and operatically declaimed, but the details were everyday and humdrum. Something similar unfolds in the best garage-group songs too. Everything is a little too hollow and raw, a little too unmediated and overstated. But there is one crucial difference in the gender dynamics: the girls have their group-support system, their union, their choirs of call and response; the boys howl alone through a barrage of fuzz. The sound of the girl groups is the sound of a cheerleader line defiantly cracking gum in the face of male oppression for ever. It's a wish-filled pillow kiss to a memory, a desire, a photo, an absence. The sound of the garage groups is a fear-fuelled empty-vessel roar in the face of female indifference, a steeling in preparation for the soul-crushing rejection to come.

In his 2001 book *Rock 'Til You Drop*, John Strausbaugh quotes *New York Press* writer Bill Repsher's riposte to the corporate-sponsored Rock and Roll Hall of Fame. In preference to all those gallery displays full of bloated tributes to rock dinosaurs he envisages an art installation. 'I'd make it just one room,' he says. 'Have a dummy made up to look like a skinny, acne-scarred kid sitting in a bedroom. There's a window in the bedroom and it looks out onto the street, where five attractive girls, the kind who would never look twice at a loser like that, are practicing cheerleader moves on a summer's afternoon. The only thing of note in the kid's room? An AM radio and a beat-up pawnstore acoustic guitar. That's rock and roll, John, straight down to the heart: loneliness and the search for pussy.'[4]

I would propose a second room, one that helps make sense of the first. Two girls sitting on a wall. They're listening to the same AM radio tuned to a different channel. It plays the Shangri-Las' 'Sophisticated Boom Boom', Martha and the Vandellas' 'I'll Keep Holding On' and the Chiffons' 'Nobody Knows What's Going on (in My Mind but Me)'. The guitarist from the first installation walks past on his way to band practice. He sees the girls but barely acknowledges them, just emits a derogatory grunt and walks on by. The girls regard him with studied indifference. 'He's a jerk,' says one, studying her nails as he walks off up the road. 'Yeah, but his brother's a hunk,' says the other.

Like the girl-group era, the garage-band sound was rarely celebrated for its intelligence. Instead rudimentary skills were promoted as a guiding principle and incompetence was fetishised, even when many garage-group records were anything but incompetent. As with punk rock in the mid-seventies a notional democracy was mooted as the music's unique selling point: the idea that anyone could do it. 'Here are three chords now go and form a band.' But not everyone can do it, otherwise almost everyone would. The fingering of A, E and G chords on a cheap guitar is still beyond the grasp of the non-musically minded, and even when you have learned these three basic positions there still remains the question of what you do with them when you have them at your disposal. Once a basic competence has been acquired that next level of aural splendour still eludes most, as 99 per cent of competently played but thrill-less, magic-less rock and roll will confirm.

The garage-band era emerged during a period when the custodians of high culture, both in Britain and America, were beginning to bequeath their patronage upon pop. This was the period when Leonard Bernstein was casting his approving eye over what he called 'this strange and compelling scene called pop music' on network TV, and Ned Rorem was stating that he never saw any of his high-brow chums at classical concerts any more because they were all at home listening to the Beatles. Bernstein's documentary *Inside Pop: The Rock Revolution* was aired in 1967 on CBS and is best remembered now for its inclusion of footage in which Brian Wilson performs a spellbinding version of 'Surf's Up', a solo masterclass that has attained retrospective poignancy given that it was shot just months before the *Smile* project imploded. Elsewhere in the programme Bernstein compares the Beatles to Schubert and praises 'Pretty Ballerina' by the Left Banke for the way in which it combines Lydian and

Mixolydian modes. 'Imagine that!' he exclaims. 'Rather unusual, wouldn't you say?' In a programme that also includes Graham Nash and Peter Noone of Herman's Hermits in animated conversation about the ability of musicians to enact change in society (they disagreed), and contributions from Roger McGuinn, Frank Zappa, Tim Buckley and Janis Ian, garage bands are conspicuous by their absence. No one is about to call upon Sky Saxon or Roky Erickson in order to validate pop's high-art credentials. As a theatrical composer, Bernstein always favoured the subtleties of harmony and the lure of syncopation over more base rhythmic impulses, and these tendencies are reflected in the music he eulogises in the programme. In his sincere passions Bernstein did what a lot of high-cultural critics did when they came to popular music: he only seemed to recognise one kind of clever. But pop music always was clever, and it didn't need the endorsements of sympathetic classicists to tell us that. Les Paul and Mary Ford were clever. Sam Phillips was clever. Phil Spector, Jack Nitzsche and Shadow Morton were clever. The Motown production line was clever. All those pushy Jewish teenagers from Brooklyn who rampaged through the Brill Building with braces on their teeth and songs coming out of their ears, they were especially clever. A lot of the dumb stuff was clever too. Lester Bangs always had a great comeback when faced with unpalatable pretension and overly complex horseshit masquerading as art: 'Yeah, but could they have written "Louie Louie"?' he would say. And there in that simple rhetorical provocation lies a universal truth so pure that it should barely need iterating. It's a standpoint that recognises that there are moments where even three chords might seem ostentatious and two will do just fine, a recognition that less truly can be more.

One of the ways in which pop critics reacted to high-cultural overstatement was to simply understate it right back and construct a trash aesthetic that said, 'This stuff isn't clever at all. It's dumb, and defiantly, unashamedly dumb at that.' Some of the biggest champions of the garage-band sound – Greg Shaw, Lester Bangs et al. – made a virtue of the music's simplicity, its three-chord thrash and low expectations. And faced with something as gloriously trashy as 'Green Fuz' by Randy Alvey and the Green Fuz, a song that sounds like a melty-headed acid casualty recorded while trapped inside a dustbin, or 'The Reality of Air Fried Borsk' by the never more appropriately

named the Drivin' Stupid, you aren't going to cite Schoenberg or Satie in their defence. You are going to cite 'Purple People Eater' and 'Surfin' Bird'. The trash aesthetes countered the patronage of high-art arrivistes by postulating the very opposite. This music is dumb, they said, and in that very dumbness lies its cleverness. But all that does is confirm the validity of the canon in the first place. They have high art, we've got the low-brow stuff. Say it loud: it's dumb and it's proud. Except that a lot of it isn't.

In his book *Sixties Rock*, Michael Hicks shows that it is possible to make a musicological case for the garage-band sound without surrendering any of its cultural virtues and validity. Hicks refuses to take ineptitude at face value, stating that such viewpoints 'imply that a small vocabulary has to do with ignorance or lack of ambition, when in fact most garage rockers could (and did) learn many chords. But their decision to restrict their harmonic vocabulary must be seen in most cases as a matter of choice.'[5] Hicks also recognises that within its self-imposed limitations a lot of garage rock is harmonically complex and not especially primitive at all. He makes the kinds of connections that an astute musicologist might make but a blinkered subculturalist could easily miss. He points out, with examples, how frequently the Bo Diddley 'shave and a hair cut, six bits' shuffle and the 'Louie Louie' riff occur during the first decade and a half of rock and roll. He notes the similarity between the Champs' 1958 hit 'Tequila' and 'Pushin' Too Hard' by the Seeds (although he doesn't mention the possible missing link, Dick Dale's 'Let's Go Trippin''). He shows how in the space of two separate versions of 'Louie Go Home' (recorded in 1964 and 1966 respectively) Paul Revere and the Raiders capitulate to the English invasion by embellishing the original with fuzz guitars, Yardbirds Gregorian background vocals and a tempo shift that moves from the Mixolydian to the Phrygian. ('Imagine that!' as Leonard Bernstein might have said.) He explains methodically and without high-art condescension the way in which purposeful oscillations between two chords were transformed into magic by a generation of garage bands, and he provides several examples of the way in which a prolonged tonic, a sustained ostinato or a sequence of falling fourths in some of your favourite garage tunes is, in fact, very clever indeed. Of Them's 'Gloria' he says: 'When the progression returns to the tonic, one hears "double plagal" motion. The subtonic loses its more common role as a lower neighbour to the tonic and becomes a subdominant to the subdominant, proceeds to the real subdominant, then to the tonic.'[6] For those unwilling to entertain such terminology, that might constitute just a little too much daylight cast on magic, but it does explain why the riff kicks ass to those who might benefit from having it explicated in this way – although it doesn't explain, nor indeed does it attempt to, how a bunch of Belfast savants created a loop that went around the world.

And so we return to where we began. Once the musicologists, the high-art proselytes and the low-art apologists have had their say, what still remains is the sheer psycho-acoustic beauty of the music, the echo grafted upon echo, the reverb storm, the sculpted salvos of fuzz-wah. It's the studio production that gives these records their sheer disorientating otherness. This is where their true savant-garde nature lies. In levels-in-the-red overindulgence we trust. 'Walk' by the Pandas turns a Roy Orbison 'Pretty Woman' riff into something altogether stranger with its crackling fuzz appliqué and its weird oscillations. The random splashes of mixing-desk colouration that producer Tom Wilson splatters all over the Models' original 1966 version of 'Bend Me, Shape Me' put a whole other mind-warped emphasis on that title and turn what would later become a pleasant pop hit for the American Breed and Amen Corner into a full-on psychedelic freak-out. It's the oscillations and add-ons of the production process that give this stuff its grain. There are noises on certain garage records – spur-of-the-moment noises, discovered-by-default noises, carelessly crafted noises – that a highly skilled exponent of musique concrète might never have come up with in ten years of dedicated lab work, despite all the tools and tuition at their disposal.

The garage-band records come from many places and draw upon many sources, and perhaps the most wonderful thing about them is that they were made at all. It's the tendency itself that casts the illuminating aura, it's the driving impulse that thrills, the fact that in America at this time people thought these were interesting noises to make. Rejoice in the fact that in 1967 a Milwaukee group called the Shaprels released a record called 'Dare I Weep, Dare I Mourn', a disc whose Shakespearean title makes teen angst heroic and perilous machismo a noble pursuit. They were probably put on this earth for that very purpose.

5

CALIFORNIA DREAMING

*At dusk we placed on the window a
notice which read 'We thank the Press
and Radio for their selfless interest
in this festival of music and people
and regret that there are no more
pieces of paper for them.' We walked
the* Time *and* Life *men to the arena
and gave them special places in the
wings; we crushed a final grabbing
arm in the lowered window, and we
said goodnight and goodbye to the
window itself and it was amazing and
wonderful to know that beyond the
badges, far from the pass system, over
and above the demands, there was a
festival. It happened at Monterey and
it mightn't have done.*

DEREK TAYLOR, press officer,
Monterey Festival[1]

The Monterey International Pop Festival, which took place during the weekend of 16–18 June 1967, was a pivotal event in the evolution of rock culture. It was the watershed moment when America (or the west coast at least) finally 'got' Jimi Hendrix, six months after he had exploded onto the English scene. The Who announced their presence in similarly volatile style. It was also the moment when David Crosby of the Byrds dropped less than subtle hints about his future intentions by putting in a guest appearance with Buffalo Springfield. Just weeks before the festival Ravi Shankar had opened his school for the study of Indian music in LA, and when he performed at Monterey rapturous waves of love rippled across the audience. In marked contrast, a large portion of the hipper than thou crowd was so affronted by Laura Nyro, who turned up in the wrong uniform – a gothy vamp number – that she and her New York-nightclub backing singers were frozen out after only three numbers. Monterey was also the moment when the rock crowd briefly endorsed soul music by going wild for Otis Redding (although in reality his set, which followed Nyro's, was only sparsely attended and was curtailed because it overran). And it was probably the last pop festival where the punters sat and watched the acts in neat rows of foldaway plastic chairs. Most of all, though, Monterey was about the power politics that were being played out between LA and San Francisco. Behind the scenes all kinds of hard-nosed negotiations were going on. The Diggers had to be appeased and assurances given that the festival would be a non-profit event, but even these concessions failed to mask the distrust felt by many in the Bay Area musical community. In his autobiography Phil Lesh referred to the festival's organisers, John Phillips of the Mamas and the Papas and Dunhill Records boss Lou Adler, as 'two LA industry types'.[2] San Francisco rock journalist Joel Selvin adopted a similarly dismissive tone in his book *Summer of Love*, calling them 'a pair of Hollywood hipsters out to galvanise their standing in the emerging rock underworld'.[3] Such withering descriptions perfectly summarised the ideological differences that existed on either side of California's cultural fault line, and they continued to be played out during the festival itself.

By the time Monterey came around the Mamas and the Papas had enjoyed five Top 10 hits during a period in which they outsold the Beatles in America. Having helped organise the event, the group spent the entire weekend digging the other acts. When they closed the festival on the Sunday night, it became apparent fairly quickly that they hadn't rehearsed for months. Cass Elliot was as unashamedly wasted as her audience, and the Mamas and the Papas, bedraggled hosts at their own party, gave a less than pristine and note-perfect performance. These were ramshackle qualities that would

have endeared the Bay Area bands to local critics. Earlier Country Joe and the Fish had performed while visibly ripped to the gills on STP, while the Grateful Dead, not for the first or last time, stumbled into a major arena and were shambolic. The difference was that the Mamas and the Papas weren't Berkeley or Haight-Ashbury. They may have been popular, but they were LA popular and, as they themselves sang on their autobiographical hit 'Creeque Alley', 'LA – you know where that's at.'

'Creeque Alley', a Top 10 hit for the group in both Britain and America, tells the story of the group's early years and rise to fame with wry and self-effacing accuracy. Probably no group apart from the Beatles ever mythologised themselves so disarmingly. The alley referred to in the title was a side street in St Thomas in the Virgin Islands, where the Mamas and the Papas first performed as a group. They had spent four months in 1965 residing on the Pacific island, taking psychedelics and, as the song suggests, living off an American Express card until Amex called in the debt and they were lured back to the west coast as a matter of expediency. Back on LA terra firma, they readily embraced the kind of pop fame that comes to those whose overnight success has taken several years. Lou Adler took one listen to their sumptuous harmonies and exclaimed, 'If you can believe your eyes and ears,' a phrase which became the title of their first album. When Adler asked the group what else they needed, John Phillips replied: 'A steady stream of money from your office to our house.'

The Mamas and the Papas' origins were as immersed in acid as those of the Grateful Dead. The four members were all tripping the first time they met: John and Michelle Phillips and Denny Doherty had all taken the drug when they invited Cass Elliot to meet them at the Phillips's apartment in Greenwich Village in 1965. 'We all had it together the same night, for the first time, and I think that formed a bond between the four of us that we just never stopped singing,' said John Phillips. 'We just went on and on and on and on, until the trip wore off, which was about four years later.'[4]

Phillips, the man scathingly described as a Hollywood hipster out to galvanise his standing in the emerging rock underworld, actually wrote some of the most distinctive songs of the 1960s. In what was possibly pop's most magnanimous gesture outside of Paul McCartney giving 'Come and Get It' to Badfinger when it should clearly have been a Beatles single, Phillips bequeathed the Summer of Love anthem 'San Francisco' to his long-term friend and former band mate Scott McKenzie to sing, even though it audibly cries out for bit-part arrangements for the group themselves. From Denny Doherty's yearning opening refrain to what should have been Cass Elliot's closing verse, 'San Francisco' is the great lost Mamas and the Papas single.

Haight-Ashbury diehards scoffed at the song's vapidity and simple-minded idealism, cautioning arrivistes not to come to San Francisco garlanded with flowers but to bring warm clothes for the cold foggy nights and sufficient funds for food in case the Diggers' meals-on-wheels service didn't show. Despite these accusations of lyrical naivety and love-shuck exploitation, the Mamas and the Papas never were about vacuous celebration. A year before the discontented and disaffected began arriving at Haight-Ashbury, the group portrayed LA's darker and more lurid lure. 'Strange Young Girls', from their second album, sings of the stoned waifs who drift along the Strip 'offering their youth on the altar of acid'. It's unmistakably an LA song, with cautionary sentiments and a melancholic heart. So too, despite its joyous, uplifting chorus, is '12.30 (Young Girls Are Coming to the Canyon)'. Its opening lines may echo 'California Dreamin''s desire to escape the east coast but the song retains more than a twitch of New York neurosis. The hallucinatory images of the final verse cast Californian beauty and abundance into shattered reflected fragments on stagnant cloudy waters. It's a song that, like much LA pop, grants shivers and shadows a foreboding presence amid daylight splendour. The young girls who parade through these songs may, as Paul Nelson wittily put it, have all looked exactly like Michelle Phillips,[5] but there is something voracious and unwholesome about their appetites. These scenarios are enacted in the unrelenting, bleached-out glare of a blood-sucking sun; they hint at vulnerability and exploitation. Even when they were being showbiz and wacky, even when Mama Cass was giving it her best Phyllis Diller/Ethel Merman-on-acid treatment, the Mamas and the Papas never sounded remotely sappy. Their intra-band bed-hopping was a soap opera played out in song ('I Saw Her Again Last Night' to name but one) and they remained both refreshingly flawed and unrepentant psychedelic hedonists for the entire journey.

They didn't particularly look like hedonists, though, not in the Haight-Ashbury sense anyway; they looked like cool folkies from an earlier era. But then the surrealists didn't look like hedonists either, and they were blowing minds thirty or forty years before the Haight hippies arrived on the scene. Subversion came in many forms and didn't always announce itself with bells, kaftans and Indian prints. When Association guitarist Larry Ramos sang a line like, 'I took off my watch / and found I had all the time in the world,' while beaming all over his genial Hawaiian face, butter would perhaps not have melted in his mouth, but as he crooned Dick and Don Addrisi's happy-go-lucky 'Time for Living' the generational subtext was obvious. The song is only a trouser crease and cufflink away from the straight life – the Addrisi brothers were jobbing songwriters and they penned plenty of stuff that was aimed at a Broadway and Christian summer-camp kind of clientele – but like all good surrealists in sensible clothing the Association transform it into something that any psychedelic convert would have understood instantly. Like the best genuinely subversive pop, 'Time for Living' had one message for the mainstream and another for the code-breakers.

The Association opened the Monterey Festival on the Friday evening with Tandyn Almer's 'Along Comes Mary', one of several US chart hits the group enjoyed between 1966 and 1968, and another of their songs that was less than covert with its colloquialisms. Like 'Mary Jane' by the Renaissance, 'Mary, Mary' by the Monkees and several other great LA pop songs (but not 'What's the New Mary Jane' by the Beatles, which is a whole other kettle of alphabetti spaghetti), 'Along Comes Mary' is sung with such heartfelt sincerity it could almost make you believe it's about a girl. Warm ocean breezes flutter through the spacious instrumental passages in the best of the Associations' music; their harmonies are delivered with all the finesse you would expect from the best west-coast pop, and although they could be cloying in the extreme, they produced some of the finest pop to come out of LA. They wore spiffy side partings and preppy collegiate clothes, but they never passed up the opportunity to rhyme 'changes' with 'rearranges', and the best of their work resounds with the spirit of the age. 'Enter the Young', 'Message of Our Love' and 'Windy' are acid flashes set to music. The latter, another of their Top 10 hits, sets overtly lysergic lyrics to a deceptively jaunty bounce. 'Pandora's Golden Heebie Jeebies', on their second album *Renaissance*, may just be one of the most accurate accounts of the acid trip ever committed to record.

Composer Gary Alexander plucks a koto while simultaneously walking paths of dark and light, endlessly reconciling and rebirthing as he orbits time and space, cleansing his soul and shedding astral bodies as he goes, sifting days of reckoning into dead ends and awakening insight, and emerging out the other side of his search knowing precisely what boxes those psychotropic keys have unlocked and what remains to be unleashed. That title, 'Pandora's Golden Heebie Jeebies', regarded by unkind critics as a feeble approximation of an acid-song title, was, in fact, unnervingly spot on. It was the Association's 'Tomorrow Never Knows', their *Tibetan Book of the Dead* for the AM radio generation. And it must have worked. On the first album's gushy pop-biz sleeve notes Gary Alexander is said to 'not smoke, drink or eat meat and would like to travel to India to study the mystic religious life there'. And that's precisely what he did. Like Richard Alpert, Steve Durkee and Darby Slick, Alexander took the Eastern route in order to reconcile his creative impulses with his growing spirituality. He was replaced in the Association by Larry Ramos, who had just finished a lengthy stint with the New Christy Minstrels. And there you have the criss-cross lineage of LA folk rock in a nutshell: 'Green

Green' and 'This Land Is Your Land' shined up into a *Diamond Sutra*.

On the back of their debut album *And Then . . . Along Comes the Association*, the quintet, dressed in Edwardian three-piece suits, pose with varying degrees of conviction beside a vintage auto. Each clutches an instrument case. It's a typical motif of the time – shades of vaudeville and a hint of *Bonnie and Clyde* and the St Valentine's Day Massacre. Before hippie threads became ubiquitous it was a common look, satirically smart and loaded with subtext. You get a glimpse of it in the sartorial mish-mash of the Monterey movie, *Monterey Pop*. Mod clothes, Old West chic, gambler chic, velvet capes, bowler hats, borrowed gowns from Granny's wardrobe, 'rags and feathers from Salvation Army counters', as Leonard Cohen put it, were mixed and matched without any concession to what the uptown boutiques were selling as this season's style. One of the many splendid things about the Mamas and the Papas was that in terms of their apparel, they looked like they had marched in from four separate bands. Spanky and Our Gang have the same off-the-peg subversion about them. When they appeared on the *Ed Sullivan Show* in March 1968, performing their Top 10 hit 'Like to Get to Know

You', they were shown in split screen. In the background the band perform the song attired in a riot of lilac, lime green and love beads. The men wear bowler hats and broad-brimmed stovepipes. In the foreground shot they act out a psychedelicised party tableau dressed in dinner jackets. The overall effect is simultaneously dreamlike, hammy and camp, one huge nudge and a wink to anyone who has ever attended a formal function while tripping their face off. As its title suggests, 'Like to Get to Know You' is a song about searching for love, more in hope than expectation. It wears its melancholy lightly, until the string-driven coda swells up and a quiet desolation creeps in.

Nearly nine months earlier, on 11 June 1967, a week before Monterey, the Mamas and the Papas had performed 'Creeque Alley' on the *Ed Sullivan Show*. Four months later the Doors would actively court publicity by defiantly screaming 'We couldn't get much higher' on the show and receiving a lifelong ban into the bargain, but here at the height of their fame were the Mamas and the Papas singing a song which made thinly veiled references to pubic lice and whose chorus repeatedly made unambiguous references to getting high. The only autobiographical liberty that John Phillips takes in

'Creeque Alley' is the line 'Cass was a sophomore, planned to go to Swarthmore,' which he used simply because Swarthmore suited the rhyme scheme better than Goucher, the college that Elliot was planning to go to. Apart from that, the narrative is accurate to the letter and tells the story of the folk and jug-band roots (and routes) of the group and their associates, namechecking Barry McGuire, Jim McGuinn of the Byrds and Zal Yanovsky and John Sebastian of the Lovin' Spoonful, as they made their way through the Mugwumps, the Halifax Three, the New Christy Minstrels and other shortlived outfits who graced the Hootenannys and New York folk clubs during 1963/4.

Despite their folksy jug-band roots, the Lovin' Spoonful rarely sounded credible when they tried to go trad. They were even less convincing when they tried to rock out. What they were was a great pop band, and a clutch of songs that John Sebastian wrote for them – 'Do You Believe in Magic', 'Daydream', 'Darling Be Home Soon', 'Summer in the City', 'Six O'Clock', 'You Didn't Have to Be So Nice', 'She Is Still a Mystery' – are among the best that anyone produced in the 1960s. Unfortunately, Sebastian was saddled with Zal Yanovsky, who, although an accomplished guitarist, clearly believed

that the greatest gift the Beatles had bestowed upon a grateful nation was permission to goof around. Yanovsky could have mugged for America in the Olympics, and he missed no opportunity to show just how adorably zany he was. His background antics on the *Ed Sullivan Show*, during which Sebastian clutches an autoharp and attempts to sing his tremulous and tender ballad 'Darling Be Home Soon', are among the most excruciating ever witnessed during a pop performance on American prime-time TV. Yanovksy did little to endear himself to the hippie heartland when in May 1966 he and bass player Stephen Boone were complicit in turning in a drug dealer to an undercover federal agent. More sympathetic elements put the act down to panic and youthful naivety, but it did much to damage the group's standing with the counter-culture, and when the information became public they were forced to pull out of a number of San Francisco dates. Grassing up their drug buddies did little to damage the group's wider acclaim, though, and 'Daydream', 'Summer in the City', 'Nashville Cats' et al. are among the great sidewalk-melting, heat-haze hits of their era. 'Summer in the City' in particular is an urban classic, full of bustle, clamour and street *vérité*, but able to turn on more bewitching charms the moment Sebastian sings 'At night it's a different world', and you can just smell the neon-lit sensuality. 'Six O'Clock' could just as easily have been the next instalment in the same song cycle, the morning-after dawn epiphany when 'the dusty light shines down on the block' and everything is shot through with memories of ill-chosen words, missed opportunities and regret. These, like the best of Sebastian's lyrics, are New York grit grafted onto west-coast topography, shot through with the new acid sensibility. 'Do You Believe in Magic', the group's 1965 debut hit, references Chuck Berry's 'Rock and Roll Music' and marries it to adult pop desires and an unambiguous promise to 'blow your mind'. By the time they get to the post-Yanovsky classic 'She Is Still a Mystery', the trepidation of the lyric could just as easily be about a trip as a love affair. By 1967 these twin desires, pharmaceutical and hormonal, have become as ambiguous and interchangeable as boy/girl lyrics were at the height of the Brill Building era.

The Mamas and the Papas and the Lovin' Spoonful were the first of many east-coast groups who migrated from east to west at a crucial point in pop's evolution. 'California Dreamin'' expressed John and Michelle Phillips's initial yearnings for that migration (particularly Michelle's), but the song was about far more than mere relocation. 'California dreaming is becoming a reality,' they sang at the end of 'Creeque Alley', but for many California never was a reality, more a rendezvous for the dream life that had always drawn people to the west, from gold prospectors to hungry Hollywood starlets. By the time they recorded 'Mansions' for their fourth album, *The Papas and the Mamas*, in 1968, the group had thoroughly mined the downside and disillusion of that dream facade. 'Wondering why this isn't like the dream,' they sing as they ponder the gentle Spanish lady who cooks their meals, but they never ask her how she feels. 'Mansions' gets right inside the gated and soulless Bel-Air palaces and anticipates the reckoning to come. 'If you play the game, you pay the price / purchasing a piece of paradise,' they sang as the dream wore off and the hits stopped coming.

San Francisco stood for ideals and a laid-back attitude; friendly strangers in the street and communal music in the park. Los Angeles was commodity and commerce, the cold hard face of rampant salesmanship and – the biggest oxymoron known to humankind – business ethics. LA was Babylon by the sea. Uptight. Insincere. Hired hands rather than artisans. Session men not craftsmen. Hollywood horror stories. Deals done and undone and sealed with a devil's knot and a forked tongue. 'Hello,' he lied. LA was pop singles, San Francisco was rock albums. The nuances of tradition were expressed differently too. The Mamas and the Papas sang showtunes and dipped into the great American songbook. They recorded three Rodgers and Hart songs: 'My Heart Stood Still', 'Glad to Be Unhappy' and 'Sing for Your Supper'. Even though the Mamas and the Papas and the Grateful Dead both did versions of 'Dancing in the Street', even though both groups had jug-band and folk-club roots, they stared at each other across a great cultural divide. The former rearranged the Shirelles' 'Dedicated to the One I Love' into a barbershop/girl-group hybrid; the latter offered renditions that were faithful in spirit to 'I Know You Rider' and 'Viola Lee Blues'. The Mamas and the Papas made something entirely new by transforming commercial pop's recent past; the Grateful Dead signified rock modernism by coveting traditionalism. Strange days indeed.

The Grateful Dead never did receive the assurances they were seeking regarding where all the money from the Monterey Festival was going, so they refused to appear in *Monterey Pop*, a decision that appeared to be vindicated when half of the money that had been allocated to minority organisations disappeared. So great was the distrust between the competing factions at Monterey that the Dead, along with Eric Burdon, Country Joe and Steve Miller, spent more time jamming in the free fields than they did at the festival proper. Although he was one of the highlights of the event and named a song in honour of that summer weekend, Burdon pronounced the tightly timetabled itinerary a drag and railed against the complex system of ticketed zones and restricted areas, which he didn't feel to be in the spirit of things. Haight-Ashbury hardliners just tsked and said, 'This is an LA thing – what did you expect?'

Monterey's fringe festival within a festival took place on adjacent playing fields and hosted clothes stalls, film shows, meditation rooms, kite-making and other practical workshops, a music-industry symposium, a Moog demonstration booth hosted by Paul Beaver and Bernie Krause, and a guitar-tuition workshop with Jim McGuinn and Mike Bloomfield. Apart from the briefest of glimpses of people making dream-catchers, none of these activities were reflected in D. A.

Pennebaker's film documentary. What *Monterey Pop* does capture, poignantly at times, is the extent to which this was still a close-knit musical community. The cameras frequently zoom in on Brian Jones, Jimi Hendrix, Janis Joplin, Mama Cass and any number of other prematurely deceased artists as they wander unobstructed about the site or sit quietly digging the other acts on the bill. The film also captures a distinctly early Summer of Love look among the audience. Hippiedom hasn't fully taken hold yet and there is an absence of long hair. A culture can recognise itself in a weekend but it takes a couple of years to grow a ponytail. There is plenty of beat chic on display, the occasional kaftan and quilted poncho, but it's still mostly boutique bell-bottoms, slingbacks rather than moccasins, headscarves rather than headbands.

Although the film captures most of the headline acts, what it doesn't capture is any of the backstage and behind-the-scenes business-as-usual shenanigans that Burdon hinted at. A revealing piece written at the time by the ever-loquacious Derek Taylor encapsulates the event in all its love–hate, cynical–innocent, deceitful–idealistic permutations. A thousand press passes were issued for an arena 'built for 250 people in faint discomfort, for 400 at a crush,

for 600 in civilian prison conditions, for 800 in boot camp circumstances, and for 1000 only in Buchenwald terms'.[6] Taylor, who was in charge of the allocation of these passes, offers a wry perspective as glimpsed from the tiny window of the backstage press box, as legions of scammers, liggers, hard-bitten hacks and innocent ingénues approach the hatch and attempt to pass the Kool-Aid accreditation test. According to Taylor, this includes everyone from 'bearded and beaded literate hippies from Haight-Ashbury and Sunset Strip' to representatives from '*Flip, Soul, Tiger Beat, Hit Parader* and *Teenscoop*, bedrock of the fan-mags'.[7] Not to mention a succession of hopeful chancers from hastily made-up publications with home-made press passes and equally inept excuses. 'The clean young man from the *Los Angeles Times* returned. "The city desk isn't answering," he said. "Really? Well can't Jim Grunt, Brian Taylor, Anatole France, Beverly Bland, Bill Johnson, Jack Hartkey, can't any of them verify you?" "Will any of them do?" "Yes," we said. "Except that we've just made all of them up. They don't exist." "I thought I didn't know them," he said. "Right," he smiled. "You're a phony but it was worth the try." "Right," he smiled, and left.'[8]

It goes on like this all weekend as an endless line of the phoney and the genuine all submit themselves to the hard-bitten LA business sass and acid-leavened generosity of the press-box window.

Despite the success of the Monterey Festival, the San Francisco/LA rift remained as entrenched as it ever was, and one group more than anyone else, simply by their absence from the event, fell foul of the ideological demarcation between Bay Area rock and Los Angeles pop. The Beach Boys were supposed to headline on the Saturday night but pulled out at the last minute, the slot being eventually filled by Otis Redding. Monterey was the moment when California divided, and the Beach Boys found themselves on the wrong side of the cultural fault line. Then again, they always were. They didn't look the part, they didn't sound the part and they certainly didn't act the part. They came from barbershop, not bluegrass. They sang about surfer girls and hot rods rather than beat girls and biker chicks. They wore charcoal and blue Pendleton shirts rather than North Beach bohemian chic. They were WASP Americana incarnate. Even when Brian Wilson was finally deemed to be hip, he never looked hip, not in the way you were supposed to look hip.

By the time Monterey came around, Wilson had all but abandoned his follow-up to *Pet Sounds*, an ambitious collaboration with Van Dyke Parks initially called *Dumb Angel* and then simply *Smile*. *Dumb Angel* was, in fact, a much better title, an accurate reflection of Wilson's complicated man–child personality. In comparison *Smile* sounds like a bland and genial sop to prevailing subcultural tendencies that were totally out of keeping with Wilson's hyperactive nature and his neurotically driven pursuit of perfection.

Wilson began to formulate the idea for *Smile* early in 1966, during the making of *Pet Sounds* and at a time when he was being widely touted as an auteur genius. A half-hearted facsimile called *Smiley Smile* was eventually released in September 1967, containing hastily recut versions of some of the tracks intended for the album ('Heroes and Villains', 'Vegetables', 'Wind Chimes', 'Wonderful'), but the sketchy and insubstantial content of the LP simply confounded those who were expecting a masterpiece. Further tracks originally intended for *Smile* trickled out on the Beach Boys' late-1960s albums ('Our Prayer' and 'Cabinessence' on *20/20*, 'Surf's Up' on the LP of the same name), but by 1970, when *Surf's Up* was released, the critical wisdom was that the Beach Boys were washed up. It is *Smile*'s absence as much as that of the Beach Boys from Monterey that tainted their reputation for many years, and despite the album's valedictory completion nearly forty years later, that is what it must necessarily be reduced to here – an absence.

Subsequently, *Smile* disappeared into myth and conjecture, and took its place alongside all the other un-realised utopian visions of the twen-tieth century: Alexander Scriabin's *Mysterium*, Vladimir Tatlin's tower, Walter Gropius's Total Theatre, Brian Wilson's follow-up to *Pet Sounds*. Hist-ory is littered with famous examples of unfinished novels and symphonies, the untimely death of the writer or composer being the usual cause. The tragedy of *Smile* was that when Brian Wilson abandoned his masterwork he was only in his mid-twenties, at the height of his fame and at the peak of his creative powers. *Smile* is pop's ultimate what-might-have-been, Brian Wilson's Icarus moment.

It was the bootleggers who filled the gaps between rumours and conjecture, and as time went by *Smile* became the ultimate under-the-counter, off-the-radar, underground text, a teenage samizdat to God. An enormous amount of *Smile* material haemorrhaged from the vaults over the years and, in the absence of any official release, those tantalising snippets became the defin-itive uncensored document of Brian Wilson's lost work. Had *Smile* been released at the time it's possible that it might have given added credence and cachet to many an unacclaimed song cycle. Conceptual continuity runs in all but name through Harpers Bizarre's quartet of albums, through the early work of Harry Nilsson, Randy New-man and Curt Boettcher, through Van Dyke Parks's solo albums and certainly through the numerous cantatas and operettas that Jim Webb gifted to all kinds of unlikely but thankful recip-ients, notably the 5th Dimension, on their *Magic Garden* album, and Rich-ard Harris, on *A Tramp Shining* and its follow-up *The Yard Goes on For-ever*. The Association's fourth album, *Birthday*, another of pop's great what-might-have-beens, was set to feature a side-long version of 'MacArthur Park' before the band foolishly turned it down and Webb offered it to Harris instead.

Like so much sweet green icing flowing down, 'MacArthur Park' drips in acid imagery. Its central metaphor, the cake left out in the rain, speaks of failure to recreate a moment. From the fleeting glimpse offered in its opening lines, which have the beauty of Jaco-bean or Elizabethan verse, to its flow-ing rivers in the sky and its paradise pastures that melt after dark, 'Mac-Arthur Park' shimmers with memories captured in reverie and vanquished in mirage. Traditional pop sensibilities would suggest that the narrator was speaking of the transient nature of love, but clearly there were other, more chemical imperatives that helped shape and interpret that temporality.

Smile might have opened up whole new vistas for the pop concept work. It could have inverted everything we thought about pop and rock in 1967. Then again, it might have sold no bet-ter in America than its predecessor *Pet Sounds*, a relative commercial failure that sent Capitol scurrying to the back catalogue and the surf hits in search of recompense. Like the first Velvet Underground LP, which at the time reached number 197 in the Ameri-can LP charts, or *Forever Changes* by Love, which peaked at number 154 when first released, *Smile* was destined to owe its reputation to endurance rather than immediate appeal. Ulti-mately, it serves as the perfect meta-phor for pop's golden age, that moment when everything seemed possible, when heaven seemed reachable. When Bob Dylan is asked about the music

he made in the mid-1960s, he answers that he doesn't know where those songs came from. It's an acknowledgement of a certain kind of compulsive energy, a blinding flash of temporary magic that can never be recaptured or replicated. That's *Smile* in a nutshell – the ultimate LSD album. One fleeting glimpse and it's gone, the cake left out in the rain.

It was another LA-based group, the Byrds, not the Beach Boys, who would indicate what pop futurism sounded like. 'Eight Miles High' broke the mould for psychedelic experimenta-tion. First recorded in November 1965 and re-recorded two months later for the version that would become a hit single, it was a moment of significant cultural fission. When Jim McGuinn transposed the short choppy clusters of Ravi Shankar's sitar sound to his twelve-string guitar and melded them to a floating phrase quoted directly from the intro to John Coltrane's 1961 composition 'India', he signposted the future. 'Eight Miles High' wasn't a sty-listic aberration, a freakish one-off; it was part of a continuum, and drew upon influences that were already deeply ingrained within the development of the west-coast avant-garde. McGuinn's inspired merging of Shankar and Col-trane was an astute recognition of the role of the two musical masters in shaping psychedelic music in America. 'India' had originally been recorded at New York's Village Vanguard in November 1961 and was Coltrane's attempt to incorporate the modalities and drone textures of north Indian music into his own rapidly expanding repertoire. The source of the borrowed melody line which McGuinn borrows for 'Eight Miles High' was a Vedic chant that Coltrane had heard on a 1952 Folkways LP entitled *Religious Music of India*.[9] Coltrane, therefore, was dipping into exactly the same folkloric influences that McGuinn, Jerry Garcia and a host of other musicians would later exploit on their own Folkways borrowings.

Coltrane was a great admirer of Ravi Shankar and expressed a desire to perform with the sitar master. The two men were formally introduced in December 1961 at the beginning of Shankar's lengthy concert tour of the US. Shankar's appearances in San Francisco during this tour were witnessed by all of the leading exponents of west-coast minimalism – Terry Riley, La Monte Young, Steve Reich, etc., as well as future members of the Grateful Dead and other Haight-Ashbury bands. Coltrane was so in awe of the great man that when his second son was born in 1965 he called him Ravi.

By 1965 Jim McGuinn was on a

similar mission to forge common ground between the Dorian modality of Indo-jazz and the unconventional scales found in many old folk tunes. The results of these experiments are most fully realised on the Byrds' third album, *Fifth Dimension*, released in the summer of 1966, but experimentation with folk, jazz and other esoteric sources remained a constant throughout the Byrds' early years. McGuinn was so taken with the techniques he exploited on 'Eight Miles High' that he repeated them on David Crosby's composition 'I See You' on *Fifth Dimension*. 'Why', the B-side of the single release of 'Eight Miles High', was Crosby's own venture into the possibilities of what would soon become known as raga rock. The early takes of both songs, recorded in November 1965, are far more experimental than the official releases. The first version of 'Eight Miles High' is taken at a marginally slower pace and is less polished than the hit single. The opening reference to Coltrane's 'India' is more studied and pronounced, the guitar line more ragged and dissonant, particularly at the end of the instrumental break, when it crashes back into the verse in a cascade of atonality. The vocal is lower in the mix and more attentive to the drone possibilities of the words. 'Why' is an equally remarkable piece of work for its time. On the early version McGuinn plays an exuberant sitar-style solo; the unresolved Eastern chord left hanging at the end of the song is clearly borrowed from the same Vedic music that Coltrane was listening to. On the later version the arrangement is more clipped and reined in, the solo more formal, tentative and tidy, and that raga chord at the end has been softened by a familiar folk-rock chime.

McGuinn and his Byrds colleague Gene Clark were both unashamed acolytes. McGuinn had his Merseybeat epiphany long before the Fab Four played the *Ed Sullivan Show*, and in 1963, at the height of the folk boom, could be found playing Lennon and McCartney songs in New York clubs. He didn't remotely look the part – photos from this period reveal him as a geek in horn-rimmed glasses, a kind of frat-boy version of Jarvis Cocker, but he grew into the role soon enough. When two would-be managers of a Beatles covers band spotted him walking down Bleeker Street they commented, 'What we need is four of *him*.'[10] When McGuinn first met Gene Clark in the Troubadour Club in West Hollywood later that year, Clark suggested they form a Peter and Gordon-style duo. Anglophile tendencies are abundantly

evident in McGuinn, Clark and David Crosby's pre-Byrds outfits the Jet Set and the Beefeaters, and they remain audible on the Byrds' 1965 debut album, *Mr Tambourine Man*, particularly on Clark and McGuinn's 'It's No Use' and Clark's solo compositions 'You Won't Have to Cry' and 'Here Without You'. The Lennon–McCartney influence endures throughout the Byrds' early years and lingers as late as 1967, when the opening Merseybeat chords of 'Have You Seen Her Face' on the *Younger Than Yesterday* album reveal an undiminished man-crush on 'Hard Day's Night'-era Beatles, even though the flirtation now comes bathed in the peak-hour blush of LSD.

To listen sequentially to the string of hit singles the Byrds made between April 1965 and January 1967 is a joyous and uplifting experience. 'Mr Tambourine Man', 'All I Really Wanna Do'/'Feel a Whole Lot Better', 'Turn! Turn! Turn!', 'Eight Miles High', '5D', 'Mr Spaceman' and 'So You Want to Be a Rock 'n' Roll Star' sketch out the mind maps and astral cartography of a generation coming of age. Listening to the quartet of great albums they made during the same period – *Mr Tambourine Man* (1965), *Turn! Turn! Turn!* and *Fifth Dimension* (1966) and *Younger Than Yesterday* (1967)

– is to experience carefully crafted folk-rock sensibilities being enveloped and immersed in something altogether more magical.

McGuinn's walk-on part on the Mamas and the Papas' 'Creeque Alley' ('McGuinn and McGuire couldn't get no higher / but that's what they were aiming at') reveals him to have been an enthusiastic pothead. He was an equally early advocate of the restorative properties of LSD, and was one of the first pop musicians to convert to Eastern religion, when he joined the Subud sect early in 1965. McGuinn made for an odd kind of mystic. Those trademark blue-tinted granny glasses that he wore during the pop-star years may have given him a charismatic aura of aloofness but for someone who was fascinated by extraterrestrials and other cosmic phenomena he remained remarkably grounded. At a time when many converts to Eastern religion were changing their name to something more fittingly exotic, Jim McGuinn changed his name to Roger because he dug aeronautical terminology.

When 'Mr Tambourine Man' was released as a single in April 1965, so sheer and shiny was the Byrds' sound that it seemed to have arrived fully formed. It hadn't, of course, and it continued to evolve throughout the 1960s, but once McGuinn locked into that flawless fusion of folk modalities and chiming twelve-string melodies the Byrds' formula sounded unimpeachable. Almost everything on their first LP proceeds at the same graceful, dreamlike pace, spooling out in endless modal loops. Their initial masterstroke was to reinvent Dylan's 'Mr Tambourine Man' as a drone poem. The folksy strum of the original is alchemised by McGuinn's ringing Rickenbaker into a chiming blur. So flawless is the rendition that you barely notice they have reduced the song to a single chorus–verse–chorus. Commencing with what in Dylan's version is the second verse ('Take me on a trip upon your magic swirling ship') nails the group's chemical colours to the mast from the outset – although McGuinn later claimed to have been channelling his new-found love of Subud. The Byrds' version expediently dispenses with verses one, three and five – the most convoluted and obtuse ones. This strips the song of much of its ambiguity and yet somehow still retains the original's beguiling mystery.

Crucial to the band's initial development (and notoriety) was their lengthy residency at Ciro's nightclub on Sunset Boulevard. The former movie star hang-out had by 1964 been taken over by an entourage of beat theatricals and oddballs who gravitated towards Vitautus ('Vito') Paulekas, a fifty-two-year-old walking art object, dancer, sculptor and boutique owner, and Carl Franzoni, who Johnny Rogan in his Byrds biography describes with admirable restraint as 'an ebullient priapic figure'.[11] Along with Vito and his wife Sue Anne, who was thirty years his junior, Franzoni was the living embodiment of the 1960s freak. Every mid- to late-sixties Hollywood movie that required a wild nightclub scene or walk-on parts for flamboyant and out-there hipsters either portrayed Vito's crowd or hired them directly. That whole demographic blur between beats and hippies is bridged by what went on at Ciro's in 1965. The Byrds played five short sets a night there, occasionally straight, but more often than not spiked to the gills. Like the Velvet Underground at the Factory, they developed their sound in a multimedia context, with flashing lights and writhing dancers and without record-company pressure. Those who witnessed those magical saturnalian escapades at Ciro's said that it was always strange to watch the Byrds on stage once their career took off, without the freak scene and the legions of interpretive dancers. Like the Velvet Underground, minus the whips and chains,

but with no less insouciance, the Byrds forged a sound and a group persona that made no concession to stagecraft. On their first tour of England in 1965 this lack of showmanship was perceived as moodiness and Yankee belligerence. It was, but it had more to do with the fact that they didn't have a game to play, not one that anyone would have recognised as a game anyway. Stripped of Vito's choreography they didn't have much of a stage act either. Bad boys in England meant the Rolling Stones pissing on a garage forecourt; it didn't mean a bunch of sulky pot-fried Americans with Beatle haircuts. Few swinging Londoners knew what to make of them, and the lukewarm reviews reflected that. But the Beatles knew.

Throughout the sixties the Byrds enjoyed a fruitful relationship with the Beatles. In a spirit of uncompetitive reciprocity the two groups exchanged acetates, instruments, influences, ideas. George Harrison freely admitted that 'If I Needed Someone' and 'I Feel Fine' were directly inspired by the Byrds, even though the latter owed just as much to Bobby Parker's 'Watch Your Step'. The Byrds introduced the Beatles to raga modalities and drones. Roger McGuinn and David Crosby introduced Harrison to the music of Ravi Shankar. Harrison had first used the Rickenbacker twelve-string in July 1964 on 'I Should Have Known Better' and it features heavily on the *Hard Day's Night* LP. McGuinn's own twelve-string chime, absorbed initially as much from the Searchers as it was from the Beatles, became the central component of the Byrds' folk-rock sound.

If the Byrds virtually invented folk rock, psych folk begins with their interpretation of 'The Bells of Rhymney'. The song was worked out in the spring of 1965 as the band rehearsed in Vito's basement, high on LSD. It was based on a Welsh lyric poem by Idris Davies, which he had written in response to the 1926 General Strike. McGuinn, who learned the song from Pete Seeger's 1959 version, had arranged it for Judy Collins in 1964, and a year later added layers of twelve-string. Each verse of the original offers politically loaded counterpoint to the children's nursery rhyme 'Oranges and Lemons'. The Byrds' version retains the radicalism but dresses it in angelic radiance. In the final verse the words don't so much end as ebb away, dissolving into an extended chorale that rises heavenwards in intonation. The blissed-out, wordless coda would become one of the key motifs of psychedelia, and the Byrds invented it on 'The Bells of Rhymney'.

'Turn! Turn! Turn!', the group's third hit single in the UK and the title track of their second album, was based on Pete Seeger's 1954 adaptation of words taken from the Book of Ecclesiastes. Seeger lifted his lyric mostly from chapter three, which begins: 'To everything there is a season and a time to every purpose under the heaven.' The phrase 'under heaven' (or 'under the sun', depending on the translation) appears twenty-nine times in the original Old Testament text. The Book of Ecclesiastes is shrouded in mystery. Biblical scholars can't say with any certainty who the Ecclesiasts were, which pretty much makes 'Turn! Turn! Turn!' the original theological Trad. Arr. Assumed to have been written approximately a thousand years before the birth of Christ, some detect the hand of more than one author and believe the book to be an open-ended meditative dialogue between a teacher/guru and a pupil. With its overriding emphasis on the cyclical nature of existence, the transience of life and the eternity of the Earth, the tone of Ecclesiastes is closer to Buddhism than Christianity. The emphasis on the seasons suggests reincarnation rather than the afterlife, while the idea that all human endeavours are based on vanity evokes another central tenet of Buddhism:

the relinquishing of ego and ambition. All of which chimed perfectly with McGuinn's experience of LSD and his modest, unpreachy Subud beliefs. It was Subud as much as the copious amount of acid that he was taking that gave his music its mystical sheen, and the two influences dovetail perfectly in 'Turn! Turn! Turn!'.

Because the Byrds' music emerged from predominantly folk origins rather than R&B ones there is an absence of misogyny in their songs – no broads, chicks or chattels, no 'Under My Thumb' or 'Yesterday's Papers'. Even when the girl done treat them wrong, as she does on several of Gene Clark's more haunted offerings, the overriding theme is courtship gone sour and sorrowful rather than the pursuit of revenge and retribution. The song that best expresses Clark's bruised and careworn sensibilities is 'The World Turns All Around Her', an album track from *Turn! Turn! Turn!* and arguably Clark's finest composition. Written at a time when the group was still in thrall to the English invasion, the best single they never released begins with the narrator expressing wonder that the woman ever considered him worthy of her attention in the first place, and he treats her loss philosophically. The payoff is worthy of Bacharach and David

at their most inspired. Addressing her new boyfriend, the narrator offers neither jealousy nor resentment. He doesn't even go through the insincere charade of asking him to take care of her. Instead he asks him to make her aware of 'everything she could be'. It's a song about the unrealised potential of womanhood, a parting shot at someone who remains uncertain of her own capabilities and might sell herself short. 'The World Turns All Around Her' describes the momentum that can be created simply by being within the gravitational pull of true love. More astonishingly, from the perspective of male loss, it suggests that momentum is endless, and if her new guy ever comes to that same realisation, he too will have no choice but to set her free. There were many ways of expressing free love in the mid-sixties, some cruder and less sophisticated than others. Most of the time they just meant free sex, not free love. 'The World Turns All Around Her' was that rare thing: a song with all the *carpe diem* sensibilities of the Metaphysical Poets, the Andrew Marvell of 'Had we but world enough and time', cast anew in the psychedelic swirl of the mid-sixties.

The October 1966 hit single 'Mr Spaceman' was a throwaway in the best sense of the word. The song acknowledges that the whole spiritual trip can sometimes best be conveyed not in philosophical tracts and dour pronouncements but in a snappy little tale about friendly space aliens, who, like Dylan's rainy day women, zap you when you're going innocuously about your business. Lyrically 'Mr Spaceman' is closer to 'Purple People Eater' than 'Purple Haze', and its tale of brief visitations is conveyed with wide-eyed cartoon wonder. 'Won't you please take me along for a ride?' reaches out to an eager and compliant audience far more readily than all those brow-furrowing encounters with *The Tibetan Book of the Dead*. Prostrating yourself before the great inscrutable godhead was one thing; telling your abductors that you'll watch your psychotropic ps and qs, while trying to wipe the toothpaste out of your beard, was a whole other way of surrendering to the void.

The Byrds' fourth album, *Younger Than Yesterday*, opens with what was arguably their last great pop single, 'So You Want to Be a Rock 'n' Roll Star'. Despite the distrust of stardom expressed by many of the San Francisco groups (some more evidently sincere than others), it was LA's Byrds who penned the definitive cynical late-1960s statement about the fame game. The song was ostensibly a response to the emergence of the Monkees, but it was also a caustic blast at everything the Byrds themselves had been part of for the past three years. Like several other great pop moments from high-minded and aloof LA bands – the Doors' 'Touch Me', Love's 'Alone Again Or' – it has a fabulous brass arrangement and the whole thing is carried on the fanfare blare of Hugh Masekela's searing trebly trumpet. The production is tinny and trebly, making the track sound as brittle as the pop process itself. The lyrics are delivered frantically, shouted hoarsely, hysterically even, into the unstoppable roar of an incoming tide. Out of the same mould, but far more foreboding in intent, was David Crosby's 'Everybody's Been Burned', a song that could only have been conceived in the city of lost angels. A brooding and fearful reflection on paranoia and distrust, 'Everybody's Been Burned' is delivered in understated tones, with minimal embellishment by the group. It is a song that anticipates the dark days to come, the sixties that would build its funeral pyres at the Manson ranch and at Altamont. The line 'I know that door / that shuts before / you get to the dream' hints not just at thwarted ambition but at something far deeper: the death of an ideal. All the more remarkable, then, that it was written in 1964.

Perhaps that's what Crosby's *Mona Lisa* smile, with its hint of malice and mischief, was about all along.

On *Younger Than Yesterday* the girls all seem to have kaleidoscope eyes. Chris Hillman's 'Have You Seen Her Face' is ablaze with sights, sounds, senses and a sorceress snare. Another Hillman composition, 'Thoughts and Words', shows that even at this late stage the Byrds' relationship with the Beatles is entirely reciprocal, with McGuinn's guitar melody anticipating George Harrison's 'While My Guitar Gently Weeps'. Maids pass gracefully in laughter in Crosby and McGuinn's 'Renaissance Fair', a song that has all the glister and glide of a good trip recalled in reverie. Crosby's lyrical evocation of an Elizabethan-themed pleasure fair observes Merry Olde England pageantry through a chemically tinted lens. Flags flutter, the sun flashes off a soda bottle, images pass in a blur, nothing is real and there's nothing to get hung up about. Eric Burdon, in the moment as ever, quoted the song's refrain – 'I think that maybe I'm dreaming' – in 'Monterey', his own acid-tinged homage to the new Elizabethan masquerade.

If *Younger Than Yesterday* was the Byrds' final acid testimony, their following album, *The Notorious Byrd Brothers*, was the sound of a group in transition. Several songs are about reminiscence. There's a version of 'Going Back', one of two Goffin and King covers on the album, the other being 'I Wasn't Born to Follow', a song whose airy country-style ambience was psychedelicised by Gary Usher's phased instrumental break and which later became iconic when given a pivotal role in *Easy Rider*. But the album kicks off in idiosyncratic style with 'Artificial Energy', Clark and Hillman's homage to amphetamine. Propelled by brash session-crew brass and Usher's vari-pitched phasing, 'Artificial Energy' comes across as a great pop-psych leftover from the Ciro's days, a song that still yearns for Vito and his bacchanalian troupe and a Mondo soundtrack. It is Hillman who at acid pop's last supper finally brings a great LSD song to the table, as 'Natural Harmony' is time-warped and phased to within an inch of its life. It's a great summer-of-1966 song cast adrift in the harsher light of a new age. The album closes with 'Space Odyssey', a fitting send-off to the Byrds' psychedelic period. McGuinn's astro-folk sea shanty ponders the perennial question, 'Was God an astronaut and have the aliens already landed?', while the composer accompanies himself on the Moog synthesizer. Elsewhere on the album country influences are to the fore. 'Get to You' reminisces about the group's first flight to London, but it skips and twirls from 5/4 to 3/4 in a gingham frock rather than a velvet cape. Folk rock makes way for country rock forty-four seconds into 'Change Is Now', at the precise point where McGuinn's lulling mantra about love's sweet plan is swept aside by a surge of pedal steel guitar. On the following track, 'Old John Robertson', Chris Hillman reminisces about an old Stetson-clad character from the small San Diego town where he'd grown up. The tune sets off at a cracking lick, as if the band are thrilled to be kicking free of all that acid-rock shit, but fifty seconds in, at the mention of the old boy's crippled wife, everything pauses for a quirky little interlude in which a string quartet plays the briefest of Beatles-baroque melodies before the barn-dance thrash recommences. A year earlier a countrified middle eight might have provided the interlude and the rest of the song would have been built around that acid baroque, but now the stylistic priorities have been inverted and the acid embellishment sounds like the interloper. No amount of phasing in the second half of the song can disguise the fact that everyone has changed partners one last time. Acid experimentation is now an onlooker, an uninvited, inappropriately dressed guest at the party.

There is a school of critical wisdom which suggests that it was the brazenly ambitious Gram Parsons who built a Trojan horse for country music and parked it fait accompli-style outside the Byrds' fortress gates, leaving an unsuspecting Roger McGuinn to happily wheel it into the compound, believing he was merely hiring a new keyboard player and not a whole new musical direction. While it was never as cut and dried as that, what is true is that McGuinn never intended initially to let country music dominate the Byrds' late-sixties output in the way that it did. Country music had always been part of the group's sound, but in 1968 it formed part of a bigger world-music project that McGuinn had in mind, a grandiose concept work intended to fuse the guitarist's folk-rock roots and enthusiasm for Indo-jazz fusions with his current obsession with Moog-led electronics. When McGuinn acquiesced to Parson's demands and dropped the electronic experiments completely, the result was *Sweetheart of the Rodeo*, a 1968 LP consisting entirely of music performed in the country style. Getting lonesome and hankering for that ol' hickory wind replaced star-gazing and meteor showers.

In abandoning psychedelicised folk rock for country the Byrds were ahead of the game. The direction their music took over the next couple of years anticipated the backwaters and dusty tracks that many of their contemporaries would explore in the late 1960s, as everyone began reinventing themselves as cosmic cowboys. The pull towards folk, blues and country roots was so prevalent by the late 1960s that bands like the Grateful Dead and Jefferson Airplane developed offshoots and side projects – New Riders of The Purple Sage and Hot Tuna respectively – to accommodate these tendencies. Folk rock begat psychedelic rock begat country rock, and apart from those whose music offered either a reaffirmation of the blues spirit or a retreat into its twelve-bar orthodoxy, the route the Byrds took anticipated the lineage of virtually every significant west-coast outfit between 1968 and 1970, and a great deal of other bands besides.

Because the great acid experiment ended when it did, it had the same effect on music as the curtailment of legitimately funded LSD research had in the early sixties – i.e. there was still so much left to do, so much left unexplored. All kinds of groups and artists who had briefly come under the drugs spell ended their dalliance and moved on. For some it had been a dalliance, a brief marriage of convenience between mind-altering stimuli (although obviously not that mind-altering in many cases) and fashionable musical tendencies. For others it hinted at hitherto untravelled pathways and opened up possibilities in their music that would have been unimaginable without acid's dreamscape. The LA-based group Spirit were acid sophisticates who on their early albums incorporated dayglo seamlessly into their virtuosic palette. Guitarist Randy California had played with Jimmy James (as Jimi Hendrix was still known then). Drummer Ed Cassidy had played with Thelonius Monk and Roland Kirk, and had been a founder member of the Rising Sons with Ry Cooder and Taj Mahal. On their debut album, *Spirit*, released in January 1968, they played jazz-tinged psychedelia with added classical flourishes, but were equally adept at lengthy improvisations and tightly arranged, sharp-edged pop songs. Steely Dan became far more acclaimed for this kind of thing several years later, but Spirit did it just as well and with far less fuss. Mac Rebennack, wearing the mask of Dr John the Night Tripper, made two startling albums of psychedelic voodoo in the late sixties. *Gris-Gris* (1968) and *Babylon* (1969) are parallel-earth fusions of gumbo variations, straight-ahead boogaloo and pre-*Super Fly* pimpsterism conveyed in Creole drug dreams, nightmare visions and Book of Revelation apocalyptic imagery, all washed down with a healthy pinch of apothecary hokum, 'boss-fix jam', 'goof-'em dust' and all. An entirely new form of psychodelphic bayou visitation music could have been conjured from the possibilities played out on the *Gris-Gris* and *Babylon* albums. It would probably have had to be performed by space Nubians, and would possibly have required Albert Hofmann to go back to the lab in order to distil a fresh batch of LSD-17 or 43 just to see if there was anything he had missed first time around, but it might have been worth the wait.

One of the few California-based outfits to forge a genuine connection between rock and the avant-garde in the late 1960s was the United States of America. Founder member Joseph Byrd had come up through the New York multimedia and performance-art scene of the early sixties. A devotee of John Cage and Charles Ives, he had worked with pianist David Tudor, Yoko Ono and artist Jim Dine before taking up an assistant teacher's post at UCLA in 1963. There he collaborated with La Monte Young, co-founded the New Music Workshop with jazz trumpeter

Don Ellis and started experimenting with primitive wave generators fed through an Echoplex. These, along with the ring modulator that fellow United States of America member Gordon Marron utilised, would become an essential part of the musique concrète bed of the group's sound when they formed early in 1967. They were joined by vocalist Dorothy Moskowitz, whose unadorned airy alto contrasted to great effect with the barrage of noise behind her. Moskowitz's singing style was often compared to Grace Slick's and to that of Jefferson Airplane's original vocalist Signe Toly Anderson. Moskowitz herself said of Slick, 'I'm grateful that she made the rock world safe for white middle-class altos like me,' but her unaffected tones also have something of the English folk singers about them, a certain Anne Briggs, Judy Dyble, Sandy Denny quality.

The United States of America incorporated Indian, Japanese and Polynesian modes into their music, as well as some fairly riotous collaging and cutting up. Byrd himself was responsible for electronics, harpsichord, keyboards and calliope, and 'The American Metaphysical Circus', the opening track on their 1968 debut album, begins with a multilayered swirl of carnival noises and marching bands, before Moskowitz's clear enunciation emerges through the pandemonium, paraphrasing Herman Hesse and promising 'the price of one admission is your mind'. 'The American Metaphysical Circus' presents a nightmare antidote to the revelry of 'Being for the Benefit of Mr Kite' and is probably one of the main reasons they weren't regulars on the *Ed Sullivan* or *Merv Griffin Shows*. It features tortured bears and children and all kinds of other sado-masochistic acts, all set to a gentle folk lilt and sung in Moskowitz's affecting middle-class alto. The best track on the album, 'The Garden of Earthly Delights', begins 'Poisonous gardens, lethal and sweet,' and offers similarly sinister and twisted visions of nightshade, ergot and deathly intent. Not so much the girl with kaleidoscope eyes as a black-hole vortex. What was most perverse about all this was not the subject matter of some of the songs but that they were often dressed in melodies of quite shattering beauty. Joseph Byrd was an unrepentant communist at a time when half of America was still in denial about its blacklists and the other half was on them. Perhaps only he (or Country Joe McDonald) could have written a lament called 'Love Song for the Dead Che', with deceptively lullaby-like lyrics and music that had it been tweaked only marginally could have been sung by Andy Williams. Williams did take acid, so you never know. Somewhere out there in another soft, velvety, cabaret lifetime he might be singing it right now.

While Dorothy Moskowitz was being compared to Grace Slick as she crooned a eulogy to a dead revolutionary, Slick's own band was grappling with barricade-rattling issues of its own. On their second album, *Surrealistic Pillow*, the Jefferson Airplane glide and shimmer as if caught in an air pocket a mile above the earth. Slick still bears traces of her Great Society apprenticeship and retains a yearning fragility in her voice that would be all but eradicated by the end of the decade. The group still sound ghostly and possess a battered grandeur as ornate as the Haight-Ashbury mansions they lived in. *Surrealistic Pillow* sounds like it was recorded in a huge cobwebbed ballroom rather than RCA's state-of-the-art studio in deepest Babylonian LA. Altogether too well-bred and too ambitious to be a garage band, they are still not above affecting an English baroque style when the mood takes them, and the album's darker, more gothic moments have a sophistication that few Bay Area bands ever attained or even aspired to. *Surrealistic Pillow* was recorded in October–November

1966 and released in February the following year. By the time its follow-up, *After Bathing at Baxters*, was released in November 1967, Jefferson Airplane had become self-appointed figureheads for the revolution. Principal songwriter Marty Balin had been elbowed aside by the Grace Slick–Paul Kantner power axis, and with that shift any remaining finesse that the group possessed all but disappeared. Slick's voice harshened into an authoritarian, hectoring howl, and her harmonising with Kantner, barked out with unceasing, bludgeoning rigidity on the on-beat, would dominate the band's sound well into the next decade. Only on 'Spare Chaynge' and her James Joyce eulogy 'Rejoyce' does Slick flicker with the literary intelligence of old. The second track on *After Bathing at Baxters*, the archly titled 'A Small Package of Value Will Come to You, Shortly', represents the nadir of west-coast rock's fleeting engagement with the avant-garde. In its one minute and forty seconds of shallow precocity it manages to encapsulate everything that had gone so wrong so quickly with San Francisco's creative spirit. Consisting entirely of ersatz musique concrète, stereo-panned screams and a mélange of tape-treated goofball dialogue, it is the sound of a group jerking off on company time. There was a precedent

for this kind of thing in '2–4–2 Fox Trot (The Lear Jet Song)', the closing track on the Byrds' *Fifth Dimension*, which David Crosby thought was at the very cutting edge of avant-garde innovation, when all it really did was presage the shape of things to come whenever rock musicians gave themselves carte blanche to go weird.

During the moments when they felt less encumbered by experimentalist *noblesse oblige*, Jefferson Airplane reverted to the familiar genuflections of bluesology. In the heavier rock passages on *After Bathing at Baxters* there are clear signs that guitarist Jorma Kaukonen and bass player Jack Casady can't wait to put the last lingering fripperies of folk rock behind them and get down to some serious boogieing.

As if to atone for the underwhelming nature of their debut album, the Grateful Dead's second LP, *Anthem of the Sun*, was much closer in spirit to most people's idea of a psychedelic record. Utilising a fragmentary and non-linear approach to the recording process that was much more in keeping with their collective consciousness, the album was assembled from live recordings and studio sessions that took place between September 1967 and March 1968. Augmented by a second percussionist, Mickey Hart, and

Tom Constanten, Phil Lesh's old Tape Center buddy on prepared piano and found sounds, the Dead approached the project in a Pranksteresque frame of mind that saw off producer David Hassinger when he objected to Bob Weir's request for a recording of 'thick air'. This legendary episode prompted Warner Records president Joe Smith to speak of *Anthem of the Sun* as the most unreasonable project the company had ever been involved with. Despite the record-company disapprovals, familiar elements, such as Pigpen's bluesy organ fills and Jerry Garcia's busy bluegrass-on-acid guitar runs, are still there, as are extended jams and sweet country harmonies, but these components are frequently subverted by the application of tape editing and collaging. At its most radical this auditory dissembling replicates the peak-hour turbulence of a dose of Owsley Stanley's finest acid. Tom Constanten's involvement in particular brings credible avant-garde input to the sound. Sections from his 1962 composition 'Electronic Study No. 3' are interwoven throughout the album and provide welcome sustenance for those who wanted more than just acid-raddled blues from their counter-cultural minstrels.

A little of *Anthem of the Sun*'s afterglow is retained on the follow-up, the palindromically titled *Aoxomoxoa*. The 1969 LP was a delicately wasted and understated affair compared with its predecessor. The gung-ho approach to production that ran rampant and unrestrained on *Anthem of the Sun* is reined in and restricted to a few choice moments, most notably Jerry Garcia's treated vocals on 'Rosemary' and his eerie, spaced-out a cappella on 'What's Become of the Baby'. Robert Hunter's increased involvement as a lyricist resulted in much of the band's blues lingua franca being jettisoned in favour of a darker romanticism more in keeping with their keenly felt sense of otherness. On *Aoxomoxoa* the folk element in the music leans more towards the transformative than the traditional. It evokes the diasporic rather than the prairie settler, the immigrant song rather than the barn-dance hoedown. *Aoxomoxoa* is the Grateful Dead's *Led Zeppelin III*.

Phil Lesh called *Anthem of the Sun* 'our most innovative and far-reaching achievement on record',[12] but the band would never again be that experimental in the studio. In his autobiography Lesh is refreshingly frank about the pragmatic nature of the Grateful Dead's subsequent gearshift. 'The problem is once you've delivered yourself of that radical a rethinking it's just not workable to keep repeating yourself in the same vein,' he says.[13] Referring to 1967 as 'our experimental period', he rationalises the new direction unveiled on the 1969 *Live/Dead* album. 'It became increasingly clear that we needed to turn away from balls-against-the-wall psychedelia towards a different mode of expression,' he says. 'It seems that music needs to periodically return to basics and build itself up again.'[14] From a musician's point of view these sentiments are entirely understandable. They spring from an acknowledgement that psychedelia was as prone to stylistic trappings as any other form of music. But from a cultural vanguardist point of view they are more problematic. Pragmatism alone doesn't explain why the music of the Grateful Dead, and of many other bands besides, evolved in the way it did in the late 1960s.

Avant-garde tendencies, absorbed intuitively in the unruly ferment of the Acid Tests, surfaced only briefly in the Grateful Dead's musical repertoire. The lengthy improvisation 'Dark Star' remained the lodestone for psychedelically inspired exploration for many years, but the *Live/Dead* album contained the last of their truly psychedelic work. By 1970 their music was anchored in tradition and they

released two albums that year which shook off the last vestiges of their Acid Test education and reacquainted them with their formative tendencies. The front-porch Americana of *Working-men's Dead* is adorned in pedal steel guitars and country harmonies, while the ten songs on *American Beauty* are described in the liner notes as 'blues, country and folk-styled originals'. Jerry Garcia stated that the title of the former album came about when he realised the full implications of the band's musical reorientation, comparing their new direction to 'a working man's version of the Dead'. Like a lot of things that Garcia said when he wasn't merely being gnomic in order to please or repel sycophantic rock journalists, this was a shrewd acknowledgement of the world that existed outside the Haight-Ashbury bubble. Garcia more than any other San Francisco musician learned his Kesey lessons well in assessing the state of the game, in realising that in fact it was all a game, a series of parts to be played, roles to be adopted and ascribed according to circumstances. Kesey didn't nickname him Captain Trips for nothing. It was Garcia who came up with one of the most succinct accounts of what could be learned from the LSD experience. Talking to Jann Wenner and Charles Reich for issue

100 of *Rolling Stone* magazine in January 1972, he was asked what effect acid had on his work and his life. 'I suddenly realized that my little attempt at having a straight life and doing that was really a fiction,' Garcia replied. A minimally adapted version of this sentiment reappears later on as 'What I got from my first trip was that my little personal fiction was just that. It was a fiction.' The first version was more directly applicable to Garcia's personal circumstances at the time, as he juggled his lifelong problem of trying to reconcile family obligations with the itinerant life of a musician, but both quotes get to the essence pretty neatly. To many who conjured its multiplicity of options the acid experience revealed that the biggest illusion of all might just be reality itself. Seen in these revelatory terms life is encountered as a sequence of charades, fictions to be negotiated, scenarios to be enacted with whatever masks and masquerades the initiate has at their disposal. In Garcia's case these blinding flashes of insight hinted at something equally profound and life-changing: the notion that in creative terms as well as workaday routine it's all a fiction, an endless progression of dream scenarios and mythical encounters, every one as illusory as the next. From a musician's point

of view the creative implications of this are immense and seriously undermine many of the fictions that pass as rock history, the biggest of all perhaps being the idea of authenticity. They certainly explain many of the scene shifts and personality transformations that took place in the late 1960s. The west-coast musical fraternity enjoyed playing with persona: guitarist John Fahey reinvented himself as Blind Joe Death; Joe McDonald prefixed 'Country' to his name; guitarist Barry Melton played gigs in his pre-Country Joe days as Blind Ebbets Field, in honour of the home of the Brooklyn Dodgers; Jefferson Airplane was a shortening of Blind Thomas Jefferson Airplane, Jorma Kaukonen's nom de plume, ascribed by a good friend as a skit on Blind Lemon Jefferson. This playfulness with persona came from the same place that a lot of the music came from: the blues. Memphis Minnie, Sleepy John Estes, Mississippi John Hurt, Muddy Waters, Howlin' Wolf – many a blues performer amended their real name. It was an old vaudevillian trick that never really went away. Just to show that there was nothing new under the sun, even Blind Lemon Jefferson released his earliest recordings in the 1920s under an earlier pseudonym, Deacon L. J. Bates. White musicians adopting black showbiz traditions in this way reveals a playfulness and flexibility that isn't always apparent in some of the more dour critical pronouncements on the blues and folk legacy. But in the late 1960s, with rock music beginning to stake its claims to authenticity, that kind of playfulness was out. Naturalism was in, and being natural was the biggest pose of all.

The Byrds didn't initiate that particular trend. Dylan and the Band probably didn't either, but they did nothing to discourage it as they went about ringing the changes up at Big Pink. 'The whole wave of the time was "burn the flag", "it's your parents' fault" and "let's put on a pink suit that glows in the dark",' Band guitarist Robbie Robertson told *Rolling Stone* magazine in 1987. 'And I was rebelling against all of it.' These recalcitrant sentiments were included in the magazine's special twentieth-anniversary issue. They gave the seal of approval to a polemic that *Rolling Stone* itself had promoted and served to confirm a legacy. 'Everybody wanted to wear paisley, yellow, red and orange clothes. I chose to wear black,' Robertson went on. 'We [the Band] looked like we were somewhere between Pennsylvania Dutch and rabbis.' The Band weren't Pennsylvania Dutch, of course, or rabbis (although Robertson was half Jewish); all of them, apart from Arkansas-born drummer Levon Helm (who was part Dutch, part Irish), were from Canada. In press publicity photos and on the cover of their eponymously titled second album the Band presented themselves as backwoodsmen, high-plains drifters, prairie prowlers, bar-room brawlers. 'I think it was kind of like, "Let's cut the crap, you know?" "Who are we kidding?" And also "Let's be cautious of ugly fads,"' said Robertson in that *Rolling Stone* anniversary valediction. As cautions against ugly fads go Ken Kesey would probably have concluded that some bands got on the wrong bus. As with Phil Lesh's earlier comments about the withdrawal from psychedelic excess, Robertson's motives were honest and honorable, but like the Grateful Dead and the Byrds all the Band were essentially doing was forsaking one mythology for another: acid for Americana. Lyrically they certainly weren't shy of presenting a fiction every bit as elaborate and rococo as that constructed by the purveyors of psychedelic pop. As musicians they had the same virtues and vices as any other contemporary ensemble – and they certainly succumbed to familiar pharmaceutical excesses soon enough – but initially they stood apart as much for their look as their music. And it was a look, and pretty soon it became the official down-home look, as the majority of musicians did indeed stop trying to look like space freaks in pink suits that glowed in the dark, preferring instead to adopt the wardrobe and demeanour of frontiersmen and panhandlers from the nineteenth century. The Charlatans had played with these sartorial possibilities up at the Red Dog Saloon as early as 1965; the Nitty Gritty Dirt Band picked up on the anti-fashion soon after and by the end of the sixties most group photos seemed to have traded in the fish-eye lens and the dayglo graphics and adopted the sepia-tinted look instead. The Nitty Gritty Dirt Band even got to act out their fantasies on the set of the movie *Paint Your Wagon*, in which they had a cameo role. But then in a way so did everyone else, as they lived out their version of mythical America on the sound stage of their own choosing. Most of the time these wild-west fantasists were simply the Charlatans with more musical nous. Even the Charlatans, when they finally did settle on a musical direction for more than five minutes, championed a rambling hybrid of acid country, until drummer and principal songwriter Dan Hicks, realising that he had hotter licks than everyone else, fled the coop and started his own country-fried combo. In 1971 there was even a self-styled 'electric western', *Zachariah*, featuring Country Joe and the Fish as a band of incompetent bank robbers, along with the appropriately named James Gang, fiddler Doug Kershaw and drummer Elvin Jones. Co-written by members of the Firesign Theatre, who have uncredited cameos in the film, *Zachariah* was loosely based on Herman Hesse's novel *Siddhartha*. Shot in Mexico and billed punningly as 'A Head of Its Time', it bombed at the box office. Thematically, though, its producers were onto a good thing. Electric westerns and cosmic cowboys were the new psychedelia.

What all this represented ultimately was a form of whiteface, a parallel version of the vaudevillian guises of blackface that had thrived in the minstrel shows half a century earlier. Not so much Americana as Americarny. The musicianship was rarely of the same high standard as that emanating from the Nashville production line, but that wasn't the point. California had been responsible for putting the western into country and western, but this new musical direction had little to do with that either. What the west-coast country rock of the late sixties acknowledged, almost by default, was the last lingering trace of LSD's influence. By opening doors of perception and initiating myriad changes in persona acid permitted musicians the freedom to don and discard masks at will. The critical currency of this particular rock dollar would eventually assure that all paths led to Hotel California, but it was still a California built, like so many Californias before it, on dreams and illusions, on dressing up and dressing down, on appropriate apparel for appropriate roles.

Two Americanas were constructed in the late 1960s: there was the homesteads and hickory-wind Americana of the Byrds, the Band, the Grateful Dead and all who followed that particular trail; and there was the modernist Americana of the Beach Boys' *Smile*, Van Dyke Parks's *Song Cycle*, Harry Nilsson's *Pandemonium Shadow Show* and Laura Nyro's *New York Tendaberry*. What those albums embody is the first stirrings of a post-psychedelic consciousness, clearly informed by acid's perceptual shifts but less enamoured of its illusions. In the late 1960s and early 1970s the great American songbook was rewritten in the light, shade and shadow play of acid's dazzling Arcadia. One is an Americana of log cabins, wood smoke, sepia tints, rose tints and quilt art; the other is an Americana forged out of electrification and Hoover Dams, an Americana of travelling shows and medicine shows,

showbands and showtunes, ferris wheels and fairy lights.

There was an equally pragmatic reason why the music changed so rapidly in the late 1960s, and it's one that afflicted many of the people mentioned in this chapter: the drugs changed too. By 1970 there was far greater use of psychedelics going on in the audience than among the bands. The sanctimonious tight-faced bravado displayed by the Jefferson Airplane on a song like 'Volunteers' was one part barricade-building to nine parts marching powder. Cocaine had been on the scene for a while but by the end of the 1960s it was really beginning to make its presence felt. 'I wasn't familiar with that until the New Riders started hobnobbing with some of the high rollers around the country,' said David Nelson of the New Riders of the Purple Sage. 'I wondered, what's everyone doing? Garcia told me, "Oh, it's coke man. Here. Try it." I remember thinking, "I don't like this . . . this is going to be another of those speed things." I had written when I was on speed, on Methedrine. I was so gung ho when I was doing it and then I'd read it back later and it was just drivel. The most self-indulgent, self-satisfying kind of drivel you could imagine. Really trivial and it had no substance and it was not soulful. And pushy to boot . . . I cautioned myself about it. Nevertheless I got bit by the same thing that everybody did. It was such a wonderful thing to have all that frontal brain activity out there.'[15]

As a summary of the direction rock music took for much of the next decade Nelson delivers as accurate a damnation as you could ever wish to read. 'Self-indulgent, self-satisfying drivel' should have been blocked out on a rubber stamp and given to all record reviewers. It would have saved them a lot of time in trying to describe what Lester Bangs nailed in three words: the 'ho hum entropy' of the early seventies. And pushy to boot. All frontal brain activity. No inner recesses. No deep soul-searching either. No depth at all, in fact. All shiny laminated surface. All the better to snort from.

Ultimately, most roads led to coke, even that celebrated lost highway the Band travelled on. In Martin Scorsese's valedictory 1976 tribute film *The Last Waltz*, Robbie Robertson eulogises the group to within an inch of its life. The overpowering stench of self-aggrandising coke bullshit hangs over the entire movie and the air lies thick with a powdery precipitation that all but threatens to clog up the lens. Cocaine, along with its buddies Jim Beam and Jack Daniels (and that insidious royal court interloper King Heroin), eventually saw off several of the musicians who feature in *The Last Waltz*, and a lot of other good people besides. History does not record how many died from putting on a pink suit that glowed in the dark.

6

UTOPIANS AND UTOPIATES

There are moments . . . when I feel I am witnessing the beginnings of new religions, that I find myself in religious mystical environments [in which] the symbolism of lights and colors are being discovered and explored . . . Something is happening and is happening fast – and it has something to do with light, it has everything to do with light – and everybody feels it and is waiting – often desperately.

JONAS MEKAS, 1966[1]

There was a movement – what we called 'the movement' – that included that whole energetic period, whether it was levitating the Pentagon or John Cage's new sound. We began to see that the traditional forms in the arts were to be, had to be, broken up . . .

These were times of pioneering. The problem is we had a utopian vision, but what we didn't have was any concept of how we get from where we were to that place.

JUDITH MALINA, Living Theater[2]

Utopia? It is indeed astonishing how little has been accomplished so far in this direction. This materialistic and practical age has in fact lost the genuine feeling for play and the miraculous . . . Amazed at the flood of technological advance, we accept these wonders of utility as being already perfected art form, while actually they are only prerequisites for its creation.

OSKAR SCHLEMMER, 'Man and Art Figure'[3]

'Suddenly the intermedia shows are all over town,' stated film-maker and underground-cinema pioneer Jonas Mekas in May 1966 in his regular 'Movie Journal' column in New York's *Village Voice*. Mekas would have known that better than most as he was responsible for staging many of them, most notably at the Festival of Expanded Cinema, which he hosted at the Film-Makers' Cinematheque during December 1965. In the same *Village Voice* article Gerd Stern elaborated on the utopian spirit inherent in USCO's current work. 'It's in the rainbow and it's in the sweep of the audio oscillator and it's in the visualization of the wave form as phosphor on the cathode ray tube that it becomes apparent to me as mystical reality,' Stern told Mekas.[4] Everybody was beginning to talk like this by 1966. Well, not everyone, obviously. Ronald Reagan wasn't. He was too busy campaigning for the governorship of California by proposing to reactivate the state's dormant capital-punishment laws. But elsewhere creative artists of every kind were challenging boundaries with utopian rhetoric and waxing lyrical about the exciting new possibilities of multimedia environments. Mekas asked Stern why he thought 'there has been such a general trend towards media mixes'. Stern replied that 'the tools are really becoming available', to which Mekas responded, 'This kind of research has been going on for at least ten years. Why suddenly all of this?'[5] As Mekas saw it, the issue was no longer how or even why, but why now. And the answer, at least in part, was LSD. Ideas that had been slowly taking shape in a number of different art forms throughout the early 1960s

177

were now being refracted through the multicoloured prism of acid. For some the newly favoured strategy for negotiating away the fourth wall and the closed flat rectangle was to hallucinate them out of existence entirely, or at least temporarily.

This strategy obviously had its drawbacks, temporality itself being one of them. 'I lay down on the floor and began to melt into the environment,' said Californian architect Eric Clough as he tested out the consciousness-expanding potential of psychedelics. 'I visualized my ego as a head sticking up above the protoplasm, trying to preserve itself . . . it just went plop and away I went.' 'Away, of course, into stereotypical grand narratives of the entire history of civilization,' says Felicity Scott, dismissively.[6] Many chose to renegotiate reality in the way Clough had done, simply by constructing dream architecture drawn from the familiar age-old tropes of the romantic imagination. Infinitesimal beauty could, it seems, only be compensated by recourse to an illusory lexicography of grand schemes and unsustainable visions. 'We had no programme,' admitted Judith Malina of the Living Theater. 'We had no ideas of constructing a new world. We knew what we wanted to destroy. We didn't know what we wanted to create.'[7]

By 1967 it was becoming clear that the avant-garde's engagement with the growing rock culture was drawing to a close. Among the rock fraternity, certainly among rock promoters, there was less talk of mixed-media events. As Charles Perry noted in The Haight-Ashbury, 'The Thunder Machines, self-interfaced TV equipment, tape recorders and other electronic toys of the Acid Tests did not survive into the dance halls.'[8] When Bill Graham had put on his first benefit dances in November and December 1965, 'the Mime Troupe was famous and the bands were the big surprise', said Perry. By the time Graham put on a benefit for the troupe in April 1967, 'the audience showed hardly any sign of knowing who R. G. Davis was'.[9]

So what became of the Neon Renaissance? What did happen to a relationship that had seemed so interwoven and fruitful only a year or so earlier? It wasn't simply a case of LSD usurping creativity's role. After all, drug-inspired music hadn't begun with the Bay Area rock bands. Terry Riley's 'Mescaline Mix', devised as musical accompaniment to Anna Halprin's theatre piece The Three Legged Stool, had been developed over a period of two years between 1961 and 1963. Inspired by Riley's own experiments with mescaline and by John

Cage's 'Fontana Mix' (the first time the word 'mix' had been used in its contemporary sense), the piece was originally known for discretionary purposes as 'M Mix', but when people asked what the 'M' stood for, Riley told them, and most of his friends knew anyway. 'Mescaline Mix' utilised tape-delay techniques to almost subliminal effect. The sound of laughter from Halprin's dancers was slowed to a low-register drawling haw-haw that resembled a Pacific fog horn. Occasional soft bursts of mournful bluesy piano notes are heard. Everything seems to slow to a subsonic white noise that drifts in and out of audibility.

By the mid-1960s there were abundant instances of underground or avant-garde artists incorporating source material from the world of rock and pop into their work. In his 1965 film *Phenomena*, which was influenced directly by *The Tibetan Book of the Dead* and the *Diamond Sutra*, Jordan Belson used a soundtrack of electronically distorted rock music. That same year Terry Riley premiered a new tape-composition piece called 'Bird of Paradise', which like 'Mescaline Mix' had begun life as accompaniment to a Halprin theatre piece. In its opening section a screed of sheet-metal noise slowly embeds itself in the listener's skull. Growing tantalisingly more recognisable with each

successive stab it slowly reveals itself to be a snippet of Junior Walker and the All Stars' 'Shotgun'. Riley subjects Walker's shrill alto sax to ever-increasing mutations as the piece continues. Drum rolls are treated with cavernous echo, dance floor-driven sax riffs become alien pulse beats.

In December 1965 Pauline Oliveros performed a new composition at the San Francisco Tape Music Center entitled 'Rock Symphony', a tape-delay collage that incorporated samples from the Beatles' 'Norwegian Wood' and 'Day Tripper', the Animals' 'It's My Life', the Bobby Fuller Four's 'I Fought the Law' and Tammi Terrell's 'I Can't Believe You Love Me'. All these songs had been released within a six-week period at the end of that year, illustrating the rapidity with which exponents of avant-garde music were prepared to appropriate and assimilate material from the pop world. With even greater prescience Oliveros incorporated *Alice in Wonderland* into one of her works – this at a time when Lewis Carroll was becoming set reading for the psychedelic generation – when she recorded 'Beautiful Soop', a 1966 piece which featured spoken extracts from Carroll's verse that were then treated with the Buchla Box and the composer's own tape-delay system.

It's easy to see how an experimental rock band might have slotted into all this activity had the spirit of creative collaboration endured. It would have been perfectly logical to chance upon the Grateful Dead or Big Brother and the Holding Company at a *City Scale*-type event or at any of the other mixed-media performances that took place when the Happenings movement was at its height. But the truth was that by the end of 1966 the role of the avant-garde had been largely usurped and the experimentalists had been driven back to the fringes. Dance went pirouetting back to the dance world. Radical and experimental theatre went off-Broadway. The Expanded Cinema continued to expand but it did so in movie theatres and on movie screens, not at the dance halls or rock concerts. And while verse continued to run freely off the page and painting occasionally ran off the walls, they did so largely within the confines of the poetry reading room and the art galleries, but not at rock gigs.

USCO's Michael Callahan offered some sombre reflections on the unfulfilled potential of mixed media. 'I could see that things were becoming more integrated in the '60s due to electronic media providing a shared experience,' he said, 'and I always assumed that these converging tributaries would come together as one. But as it happened, even when they did cross, they kept going their separate ways'. Callahan maintained that 'in 1968–69 we were as electronically "together" as we were going to get'.[10] This retreat coincided with the rise of the rock dollar, but not all of the blame can be apportioned to the money men and the rationalists. Part of the problem lay with the avant-garde itself. Everything can be reduced to its idioms soon enough, and experimentalism was as prone to overworked devices and clichés as any other form of creative activity. Even Allan Kaprow, the man who coined the term 'Happenings', acknowledged that this was precisely what had happened to the movement he championed. It is sobering to observe that Kaprow was offering this critique in 1966, at a time when rock culture was only just beginning to fully explore the polysensory possibilities of the performance environment and the counter-culture was still in its infancy. It is equally salutary to be reminded that a particular phase of late-modernist experimentalism may have been effectively over by the time the Jefferson Airplane recorded their first LP. But Kaprow was right: radical theatre, performance art and Happenings, for all their boundary-shaking rhetoric, often fell back on familiar techniques and strategies (for instance, multi-layered imagery, simultaneously occur-ring events) and an equally predictable repertoire of shock tactics (loud atonal noise, nudity). As early as 1964 Ramon Sender was suggesting that 'I often felt we were expected to perform amusing antics during concerts, and that some in the audience were disappointed in not witnessing some sort of scandalous behaviour on our part. Avant-garde is coming to mean a comedy act.'[11]

At the Golden Gate Be-In in January 1967 poet James Broughton turned to dancer Anna Halprin and said, 'They've caught up with you. Now how do you define your task?' In other words, the audience speaks the same language now, it has absorbed the information – where do we go from here? Richard Kostelanetz asked Halprin the same question. 'What I'm against,' Halprin replied, 'is a personal statement that remains so introspective, private, eso-teric, that it leaves an audience play-ing guessing games.'[12] Halprin called for 'a collective statement based on the need for audiences and performers to be assembled; so that what occurs is a process that evolves out of both the movement and all the people there'.[13] Anyone looking for an enactment of that philosophy during the latter part

of 1966 and early 1967 was increasingly less likely to be seeking it at the Hap-penings and the Expanded Cinema. Instead they were discovering it in the visceral absorption of the rock concerts and the impromptu picnics in the park. The rock dance was becoming one of the few arenas where genuine sponta-neous joy might be found. 'I thought the rock scene was magnificent, and I was very excited to be invited to par-ticipate with them,' Halprin told David Bernstein.[14] 'It appears to me that art-ists and audience are at a threshold of a most exciting period,' she told Richard Kostelanetz.[15] But that spirit of collab-oration proved to be relatively short-lived. Something was already shifting in the relationship between bands and audiences. 'The whole character of the thing changed,' noted Owsley Stanley. 'Instead of people just having a good time and dancing and everything, they stood around mesmerized, staring at the stage as if they were going to miss a stroke of the guitar player's pick or some-thing . . . Eventually they even started sitting down and staring at 'em.'[16] Stan-ley suggested that rock audiences were becoming increasingly supine (and, he could have added, stupefied by the mammoth doses of lysergics that he had manufactured and distributed to them), but there was more to it than that.

Speaking to *Artforum* magazine in 2008, Michael Callahan offered a more pragmatic take on the inactive audience. 'I wanted a little more direction or substance rather than just "heightening consciousness",' he said. 'Heightening, well, why? What's the point? Maybe people were happy the way they were.'[17] Such a viewpoint hints at something inherently conservative and herd-like in the rock audience, but it also perceives something combative, hostile and a tad too macho in the anarchic techniques unleashed by the Acid Tests and those who followed in their wake. Even hardened heads like Grateful Dead manager Rock Scully could see the drawbacks of the no-safety-net approach to set and setting. 'LSD can be a razor-edged kind of deal sometimes,' he said. 'It takes away your defenses and then leaves you vulnerable.'[18] Warhol biographer Stephen Koch concurred and offered a damning critique of the *Plastic Exploding Inevitable*. 'The effort to create an exploding (more accurately, imploding) environment capable of shattering any conceivable focus on the senses was all too successful,' he said. 'It became virtually impossible even to dance, or for that matter do anything but sit and be bombarded – "stoned", as it were.' Koch saw in certain aspects of the drug culture deep-seated issues that weren't necessarily going to be resolved with sensory bombardment. 'It came home to me how the "obliteration" of the ego was not the act of liberation it was advertised to be, but an act of compulsive revenge and resentment wholly entangled on the deepest levels with the knots of frustration. Liberation was turning out to be humiliation; peace was revealing itself as rage.'[19]

It was also revealing itself as profit and entrepreneurialism. The most ambitious and certainly the most publicised of USCO's shows was *Murray the K World*, a huge multimedia discotheque they designed for the self-styled 'fifth Beatle', New York DJ Murray Kaufman. *Murray the K World* opened in April 1966 at Roosevelt Field, a huge abandoned aircraft hangar in Long Island, and was financed in part by sixty-year-old Michael Myerberg, a former Broadway director and producer whose credits included working with Tallulah Bankhead and a young Montgomery Clift in the 1942 stage production of *The Skin of Our Teeth* and, most famously, producing *Waiting for Godot* at the John Golden Theatre in 1956. Andy Warhol and his Factory entourage had originally been invited to be part of the set-up, a request which led directly to Warhol encountering the

Velvet Underground for the first time when he went in search of a band. 'However, there was let's say an Italian influence in this club and I think they had their own plans for the opening,' said Warhol's assistant Paul Morrissey. 'About a week before they were scheduled to open, this lawyer said, "They've changed their minds, they're going to open with the Young Rascals."'[20]

Murray the K World was unlike anything USCO had been involved in before, a head-on collide-oscope (to borrow a McLuhanism) between hip thinking and straight (and criminal underworld) finance. The opening night's acts were the Young Rascals and the Hollies, with appearances promised in forthcoming weeks from Del Shannon, the Isley Brothers and Mitch Ryder and the Detroit Wheels. USCO's contribution was to provide two and a half hours of 16mm film and twenty-one slide projectors and screens, all of which were controlled from a central console built out of Michael Callahan's scavenged IBM mainframes. True to the USCO ethos, the venture also utilised surplus equipment acquired from the 1964 New York World's Fair, including the Eidophor video projector, which had been devised in the 1940s to create theatre-sized images of remarkable clarity and which NASA

later acquired for use at Mission Control during the Apollo missions. USCO utilised its innovative optical system – a slowly rotating mirrored dish coated in thick transparent oil – to provide disorientating visual mixes of superimposed images of the crowd and Murray the K's specially hired go-go dancers. In addition there were experimental films by Stan Vanderbeek, Jud Yalkut and Gerd Stern, and Robert Indiana-style graphics reading 'ACT', 'SLIT', 'IS', etc. These were interspersed with fetishistic images of leather boots, choreographed to Nancy Sinatra's current Top 10 hit 'These Boots Were Made for Walking'. There were also closed-circuit TVs and self-operating cameras tracking the audience. At first the cameramen took conventional TV shots of girls in miniskirts, à la *Where the Action Is* or *Shindig!*, until Stern encouraged them to loosen up and synchronise their zoom shots in time with the music.

'It was more teenybopper than stoner,' remembers Michael Callahan. 'But it was strange because it was so suburban, pretty straight, and we were dropping this pseudo-psychedelic event.'[21] On 27 May 1966 USCO found themselves on the cover of *Life* magazine. 'New Madness at the Discotheque' blared the headline, above a photo of two young hipsters throwing geometric dance shapes as a bevy of dress code-observing, clean-cut suburbanites looked on. 'At "The World" dancers gyrate amid far out movies and flashing light,' read the accompanying caption. The *Life* magazine piece was also the first to feature the phrase 'Be-In'. After that an increasing number of people wanted to be at the Be-In.

Also making the cover of *Life* magazine that year was Richard Aldcroft. In June 1965 Aldcroft had contributed to the *Psychedelic Explorations* event with USCO and Leary's Castalia Foundation. In September 1966 he was on the cover of *Life* magazine, under the lurid caption 'LSD ART: New Experience that Bombards the Senses', where he could be seen modelling his patented 'Infinity Machine'. The device was a headset hybrid of Moholy-Nagy's Light Space Modulator and Wilhelm Reich's orgone accumulator. By the winter of 1966 Aldcroft had turned his attentions to architecture, and specifically towards new ways of housing his Infinity Machines. The structures of the future, he announced, would be floating cities of transparent geodesic spheres. These dodecahedron structures would also provide air conditioning and generators, storage equipment to provide anchorage, and a nuclear generator. 'And you think this can all

come about through heightened consciousness through LSD?' Jonas Mekas asked him. 'Yes, that's right,' responded Aldcroft.[22] This prompted George Maciunas of Fluxus to comment. 'This scheme, if inspired by LSD, should be the best argument why engineers should not take LSD.'[23]

It's just a light show, but it comes on heavy.[24]

'What are all these lights doing? What is the real meaning of the strobes?' Jonas Mekas asked Steve Durkee in 1966. Durkee suggested that they encouraged the dissolution of ego. Strobes, he said, 'created a continuance . . . loss of who you are – because all you see are fragments of yourself'.[25] Whether working with back projections which cast pretty colours on the wall or immersing the audience in what Durkee called 'electrical showers', the light-show practitioners were integral to the formation of the west-coast rock experience, so integral that in the early days at least it was impossible to imagine psychedelic music being performed without them. The very genetic coding of the Grateful Dead had been shaped by the bombardment of liquid sub-particles at the Acid Tests. Everyone who played the Fillmore and the

Avalon was subjected to the celestial embrace of abstract light. The San Francisco dance-hall concerts brought together all the different lighting techniques that had been quietly fermenting in the Bay Area since the days when Seymour Locks first dripped heated gelatin into a clear convex dish. Tony Martin of the Tape Music Center showed his multiprojector light paintings at Bill Graham's Fillmore events; Bill Ham, Glenn McKay and Ben Van Meter worked Chet Helms's Avalon Ballroom concerts. Hard-edged geometry and multilayered slide projections met the amorphous swirls of the liquid shows. Non-figurative drips and blobs blended with distressed film stock and library footage. Alpha waves and ultraviolet rays formed huge rolling washes that ran like gravity-defying waterfalls up, down and across the walls in a polysensory celebration of everything that Moholy-Nagy had anticipated in the 1940s.

'How long . . . can any rotating, vibrating, whirring contrivance together with an infinite variety of forms, colors, and lights sustain the interest of the spectator?' Oskar Schlemmer had asked in *Theater of the Bauhaus* in 1925.[26] The answer, as it turns out, was until August 1969. That was when the grandly named Light Artists Guild decided to strike for parity and to picket the Fillmore West and Winterland ballrooms. In addition to the $750 a night they were receiving from Bill Graham they demanded a percentage of the door takings too, a request that Graham rejected out of hand. In the midst of counter-culture utopianism this was a good old-fashioned labour dispute. The light-show operators reasoned correctly that as their craft was labour-intensive, it deserved appropriate renumeration. They surmised less accurately that people were coming to the concerts as much for the light shows as they were for the music. Graham's freeze-out disabused them of such a notion. Stripped of the visuals the punters still poured through the doors. Light show or no light show they were there for the music. What had once seemed an integral part of the culture evaporated almost overnight, like so much heated liquid oil. Jerry Garcia, whose grandmother had been a co-founder of the Laundry Workers Union, refused to cross the picket lines – other members of his band had no such scruples – but even Garcia could see that the light operators' profits were a result of what he called 'largesse from the promoters', and he reasoned correctly that 'nobody was going to pay more money on their ticket just to get a light show'.[27] As

Garcia pointed out, 'The light shows, which were not exactly thriving up to that point, but at least were existing, created their own doom. That was it for them.'[28] And it was. Chet Helms's Family Dog organisation downsized and put on a few small-scale events run by co-operative before disbanding completely, and many of the other light-show outfits disappeared overnight. In their absence spotlights and traditional stage lighting reasserted themselves, and so to a certain degree did traditional stagecraft. Hierarchical presentation values reasserted themselves too – appropriate lighting for appropriate stars.

Detecting that an entire movement's visual iconography was succumbing to vulgarisation and commercialisation, Matthieu Poirier called psychedelic art 'a misappropriated and diminished realization of an avant-garde intention'.[29] Its only function, as he saw it, was to replicate the visual patterns and enhance the experience of those who had taken psychotropic drugs. There were those who continued to make claims for the artistic integrity of the light shows, pioneers and practitioners who argued that the lights were not just there to serve as a decorative effect, they were a vital creative component of the entire immersive experience,

but for all too many this merely translated into trippy visuals of the most idiomatic kind as light projections began to form a kind of fractal orthodoxy and settled down into a recognisable style. Audiences came to expect the same amoeba-like blobs again and again. In the end this was the crucial factor that psychedelia's dominant aesthetic hinged upon, and ultimately what it was impaled on. If temporality was built into the very fabric of liquid light technology (and indeed the neurobiology of the acid trip), what was there of substance to cling to, what could be replicated, what might endure, what came after the afterglow?

In the International Times editor Tom McGrath was addressing this question as early as February 1967. In issue 9 of the newspaper he asked, 'What are you doing to those walls when you project hallucinations onto them? Why not go out and paint a mural instead?'[30] Proselytes would have answered that with: 'At least the hallucination belongs to you, whereas the mural belongs to the council or city hall or whoever owns the building.' But McGrath at least raised a necessary question about the limits of the drug culture, one that was beginning to exercise advocates and cautionary voices alike. In fact, the question had lain latent since Aldous

Huxley first broached the issue in *The Doors of Perception*. 'This is how one ought to see, how things really are,' he had exclaimed as he marvelled at his trouser folds and his Van Goghian chair. 'And yet there were reservations,' he added. 'For if one always saw like this, one would never want to do anything else.'[31] This was an issue an entire subculture was now having to grapple with: how to face the comedown.

Like the light shows, the immersive environments had fallen on hard times by the late 1960s. Unable to sustain their initial energy and impetus they rapidly descended into kitsch. One such operation, Cerebrum, opened in New York in November 1968 and generated considerable media publicity. A 'super, electric, turned on, far-out fantasy land', promised the enticing late-night ad on WNEW-FM. Cerebrum hosted two three-hour sessions nightly, 8 to 11 p.m. and 11.30 p.m. to 2.30 a.m. Upon entering visitors paid their admission fee – anywhere between $1 and $7, depending on the night – took off their shoes and were led into an 'orientation room', where they were regaled by a cod-futuristic environment (later immortalised in Woody Allen's film *Sleeper*) full of white diaphanous robes, glowing orbs and huge helium inflatables. 'Eventually they break out

the parachute, with patrons grabbing each side and watching as the white billowy fabric flaps back and forth in the air,' noted one eyewitness. 'Like what you did in elementary school, except with lots of stoned adults.'[32] Water and marshmallows were served by so-called 'Cerebrum guides'. Co-founder Ruffin Cooper explained to *Time* magazine that Cerebrum was 'trying to overturn every entertainment convention – the "sit here," the "look that way," the "dance over here".' But for all its talk of 'an electric studio of participation' the overall ambience was more akin to a swingers' party, minus the actual swinging. Gene Youngblood eulogised Cerebrum in his book *Expanded Cinema*; Alvin Toffler spoke approvingly of it in *Future Shock*; *Rolling Stone* magazine gave it a rave review. In the end it mostly attracted stoners and would-be promiscuity-seekers. *New York* magazine referred to it in March 1969 as a 'place implicitly geared to voyeuristic impulses'. The whole venture closed just five months later.

As Cerebrum amply demonstrated, hippie infantalism could impose itself upon the most potentially liberating of circumstances. Peter Douthit (aka Peter Rabbit), who was part of the short-lived Drop City commune in southern Colorado in the late 1960s, described Clard

Svenson's circular geodesic structure the *Drop City Spatial Paradox Painting* as 'a spinning spherical disc almost six feet in diameter with strobes on it. You can make it stand still, move slowly forward or backward, all the time pulsing. It's a mind blow.'[33] It might have been 'a mind blow' to those caught up in the moment, but whichever way you look at it it was a big balloon inflatable, a children's toy by any other definition. If the *Drop City Spatial Paradox Painting* was art, then it was art that all too pointedly illustrated the scaling down of utopian dreams. Never mind painting with light. The Frisbee generation was coming.

Before they ditched him Jefferson Airplane manager Matthew Katz had big plans for the band. As well as printing up business cards with 'Fojazz' on them, he envisaged a fan club full of cuties called 'Jefferson Airplane Stewardesses' who would attend concerts and shower the audience with complimentary goodies. He also wanted the band to back topless dancers at strip joints. Such entrepreneurialism seemed to belong to an earlier, more sleazy age and revealed the apparent disparity between old-style showbiz promotion and the new breed of artists, but it does offer a tantalising glimpse of what could have transpired

in a parallel psychedelic universe. The phased-up, fuzzed-up, R&B bump-and-grind favoured by many outfits lent itself readily to the more raunchy scenes of psychsploitation movies, and in years to come would feature equally prominently in both soft- and hardcore porn-movie soundtracks. One man who understood that world's curvature perfectly was Hugh Hefner. His *Playboy After Dark* TV series was aired throughout 1969 and 1970 and incorporated psychedelic ambience effortlessly into its penthouse-and-playmates shtick. *Playboy After Dark* captured perfectly that period when floaty, trippy, gossamer-light psych was giving way to the hardcore sound of heavy rock. Musical guests on Hefner's show included the Grateful Dead, Deep Purple, Joan Baez, Harry Nilsson, Steppenwolf, Three Dog Night and Ike and Tina Turner. The programme repositioned the immersive environment as a slightly upmarket burlesque, with table service and an A-list of celebrity guests, including Sammy Davis Jnr, Roman Polanski and Sharon Tate, who came on as high as a kite. It was simultaneously louche, gauche and grown up in a way that the infantalised love puppies of the Golden Gate gatherings would have flinched at. *Playboy After Dark* revealed the very thin line that existed between the super-realism of *Beyond the Valley of the Dolls* and the surrealism of the Acid Tests. One of the best musical moments occurs when Iron Butterfly perform 'In-A-Gadda-Da-Vida', the seventeen-minute title track of their 1968 debut album. The song owed its title to a stoned conversation in which singer and keyboard player Doug Ingle couldn't say 'in the Garden of Eden'. It was one of the indisputable psychedelic rock classics of the era, an organ-led slab of heaviosity with crashing guitars and growled, graunchy vocals. When they performed it on *Playboy After Dark*, a conversation between Hefner and a church minister about the place of God and religion in society segued seamlessly into the music. 'Sounds churchy,' says the minister as the opening organ riff crashes their theological small talk. 'Well, now it doesn't sound churchy,' he adds as the guitars come in. Hefner and the minister continue their conversation as they stroll casually over to a windowed partition. The host boasts about his mansion's abundant gadgetry, to which the minister responds: 'Well, next time I visit I wanna use that sauna.' The chat fades into the music with that perfectly timed precision that only American TV could manage. The band mime a truncated version of their seventeen-minute epic to an accompanying bacchanal of writhing bodies. Afterwards Bill Cosby and Hefner grill Doug Ingle about the band's name. 'Well, we wanted something that was heavy,' he says. The truth is, they were pussycats. In the *Playboy After Dark* footage they look the most innocent people in the room, the look-don't-touch house band at an orgy. Strip away the Doorsy affectations and bluesy growls on their debut album and most of the songs are about compliance with your best gal's desires. Typical of these was 'Flowers and Beads', a smoochy singalong about true love. 'Flowers and beads are one thing / but having a girl is something,' they sing in a style that wouldn't have offended the most prissy programme director, which was more than could be said for *Playboy After Dark*, whose mixed-race gatherings of raunchy dancers didn't play well in markets where Jim Crow still ruled. *Playboy After Dark* was indisputably of its time and was gone by May 1970, but in its brief lifespan it offered an X-rated option for those who had outgrown or outlived hippie innocence, a pornotopia to replace all those infantilised kindertopias.

7

I AM THE BLACK GOLD OF THE SUN

The Negro performers, from James Brown to Aaron Neville to the Supremes to the Four Tops, are on an Ed Sullivan *trip, striving as hard as they can to get on that stage and become part of the American success story, while the white rock performers are motivated to escape from that stereotype. Whereas in years past the Negro performer offered style in performance and content in song – the messages from Leadbelly to Percy Mayfield to Ray Charles were important messages – today he is almost totally style and very little content.*

RALPH J. GLEASON[1]

When you start talking about the fact that the black man is still hung with status symbols, man, don't forget that he's trying to grab onto exactly the things that the white kids are trying to give up. Drop out? Wow, man, what we got to drop out of anyway? You don't want your fancy house or your good job? Shit, let me have it, man, 'cos I've been trying to get something like that all my miserable life.

UNNAMED MEMBER OF THE FIFTH DIMENSION[2]

In Chapter 18 of *The Electric Kool-Aid Acid Test*, Tom Wolfe's seminal first-hand account of the Merry Pranksters' frolics at the new pharmaceutical frontier, he introduces us to a character called Big Nig. Big Nig, we learn, is 'a local boho figure' who loaned Ken Kesey his house for what would become the second Acid Test. The event took place on 4 December 1965 and it would appear that Big Nig's main contribution was to deem himself terminally uncool by hustling the Grateful Dead for a contribution towards the rent. Or, as Wolfe put it, 'A new star is being born, like a light bulb in a womb. And Big Nig wants the rent – a new star being born, a new planet forming, Ahura Mazda blazing in the world womb, here before our very eyes – and Big Nig, the poor pathetic spade, wants his rent.'[3] From the little that we learn during this brief

encounter 'the poor pathetic spade' has, in fact, presented his case entirely reasonably and with cogent logic. 'I mean, like, y'know,' says Big Nig to Garcia, 'I didn't charge Kesey nothing to use this place, like free, y'know? And the procedure now is that every cat here contributes, man, to help out with the rent.'[4]

Big Nig's give-a-little request wasn't particularly new. Similar down-home economics had been sustaining the jazz avant-garde since the late 1940s, when loft parties and other small gatherings were funded by everyone throwing a few coins into the hat so that the next event might take place. But in *The Electric Kool-Aid Acid Test* Big Nig is not portrayed as an adroit sponsor of cutting-edge performances; he is presented as some sort of adversary, an unbenevolent spirit, an irritant even. He is a terminally unhip bread-head landlord completely out of touch with the prevailing spirit of the age. 'A freaking odd thought, that one,' concludes Wolfe. 'A big funky spade looking pathetic and square. For twenty years in the hip life, Negroes never even looked square. They were the archetypal soul figures. But what is Soul, or Funky, or Cool, or Baby – in the new world of the ecstasy . . .?'[5]

In the garbled prosody of new journalism Wolfe never does take the time to pause, draw breath and reflect on his rhetorical question. So what does constitute 'Soul, or Funky, or Cool' in the new groovy world order? All we can ascertain for certain is that it sure ain't a black landlord who has the temerity to ask for a contribution towards wear and tear and blown fuses. The other great unspoken, of course, is that nickname. If we are to assume that the landlord isn't a man of exceedingly large stature called Nigel, then there is only one thing that Nig is short for. And if we are also to assume that Big Nig didn't bestow the nickname upon himself, then we are into a whole other ethical universe, one where some stars burn more brightly than others and the dark ones don't burn at all. I've endeavoured to find out more about Big Nig. I've trawled all the dedicated Grateful Dead and Haight-Ashbury websites

and not found a single mention. I've visited chat forums and bulletin boards populated by music obsessives who can tell you to the very demi-quaver where two Jerry Garcia guitar solos were spliced together on any given album. They can detect from the audience ambience alone where a live Grateful Dead bootleg was recorded, but they somehow draw a complete blank when it comes to revealing the identity of our spunky, hunky, deeply unfunky rent-grabbing brother of another colour. Like most African Americans, Big Nig merely has a walk-on part in the new Aquarian escapade, and his anonymity speaks volumes. A similarly salutary reminder of the role served by African Americans in the new-age pageant is provided by Charles Perry, who offers the following seemingly incidental detail from the conclusion to the legendary Golden Gate Park Be-In in January 1967: 'At the end of the event a few knots of hostile teenagers from Mission High School and Polytechnic High, Latins and black, got into confrontations with trippers.'[6] Latins, blacks and Hispanics, as so often, are an aside, an afterthought. They are presented as begrudging bystanders, footnotes to the larger narrative.

That same ethnic anonymity can be seen in numerous accounts of the rise of the counter-culture, an absence that is evident whenever and wherever white affluence rides roughshod over the aspirations of the dispossessed. In March 1967 disc jockey and Autumn Records boss Tom Donahue approached Leon Crosby, the owner of ailing San Francisco radio station KMPX, with a view to giving more airtime to the underground rock community that was by now thriving in the Bay area. KMPX had been a jazz station in the 1950s (when it was known as KHIP), but when Crosby bought the station for $147,000 from the owner of a local San Francisco basketball team he changed its name and the format to middle-of-the-road music. By 1967 KMPX was basically a leasing facility, renting the majority of its airtime to small Portuguese, Spanish, Italian and Armenian businesses. Financially it was barely keeping its head above water. The station's only contacts with the white youth audience were Roy Trumbull's folk-music programme and an all-night show hosted by Larry Miller. Donahue would subsequently base his entire programming philosophy around Miller's eclectic mix of folk, jazz, classical and rock music. Initially he was handed the 8 p.m. to midnight slot, replacing one of the ethnic-community shows, a Chinese-language programme whose

sponsors had been unable to pay their bills. As other ethnic-minority contracts expired their slots were replaced in the KMPX schedules by free-form music shows. By August 1967 only a few ethnic programmes remained on Sundays, with rock now the dominant sound on the KMPX airwaves.

In the same way that I have unsuccessfully pursued the identity of Big Nig, I have been unable to ascertain any information about the Chinese-language programme or any of the other ethnic shows that made way for Donahue's more lucrative rock format. They remain invisible others, displaced by the affluent forces of hip capitalism. By 1967 the same displacement was occurring all over Haight-Ashbury, but it received little attention from the hip community. These unsuccessful ethnic initiatives and the cultures they represented were merely incidental to the main event. Physically and geopolitically they stand, like those Latins and blacks at the Be-In, on the periphery of things, lurking on the fringes, outside looking in.

'Haight/Ashbury is the first segregated Bohemia I've ever seen,' wrote Chester Anderson in a scathing broadside that he distributed on the streets of San Francisco in February 1967. With rents rising and lower-income residents being driven further out into the Fillmore district ghetto, Anderson offered a cautionary take on the new economic balance of power: 'Dear all my brethren, we have a race problem. Along with all the other things we're developing, we have developed new patterns of prejudice . . . I brought this up at the H.I.P meeting last night causing a furor (through which, clear as a bell, rang the complaints of a very few merchants that these little kolored kids – too genteel to say either spade or nigger – shoplift shoplift shoplift, which is mere profiteering bullshit) . . . Spades probably resent us because we have so lightly abandoned exactly what they (and many of us with them) have worked and fought so long, so hard with so many dead and wounded to obtain. They resent us dipping so blithely into their ghetto. We can get out by cutting our hair, most of them can never get out.' Anderson thought that the drug culture should shoulder at least some of the blame. 'Lots of our new young hippies have entered the scene by the acid route, bringing all their deeper straight prejudices with them uncorrected. They're little more than freaked-out WASPs,' he said, and warned: 'If the Fillmore erupts again this summer – and it most likely will – and we haven't re-established ourselves with the Fillmore's people, then they'll erupt against us as well as against the man AND WE WILL BE BURIED.'[7]

The Diggers, as always, were hip to the situation right from the start. Emmett Grogan noticed that when the Haight Independent Proprietors Job Co-Op made jobs available for the unskilled, they went to white kids with a good education rather than the unemployed minorities who needed them. 'Even the post office jobs promised to San Francisco's blacks during the "riots" were given to the newly arrived hippies,' he noted. 'This aroused the black and Chicano communities, causing friction and animosity between them and the longhairs who began arrogantly to consider themselves the new niggers.'[8] When he relocated to New York, Grogan found the same thing occurring in the slums of the Lower East Side. 'The sight of a pair of well-fed hippies walking through the neighbourhood, panhandling change against a backdrop of desperate bleakness, may have appeared farcical to strangers but to the people who lived their entire lives in the area, grew up there it was a mockery, a derisive imitation of their existence, and it got them angry. Plenty angry.'[9] Just how angry was illustrated in October 1967, when teenage socialite Linda Rae Fitzpatrick and her twenty-four-year-old boyfriend James Leroy Hutchinson, known as 'Groovy', were brutally murdered in the basement boiler room of a tenement block on Avenue B. The eighteen-year-old Fitzpatrick had been raped, and both had had their faces stomped on beyond recognition. Press coverage made much of the fact that they were Aquarian innocents abroad, the kind of naïfs and waifs that can be seen in Haight-Ashbury TV footage wandering unencumbered and fancy-free, blithely unaware of what might happen should they ever get lured out of their safety zone, as these two were. Groovy was by all accounts a semi-literate dispenser of drugs and hippie wisdom, and he elicited pitiful testimonies from those who knew him. 'Groovy freaked out in such a beautiful way,' his friend Galahad told the *Village Voice*. 'He would walk up to you and give you a pop bottle cap. If you asked him what it was for, he'd say, "It's yours because I gave it to you." It didn't have to be a thing of value. It didn't even have to mean anything to anyone. It was just the idea that he'd given you something.' In a piece appropriately entitled 'A Groovy Idea While He Lasted', Richard Goldstein, senior editor at the *Village Voice*, wrote a telling obituary. It was a sombre farewell not just to Groovy but to everything

he represented. 'Flower power was a summer vacation,' he reports one disenchanted hippie as saying. 'In San Francisco they staged the death of the hippie. Here we got the real thing.' 'The mindblower is not that love is dead in the East Village,' says Goldstein, 'but that it has taken this long to kick the bucket.'[10] Goldstein accurately captured the simmering hostility that existed between residents and arrivistes. This was no place to be living out your turn on, tune in, drop out fantasies. From a black perspective you couldn't drop out if you'd never been invited in in the first place. From a wealthy white perspective dropping out was an indulgence; you could always drop back in further on down the line once you'd had enough of voluntary poverty. 'The flower children brought their material feast to areas of constant famine, and then went on a hunger strike. Even in rags they seemed wealthy,' noted Goldstein. "The hippies really bug us," a young black East Sider told the *New York Times*. "Because we know they can come down here and play their games for a while and then escape. And we can't."'[11]

Emmett Grogan spelled out the message more forcefully: 'You see most of these people want, more than any of you could ever not want, things like a pre-fab house out on the suburbs, or a pre-fab house or bungalow back in Puerto Rico. They're just like all the other lower classes that came before them, dreaming of becoming middle class with all the trimmings that come with it.'[12] He poured scorn on those who came to slum it among the rat-infested, needle-strewn streets of the ghetto. 'To these people and their sons and daughters who've had no choice but to live their lives in the disaster of the Lower East Side, there ain't nothing hip about junk or poverty or violence and they have nothing but contempt for young educated fools who think it's exciting to live in a world they really know nothing about, the kind of world these kids' middle-class parents built the suburbs to protect them from.'[13]

It was that last line that delivered the *coup de grâce*. Out there in those much-derided suburbs affluence and complacency were busy being born, but few were busy dying. It was a different matter in the poor parts of the cities, especially in those zones where the First World's well-fed inhabitants rubbed up against the resentment and the abandoned aspirations of the desperate and the dispossessed.

In 1966 less than 1 per cent of California's student body was black. That simple statistic speaks volumes about

the paucity of ethnic access and representation at the height of the civil-rights struggle. In April 1967 100,000 people marched from Second and Market Streets to Kezar Stadium in Golden Gate Park, an event sponsored by the Spring Mobilization to End the War movement (MOBE). A similar gathering in New York drew a crowd of 400,000. In his report on this day of action Charles Perry noted the political in-fighting and factionalism that beset the San Francisco event. He bemoaned the fact that there were too many pacifist and trade-union speeches and not enough music – the only musicians billed to appear were Judy Collins and Jon Hendricks ('tame humanitarian stuff', as Perry describes it). The only rock and roll was provided by Country Joe and the Fish, who performed on the back of a flatbed truck after the Diggers had broken the locks on the gates and let them in. Once their performance was over the crowd quickly dispersed. By the time the star turn of the afternoon, Mrs Martin Luther King, got up to speak, Perry reported that 'the stadium was less than half full and emptying fast'.[14]

What was becoming clear from these gatherings was that the counter-culture preferred its spokespersons to be rock and rollers, not political activists and esteemed civil-rights leaders. Phil Lesh confirmed the point in his celebration of the Golden Gate Park Be-In. 'We even had some leftist politicos from Berkeley ranting, the only bring-down of the day,' he said.[15] Without discernible irony his very next sentence reads: 'The sense of timelessness was even stronger as we kicked into our opener, "Dancing in the Streets".' The Marvin Gaye, William Stevenson and Ivy Jo Hunter composition, recorded by Martha and the Vandellas in 1964, was a celebration of black identity that became as much of a civil-rights anthem of defiance as 'We Shall Overcome'. The song took on more militant connotations in the aftermath of the Watts riots in LA, but here it was being stripped of its militancy in Golden Gate Park by performers who actively despised commercial pop music and by a good-time crowd that had little sympathy for 'leftist politicos' and 'tame humanitarians'.

It's a curious anomaly of the 1960s that while the blues was revered, soul music was despised or ridiculed for its showbiz aspirations. Even the more politically enlightened members of the Bay Area fraternity – even those Berkeley politicos, no less – were prone to caricature when it came to black music. Just glance again at the Ralph J. Gleason quote that heads this chapter. It tells you all you need to know about black music's role in the scheme of things. This was an era when everything from a Diggers communiqué to an interview with Jimi Hendrix would contain the word 'spade'. The casual racism of the term carried all kinds of casually racist assumptions in its wake. In a November 1966 interview with Country Joe and the Fish carried out by Greg Shaw for his magazine *Mojo Navigator*, the band's manager Ed Denton informs Shaw that the B-side of their new single will feature a song called 'Thing Called Love' – 'Which is a song Barry sings and [he'll] spade it up.' Barry Melton elaborated: 'I want 40 nude spade chicks singing "Whoo, he's got love" in back of me.' 'The Otis Redding trip,' concludes Denton. 'Spaded up so we can get the spade stations.'

Country Joe and the Fish regularly ventured into Stax/Atlantic territory, particularly on their later LPs. The self-explanatory 'Rock and Soul Music' on their third album *Together* was one of the highlights of the band's set at the Woodstock Festival in 1969. Critic Joel Selvin described the song as 'a brilliantly realized parody of James Brown',[16] and for that portion of the audience who thought a James Brown parody was just what the world needed in the era of 'Say it loud, I'm black and

I'm proud', it more than adequately served its purpose. Country, blues, jug-band songs and folk were deemed to be a necessary part of a Bay Area musician's apprenticeship and were treated with dignity and respect – licks to be mastered, traditions to be learned. Soul music, it would appear, was there to be parodied and pastiched.

In December 1968 Janis Joplin and her recently formed Full Tilt Boogie Band were invited to play the second annual Stax/Volt Christmas party. Joplin was the only out-of-town act on a bill that also included Booker T. and the MGs, the Staple Singers, Johnnie Taylor, Eddie Floyd, Albert King, William Clay and Judy Bell, and Rufus and Carla Thomas. The Full Tilt Boogie Band blew it by not only being under-rehearsed but also by bringing their hey-let-it-all-hang-out credo of onstage slackness live and direct from the Fillmore. What worked in San Francisco died a thousand deaths among the leopard-print couches and lavishly laden supper-club tables of the Memphis Coliseum, a venue named somewhat appropriately after the Roman arena where believers of a dissenting faith were thrown to the lions. 'Everybody did those dance steps and shit,' Joplin complained, 'and our thing is selling sincerity, and they aren't buying it down there . . . I'm used to playing for people who want to feel what I feel. They don't give a shit about feeling – they just want to see a few dance steps, a nice boogaloo beat and go home. It's not my crowd.'[17] As sanctimonious horseshit goes from someone raised on Bessie Smith and Etta James, Joplin's account of 'selling sincerity' was right up there. Stanley Booth's *Rolling Stone* feature on the event put a more insightful spin on the story. 'A stage act in Memphis, Tennessee (or, as the famous Stax Marquee puts it, "Soulsville USA") is not the same as a stage act in San Francisco, Los Angeles or New York,' he said, launching into a thinly veiled pop at Jim Morrison. 'These days a lot of people think if a fellow comes on stage wearing black vinyl pants, screams that he wants to fuck his poor old mother, then collapses, that's a stage act; but in Memphis, if you can't do the Sideways Pony, you just don't have a stage act.' Booth reported that Joplin's band watched the other acts from the wings, shaking their heads not in appreciation but dismay. 'The crowd at the Fillmore, East or West, expects to see a band shove equipment around the stage for ten minutes or more "getting set up" – not being showbiz, in that context, is accepted show-biz practice,' said Booth astutely. 'But in Memphis this is not what the people come to see.'[18] As Joplin discovered to her cost, a shambling, under-rehearsed stage act and a few half-hearted shimmies, apoplectic shakes and praise-de-Lord glad hands didn't really cut it with an audience versed in slick patter, sharp attire and even sharper choreography. They just didn't buy the brand of sincerity she was selling.

It's instructive to compare the way soul and R&B music were treated by white critics in comparison with the reverence afforded the blues. At a time when an entire generation of white musicians was bestowing patronage on the blues and critics were admiring its integrity and endurance, soul and R&B were being disdained for their showbiz tendencies. The influence of the blues remained steadfast throughout the psychedelic sixties, not merely as a musical style but as a badge of authenticity and a confirmation of the solid bonds of tradition, even if much of that tradition was rooted in myth. Wherever you look in the second half of the sixties the blues myth ran the game. This was a period when a generation of old-time bluesmen were being recast as exotic others as they were rescued from remote pinewoods and homestead shacks and wheeled out in front of a receptive new audience. Now

in their sixties and seventies, some of these Mississippi and Tennessee rediscoveries – Sleepy John Estes, Furry Lewis, Fred McDowell, John Hurt, Bukka White – hadn't played for twenty years or more, but every one of them was guaranteed a warm response when they played the folk and blues festivals and college campuses. They were seen to be the living embodiment of an oral tradition that had its roots in the Mississippi Delta of the nineteenth century, from where the music was supposed to have emerged, even though the Delta at this time consisted almost entirely of uninhabited swamp. However, in more recent years a whole new school of thought has emerged which posits that the blues was entirely a twentieth-century invention and that its roots lie not in the mists of mystic time or the post-diasporic consciousness of slavery but in minstrelsy, the medicine shows and vaudeville.

The twelve-bar blues sung by a solo singer (i.e. the form we now recognise as the classic blues archetype) only emerged in the third decade of the twentieth century and yet this is the style that has been selectively plucked from tradition and served up as the entire tradition. Among fundamentalists any questioning of the 'immemorial spirit' of the blues is considered blasphemy. Tradition, they suggest, is an indestructible unifying force that has somehow survived the slave ships, the cotton fields and the barbarity of the Jim Crow laws in the deep south. African American people have somehow endured tyranny and hardship not only with their dignity intact and untainted but, equally remarkably, their culture too. To suggest otherwise is to denigrate the core identity of an entire continent. In fact, a case can be made for a diametrically opposite scenario. That is to say, the enforced discontinuities and dispersals brought about by centuries of slavery were so brutalising that they all but abolished any sense of tradition or folk memory and forced black people instead to develop America's first modernist consciousness. Twenty years before abstract expressionism, jazz emerged as America's first avant-garde art form. While folklorists went in search of slave songs and plantation survivalists, black America shook off its manacles and went about inventing itself a future. Or, as Nelson George put it in *The Death of Rhythm and Blues*, 'The most fanatical students of blues history have all been white. These well-intentioned scholars pick through old recordings, interview obscure guitarists, and tramp through the Mississippi Delta with the

determination of Egyptologists . . . Blacks create and move on. Whites document and then recycle.'[19] Miles Davis put it more succinctly. 'The subject of the blues was once mentioned in a conversation,' recalled Alexis Korner. 'Don't talk to me about that slavery shit,' replied Davis.[20]

'If it is perceived to be relevant at all, the history of slavery is somehow assigned to blacks,' notes Paul Gilroy in his book *The Black Atlantic*. 'It becomes our special property rather than a part of the ethical and intellectual heritage of the West as a whole.'[21] As a result of this assignation successive generations of folklorists, musicologists and music critics have found it hard to embrace, or at times even comprehend, developments in African American creativity which display modernist rather than survivalist (or revivalist) tendencies. From bebop to hip hop, and at several intersection points in between, critics have been baffled by or downright hostile to any manifestations of black creativity that do not bear some trace of the noble savage ancestry. Such thinking simply does not allow for the existence of a black avant-garde; it certainly doesn't allow for the existence of a black psychedelia. And what is black psychedelia anyway? Is it Sun Ra and his Arkestra inviting us to 'travel the spaceways from planet to planet', calling out 'next stop Jupiter' like an interstellar tour guide while his brightly bedecked band, resplendent in Afro-futuristic costumes, enact vaudevillian theatrics and explore the outer reaches of the omniverse? Is it Impulse Records optimistically adorning the sleeve of the *Albert Ayler in Greenwich Village* LP in bright colourful swirls and a bubble fount that resembles a Stanley Mouse handbill? Or is it John Coltrane, who, unlike Sun Ra, did experiment with LSD in order to further his understanding of the molecular structure of music? If the 1963 interview he gave to Jean Clouzet and Michel Delorme is anything to go by, he gained much from the experience. 'I would like to discover a method so that if I want it to rain, it will start right away to rain,' he said. 'If one of my friends is ill, I'd like to play a certain song and he will be cured . . . but what are these pieces and what is the road to travel to attain a knowledge of them, that I don't know.'[22] It was Albert Ayler who would actually name an album *Music Is the Healing Force of the Universe*, and it was Ayler, with lyrics provided by his girlfriend, Mary Maria Parks, who would make the most conscious effort to bridge the gap between new-thing jazz and psychedelic rock in the late 1960s. But it was

John Coltrane who lived and breathed the connection explicitly. Several of the recordings that he made in his final years were directly influenced by his acid experiences. The *Expression*, *Interstellar Space* and *Live in Japan* albums he recorded between June 1966 and March 1967 all bear witness to an expanded LSD consciousness at work. On *Om*, recorded on 1 October 1965, the entire band was allegedly tripping. The album features group chanting from the *Bhagavad Gita* and there is similar spiritual prayer song in the version of 'Afro-Blue' featured on the posthumously released *Live in Seattle*, taped the day before the *Om* sessions. The entire unit is said to have been tripping on this date too. There are also group chantings and prayer recitals on another posthumously released LP, *Cosmic Music*, recorded in February 1966.

The idea of departure, escape, interplanetary exploration takes on a whole other perspective in the context of black American music, particularly black American music recorded during the 1960s. Much of it could not help but be influenced by the civil-rights campaign, the ghetto unrest that took place in several American cities and the rise in black militancy. Truth was indeed marching in. In such circumstances the desire to escape was no longer solely a hedonist quest or a pursuit of chemical obliteration; it took on a more politicised hue. Which brings us to Jimi Hendrix. To many who witnessed his arrival in London during the late autumn of 1966 he seemed to have been beamed down from outer space. In fact, he'd played lengthy stints with Little Richard, the Isley Brothers, Curtis Knight and a host of lesser-known combos. He'd learned just about every standard and crowd-pleaser in the R&B repertoire and had watched every famous name in black American music from the wings. He'd picked up on all their showbiz tricks too. He learned to twirl and thrust and ride his guitar without missing a note, and he played it behind his head like Charlie Patton had forty years earlier. He executed that age-old conjurer's trick of pretending to play it with his teeth too. When he concluded his Monterey set with the lighter-fluid immolation of his guitar, the audience was aghast, but English pop fans had been watching him do that at provincial Gaumonts and Granadas for several months, usually with uniformed safety officers in attendance and sand buckets at the ready.

Everyone seemed to want a piece of Hendrix and everyone interpreted him according to their notion of what he represented and where he should fit in. Probably no other artist in the modern era, apart from Dylan, had to shoulder so much responsibility and expectation. Hendrix was ascribed multiple roles. Blues man. Showman. Shaman. Hendrix 'the wild man of rock'. Hendrix the exotic other. Hendrix the astral traveller. Hendrix the cosmic troubadour. Hendrix the cosmic buffoon. Hendrix the minstrelsy throwback. Hendrix the honorary white man. And ultimately, of course, because he died so young, Hendrix the museum piece, embalmed in myth. Just as everyone laid claim to the image rights when he was alive, in death he continued to suffer the slings and arrows of idle hypothesis. All of which does him a great disservice and ultimately detracted from what he was attempting to achieve as a musician, which was to liberate rock music from its roots and use the blues not as a safe haven but as a launch pad via which rock might fruitfully explore previously uncharted territory. Hendrix never fully resolved this issue, and all those clashing identities and parallel musical pathways were still in evidence right to the very end, but the journey was rarely less than eventful. On the first Jimi Hendrix Experience albums, *Are You Experienced* and *Axis: Bold as Love*, both issued in 1967, two distinct musical directions are already emerging. One is aligned with tradition; the other jet-packs psychedelia into another realm. Tracks like 'Foxy Lady', 'Fire', 'Can You See Me', 'I Don't Live Today', 'Love or Confusion' and 'Remember' offer bump-and-grind riffs that would influence heavy rock for a generation. They frequently threaten to break free of formula and expectation – 'Fire', for instance, is nimble and quick in a way that makes almost everything on Cream's debut LP sound leaden in comparison – but for all their surface flash they remain tethered to the blues.

Alternately, about as alternate as it gets actually, the two longest tracks on that debut album, 'Third Stone from the Sun' and 'Are You Experienced', explore the spaceways by utilising the performance dynamics of avant-garde jazz. Both tracks make extensive use of studio stratospherics, backward tape, stereo-panned echo, slowed-down distorted vocals, etc. In less capable hands this would have been mere psychedelic embroidery, but Hendrix was clearly aware of and attuned to the innovations of John Coltrane. 'Third Stone from the Sun' is modelled on Coltrane's classic quartet workouts of the early sixties. It doesn't really belong in rock, but neither does it belong in jazz. In the introduction Hendrix attempts to emulate 'Trane in Eastern mode, while appearing to inhale some sort of foggy oxide that induces the opposite effect to helium. It's all tape-slowed trickery, of course, but the effect, previously unheard in rock and roll, is startling. The track's central melodic theme is stately and anthemic but is used sparingly – at forty-five seconds in, at the two-minute mark and in a final majestic reprise at 5.15. 'Third Stone' rapidly jettisons any lingering adherence to conventional pop structures at two minutes thirty. Drummer Mitch Mitchell, who along with Ginger Baker was the nearest rock music had to an Elvin Jones-style pyrotechnician, suddenly begins to skitter restlessly about his kit, while Noel Redding locks into the kind of repetitive bass line that Dr Feelgood would later build an entire career on. Over the top of this Hendrix explores atonality and abstraction with reverb shrieks and feedback-riddled glissandi. Submerged deep in the mix at 4.30 he informs us that we will never hear surf music again, but surf music is precisely what we are hearing – surfing of the astral plane rather than the Pacific crest.

Are You Experienced's title track builds its rhythmic pulse on the bold premise that the coda to 'Strawberry Fields Forever' was a starting point, not a fade-out. Hendrix leads the listener gently by the hand into the star clusters of the night with one of LSD's most enchanting chat-up lines, one which all trippers still capable of smooth talking should have tried out at least once in their lives. 'We'll hold hands and then we'll watch the sun rise from the bottom of the sea,' he sings, while making it perfectly clear that more earthbound urges are at the forefront of his trousers and what remains of his mind. Although the lyrics turn a little pimpy, the music builds an atonal tapestry out of tape hiss and reversed guitar. And all this time the rhythm bed of that 'Strawberry Fields' coda continues to clang away relentlessly, before riding off into the aquatic sunset. Necessarily stoned and beautiful.

On his second album, *Axis: Bold as Love* (one of the most beguiling unexplained LP titles of the 1960s), Hendrix can still be heard hard-rock riffing and blues vamping on 'Up from the Skies', 'Spanish Castle Magic', 'Ain't No Telling', 'If Six Was Nine', 'You Got Me Floatin'' and 'Little Miss Lover'. 'Wait Until Tomorrow' (complete with feeble backing vocals) lays the boogie-funk trail that outfits like the Doobie Brothers and Little Feat would follow during the next decade. 'Castles Made of Sand' injects subtle flourishes into tired riffology, and

nails down the rhythm that the Band would borrow lock and stock for 'The Weight'. 'Little Wing' and 'One Rainy Wish' introduce us to the sea-breezes balladeer who would soar to new lyrical heights on his later recordings. They give us a first real glimpse of the man's poetic sensibilities, an aspect of his work that often gets overlooked in the rush to worship at the altar of the new phallic rock god. When the lyricism of his images is in harmony with the flow and fluidity of his guitar-playing (which it is by the time he records 'The Wind Cries Mary' and 'Burning of the Midnight Lamp' in the summer of 1967) it is possible to see Hendrix as heir not to Muddy Waters or B. B. King but to Dylan in his Baudelairian pomp. Hendrix can do allegorical Dylan. He can do symbolist Dylan. He can even do absurdist Dylan. And on 'All Along the Watchtower' he showed that he could do Dylan better than Dylan. For someone who initially displayed a reluctance to sing in the studio, Hendrix was an unabashed purveyor of florid romantic verse. His lyrics spin courtship sentiments in endless unravelling skeins of interstellar imagery and mutated blues Esperanto. Even when they dribble out in flappy ribbons of euphoric space jive they still sound affectionate and unaffected. Beautiful lines leap out of the purple haze all the time, some of them gossamer gentle ('If we travel by dragonfly' on 'Spanish Castle Magic'), some tender ('And when the day melts down into a sleepy red glow' on 'You Got Me Floatin''), some desolate and apocalyptic ('I come back to find the stars misplaced / and the smell of a world that has burned' from 'Up from the Skies'). He also did a fine line in sci-fi hokum. Traditional lust scenarios are never more than a star twinkle away. Noah might be sailing his ark on lunar seas of tranquillity, with Neptunian mermaids at the helm, but there's a cosmic come-on and corny chat-up line ready and waiting when you reach those distant shores. Best of all are the lines from 'The Wind Cries Mary' that evoke after-party scenes and darkness-before-dawn images of the night outside, as lost souls aimlessly drift by your window as you sleep. When the muse struck, words, as Jim Webb put it in 'MacArthur Park', were like tender babies in his hand.

Electric Ladyland was Hendrix's sprawling masterpiece. Featuring an extended ensemble for the first time, the majority of the double album's tracks were recorded between April and August 1968, with sessions frequently squeezed in between tour dates, as the Experience criss-crossed America with the Soft Machine. *Electric Ladyland* is a montage of exquisite miniatures, messy splashes and exploratory abstract impressionism. It features several extended workouts but few of the longueurs commonly associated with rock double LPs. By the time he came to record his third album Hendrix had started referring to his sound as 'electric church music'; he described the LP's opening track, 'And the Gods Made Love', as 'a ninety-second sound painting of the heavens'. Taking his cue from Coltrane's expanded unit he augments his basic trio line-up with members of Traffic, Jack Casady of the Jefferson Airplane, Buddy Miles of Electric Flag, Al Kooper and the Sweet Inspirations. On 'Rainy Day, Dream Away' and 'Still Raining, Still Dreaming' he assembles an impromptu pick-up band, plucked from the studio next door to create a mellow vibe that could have been borrowed from any Blue Note album of the period. He tells organist Mike Finnegan, 'You be like Jimmy Smith and I'll be Kenny Burrell,' as they embark on a blues shuffle in D, complete with talking wah-wah. On the title track Hendrix is inhabited by the spirit of Curtis Mayfield as he finally sheds all inhibition about his singing. The light-bulb moment probably occurred when he heard 'I want to show you different emotions' on the playback and it dawned on him that he could. An audible Mayfield influence settled on his best vocal endeavours from this point onwards and never left him. The other clear indication that he was heading in a more soul-driven direction was 'Burning of the Midnight Lamp'. Aside from containing the most exquisite wah-wah sound ever captured on record and one of the best requiem-blues lyrics he ever wrote, 'Burning of the Midnight Lamp' also features the Sweet Inspirations as backing singers. Led by Cissie Houston, the Atlantic Records house trio provided electric church music with a soaring chorale that was only ever matched in the 1960s by Jack Nitzsche's arrangement of 'You Can't Always Get What You Want' for the Rolling Stones.

On his first two albums Hendrix was guided by Chas Chandler's parsimonious production values and usually recorded in one or two takes with minimal overdubs. On *Electric Ladyland* he began to realise the full potential of the facilities at his disposal. Not only did he begin to utilise the full potential of the mixing desk, he also explored as never before the guitar as a prepared instrument. In a live setting Hendrix had been the first rock guitarist to make full use of overamplification, effectively turning his guitar into a network of responsive circuitry. Elements like sustain, delay, decay, distortion and feedback could be utilised simply by tapping the neck or scraping the bridge. Along with his kleptomaniac accumulation of state-of-the-art pedals Hendrix now had an abundance of sound-colouration tools at his disposal. Ten-hour playback sessions were not uncommon as he and his colleagues conjured magic from the mixing desk. The most intricate example of this close attention to detail is the interweaving cluster of guitar overdubs that rise and fall in choreographed unison during the second half of 'All Along the Watchtower', but it's not a one-off. He reprises the trick throughout the album, frequently creating textural colouration with exquisite washes of overlapping sound.

The most adventurous sound painting to emerge from these lengthy explorations was '1983 . . . (A Merman I Should Turn to Be)'/'Moon, Turn the Tides . . . Gently Gently Away'. Launched by a military drum roll and one of Hendrix's most memorable soaring melodic themes, '1983' was a thirteen-minute work that took up all of side three of the original double LP and was the nearest he ever got, perhaps the nearest rock ever got, to fully exploring its improvisatory possibilities without lapsing into ego-ridden indulgence or overstatement. '1983' is all the more remarkable when you hear the early exploratory takes and realise that Hendrix had most of the components worked out long before the final take was recorded. '1983' is essentially a quartet recording: Mitch Mitchell on drums, Chris Wood on flute and Hendrix augmenting himself on bass and multiple guitar parts. The fourth member is, of course, the mixing desk, which fully deserves a sleeve credit of its own. A generation of space-rock bands were spawned by the pan-galactic possibilities of '1983''s 'Moon, Turn the Tide' section. You can practically hear Daevid Allen's Gong being invented between the six- to seven-minute mark. The multilayered deep-space explorations of this pivotal tone poem are without peer or parallel in rock and roll. Its nearest equivalent is to be found in the more ego-free moments of free jazz, in which frantic fire music gives way to cosmic grace. The 'Moon' section contains moments of sumptuous beauty, in particular the delicate dialogue that takes place between Chris Wood's flute and the infinitely echoing omnipresence of the mixing desk. Like Coltrane's 'India', everything revolves around a single pedal note that floats weightlessly until Hendrix gently reintroduces his blues

runs at around the nine-minute mark and the whole thing turns earthbound once more. It's tempting to say that after this sublime moment everything he did was earthbound.

At Woodstock a tired, bedraggled Hendrix delivered his valedictory statement to a tired, bedraggled crowd amid mounting acres of garbage. Tracer-fire elements of 'The Star-Spangled Banner' can be heard in numerous live performances long before the festival took place; it's there in all its dive-bombing glory at the end of 'House Burning Down' on *Electric Ladyland*. At Woodstock the American national anthem was transformed into an eloquent 'Hell no, we won't go'. It was one of those rare iconic moments when music says much more than any words can express. Anyone who hadn't witnessed that live performance or had only heard the soundtrack LP without first seeing the film (i.e. most of the world at the end of 1969) would have assumed from hearing the incendiary rendition that Hendrix must have been flailing around the stage in full poster-boy rock-god mode, throwing shapes, thrusting his guitar towards the amp for feedback, strafing the audience theatrically, knee-bending with every cluster bomb of notes. But as the movie footage confirms, he just stands there, nailed to his pedals, his only armoury, and delivers one of the most dignified refusals in rock history. It's his 'Alabama' moment. John Coltrane was said to have written 'Alabama' in response to the killing of four young children in 1964, when the the Ku Klux Klan fire-bombed a Baptist church. It's opening recitative was reputedly based on a speech by Martin Luther King. Neither connection is true. Coltrane's composition simply illustrated what the most powerful music is capable of in those rare moments when the instrument proves mightier than the sword. Before Woodstock anti-Vietnam protest was signified by draft dodging and flag burning. After Woodstock the atrocities of carpet-bombing and village-burning were soundtracked by the symbolic flag-shredding that takes place during Hendrix's extraordinary rendition of 'The Star-Spangled Banner'.

After that it was mostly vapour trail, meteor dust and diminishing returns. Various musical line-ups were tried out, numerous new initiatives sketched out. Hendrix spoke of a proposed new album called *First Rays of the New Rising Sun*, some of which did eventually appear on the hastily assembled posthumous album *The Cry of Love*, but that patchwork of possibilities only gave a glimpse of where Hendrix might

have been heading next. The fact that his momentum stalled in the final months of his life is indisputable. There are flashes and glints of gold dust, but there is an awful amount of silt and sludge to sift through too. Some suggest that he'd simply gone as far as he could, and that brief liberating period when he broke free of the shackles of pick-up bands and other people's endeavours had been just that, a brief liberation, and now it was over. Others suggested that the silt and sludge he was putting in his veins might have contributed to his decline too. By September 1970 Hendrix was either irreparably burned-out or on the verge of some new cosmic dawn, depending on which story ending you subscribe to. Because he died when he did, Hendrix came to embody one of the great What Ifs, a set of unrealised possibilities on which you could have hung the musical development of the next ten years. At the time of his death he was all set to collaborate with Gil Evans on an album of orchestral arrangements of his work. He had jammed informally with a nucleus of musicians – John McLaughlin, Tony Williams, Dave Holland, etc. – who were all connected to Miles Davis. A collaboration with Davis himself was said to be on the cards. In one of his final interviews, given just weeks before he died, Hendrix spoke to Roy Hollingsworth of *Melody Maker*. He talked enthusiastically about his ideas for a new expanded ensemble. 'I want a big band,' he said. 'I don't mean three harps and 14 violins. I mean a big band full of competent musicians that I can conduct and write for. And with the music we will paint pictures of earth and space, so that the listener can be taken somewhere.' He didn't know what form this music was going to take, referring enigmatically to 'western sky music' and, more problematically, to 'sweet opium music', and predicted that 'when there are vast changes in the way the world goes, it's usually something like art and music that changes it. Music is going to change the world next time.' He spoke earnestly about his desire to become a composer and his need to improve as a guitarist. He still thought he had a lot to learn.

Had that touted Miles Davis collaboration actually happened it might have taken both jazz and rock (as opposed to jazz rock) in directions that could have dictated the way ahead for both forms. Davis spent the first half of the 1970s filling his albums with an ever-changing array of Hendrix clones while he laid the voodoo down. Then again, Hendrix might easily have settled for a more sedate path, noodling out polite and polished jazz pop like another former Davis collaborator, George Benson. 'It's all turned full circle. I'm back right now to where I started,' Hendrix stated in that last *Melody Maker* interview. Whether he meant musically (enslaved by the audiences' desire for hard-rock showmanship) or geographically (happy to be back in London, where his reputation first blossomed) he didn't make clear, although he does suggest the former when he says, 'I still sound the same. My music's the same, and I can't think of anything new to add to it in its present state.' No evidence of the first rays of a new rising sun in that frustrated statement, or indeed in the knowledge that he spent those last weeks in England just hanging out and jamming. Perhaps the most poignant of the final recordings he made was 'Drifting', with its beautiful floating Curtis Mayfield melody and its simple thirty-two-word eulogy to purposelessness. 'Drifting on a sea of forgotten teardrops,' he sings. 'On a sea of old heartbreaks.' Perhaps the 1970s would simply have presented him with a succession of concentric circles and restricted choices. An anonymous guest spot under a thinly veiled nom de plume on an Isley Brothers album. A fellowship-of-the-cokeheads collaboration with Sly Stone. Perhaps. Perhaps.

Meanwhile, there is the music he did make, the best of which still sounds like a time capsule blasted into the deepest recesses of outer space, still shattering into starbursts and turning distant civilisations on as we speak.

At about the time that Jimi Hendrix was making his mark in England, back in Chicago, home of the electric blues, a band called Rotary Connection was being put together. The band was the brainchild of Marshall Chess, son of Chess Records founder Leonard. Marshall had been put in charge of the Chess spin-off label Cadet Concept and instructed to expand the musical brief of the original imprint beyond its trademark blues and R&B output. Having decided to venture into more experimental territory he recruited orchestral arranger and classically trained vibraphone player Charles Stepney, gospel singer and future northern-soul legend Sidney Barnes, Chess receptionist, backing singer and former member of vocal group the Gems Minnie Riperton, gospel singer Judy Hauff and a rhythm section drawn from a little-known Chicago rock band called the Proper Strangers. This basic nucleus was augmented by an ever-changing pool of Chicago session men, handpicked from the cream of local musicians. At one time or another

the Rotary Connection crew included such notable names as guitarists Phil Upchurch and Pete Cosey, drummer Morris Jennings and percussionists Henry Gibson and Bobby Christian. The sheer wealth of experience and expertise that this group of musicians brought to the party was breathtaking. Bobby Christian had played with Paul Whiteman in the 1930s and was also a member of the Chicago Symphony Orchestra. After Rotary Connection broke up Pete Cosey joined Miles Davis when his electric experimentation was at its peak; he can be heard playing the surrogate Hendrix role on the *Get Up with It*, *Dark Magus* and *Agharta* albums. Phil Upchurch played with everyone from Cannonball Adderley to Ramsey Lewis, and, with his own Phil Upchurch Combo, was well known to English mods for the early 1960s Sue label instrumental 'You Can't Sit Down'. Along with Upchurch Henry Gibson also played in Curtis Mayfield's group, and it is his conga work that distinguishes Mayfield classics like 'Pusherman' and 'Freddie's Dead'. Judy Hauff, who left after the first Rotary Connection album, would become a singer and composer and leading exponent of Sacred Harp music, shape-note songs and psalmody from the nineteenth century. These astonishingly gifted alumni span everything from the ancient to the avant-garde, and between 1967 and 1971 they provided the Rotary Connection sound.

Despite regular fluctuations within the line-up the key components of that sound remained constant from album to album and revolved around Minnie Riperton's four-and-a-half octave voice, Charles Stepney's innovative and idiosyncratic arrangements, and the heavy-funk velocity of Bobby Simms's lead guitar. Riperton's singing voice was a thing of awesome majesty. It had an upper register as eerie as a theremin and a baritone that could fathom hell and soar angelic. Before she joined the band she had sung commercials for everyone from Coke to Clearasil and had also served time as a Chess Records office clerk, helping the Rolling Stones select material from the vaults when they came to town in 1965. Once Judy Hauff left the group Riperton became its one-woman gospel chorus. In addition to his Rotary Connection duties Stepney was also in-house arranger for Chess soul acts like the Dells and the Radiants. His classical flourishes and chamber-soul experiments are all over their output. The Dells' 1968 single 'Wear It on Our Face' must be the only northern-soul anthem to commence with the sound of a prepared piano,

while the gothic melodrama of Radiants cuts like 'The Clown Is Clever' and 'I'm Glad I'm the Loser' is cast in CinemaScope by Stepney's unconventional orchestral colouration. His colour palette also transforms the Dells' medley of 'Love Is Blue'/'I Can Sing a Rainbow' from soul balladry into an Age of Aquarius anthem.

Rotary Connection's eponymously titled debut album begins with 'Amen', a wordless space spiritual. It's introduced by a sitar and Riperton and Hauff's high-register duet. Four minutes of orchestrated gospel bliss is followed by a thirty-eight-second avant-garde interlude of pizzicato violins and plucked piano strings before the Sidney Barnes composition 'Turn Me On' issues an unambiguous clarion call. 'Turn me on / I want to know what it's all about,' the Connection croon over the gentle lilt of Stepney's strings. The other track to feature sitar is 'Memory Band', a joyous skip-along of a song in which Riperton la-la-las to herself while Stepney fleshes out her ditzy childsong with a sumptuous wide-screen score. Elsewhere on the album he adds snippets of collaged concrète that anticipate the later innovations of turntablism. Snatches of 'Hello, Good-bye''s Hawaiian coda go floating by on 'Black Noise'. 'Sursum Mentes' evokes a

North African souk, while the concluding track, 'Rotary Connection', features fragments of the preceding twelve cuts in brief hallucinatory bursts. The idea is hardly unique and rudimentarily executed but it signposts a future in which songs will no longer be end products but raw material, ripe for transformation and recontextualisation.

On their second album, *Aladdin*, Rotary Connection parade themselves in an array of carnival masks: comic and grotesque, exotic and voodoo-esque. The two sides of the band's eponymous debut were labelled 'Trip 1' and 'Trip 1 Continued', and they repeat the theme on *Aladdin* with 'Trip 2' and 'Trip 2 Continued'. If anything, *Aladdin* is the trippier album. The ten tracks oscillate between 'Venus in Furs'-style cabaret for the soul-food generation and vaudeville blues for acid heads. 'Teach Me How to Fly' layers synth tones over the kind of busy big-band arrangement that Stepney was tearing off by the yard for the Dells at the time. 'VIP' commences with a Chinese gong and a string arrangement that references the Lemon Pipers' 'Green Tambourine'. It features a bittersweet lyric about a nobody who wants to be a somebody. 'Maybe I'd become a president / hear my name wherever I went,' sings Sidney Barnes as he dreams unfeasible dreams

in 1960s America. 'I Took a Ride (Caravan)' has appropriately Middle Eastern flourishes in the arrangement but ends in a freak-out crescendo of harps, strings and sitars. And in the midst of all this they plant the most beautiful song they ever recorded. '(I Live in a) Magical World' builds utopia out of a simple love sentiment. Riperton at her most prelapsarian sings of a reluctance to be awakened from what could be nocturnal slumber or a hashish-induced meditation. Either way, it's a world where joy can only be experienced in dream sleep or drug state. The real world can't compete.

Aladdin concludes on a polemical note with 'Paper Castle', a reality check set to a barrage of squalling heavy-rock guitars and a militantly nihilistic message, where the only solution to population explosion is to send everyone to live on the moon and where putting money into education is no good if people don't have enough to eat. 'Living in a paper castle / the wind is gonna blow it down,' goes the chorus, putting an end to the flights of fancy that characterise the rest of the album.

Rotary Connection followed the tripped-out theatrics of *Aladdin* with the first psychedelic Christmas album – indeed what is possibly the only psychedelic Christmas album to date. Entitled

Peace, its cover depicts a wigged-out Santa smoking a long clay hookah pipe, while miniatures of the band members are disported randomly about his costume. The music is equally wigged out. 'Peace at Least' begins innocuously with soft chimes and the kind of mellifluous tones that suggest Johnny Mathis has just seated himself by a blazing log fire dressed reassuringly in a hand-knitted sweater. The song ponders the age-old question of why Father Christmas rides at night and comes down the chimney rather than through the front door. 'I know why,' comes the reply. 'Because he's high / because he's stoned / he's smoking that old mistletoe.' The album contains three separate versions of 'Silent Night'. The first commences with a blissful string crescendo and an exquisite duet between Sidney Barnes and Minnie Riperton, before giving way to a lengthy freak-out duel between lead guitar and sleigh bells. The song has two truly miraculous moments, both featuring Riperton. The first occurs when Barnes drops out after the introductory verse, leaving her hushed, awestruck baritone to carry the next verse. The second is after the guitar solo, when Riperton returns to sing of quaking shepherds and heavenly hosts. The other two versions of 'Silent Night' on the album are just as eventful. One

features a 'Star-Spangled Banner'-style apocalyptic freak-out for solo guitar, a year before Hendrix did the same thing at Woodstock. The other sets a group chant of 'Silent night / holy night' to a twelve-bar-boogie beat, complete with reverb overload. Everyone sounds like they are having a thoroughly stoned good time.

Elsewhere on *Peace* there are Yuletide messages of a less reassuring kind. 'If Peace Was All We Had' asks the uncomfortable question, 'Why can't we always live like this?' 'Sidewalk Santa' ponders what the old guy in the red fancy dress does the rest of the time when he's not acting out his Yuletide masquerade. In less sensitive hands the song would have turned into mawkish slush, but this is black America in 1968 and this sidewalk Santa is a homeless ghetto drifter for the rest of the year. Loneliness surfaces frequently amid the merriment. Sleigh bells ring out throughout the album, initially sounding a joyous Noel, but as the album progresses they toll increasingly in requiem for the mounting body count in South-East Asia.

The band's next album, *Songs*, was released in 1969, and was given over entirely to cover versions. Rotary Connection excelled at covers, their bold interpretations often transporting the originals into unknown realms. The version they did of Jagger and Richards's 'Lady Jane' on their debut album retained the Elizabethan-courtship sensibilities of the original, but Stepney interspersed bursts of dramatic orchestration throughout the song, over which Riperton and Hauff laid a caravan trail of exotic harmonies. Their version of Dylan's 'Like a Rolling Stone' dispensed with the verses and turned the song into a moody five-minute instrumental save for the choruses, in which 'How does it feel?' became imbued with a soulful yearning completely absent from the bitter and recriminatory original. By stripping the song of its cluttered symbolism Rotary Connection revealed the true nature of the ghost of electricity that howled through Dylan's bones. The original concentrated on comeuppance and bad karma; Rotary Connection emphasised the comedown, the loneliness, the no-direction-home. It's Dylan in dub version.

Ironically, the ones that work least well are the soul covers. As their version of Isaac Hayes and David Porter's 'Soul Man' on their debut had shown, the band were at their least inspired when presented with a basic sock-it-to-me formula. 'Got My Mojo Working' and Stevie Wonder's 'This Town' suffer from the same lack of spirit on *Songs*,

while all they can do with Otis Redding's 'Respect' is slow it down, make it less Staxy and give the session men an excuse to exercise their jazz chops. But when Rotary Connection covered rock songs the results were remarkable. The stand-out cuts on *Songs* were 'Burning of the Midnight Lamp', where Hendrix's delicate wah-wah is replaced by Riperton in full-on Yma Sumac mode, and a trio of Cream covers: 'Sunshine of Your Love', 'Tales of Brave Ulysses' and 'We're Going Wrong'. On 'Sunshine of Your Love' the rigid staccato of Jack Bruce and Pete Brown's original is replaced by a fluid, funky bass line and John Barry strings. On 'Tales of Brave Ulysses' they are sensible enough not to meddle with one of Cream's most adventurous and unconventional arrangements, and simply opt to replace Jack Bruce's low-register growl with delicate counterpoint between the male and female voices. 'We're Going Wrong' retains the intensity of the original but adds an element of swingbeat to Ginger Baker's menacing rumble. It is testimony to the power of Baker's polyrhythmic blueprint that the finest Chicago session drummers can barely match its sheer dynamic force. The ominous portents of the lyrics are transformed utterly. In Rotary Connection's hands they reverberate to the sound of civil unrest, ghetto riots and Vietnamese village massacres.

There is YouTube footage of the band miming to 'Lady Jane' on Jerry G. Bishop's TV show, filmed in Chicago in 1969, shortly before the release of *Songs*. Minnie Riperton, resplendent in her Afro and looking decidedly heavy-lidded, is interviewed by the show's host. He asks her where the band's name came from, and she mumbles, 'Yeah, well, you see it was like this and that's where it's at.' The moment where it becomes obvious just how truly ripped she is occurs when Bishop hands her a copy of the new album. 'Do you know what this is?' he says. 'Yeah,' she replies. 'It's an album.' Bishop asks her to name a couple of tracks, and Riperton pauses for thought, her memory temporarily adrift. The host politely points out that she might want to consult the sleeve.

After 1970's disappointing *Dinner Music*, which was redeemed only by Charles Stepney's electronic abstractions and musique concrète interludes, the band briefly split up and Riperton went off and made her first solo album. They reconvened in 1971 for one more record. Billed as New Rotary Connection, *Hey Love* features Stepney at the top of his game, combining the Brill Building classicism of Burt Bacharach,

the acid baroque of Jim Webb and his own expansive orchestral pieces, which sound like they have been written for some futuristic astro-black Las Vegas. The same tricksy prepared-piano motif that Stepney showcased on the Dells' 'Wear It on Our Face' recurs throughout the album. There's also a lot of Spanish guitar and more than a hint of the summer-breeze mellowness of the early 1970s. *Hey Love* is more overtly soulful and jazzy than Rotary Connection's earlier material. It also contains the most extraordinary song they ever recorded. 'I Am the Black Gold of the Sun' is Afrocentricity taken to new levels of luminosity. It begins with a plangent Spanish-guitar figure and a snatch of Afro-Cuban dialogue between jazz piano and conga drums. Then an incantatory gospel chant of the song's title line joins the throng. Everything locks into a jungle-funk groove. The God spell chorale continues, with Riperton soaring angelic. Then suddenly, just when you're least expecting it, the groove dematerialises at the stroke of a harp and the song bursts into celestial flames. A male voice appears like a vision in the clouds: 'I am the tall oak tree / I am the jungle stream / I am the morning sun / smiling on everyone / I am the silent sea / I am the mountain high / I am so free.' He lets out a laugh after 'the morning sun', a peace-that-passeth-all-understanding laugh, a revelatory laugh at the preposterous nature of all the earthly endeavours going on down below. It's delivered with the twinkle of a ghetto Buddha perched on solid air. The groove returns. Riperton riffs on wordless bliss, her rhythmic scat spirals skywards. Heavily reverbed guitars weave in and out as they have done since day one, track one. 'I Am the Black Gold of the Sun' is the sound of a black avant-garde urban sensibility that has been psychedelicised and born anew. Its counterparts are to be found not in acid rock but in Albert Ayler's *Spirits Rejoice*, John Coltrane's *Ascension*, Alice Coltrane's *A Monastic Trio*. It's the sound of black America having its psychedelic sixties in the early 1970s.

The song that gave the world the word 'psychedelicised' was the Chambers Brothers' 'Time Has Come Today'. Originally from a poor sharecropping family in Mississippi, the brothers first performed in church gospel competitions before relocating to southern California in 1952, when oldest brother George finished serving in the army. They continued to sing gospel a cappella in LA folk clubs and coffee houses before picking up instruments and becoming a fully fledged musical unit. At this time the band consisted of Joe and Willie Chambers on guitars, George on washboard bass and Lester on harmonica. In 1964 they were joined by white drummer Brian Keenan. Signed to ABC Paramount for a three-record deal they were embraced by the east-coast folk community, and in 1965 played the Newport Folk Festival, where their electric set was greeted with less hostility than Dylan's. During this time they made their living playing the nightclub circuit, performing cover versions of rock-and-roll and R&B numbers. The material on their early albums reflects this eclectic apprenticeship: energised versions of bar-band staples like 'Long Tall Sally' and 'Bonie Maronie', and covers of Otis Redding's 'I Can't Turn You Loose' and the Impressions' 'People Get Ready', alongside faithful renditions of folk-club favourites like 'Go Tell It on the Mountain' and 'Pack Up Your Sorrows'.

The turnaround came when they recorded two albums for Columbia: *The Time Has Come* in 1967 and its 1968 follow-up *A New Time – A New Day*. The stand-out cuts on both albums were the title tracks: the eleven-minute heavy-rock freak-out 'Time Has Come Today' and the seven-minute 'A New Time – A New Day'. Both titles tapped into the new black militancy. African American music's engagement with nowness and anticipation had a long tradition and it carried deep political resonance. Sam Cooke's 'A Change Is Gonna Come' and Curtis Mayfield's 'People Get Ready' both spoke of the new urgency. Up till now, though, it had been most commonly expressed in jazz. Charlie Parker's 'Now's the Time' (1945), Dizzy Gillespie's 'Things to Come' (1946), Ornette Coleman's *The Shape of Jazz to Come* (1959), Max Roach's *Freedom Now Suite* (1961) and Jackie McLean's *It's Time!* (1964) and *Right Now!* (1965) all allude to the cultural and political circumstances in which they were made. The precise intent of those commentaries, though, has always divided critics.

In the 1960s jazz polemicist Frank Kofsky became embroiled in an argument with *Downbeat* magazine editor Ira Gitler about the cultural significance of Parker's 'Now's the Time'. Kofsky maintained that it stood for 'Now's the time to abolish racism, discrimination, oppression and Jim Crow,' and pointed out that the tune was composed against a backdrop of 'Afro-American workers [organising] for a massive March on Washington for equal employment opportunities; the insurrections in Harlem and Detroit; the "Double V campaign" for victory over racism at home as well as abroad;

innumerable clashes both on and off the military posts . . .' etc., etc.[23] Gitler's response was, as Kofsky observed, 'instructive'. 'I deny the obvious social implication,' he said. 'The title refers to the music and the now was the time for the people to dig it.' This divergence – 'It's all about the music' versus 'It's also about the context' – gained momentum during the psychedelic era and came to define two critical approaches towards the counter-culture. A radicalised stance of 'context is all' was more often than not countered with an apolitical 'It's just about the notes'. Amid the ferment of the 1960s it remained 'instructive', as Kofsky put it, to see just how many cultural commentators, and indeed musicians, would adopt the Ira Gitler line, depoliticising the musical soundtrack of the times in a similar fashion. 'Hey, man, don't try to pin an agenda on us, we're just doing our thing' was aired in many group interviews, often by the very figureheads of the counter-culture. LSD, of course, introduced its own distinctive take on *tempus fugit*. Acid had a whole other way of exaggerating the immediacy of now, the simultaneity of everything and the illusory spectacle of seconds, minutes, hours, expanding and contracting at will, but it was noticeable during a time when cops were busting heads, tear-gassing peaceful marchers and shooting people on college campuses, while the government was drafting them halfway across the world to die, that the 'Feels-Like-I'm-Fixin'-to-Die's, 'For What It's Worth's and Ohios of this world remained the exception rather than the rule. When the Grass Roots invited us to 'La-la-la-la live for today', they reflected a grab-it-now gratification that spoke directly to the denizens of Haight-Ashbury, but to the majority of impoverished Americans they might as well have been singing about la-la land itself. When the Blues Project evoked immediacy in 'No Time Like the Right Time', they were singing about carnal urges and the desire to get it on. When Chicago Transit Authority (who dedicated their first album to the revolution) sang, 'Does anybody really know what time it is?', they offered a ponderous discourse that sneered at office workers on their lunch breaks and evoked only a drug-fuzzy sense of *carpe diem* (albeit set to a terrific brass rock beat). But when the Chambers Brothers sang 'Time Has Come Today', they locked into a whole other tradition of seizing the moment.

'Time Has Come Today' gets right to the point and stays there for eleven minutes. Introduced by a metronomic tick-tock beat and nailed down by a killer guitar riff, the song is propelled by militant urgency. 'I've been lost and put aside,' sings George Chambers. 'I've been crushed by the tumbling tide.' There was an obvious nod to the love generation in 'Young hearts can go their way,' but there was always something deeply ambivalent about the key line, 'My soul has been psychedelicised.' There's a mocking tone in the way he sings it that suggests both 'Oh well, go with the flow, brother' and 'They've taken our music and drugged it up.' The majority of the lyrics are spat out in anger. 'I don't care what others say / they say we don't listen anyway' is an anthem to refusal rather than love-generation allegiance, as is the rootless and nothing-to-lose former slave refrain of 'I have no home / I have no home.' The pay-off line comes in the shape of a Panthers fist: 'Time has come today.' At this point in proceedings the AM radio-friendly single version grinds to a halt with a heavily reverbed cowbell and an echo-treated chant of 'Time–time–time'. After the briefest of breakdowns it gathers momentum once more with a reprise of the opening verse and a truncated finale. On the full-length LP version the mid-song breakdown is the point at which things are only just getting started. Three minutes in everything plummets into an echo-laden pool of percussion, re-emerging forty-five seconds later through a barrage of fuzz and launching into full-on 'Sister Ray' mode with five and a half minutes of guitar-driven intensity that never lets up. Through the fizzes and sparks you can almost hear Lou Reed's amphetamine mantra drawl. Towards the end of the guitar solo piercing diabolic screams and hollow laughs ride the barrage of fuzz, before the band lock into that killer riff once more and drive everything towards that final defiant chant that echoes down the ages. Time. Time. Time.

Although the song reached number 11 in the American *Billboard* singles chart during the incendiary autumn of 1968, it had an uneasy gestation. 'Our style of music scared all the executives at Columbia because we were crazy hippies playing an unusual style of funk, blues, rock, and gospel all combined,' said Lester Chambers. 'We were told by the president of Columbia records that we weren't going to even think about recording "Time Has Come Today" and that we must sell it to a white group on Columbia.'[24] The Chambers Brothers stuck to their guns and the stripped-down version of 'Time Has Come Today' spent thirteen weeks in the Hot 100. They repeated the trick with 'A New Time – A New Day'.

Structurally it reprises 'The Time Has Come Today''s highlights, while melodically it owes more than a little to 'Purple Haze'. 'A New Time – A New Day' is taken at a slightly slower pace but it has the same extended guitar break between verses. The soloing is more subtle and melodic, the breakdown is briefer, a boogie guitar slam-ricochets off a wall of drum echo, but those same brain-frying effects psychedelicise the song. That mocking demonic scream is there again and the lyrics speak of the same impending day of awakening: 'It's a new time / a new day / strange vibrations keep coming my way.'

As Lester Chambers indicated, the group didn't really fit in. The record company didn't know what to do with them. Soul stations rarely played their music, while most FM rock stations regarded them as a one-hit novelty. And they most definitely did not do the sideways pony or the boogaloo, but unlike Janis Joplin, alas, they did not have Albert Grossman to look after them. 'Our career really suffered from our refusal to do what the white man said we could do,' said Lester Chambers.[25]

'You've been living in disguise / it's time for laughter, so dry your eyes,' they sing on 'A New Time – A New Day'. 'Take off that purple mask of sorrow / get rid of your plastic pride.'

There's more than a suggestion in all of this that whatever strategies you adopt, it's all an act, a bunch of see-through stances, appropriate responses for appropriate circumstances. Throughout 'Time Has Come Today' there is an underlying sense of scorn; from the quietly mocking cry of 'Cuckoo' in the intro to the diabolic cries there is the sense that none of this role play adds up to a heap of shit unless everyone gets their act together. They aren't laughing at the audience but they are mocking the notion that utopia is within easy reach and that the Jefferson Starship is about to be launched or David Crosby's 'Wooden Ships' are about to arrive any day soon to free us from our social conditions. Like almost all black psychedelia, 'Time Has Come Today' and 'A New Time – A New Day' are predicated on the understanding that the drugs will eventually wear off and the ghetto will still be there tomorrow.

There is another critical take on all this, of course, one that bears little trace of reverence, one that sheds the white man's burden and the liberal guilt trip and just tells it like it is, or at least how Lester Bangs tells it like it is. Here's his take on Sun Ra: 'Like I saw Sunny and his entrudge at a great concert in Berkeley awhile back, and the most interesting part was scoping out this date sitting on the rail right in front of us: Here's this big black dude with this white coed in pigtails, and she's all agog openmouthed in wonder turning to him saying *"Oh wow, isn't this INCREDIBLE!?"* And the black dude's just sitting there half asleep with a big grin on his face cracking up at the whole thing, yeah, sure sweetmeat, it sho do be just as funky and far out as you dare, whoee the jive these joans'll lap up, I'd lay some Lou Donaldson on you but I know you woudn't relate to it becuz it jes ain't heavy enough . . .'[26]

Bangs, with his inimitable capacity for Yiddish 'yo' mama' speed jive (which at times is as damn near impenetrable as some of the music he is describing), refers to Sun Ra as 'this old spazzdome coot who hangs around in his robes' and suggests that the good Mr Blount has been 'spooning out this clank for years'. He describes Sun Ra's 1966 LP *Heliocentric Worlds* as 'a lot of brdreegleblat and kfweet with plenty of static rustling silences between, and it was tailor made for the real blacklite space-out potso aficionados. In other words, it was boring as shit, but you didn't care because it was Sun Ra and he's earned the right to get away with it by being the grandaddy of all this stuff.'[27]

The comments tell us as much about Lester Bangs (and his need for a co-ed in pigtails to soothe his restless heart) as they do about Sun Ra's lifelong explorations at the frontiers of astro-black infinity, but they do hit upon a few inconvenient and impolite truths. And whether you agreed with him or not, Bangs, like Sun Ra, by virtue of being the granddaddy of his own particular school of splenetic sacrilege had earned the right to get away with it. Or as Bangs himself put it as he paused just long enough to qualify his vitriol and wipe the cough syrup from his chin, 'Besides he's gotta real theatrical troupe swaddling his live sluice, they all stalk through the audience replete with near bare dancers swirling around like they was at the Trips Festival and sax cats facing off in sweatbrown honko blat battles, and it worx fine lined and gets all the collegiates real razzed up and goo goo goo joobing.'[28]

Getting the collegiates real razzed up and goo goo goo joobing was half the battle, and some managed it better than others. The Chambers Brothers realised that as well as anyone as they laid their heavy-rock gospel on the Fillmore faithful. And even if you did manage to get the collegiates real razzed up, that was only part of the job done. Further critical opprobrium was waiting in the shape of a new militant aesthetic that decried white hero worship of black role models, and positively scorned ofay approval. Quoting LeRoi Jones's allegorical 1964 stage play *Dutchman*, Frank Kofsky offered a lacerating fuck-you to the denizens of blues patronage:

Old bald-headed four-eyed ofays popping their fingers . . . and don't know yet what they're doing. They say, 'I love Bessie Smith.' And don't even understand that Bessie Smith is saying, 'Kiss my ass, kiss my black unruly ass.' Before love, suffering, desire, anything you can explain, she's saying, and very plainly, 'Kiss my black ass.' And if you don't know that, it's you that's doing the kissing.[29]

LeRoi Jones, as Amiri Baraka was still known then, was as close to the mark as any reverential blues fan and folklorist. In the white man's world of 1920s America Bessie Smith had entire railroad wagons to move her and her entourage around. She showered expensive gifts, expensive cars and all manner of conspicuous wealth on her husband, and when the vogue for vaudeville blues ended in the mid-twenties she moved with the times and adapted her material accordingly. She appeared in Hollywood movies. She was showbiz to her much petted derriere. The message here was clear: it's all showbiz, every vestige, every trace; even the bits of your rarefied and selective tradition that you choose to assume aren't showbiz, they are.

In black psychedelic terms, as in any other terms, it became a case of choose your fiction and don the appropriate apparel. The blues wore many faces. It had its po' boy misery-of-the-ages face. Its voodoo face. Its carnival face. Its medicine-show snake-oil face. Its kiss-my-big-black-ass face. Its humble face. Its funny face. Its sardonic face. Strip away all the layers and the last mask left, the one closest to the skin, is the one that was worn on all those vaudeville stages back at the start of the twentieth century. It's the one that was worn by comedians as they performed blues songs that parodied melancholy; it's the one that didn't in fact spring from some deep dark well of human suffering. African Americans were busting out of 'all that slave shit' long before Miles Davis gave some poor nervous interviewer the evil eye. The blues from the very beginning was wrapped up in role play and costume drama. To acknowledge that is to open up a whole other line of tradition and critical enquiry, one that helps make sense of a black psychedelic consciousness compelled to operate in a white man's market place. Dogmatism frequently overrides pragmatism in these matters, and dogmatic definitions of the blues largely ignore these notions of showmanship and entertainment, even though they were integral to the music's development.

Purists see no linkage whatsoever between George Clinton and his Mothership Connection dancing their way out of their constrictions and the output of earlier African American refusenik entertainers, who unconscientiously objected to a prescribed legacy of noble savagery and manacled muse. It was P-Funk in all its multifarious incarnations and multiple personae that was black psychedelia's true heir to this theatrical tendency. George Clinton and his crew were as entitled to the mantle as the San Francisco Mime Troupe or the Merry Pranksters or any of the other groups who engaged with the liberating possibilities of play power. George Clinton, Bootsy Collins, Bernie Worrell and their fellow intrepid travellers spawned a multiplicity of contract-busting hybrids – Funkadelic, Parliament, Bootsy's Rubber Band, the Brides of Funkenstein, Parlet, the Horny Horns, etc. – and a list of alter egos as long and creatively playful as any since the Pranksters stepped onto the Furthur bus. These noms de plume grew more elaborate and fanciful with every album release – three or more albums a year at their prolific peak – and each LP came adorned with distinctive artwork and accompanied by cartoon booklets full of cosmic doodles and grand-goof narration. The whole enterprise was a huge cosmic cartoon, in fact, and LSD played no small part in that. The P-Funk entourage went on providing the full conceptual package long after all the Bay Area bands had dismantled the light shows, abandoned the multimedia finery and settled down to a life of country rock. It took a shambling entourage of cosmic jammers and space clowns from deepest, darkest industrial Detroit to remind us of what rock music had jettisoned in its tedious pursuit of roots and authenticity.

George Clinton has remained loyal to his quest for nigh on half a century, yet still retains a pragmatist's understanding of where his music sits within the grander scheme of things. Or, as he once put it in an interview, 'Hey, if my records stop selling remind me to take all this shit out of my hair.' I think of that comment every time I gaze at the cover of the Temptations' 1969 LP *Puzzle People*, which depicts them posing on the stoop of a flaking tenement block festooned in their full colour-clashing array of contemporary chic. They are modelling pimp clothes, hustler clothes, hippie clothes, headbands and kaftans, purple flares and Afro hair, but the expression worn by every member tells the same story: 'Hey, if that eleven-minute version of "Papa Was a Rolling Stone" doesn't outsell the three-minute single and if that twelve-minute version of "Stop the War Now" doesn't actually stop the war, then get us back into those matching waistcoats and cravats and book us into the Copacabana pronto.'

Motown read the sea changes of the late sixties as well as anyone and shimmied effortlessly from the sideways pony into psychedelic soul. It was the Temptations who got the whole thing rolling with 'Psychedelic Shack' and 'Cloud Nine'. They started to stretch out on their LPs too, recording lengthy versions of their hit singles and adding fuzz and wah-wah to the showmanship and the slickness. Many of the records that Holland, Dozier and Holland made when they left the Motown operation and set up their Invictus and Hot Wax labels in 1968 continued these principles, and that distinctive psych-soul production sound, pioneered by Norman Whitfield, can be heard all over their post-Motown output. They were responsible for putting out Parliament's freaky-deaky debut album *Osmium* in

1970, and in the Politicians, a group consisting of past and future members of Funkadelic and the Dramatics, they had a house band every bit as versatile as the Funk Brothers. The Politicians were their MGs, Bar-Kays, Mar-Keys, MFSB, NRBQ and Wrecking Crew rolled into one.

Norman Whitfeld's production work with the Temptations and subsequently with the Undisputed Truth took psychedelic funk to new heights. Albums like *Method to the Madness* and *Cosmic Truth* merged Mothership sensibilities with tightly crafted musicianship to form a whole new hybrid. The Undisputed Truth revolved around an ever-changing nucleus of hired hands who at any one time included Joe Harris, Dennis Coffey, Melvin 'Wah-Wah' Ragin, Tyrone Barkley and Chaka Khan's sister Yvonne Stevens, along with the usual posse of under-acknowledged bit-part heroes who shaped the sound of everyone from the Love Unlimited Orchestra to the Pointer Sisters. Tracks like 'Cosmic Contact', 'Take a Vacation from Life (and Visit Your Dreams)', 'UFOs' and 'Spaced Out' explored the full cosmological possibilities of space funk while retaining a shrewd awareness of all the less-than-fabulous ghetto shit that was being left behind.

The other Motown group that happily surfed psychedelia's second wave was the Isley Brothers. By the time they came to record their classic run of rock-infected soul tracks in the early 1970s – 'That Lady', 'Summer Breeze', 'Highways of My Life', 'Harvest for the World', etc. – they had already ridden the changes of three previous musical eras. They recorded the original versions of 'Shout' (1959) and 'Twist and Shout' (1962) during their R&B days; during the mid-sixties era of classic Motown they had hits with 'Behind a Painted Smile' and 'Put Yourself in My Place'; and in the late sixties they reinvented themselves again with the skeletal funk of 'It's Your Thing' and 'I Turned You On'. During this latter period the family unit of Rudolph, O'Kelly and Ronnie Isley was joined by younger brothers Ernie and Marvin. The family elders stand resplendent in orange monk cowls on the cover of the 1969 album *The Brothers Isley*, and again there's more than an element of 'Hey, if this shit ain't working' in their expressions. By the time they recorded *Givin' It Back* in 1971 the transformation into ghetto prophets was complete. *Givin' It Back* contains versions of Stephen Stills's 'Nothin' to Do but Today' and 'Love the One You're With', and extended workouts of James Taylor's 'Fire and Rain' and

Eric Burdon's 'Spill the Wine', and a ten-minute take on Dylan's 'Lay Lady Lay'. It commences with a nine-minute medley of Neil Young's 'Ohio' and Hendrix's 'Machine Gun'. The 'We're finally on our own' sentiments of the CSN&Y original are slowed to a funereal crawl as the brothers Isley adopt the Vanilla Fudge approach to stretching every nuance to breaking point. On the 1972 LP *Brother, Brother, Brother* they do the same with Carole King's 'It's Too Late'. On subsequent albums they proved as adept at innovative adaptations as Rotary Connection, and Seals and Crofts' 'Summer Breeze' and Todd Rundgren's 'Hello It's Me' both got the psychedelic-soul treatment, complete with the recently acquired armoury of the ARP synthesizer.

George Clinton and his entourage remained the most dedicated inhabitants of the territory, but psychedelic space funk could be heard everywhere during the 1970s: on Kool and the Gang's 'Mother Earth' and 'Cosmic Energy'; on Stargard's 'Three Girls (from Another World)'; in Labelle's decades-spanning display of gospel-girl soul and hippie-gumbo variations. Soul mannequins shed the sequins and the well-drilled dance steps and donned spangly space suits and jet-wing collars. Black psychedelia spread its inky tentacles into all kinds of new and uncharted waters. And while many of the original west-coast pioneers now sound indelibly rooted to a particular moment in time (an assessment that only the most time-bound advocates of that music would dispute), the music of P-Funk, Rotary Connection, the Chambers Brothers, the Undisputed Truth and all the other space-age funkateers, music that was either ignored or derided by the taste-makers of the time, continues to thrive, gaining a new lease of life, and a new life of lease, every time a hip-hop artist embeds a fragment of its textures into a twenty-first-century composition.

At the time of writing George Clinton has not yet been required to take all that shit out of his hair. His reputation, ironically enough, now seems as assured as that of those old bluesman who were once paraded before the Newport Folk faithful. Like Memphis Slim or Sleepy John Estes in 1965, Clinton no longer needs to do very much. Just being there is enough. Vaudeville showman. Psychedelic shaman. Hall-of-fame spaceman. If you live long enough, you get to wear any mask you want.

8

CONCENTRATION MOON

The Dark Side of Psych

The Haight-Ashbury was appealing. It was much more open than any other place. But the air was so thick with bullshit you could cut it with a knife. Guys were running around saying, 'I'm you and you are me so get down and suck my dick.' These young middle-class kids were just too dumb about it. It was just too silly. It had to be killed. You'd see them skipping through the park with their bamboo flutes and their robes, calling themselves things like Gingerbread Prince. And they had an irritating, smug, superior attitude. If you didn't have long hair, if you didn't have a bamboo flute, they just ignored your existence.

ROBERT CRUMB[1]

I was sitting in the shallow end of my sister-in-law's pool in Beverly Hills when she received a telephone call from a friend who had just heard about the murders at Sharon Tate's Polanski house on Cielo Drive. The phone rang many times during the next hour. Those early reports were garbled and contradictory. One caller would say hoods, the next would say chains. There were twenty dead, no, twelve, ten, eighteen. Black masses were imagined and bad trips blamed. I remember all the day's misinformation very clearly, and I also remember this, and wish I did not: I remember that no one was surprised.

JOAN DIDION[2]

Among all the documentary and newsreel footage that was shot in Haight-Ashbury during the spring and summer of 1967 two sharply contrasting scenarios stand out. One conveys the apparent childlike innocence of it all. The air peals with shrieking laughter. People link arms, form figures of eight and dance across Golden Gate Park. The mood is not one of an alternative society being constructed; it's more like an extended summer camp. The other scenario captures fresh-faced young boys and waif-like flower girls wandering about the Haight and surrounding streets begging passers-by for small change. It's not so much Robert Crumb's 'air thick with bullshit' that assails the senses here; it's the potential for exploitation, physical harm, betrayed trust, hidden dangers in forbidden zones after dark.

By the time the Summer of Love was officially declared open for business, kids – young kids, some not even out of high school – were arriving in San Francisco by the Greyhound busload. What were they expecting to find, these puppies being born by the truckload, as Bill Graham called them? What were they leaving behind? 'All gone to look for America,' as Paul Simon put it. Yes, but which America?

Existing drug laws would have told them that the Marlboro man was good but the Reefer man was bad, and that there were legally prescribed palliatives for every ailment. Plenty begged to differ. 'And the ones that mother gives you don't do anything at all,' sang Grace Slick, clearly no fan of four-in-one pain relief. 'America drinks and goes home,' sang the Mothers of Invention, as they offered the bleary-eyed view from the bandstand, with the crooner shoo-be-dooing and the audience downing their parting shots. Frank Zappa was no fan of the drug culture but he knew the stench of hypocrisy when he sniffed it. This hypocrisy was reflected in the darker aspect of the psychedelic muse, the stuff that didn't concern itself with flowers in the hair or gingerbread princes or cutely cloaked flautists fol-de-rolling around Golden Gate Park while busloads of newly arrived truth-seekers spread their bed rolls and frolicked in the grass. There was always a more sinister side to the LSD experience, one that led the unsuspecting to a ringside seat by the abyss, and to others opened up a gateway to a less than welcoming void.

The first and only issue of *Psychedelic Oracle Frisco* came off the presses on 2 September 1966. One of its cover stories was about Vietnam GIs speaking out against the war. The other was headlined 'Concentration Camps Ready for Subversives' and concerned the dozen or so internment camps in California where over 100,000 Japanese Americans were incarcerated during the Second World War. The article suggested that these camps were being readied for 'subversives and revolutionaries'. Anyone who lived in America while Edgar J. Hoover was head of the FBI,

especially those who have since gained access to their personal file under the Freedom of Information Act, will know that the country's capacity for domestic witch-hunting had never really abated since the McCarthy days and that central intelligence still had a fairly flexible definition of the terms 'subversive' and 'revolutionary'. The *Oracle* article was chiefly a product of Progressive Labour Party paranoia but many in America would have agreed that there was still plenty to be paranoid about. 'Paranoia strikes deep / into your heart it will creep,' sang Stephen Stills on Buffalo Springfield's 'For What It's Worth', a song written in response to the police brutality waged on those young longhairs who broke curfew on the Sunset Strip in November 1966. 'What a field day for the heat,' sang Stills, in anticipation of things to come. 'Step out of line and the man come and take you away.' Given that by 1966 many Americans were increasingly inclined to believe that their own recently assassinated president had been taken out by more than one assailant, there was no reason why some of them wouldn't also believe that former internment camps were being readied for their arrival. Frank Zappa certainly thought that there was credence to the theory and said so in 'Concentration Moon', a song on the

Mothers' 1968 LP *We're Only in It for the Money.* Zappa satirised the hippies remorselessly on the album – Zappa satirised everything remorselessly, everyone from plastic hippies to their plastic parents got their share – but amid the mockery he could also see what was really going down. Buffalo Springfield began 'For What It's Worth' with a wary 'Something's happening here / what it is ain't exactly clear.' Zappa was far less uncertain in his appraisal of political realities. William Burroughs defined 'the naked lunch' as that 'frozen moment when everyone sees what is on the end of every fork', and there are frequent naked-lunch moments on those early Mothers albums, moments when Zappa casts an unsparing accusatory eye on modern America in all its farcical manifestations. The Zappa who sneered that 'Every town must have a place where phoney hippies meet / psychedelic dungeons cropping up on every street' in 'Who Needs the Peace Corps?' also railed against those who railed against 'the left behinds of the great society' in 'Hungry Freaks, Daddy', the opening track on the Mothers' debut album *Freak Out!* The same album contains 'Trouble Every Day', Zappa's response to the 1966 Watts riots. Singing 'I'm not black, but there's a whole lotta times I wish I could say

I'm not white' in response to the water cannon, baton charges and beatings is probably the closest the notoriously sardonic Zappa was ever going to get to liberal guilt, but somebody had to be saying these things on an LP in 1967. Better still that they were uttered by someone watching events unfold on the evening news, where insurrection (if not the revolution) clearly was being televised.

Another group that knew a thing or two about FBI surveillance and the strategic uses of satire was the Fugs. Founded by free-sheet poets Ed Sanders and Tuli Kupferberg in 1964, the Fugs were the genuine East Village Others. Like the Mothers, their name was a euphemism, in their case taken from Norman Mailer's *The Naked and the Dead*, and their entire existence was one huge 'Fug you' to Amerika and all that it stood for. The Fugs were there before the beginning, hanging out in Lower East Side coffee houses and bars with Ginsberg and Burroughs and the underground film-makers, busy talking themselves up in a voice that was very different to the one coming out of the west coast. In February 1962 Ed Sanders issued *Fuck You: A Magazine of the Arts*. Tuli Kupferberg, meanwhile, was putting out mimeo broadsides with titles like 'Birth' and 'Yeah'. In 1964 they pooled their energies and started writing scabrous doggerel at a prolific rate, which they recorded samizdat-style on three- and six-inch reels. Early in 1965 they were joined by percussionist Ken Weaver and, augmented by two members of the Holy Modal Rounders – Steve Weber and Pete Stampfel – they began playing gigs. Between 1965 and 1970 the Fugs released seven albums of vituperous and licentious vitriol, targeted directly at buttoned-down, placebo-driven, nucleared-up America. Jack Newfield wrote about them in *Village Voice* in September 1965, calling them 'The Rolling Stones of the Underground', a description they proudly displayed in their promotional material. 'YOU ARE ALL A FUG GENERATION,' they proclaimed. 'THIS IS THE ERA OF THE CIVIL RIGHTS, SEXUAL AND CONSCIOUSNESS EXPAN-SION REVOLUTIONS & THOSE ARE THE BANNERS UNDER WHICH THE FUGS ARE GOING TO PRESENT THEMSELVES TO AMERICA.' They described them-selves as 'the Lower East Side's most fantastic protest rock 'n' roll peace–sex–psychedelic singing group', and flyers for their gigs promised 'dope-grope rock 'n' roll meat-shrieks and rice paddy frenzy' and 'the Lower East

Side's most unbelievable Hallucination'.

The Fugs played the first Mime Troupe benefit with the Committee, Lawrence Ferlinghetti, the Family Dog and Jefferson Airplane. They played Washington Square Park with USCO, Ginsberg and Gary Snyder, the one where everyone was instructed to bring 'Mothers, lovers, babies, balloons, flutes, flowers, whistles, rollerskates, and other beautiful things'. They played Lenny Bruce's memorial service in August 1966 and provided the Ben-ediction at the failed attempt to raise the Pentagon in October 1967, when the expectant gathering chanted Ed Sanders's 'Out, demons, out' exorcism at the unmoveable object. In February 1968 they performed a less publicised exorcism at the Wisconsin graveside of Red-baiting, career-destroying senator Joseph McCarthy. They wrote songs with titles like 'Slum Goddess', 'Coca-Cola Douche', 'Johnny Pissoff' and 'War Kills Babies', titles clearly guar-anteed to get them plenty of AM radio airplay and *Ed Sullivan Show* action. The FBI and the Justice Department had files on them and they attracted death threats and parcel bombs. When the police raided the Peace Eye book-store on New Year's Eve 1965/6, Sand-ers's publications were impounded. Their second LP, entitled *The Fugs'*

Second Album, reached number 89 in the US album chart (one place above Martha & the Vandellas *Greatest Hits*, they noted proudly). Sanders made the cover of *Life* magazine in February 1967 under the headline 'HAPPEN-INGS. The Worldwide Underground of the Arts Creates THE OTHER CULTURE.' As a result of this exposure they were invited to appear on the *Johnny Carson Show*, which they turned down because they weren't allowed to sing their anti-war anthem 'Kill for Peace'.

They were out on the streets performing from flatbed trucks as often as they were playing paid gigs. Even when they were in the studio, augmented by proper musicians from the Wrecking Crew, they still sounded like one long rabble-rousing howl recorded live in Washington Square Park. When acoustics and bongos were replaced by electrified instruments, the anarchic stoned strum didn't miss a beat. It was as if someone had prised one set of instruments from their grip and set Fenders in their laps, and they hadn't even noticed the switch and just ranted on regardless. They claimed that everything they did, every note they played was a reaction against the Vietnam war. 'All through the history of the Fugs in the '60s, the war in Vietnam throbbed like an ever-suppurating wound of the soul,' said Sanders. 'However much we partied, shouted our poetry and strutted around like images of Bacchus, we could never quite get it out of our minds. It was like that Dada poetry reading that Tristan Tzara gave in 1922 in Paris, with an alarm clock constantly ringing during the reading. The Vietnam War was THE alarm clock of the late 1960s.'[3]

And the polemic just never let up. They sounded like Ferlinghetti's 'Big Fat Hairy Vision of Evil' set to music. They sounded like firebombed, phone-tapped dissidents (which they were). They sounded like City Lights shoplifters who had decided to lift the entire shop. This is Ed Sanders introducing 'Crystal Liaison' at the Fillmore East on 31 May 1969:

[mumbled – 'Jack-Off Blues'?] 'This is a song dedicated to the Maharishi freak puke and the Zoroastrian dope squad. You know the last Donovan record jacket? It shows a picture of the Maharishi. It looks like he's on a leukaemia ward there and he's got Donovan slipping him some dope-covered gardenias. It's really wonderful. And it gives you spiritual spine tingles. Salvationgasms!' [Recites opening

lines of 'Crystal Liaison': 'In the great bowling alley of your mind I am your pin boy . . .']

They were like that all the time.

Someone else who shouted his poetry and strutted around like an image of Bacchus was Jim Morrison. It has been said, both of Marlon Brando and Richard Burton, that the barely concealed contempt they brought to many of their cinematic roles came about because they had realised how easy it was to get away with it. Brando, a product of the Method school, and Shakespearean high classicist Burton, as anti-Method as an actor could get, were both consummate artists, comfortable in their skins, at ease with their abundant talent, but both took the king's shilling when it came to trading in effort for mannerisms. As a result the greater portion of their celluloid lives was played out as a charade among a carnival of fools. There was an air of that same travesty of posturing in Jim Morrison too. Like Frank Zappa, he played the role of big fish in a little pool with aplomb, although in Morrison's case the satire was frequently cloaked in European symbolist sensibilities and a romanticised vision of mythical America. Zappa conveyed his distaste with a sneer. Morrison

conveyed his with a snarl. The Doors' singer was a film-school drop-out and lived out his entire creative life as if it were a movie. He had desires to be a bard, but once he was ascribed the role of rock poet, and seeing how low the bar was set for that particular appellation, Morrison, like Burton, indulged himself all the way to self-destruction. During his rare periods of sobriety he was only too painfully aware of the limitations of indulgence as a strategy – hence, like Burton, like Brando, the rapid recourse to self-loathing and the loathing of others. Morrison's tragedy, like Burton's, like Brando's, was that he turned into his masques. His creative decline began the moment he started to believe his own publicity, when the world view became an extension of the act, rather than vice versa. There is no shortage of biographical and anecdotal evidence to suggest that he could be a belligerent frat boy of a drunk, the kind of guy who used to pin people down at parties, squat on their faces and fart. He was, according to some accounts, a violent acid head too, trashing recording studios and leaving others to pick up the bill. That spoilt-brat demeanour (like Brando he was pudgy-faced even in his prime) came from privilege. His father was a rear admiral in the US navy, while his mother worked for the

Navy's public-relations department. Both were on the Pentagon payroll and both had witnessed the invasion of Pearl Harbor. Their son hated them equally and often pretended they were dead. He was, then, singularly suited to the role of Oedipal wreck and his songs became one long purgation, an exorcism of the American id. When such strategies became too raw to sustain, he desensitised himself by chewing on a huge lump of hash and heading for the next whisky bar.

The Dionysus or drunk/Bacchus or bar-room bore debate divided audiences, and still does. There were always dissenting voices amid the hype and the hagiographies. 'I remember when Jim Morrison came into the house and started talking about Dionysus. I thought that was the most ridiculous conceit that a guy could come up with in my presence,' said Van Dyke Parks. 'I just knew that he was a philanderer and I was quite amazed that anybody inferred anything of depth out of the man, who just seemed to me the perfect party animal in his black leather pants.' Lester Bangs crowned him the Bozo Dionysus and recalled the Berkeley FM DJs who used to take the needle off the record halfway through 'The End' just so they could offer choice comments about Morrison's general preposterousness and poetic pretensions. Bangs also rounded on the hangers-on who encouraged the singer in his bad behaviour, that 'offensive myth', as he called it, 'which holds that artists are somehow a race apart and thus entitled to piss on my wife, throw you out of the window, smash up the joint and generally do whatever they want'.[4] In one of the most morally astute summations he ever wrote, Bangs said of such behaviour: 'It always goes under the assumption that to deny them these outbursts would somehow be curbing their creativity when the reality as far as I can see is that it's exactly such insane tolerance of another insanity that also contributes to them drying up as artists.'[5]

The Doors rehearsed solidly for a year before they were signed by Elektra, and it shows. By the time they came to record their first LP in 1966 they already sounded way too polished. They did a fine line in glacial shimmer and southern gothic; they were also adept at flamenco and samba, welcomingly airy elements that counteracted all that mannered cool. But they rarely sounded convincing when they rocked out. It was only when session strings and brass were added to their fourth album, *The Soft Parade*, that their music acquired any genuine degree of warmth, and only on their penultimate album, *Morrison Hotel*, did they develop a feel for funk and swing. Producer Paul Rothchild declined to work on their final LP, *LA Woman*, calling the demos 'cocktail music', but in a way it was all acid cocktail music right from the start.

For all his theatrical prowess Jim Morrison displayed remarkably little variation in his singing style. Because his favoured medium was poetry rather than pop music he had a tendency towards the declamatory and the recitative. Despite all the eulogising (which is usually about his aura and rarely about his talent) he had a surprisingly limited range as a singer, barely rising above a two-octave baritone. He never used vibrato and restricted his use of sustained notes to a languid descending glide at the end of a line, which he utilised to the point of cliché. He had no falsetto to speak of; high notes were usually shouted rather than sung. His lyrics were delivered in one of two registers: a spaced-out low-key croon (at which he was highly effective) and a sermonising growl – which more often than not grounded his carefully crafted versifying into dust. Pitch shifts in emotion were conveyed by shouting a bit louder in the final verse (e.g. 'Light My Fire', 'The Crystal Ship', 'End of the Night', 'My Eyes Have Seen You', 'The

Soft Parade') or by unleashing a strangulated yelp ('Strange Days', 'Touch Me', 'Waiting for the Sun') or scream ('The End', 'When the Music's Over').

It was also hard to detect any discernible sense of humour in his outpourings. Perhaps only Jefferson Airplane in their po-faced, coked-up prime displayed such an absence of levity. Even when humour was intended Morrison's hectoring injunctions and earnest delivery meant that comedic sensibilities were all but buried in sanctimony. Humour was there – it's just that most of it was unintentional. The moment when Morrison introduces 'The Soft Parade' with the admonishing preacher cry of 'You cannot petition the Lord with prayer' is just one of many occasions when his summoning of the apocalyptic comes across as high camp, the foot-stamping petulance of a drama queen. As further prosecuting evidence Lester Bangs cited the mock portentousness of the 'Do you remember when we were in Africa?' coda of 'Wild Child', which he calls a great Bozo moment. In Morrison's defence, Bangs maintained that we shouldn't separate the drunken clown from the poet and he likened the singer's delivery on the *Absolutely Live* version of 'The Soft Parade' to Lenny Bruce's preacher-baiting on 'Religions Inc.'.

Bangs also regarded the intro to 'Close to You' on the same live album (where Morrison alluded to his infamous Miami obscenity bust) as one of the great comic monologues.

When he wasn't trying to change the mode of the music by getting his cock out on stage, the Doors' vocalist painted a psychological landscape as bleak as LA's underbelly. *Strange Days*, the Doors' second and best album, is an unsettling and spooky work full of epitaph and elegy. Joel Brodsky's cover photo depicts fairground freaks, a circus strongman, a trumpeter, a juggler, a pierrot and a pair of dwarfs. The music parades similar carnivalesque tendencies while also cradling the burnt embers of alienation to its torn bosom: a *non, je ne regrette rien* death wish here, a torch-song requiem there. There are songs for lost lovers, lost innocence, lost identity and lost Angeles. That well-aired story about Morrison walking along the beach in 1965 crooning 'Moonlight Drive' to Ray Manzarek in Sinatra-like tones suggests that in some alternative Vegas life that he lived in his head he could have started the new lysergic Rat Pack. And what was 'The End' anyway, other than 'September Song' for the *Apocalypse Now* generation? Indeed, what was Morrison's entire career other than

a playing out of Johnny Mercer and Harold Arlen's 'One for My Baby (and One More for the Road)', rendered in leather pants and doom-scenario chic? He presented himself as the Lizard King, but he ended his days as a louche and paunchy lounge lizard. Had he lived he might have nailed his fixation with an album of Sinatra covers – preferably with Gordon Jenkins looking after the arrangements. It would have done him the world of good. It might even have saved his life. On *Morrison Hotel*, in a rare moment when he's not just blues bellowing, he segues out of the barricade-rattling 'Peace Frog' into a beautifully crooned 'Blue Sunday'. It is the most acutely rendered realisation of that Sinatra fixation he ever recorded and hints at what might have been had he not succumbed to his myth.

Morrison was painfully aware of the rock-and-roll Babylon in which he was immersed and of the Garden of Eden that lay beyond. There was enough clarity and rationale in his make-up to suggest that he knew full well that paradise was always out of reach. 'Oh, tell me where your freedom lies,' he sang plaintively on 'Crystal Ship', and he wasn't being rhetorical or playing mind games. It's a direct, penetrating question, not a Dylanesque riddle. Like many rock utopians he lived in a permanent state of disappointment and had a keen sense of the unobtainable. Like many a tragedian turned joker he knew what temptations lay all too easily within his grasp. When he sings 'Five to One', it sounds like a put-on, just so much bullshit sloganeering. When he sings 'Twentieth Century Fox', you can smell her perfume and his disdain. Ditto the inquisitive/indifference dualism of 'Love Street'.

By the time *Morrison Hotel* was released in 1970 the gliding, graceful crystal ship of the Doors' debut album has become a ship of fools, the Pilgrim Fathers recast as reckless drunkards, with 'Land Ho!' as their gung-ho theme. On the *Morrison Hotel* out-takes you can hear the singer belittling and berating his fellow band members, himself, everyone in his orbit, audibly bloating into the belligerent asshole drunk that everyone says he was. In contrast, *LA Woman*, the Doors' final album, is a redemption suite. The LP is one long moonlit night drive across a nation, full of ghostly beauty and flickering silhouettes. Morrison, by now 'half in love with easeful Death', as Keats put it, cruises through a sensual landscape, at one with the mystery of fate, as he heads not entirely unknowingly for pop's own funeral pyre. At the end of it all, six albums and five years down

the line, all the random inchoate urges he displayed in his music betray a stark sense of something left incomplete. A third act truncated and a soul unsatiated. In 1971, done with existentialist slumming on rock albums, he thought he might find fulfilment in the old Europe of his dreams and so he fled to Paris to be dead. Although he still possessed a poetic sensibility, his accomplishments as an actual poet remained as slender and insubstantial as the brief volumes of verse that appeared in his name. That realisation gnawed at him to the grave. In his departing he lived out another fantasy – the fantasy of an early demise, every symbolist's death-wish dream. And now, his admirers would tell you, his drunken ghost swaggers down dawn-lit boulevards, still in pursuit of the spirit of Baudelaire and Rimbaud, still trailing in their shadow. Meanwhile, fans make pilgrimage from all over the world to come and litter his graveside and graffiti his headstone.

In the greater Sunset Strip-billboard marketing scheme of things the Doors displaced Love as the darlings of Elektra. This bloodless coup was accomplished the moment they proved compliant with the niceties of promotion and allowed their record label to release an AM-friendly edit of 'Light My Fire'. It was the Doors who made paranoid LA pop palatable but it was Love who lived the city of light's insularity to the full. The most ironically named band in the history of hippiedom, Love spent most of 1966 holed up in an old mansion house midway between Silver Lake and Hollywood so that they could spend more time with their drugs. They called this habitat the Castle and wrote a song about it. They partied there all the time and refused to tour. As far as gigging went they made occasional forays into San Francisco, where they were adored, but otherwise they pretty much refused to budge from the Sunset Strip, where they were regarded as gods. Even the Monterey Festival was deemed to be a commute too far.

Jim Morrison was self-contained but his inner world was accessible. His symbolism was accommodating and relatively unambiguous, displaying all the regular sex–death polarities necessary to make him a nihilism-by-numbers campus darling and a figurehead for rock's poetic aspirations. Love made no such concessions. Instead of storming rhetorical barricades they built an enclave. Morrison hinted at 'speaking secret alphabet' in a stern, foreboding growl, but it was a translatable lexicon that could be readily acquired and indulged. Break on through? Sure, Jim,

the psychedelic storm troops are gathered and ready. Just give us the sign. In stark contrast Love's Arthur Lee issued opaque aphorisms and puzzling non sequiturs in a beguiling lilt that sprang from a more fractured vernacular. He littered his songs with cryptic clues about commonplace things and dressed even the simplest sentiments – A my love, B my love, so hard to choose – in in-jokes and hip idiolect. While the rest of the band sat in their mansion rooms tripping, Lee took his dog, Self, for a walk. He'd head down to Hollywood Boulevard and then come back and versify about what he'd seen, or imagined he'd seen. Less self-consciously poetic than Morrison, Lee was just as gifted. Unlike Morrison he possessed the nimble melodic acumen of a Broadway writer, a Brill Building nine-to-fiver, Bacharach and David rolled into one, but he doused this abundant lyricism in word spillage that was at times so enigmatically impenetrable that it guaranteed *Forever Changes*, a work of eloquent craftsmanship and one of the greatest achievements in rock history, a place no higher than number 154 in the US album charts when it was first released in November 1967.

Love's second and third LPs, *Da Capo* and *Forever Changes*, are tenderly orchestrated gems full of jazz-folk cadenzas, mariachi grace and dark foreboding prophecy, but their early music is grounded in garage punk. Their eponymously titled debut album, released in the early spring of 1966, is brash and Byrdsian, with just a hint of the British invasion thrown in for good measure. From the opening tambourine beat of their garage-punk take on Bacharach and David's 'My Little Red Book' they displayed a three-chord grandeur all of their own. The arrangements, when there is anything to arrange, are sparse and spiky. Johnny Echols's abrasive electric guitar is right up front in the mix. They offered a punked-up 'Peggy Sue' on 'My Flash on You' and '7 and 7 Is', and as with a lot of garage bands during the *annus mirabilis* of 1966 they liked 'Hey Joe' so much they rewrote it endlessly. Arthur Lee, a black hippie resplendent in hip threads, dug Sam Cooke but he dug Bobby Darin too. Where Morrison nursed Sinatra-esque aspirations, Lee cast himself as a psychedelicised Johnny Mathis. His songs, even his early rudimentary ones, were delivered in a strong vibrant tenor offset by a quivery vibrato. Love's other principal songwriter, Bryan MacLean, offered sweetly sung and simply expressed counterpoint to Lee's more convoluted digressions. Folk-baroque compositions

like 'Softly to Me', 'Orange Skies' and, most famously, 'Alone Again Or' reveal that MacLean was no slouch as a lyricist either. 'Softly to Me''s 'How come so suddenly / everything depends on you?' showed that he was just as well versed as Lee in the Hal David school of expertly calibrated cadence.

The only real hint of self-absorption on that debut LP appears on Lee's acid travelogue 'You I'll Be Following' ('Tripped in the Canyon / my head is still there'), with its namechecks for fellow band members. But it's on Love's second album *Da Capo* that the lyrics start to get opaque. '¡Que Vida!' has a lush flute-led arrangement and Lee sings in deceptively beguiling tones, but he offers increasingly unsettling glimpses of his inner visions ('It's dark there they say / but that's just superstition') before concluding with the militant bad karma of 'And things to kill your brother / but death just starts another'. '¡Que Vida!' is the first of many Lee songs that will end in quiet menace and unsettling incantation. Even their song titles were oblique: they are only mentioned in the lyrics on three occasions on *Forever Changes* ('Andmoregain', 'Old Man' and 'Bummer in the Summer'); the rest are cryptic signifiers, misnomers and, in the case of 'Live and Let Live', caustically ironic.

In Arthur Lee's world nothing quite adds up to the sum of its parts. Narrative voices shift and intertwine. Perceptions fragment, elide and overlap. On 'The Daily Planet' 'I can see you with no . . .' concludes with the simultaneous chanting of 'hands/face'. Lee repeats the trick on 'The Red Telephone', with 'And if you want to paint me / paint me (yellow/white)'. On 'Between Clark and Hilldale' the last word of each verse becomes the first word of the next. Onomatopoeia (which Lee first utilised on the 'ooh-bip-bip-yeah' of '7 and 7 Is') resurfaces on 'Andmoreagain''s 'Can you feel your heart beating / bom bom bom bom.' These are old showbiz tricks given redemptive energy by psychedelia's very own Johnny Mathis.

Jim Morrison mixed up the 'mysterious union' with more priapic urges and concocted a winning recipe out of the basic primal ingredients of sex and death. Arthur Lee was rarely as linear or as binary. He could go toe to toe with Morrison in the paranoia stakes, matching 'This is the strangest life I've ever known' with 'Sometimes my life is so eerie,' but he could obliterate his ego in ways that Mr Mojo Risin' would never have entertained. When Lee writes an acid song he often eradicates the self completely. 'When I was invisible / I needed no light,' he sings on 'She Comes in Colors'. On 'The Red Telephone' he sings, 'And if you want to count me / count me out.' There's far more death than sex in Lee's songs. His love sentiments are flirtatious and teasing, but they are as codified and convoluted as everything else he wrote. When he sings about death he enters another realm entirely; regeneration to degeneration and back again in the blink of an eye. Violence rears up in unlikely places ('There's a bluebird sitting in a branch / I think I'll take my pistol') and portents are delivered through the barrel of a gun. The opening of 'The Red Telephone' – 'Sitting on a hillside / watching all the people die' – is as far removed from the Summer of Love as it was possible to get. It's a black snapshot drawn from events still fresh in the memory: race riots and curfews. Watts burning. Trouble every day. Denouement can't wait till the end of the song; it's delivered in the very next line – 'I'll feel much better on the other side.' Mortality stalks Lee's songs with stealth and presents itself in multiple guises. 'The Red Telephone' ends with the Kafkaesque 'I wonder who it will be tomorrow, you or me,' and the mocking preacher tones of 'All God's children gotta have their freedom.' Love and peace platitudes are delivered with palpable derision.

By the time Lee came to write 'The Red Telephone' he was sick of the Castle's squalor, the endless guests and the constant partying ('I don't need you using up my time'), so he moved out and found himself a new enclave high up in Laurel Canyon. The house, somewhat appropriately, had been used for the filming of Roger Corman's movie *The Trip*. Here, with a panoramic view across the entirety of LA, from Watts and Compton to the Hollywood Hills, Lee pursued his very singular trip imperiously and without distraction. 'A House Is Not a Motel' is a parable about that new-found seclusion. It begins with a hallucinogen-tinged description of mansion hallways lit like Vermeer paintings and invokes party guests who may just be apparitions. When the song re-emerges on the other side of the instrumental break, the spell has been recast; the bells of war are ringing and blood is flowing from the taps. It's a Vietnam-bad trip, chickens brought home to roost, with a shrewd 'The news today will be the movies for tomorrow' thrown in. The shifting of psychic scenery in this manner was another sleight of hand that Love executed frequently. 'The Daily Planet' pulls off a similar trick. It begins with routine and repetition. Lee walks his dog down to 'Go-Stop Boulevard', watches sirens

and accidents and mothers buying plastic guns for their children – 'To keep in practice / waiting on the war.' But after a brief Spanish cadenza everything mutates. There's a cryptic dig at Bryan MacLean, who Lee accused of writing ice-cream songs ('Hope he finds a rhyme for his little mind'), followed by a drug-weary 'Look, we're going round and round', then everything whirls off wordlessly into an extended coda. It's an acid song about ho-hum routine and disillusion, about how drugs just make things more shimmering and sparkly. Everything changes. Nothing changes.

The fictitious newspaper *The Daily Planet* was the place where mild-mannered Clark Kent plied his trade when not travelling faster than a speeding bullet. It's a fitting metaphor for Lee's dual identities and persona shifts. *The Daily Planet* would have made a good Love album title (as indeed would *Go-Stop Boulevard*). When he wasn't being ace reporter Clark Kent, Lee could turn in delightful city pastorals like 'The Good Humor Man He Sees Everything Like This'. It's another perfect (stationary) vehicle for his tangential observations: the view from the ice-cream truck and the world that passes by the vendor's window. Its opening lines – 'Hummingbirds / why do they hum / little girls wear pigtails in the morning,' cast in that trademark tremulous lilt – are as beautifully disconnected as anything Lee ever wrote, observations from separate songs conjoined seamlessly, and we're only two lines in.

'And I'm lost in confusions,' he sings on 'Andmoreagain', another acid song cloaked in astral visitations, another love sentiment with spells cast darkly ('And you wish and you are here'). 'Do you like the part you're playing?' he asks on *Forever Changes*' closing track, 'You Set the Scene', a question he has been building up to for the entire album, an acknowledgement that life is but a play. 'You Set the Scene', like Lennon's 'Happiness Is a Warm Gun', was stitched together from three separate sketches, but many of Lee's best songs sound like that anyway. Each one offers tantalising jigsaw pieces from a bigger puzzle. Sense, identity and self-worth are always shifting, rearranging, forever changing. There's no sense of the sequential; everything happens in an eternally evaporating now. *Forever Changes* is a deeply ambiguous title, paradox dressed up as permanence, the universal instability of things. 'I thought I'd love you for ever, that everything would stay the same for ever.' Yeah, but forever changes. That's what it's like in Arthur Lee's world.

Everything seems to be simultaneously beginning and ending. *Da Capo* literally translates as 'from the beginning', but in musical terms it suggests something more cyclical: go back to the beginning and repeat, repeat selective sections, repeat to the coda, continuum in all its variants, more forever changes. 'There'll be time for you to start all over,' sings Lee as 'You Set the Scene' fades on a mariachi air. At the very end he chants the familiar refrain of the psychedelicised African American: 'Time–time–time–time.'

Forever Changes was a work of bold intent and tarnished beauty; its orchestral splendour is undercut by unsettled and unsettling sentiments. Elegant requiems, death and resurrection, and dark, sardonic doomscapes loom out of the sickly LA fog. Bold intent and tarnished beauty are themes that the counter-culture knew all too well by the late sixties. A little-aired record by Ted Anderson called 'House on the Hill' encapsulates the entropy, fear and loathing perfectly. Released in 1967 on Columbia, the song doesn't reveal its hand until the final verse. It starts off as a 'Little Boxes'-style satire about the strange folks who set the townsfolk's tongues wagging by moving in, keeping themselves to themselves and not observing local pieties. They don't mow their lawn or wash their car. They don't take the local paper and they don't go to church on Sunday. They stay up all night and, horror, one of them is growing a beard. The indiscretions mount up with each successive verse – 'Everyone's alarmed but no one has been harmed' – until a shocking denouement arrives in the form of late-night vigilantes who go up there and burn the place down.

By the late 1960s a chain of hate every bit as durable as the bonds of love was spreading across America. Rednecks hated hippies. Hippies hated straights. Cops hated hippies. Cops hated blacks. Blacks hated hippies. Hippies hated cities. Hippies fled the cities. Hippies bought land. The newly dispossessed land-dwellers hated the hippies. 'Every time a white hippie comes in and buys a Chicano's land to escape the fucking city, he sends that Chicano to the city to go through what he's trying to escape from, can you dig it?' said an unnamed Chicano in Hugh Gardner's *The Children of Prosperity*. 'What can you do with that bread out here, man? Nothing. Then when that money's gone, see, the Chicano has to stay in the city, 'cause now he ain't got no land to come back to. He's stuck and the hippie's free. That's why they don't dig the fucking hippies, man.'[6]

Alistair Gordon reports how communards were torched, raped and pillaged out of their temporary geodesic Edens in New Mexico.[7] Those who weren't forcefully made unwelcome were offered an equally harsh dose of reality by the onset of winter, the crop failure and the collapse of badly constructed, difficult to maintain domes. Others were defeated by more pragmatic considerations and the growing realisation that perhaps there was something to be said after all for non-communal space, separate cooking and sleeping areas, and rooms with alcoves, nooks and crannies.

On a prosaic level constant LSD use might have encouraged mind expansion, but it encouraged squalor too. At Politics of Ecstasy Central the dream life had been crashing for some time. Returning from India, where he had attended Timothy Leary's marriage to his third wife, Nena, Ralph Metzner found that the sixty-four mansion rooms at Castalia HQ had turned into what Jay Stevens called 'a playground for rowdy omnisexuals'.[8] 'Metzner thought he had stumbled into an occult version of hell,' said Stevens. 'The walls had turned into bizarre frescos, covered with glittery shards of mirror and grotesque faces.'[9] In Metzner and Leary's absence the Foundation had divided into two competing factions: those who wished to at least keep the place clean and tidy, and those who advocated permanent tripping. 'Charles Slack, unaware that his old friend was honeymooning in India, had dropped by one Saturday and had found the place full of Greenwich Village hustlers "lying naked and freaked out all around the mansion",' said Stevens.[10] Slack went into the kitchen to try and find Leary's two young children, but instead found a sink piled shoulder-high with dirt-encrusted dishes. 'It was hard to understand how people who had witnessed the splendors of psychedelic vision could be so aesthetically blind as to live in relative squalor, with perpetually unmade beds, unswept floors, and hideously decrepit furnishings,' said Alan Watts. 'It could be, I suppose, that being turned on all the time is like looking through a teleidoscope: it makes far more interesting patterns out of messes (such as dirty ashtrays) than out of such orderly scenes as neatly arranged books in shelves.'[11]

Of all the myths that sprung up around the counter-culture in the sixties perhaps the most enduring one was the idea that a temporary township of canvas tents pitched for a long weekend in a hired field somehow represented a microcosm of how people might live permanently. Rather than recognising such circumstances for what they were – the chance to get blasted in guilt-free surroundings while watching some half-decent bands – these events became enshrined in hippie lore as role models for communitarianism, and none more so than the three-day Woodstock Festival that took place on 15, 16 and 17 August 1969. 'Woodstock Nation' rapidly became a tenet of good faith, a you-had-to-be-there confirmation of a vibe that spread from coast to coast. Most mainstream reportage of the festival concentrated on the logistical problems of half a million people gathering in one place – the gridlock, the blocked freeways, the deluge of rain – and in England the festival was hardly reported at all. But Danny Goldberg in *Billboard* glowed euphorically, calling it 'the dawning of the age of Aquarius'. 'One of the effects of underground music has been the emergence of performers and entire record companies the same age as the audience,' he gushed uncritically. 'The promoters of the festival, Woodstock Ventures, Inc., consisted of four under-39 music entrepreneurs whose only fault was their vastly low estimate of the mass attraction they offered. What other branch of the music business would suffer because of understatement? It is honesty as well as quality which gives the music its appeal.'[12]

As it turned out, Woodstock Ventures Inc. did not suffer unduly. The film of the festival, made on a budget of $600,000 and released in April 1970, grossed over five times that amount during its first week and would go on to make $50 million in America alone. It was Michael Wadleigh's three-hour cinema feature and the accompanying triple-album tie-in that cemented the festival's legendary status and, indeed, the reputation of many of the acts who performed that August weekend. But among the eulogies there were other more dissenting voices, and they came from some of rock music's most uncompromising sources. Frank Zappa called the Woodstock army 'sheep'. Jim Morrison watched TV coverage of the denim-clad hordes and said they looked like 'dupes' marching to the tune of some bogus cause. Like almost all large-scale rock festivals, Woodstock was profoundly anti-ecological. It took half a million people and a deluge of rain approximately twenty-four hours to turn farmer Max Yasgur's arable pastures into a disaster area. The National Guard had to be called in. Artists had to be ferried around by helicopter as all the surrounding freeways were clogged (a life-endangering catastrophe waiting

to happen that was announced in awed tones from the stage like it was some kind of achievement). One of the recurring motifs in Wadleigh's film is the sound of stage announcements being drowned out by the choppers. Amid the great gathering they served as an uneasy reminder of military operations that were taking place 3,000 miles away.

The film itself doesn't tell anything like the full story. 'In light of all the real things that were happening, it is interesting that Woodstock, the film about the festival, served only to solidify and perpetuate the myths,' claimed New York Times reporter Mike Jahn. 'As a documentary, it's terrible. Almost nothing happened the way it's depicted in the film. The film chose to live off the love, peace, eternal beauty, hopes and fantasies of Woodstock Nation, rather than explore its human struggles.' Jahn's piece, entitled 'Recollected in Tranquility: Woodstock Music & Artists', was written for Music & Artists, to coincide with the release of the film. Published in June 1970, it was one of the few appraisals written at the time that attempted to put the festival's highs and lows into some kind of perspective. 'I thought about the news reports,' Jahn reflected. 'Drugs rampant, some sex and a good deal of nudity. This all was true. Rock music, mud, rain, sleeping on blankets and in trees and under cars parked in the middle of Route 17B. This also was true. Drug use was fairly heavy, and although there supposedly were 3,000 bad trips, that's not such a large number out of a population of 500,000 stoned groovers. There was a good deal of nudity. Also the distinct impression that the best-looking people were not the ones without clothes. But though some of the choicer vices were explored at will, I felt there was less actual freedom than fascination with the *availability* of freedom. We can if we want to, and that's enough.' Abe Peck, who also attended the event, offered a more acerbic analysis in *Uncovering the Sixties.* 'Woodstock was El Dorado, shimmering, illusory,' he wrote. 'Had helicopters not airlifted food and doctors, had water purifiers not been hastily installed, had the locals not caught the sharing spirit Woodstock would have become *Lord of the Flies.*'[13]

The event that did turn into *Lord of the Flies* took place a little under four months later, on Saturday 6 December, at the Altamont speedway track. Woodstock Nation spread its bed rolls and tents amid the lush rolling hills of upstate New York. Altamont took place on sun-baked, brown-hilled,

cinder-pathed asphalt on the edge of the California desert. It was here that self-policing would descend into rule by thuggery. At Altamont nebulous anarchy floundered in the face of brutal enactments of social Darwinism.

The initial idea was that the Rolling Stones were going to play 'a free concert for the people' in San Francisco at the end of their 1969 US tour. The Band were pencilled in to appear, as was Ali Akbar Khan, which in the cold light of hindsight could only have been more shiver-inducing had the organisers promised Melanie Safka, Tiny Tim and the Incredible String Band. The original intention was to play Golden Gate Park. Performances from radical theatre groups were promised, although the Mime Troupe pulled out when they failed to receive assurances that all proceeds would be donated to the Weathermen's defence fund. In the middle of all these hasty piecemeal negotiations no one thought to formally approach the San Francisco Parks and Gardens department, and by late November they had left it too late anyway. Four days before the free concert was due to take place it was announced that the location would be the 1,000-acre Sears Point Raceway, an hour's drive north of San Francisco. Sears had adequate access roads, parking, sanitation and medical-aid facilities. Sam Cutler, the Rolling Stones' tour manager, reputedly took one look at the site and deemed it 'aesthetically unpleasing'. The parent company that owned Sears Point played their part in the abandonment by demanding distribution rights for an intended concert film and a significant cut of any profits. At less than twenty-four hours' notice everyone settled for a stock-car racetrack in a steep-sloped arena surrounded by bleached barren hills, and a site full of wrecked cars and garbage left over from the previous demolition derby. Ralph Gleason, who had penned his Friday-morning piece for the *San Francisco Chronicle* on the understanding that the gig would be held at Sears Point, advised concert-goers to 'forget flowers. Bring plenty of food and water.' Emmett Grogan, his finger on the quickening pulse as ever, left a message on the bulletin board at Alembic Sounds, where the Grateful Dead were rehearsing. It read: 'First Annual Charlie Manson Death Festival'.

Anyone with reasonably tuned antennae could sense what was going on from the moment they arrived. Grateful Dead bass player Phil Lesh reported that the air was full of grit and smelled of burning tyres, which turned out to be farmers downwind in the central valley burning their chaff at the end of growing season. As omens go, having the air smelling like a funeral pyre is right up there. The Grateful Dead took one look at what was going down, retreated to their truck and refused to play. A reporter from *Rolling Stone* magazine noted that he arrived at the site to hear KSAN radio DJs 'joyously proclaiming "good vibes" and "peaceful gathering" while Hell's Angels beat dozens into the ground before your eyes and the crowd around you pushed shoved and cursed your very presence'. *Newsweek* and *Life* chose not to run any coverage at all once it became clear that the photographic evidence was destroying any notion that this was going to be 'Woodstock West'.

Many things became crystal-meth clear at Altamont. One was the inability of these large gatherings to police themselves or offer a sustainable model of community. Altamont was a feral free-for-all, with some more free (and more feral) than others. The decision to 'hire' the Hell's Angels as stewards backfired spectacularly, the main reason being that the Hell's Angels cannot be bought or hired in any conventional sense of the words. Placating bikers with crates of beer is not an organisational strategy that Bill Graham would have recognised or readily endorsed.

There is a telling moment in the *Gimme Shelter* movie where the Rolling Stones are performing 'Under My Thumb' on a stage overrun by bikers who glare accusingly into the crowd. Right beside Jagger a denim-clad longhair of quite stunningly anthropoid mien executes the most spectacular drug-induced gurn ever captured on film. He grips his jacket tightly and pulls the kind of face that can only be expressed when pharmaceutical overload has turned both upper and lower jaw into megaton granite cliffs that grate upon each other with all the force of a San Andreas fault line about to blow. Jagger casts him the briefest of glances and carries on singing his misogynistic lyric about a dog that's had her day. He's probably seen similar gouging at any number of Chelsea-set gatherings. It's a scene he had soaked up and coolly regurgitated on *Their Satanic Majesties Request*, the Stones' dark-side response to the fripperies of *Sgt Pepper*, but he's never encountered anything as extreme as this, or as close up. The guy is literally in his face. Eventually the Hell's Angel beside him notices the grotesque apparition and hurls him forcefully into the front rows. Just under a minute later, as 'Under My Thumb' is coming to an end, the crowd parts about ten yards in front of the stage and Meredith Hunter, high on methamphetamine, is stabbed to death. 'Look, we're splitting if those cats don't stop beating everybody up in sight. I want them out of the way, man,' yells Jagger, clearly unaware that he's seen anything more nasty than another vicious scuffle.

At Woodstock there was peaceful survival and coexistence under the stars. At Altamont there was little but threat-filled endurance, with no assistance from the stars whatsoever. Watching Jagger pleading with the crowd at the end of 'Sympathy for the Devil' is one of the most pitiful sights in rock and roll, the precise moment when libertarian rhetoric is hoisted by its own petard. 'I mean, like, people, who's fighting and what for?' he cries in a shrill voice. 'Who's fighting and what for?' he repeats. 'Why are we fighting? Why ARE we fighting?' The Hell's Angels just look at him like he's shit.

Earlier in the day Jefferson Airplane singer Marty Balin had been beaten unconscious by bikers when he had the courage, or blatant stupidity, to intervene when another violent episode was enacted in front of him. As Balin disappears beneath a phalanx of leather and death crests, Grace Slick begins to chant 'Easy' and makes calming gestures with her hands. What might have worked on a bad tripper in a Haight-Ashbury mansion pad fails miserably in the parched daylight of Altamont. When appeasement fails, Slick retreats behind the drum stool and repeats her feeble mantra. 'Easy,' she says. 'Easy times.' Paul Kantner is more forthright. 'Hey, man, I'd just say that the Hell's Angels punched Marty Balin in the face and knocked him out for a bit. I'd like to thank you for that.' This elicits menacing stares from the Angels, and one jumps up on the stage clearly willing to take the discussion to the next level. Still attempting to restore peace, Slick issues another inadequate request. 'You've got to keep your bodies off one another unless you mean love,' she says. 'People get weird and you need people like the Angels to keep people in line. But the Angels, you know, you don't bust people in the head for nothing. So both sides are fucking up temporarily. Let's not keep fucking up.' Perhaps the most revealing aspect of her testimony is the phrase 'both sides'. The Jefferson Airplane had kicked off their set with 'We Can Be Together', but after Altamont there was no further pretence that this was the case. For all their gotta-revolution/ Volunteers of America sloganeering the Airplane saw their dream undone not by guns, but by blades, chains and pool cues. It's easy to put a flower down the

barrel of an uncocked rifle. It takes a lot of nerve and a steady hand but it can be done. It's not so easy to wrap a daisy chain around a beating stick when it's being wielded by a San Jose biker who has been necking Owsley sunshine and complimentary beer all morning.

Ultimately, Altamont was the end of psychedelic theatre, the defining moment when the legacy of the *City Scale* Happening, Anna Halprin's joyous and liberating physical meditations, the Mime Troupe's mimicry and the playful antics of the Acid Tests came to grief in a blood-flecked cinder pit at a demolition-derby site. 'I'm the prince of darkness,' Jagger suggested as he toyed with diabolic imagery in his songs. 'Oh no, you're not,' said the Hell's Angels, only too happy to show the man of wealth and taste what darkness really looked like. All through the Stones' shambolic set Jagger issues broken pieties to a shattered dream. 'Something very funny always happens when we start that number,' he says initially, attempting to make light of circumstances as 'Sympathy for the Devil' falls apart for the first time. 'Brothers and sisters, brothers and sisters, come on now! That means everybody just cool out!' he says, admonishing the pit of Hades in sixth-form prefect tones. He continues to prance and preen for a while, singing about the street-fighting man and the midnight rambler and about how it's all just a shot away. How small he looks. How little he knows. Out there at the perimeter people may be stoned but they are less than immaculate. Gun-toting Meredith Hunter is pronounced dead at 6.20 p.m.

Altamont hadn't even been the first music event that year to descend into violence. Only a month before Woodstock the long-established Newport Jazz Festival had to be temporarily halted when thousands of aggrieved fans without tickets stormed the main arena. Fences were torn down, seats were smashed and the VIP area and stage were invaded. In the festival's aftermath several acts agreed to forego their fee in order to minimise the anticipated financial loss; others who had already been paid sent back donations. The disturbances were widely reported in the music press, both in the UK and US. *Melody Maker* made Newport its front-cover story. Organiser George Wien regarded it as the nadir of his career, and over a hundred people were hospitalised. What shocked everyone was the sense of entitlement the gate-crashers felt as they mob-charged the fences and ransacked the main arena. This sense was increasingly abroad in 1969. Joan Didion, who saw more

portents than most during that long hot summer, spoke of 'boys who majored in shop and worked in gas stations and later held them up . . . children who grow up absurd in the West and Southwest, children whose whole lives are an obscure grudge against a world they think they never made. These children are increasingly everywhere and their style is that of an entire generation.'[14]

Didion saw warning signs where more complacent spirits didn't venture. She detected them in the rock culture itself, in the non sequiturs that pass for communication among stoned musicians, when she sat in, bored *in extremis*, on a Doors recording session. Ultimately, Didion detected them in the stultified reaction to the Manson slayings up on Cielo Drive. You see that same passé and drug-numbed reaction in some of the Altamont photos. There are a couple in particular that say more than any hand-wringing underground-press post-mortem ever could. One shows the 300lb naked man. Everyone who was there remembers the 300lb man. He seems to crop up in almost every reminiscence of the event. Some remember him disrobing and running down the hill. Others recall him, still in his Bermuda shorts at this point, drunkenly sitting on a guy and fondling his girlfriend's breasts, while everyone around him felt either too damn cool or too impotent and powerless to intervene. Even a brief cautionary 'back off, man' beating from the Angels failed to have any effect on his behaviour. And there he is in the photos, captured in all his spaced-out, boozed-up, corpulent glory, swigging ale from a huge jug, the kind the Bay Area bands used as percussion before they all went psychedelic. Everyone around him seems to be affecting a let's-pretend-this-isn't-happening stare.

The other key photo was taken from the stage during the Jefferson Airplane melee. The crowd clears a fearful circle around the violence. One woman clings to her boyfriend in shock. Another clasps her hand to her head in obvious distress. A couple of front-line photographers with jobs to do frame their shots within hitting range of the raised pool cues. Two women, positioned directly in front of the violence, look either oblivious or unconcerned; one appears to be fiddling with her earring. It may be a trick of the frozen moment. The camera can lie. But one thing it can't lie about is the look on the majority of faces. They look blank-eyed, not necessarily indifferent, but immured certainly. Powerless to intervene, and with no coherent philosophy at their disposal that might make sense of the

unfolding malevolence, they just gape and gaze, immobile and uncomprehending, or perhaps comprehending only too well. A couple of ringsiders crane their necks for a better look. Welcome to the First Annual Charlie Manson Death Festival.

Bill Graham, a concentration-camp survivor, likened Altamont to the Holocaust. Ken Kesey said he had long suspected that Altamont would happen; he just didn't know where or when. Lester Bangs referred to Altamont not as the death of Woodstock innocence, but as a 'facing up', as he called it, a reckoning that could have taken place at any time in any place. 'I remember the naked sobbing girl who came stumbling down past us, shoved by some irate redded-out boyfriend up the hill, everyone ogling her and snickering, and her attempts to cover herself as she dazedly picked her way back to her friends, stumbling as she stepped uncertainly through the tribal circles of beatified freaks who dug it all laughing and grabbing.'[15]

Meanwhile, out there in the hinterland, the slouch towards Bethlehem had already begun. A week before Woodstock, the inhabitants of Terry Melcher's old place up at 10050 Cielo Drive were slaughtered by members of the Manson family. The following night Charlie's Angels drove up to Los Feliz and killed supermarket executive Leno LaBianca and his wife Rosemary. Manson had been a resident of Haight-Ashbury during 1967. He bought the old Spahn Movie Ranch near Topanga Canyon Boulevard in August 1968, where episodes of *Bonanza* and *The Lone Ranger* had been filmed, and set about constructing his own Wild West adventures. When they weren't out robbing autos and converting them into dune buggies, Manson and his followers were devoted adherents to the trip-all-the-time acid diet, as practised by the residents of Leary's Castalia mansion during the Foundation's last day. There the similarities ended.

The degree to which Manson himself was involved in the slayings and the extent to which he got his disciples to do his bidding is still hotly disputed, especially among Manson groupies and acolytes, who keep his tarnished name and his charitable deeds alive on dedicated websites that all but erect cyber-shrines to the holy church of Helter Skelter. Manson was as much a product of the American prison system as he was of the alternative society. He saw an opening in the lapsed morality and exploited it. Tinseltown was a florid gossip grapevine, drugs and sex parties were rife and news travelled fast.

A dishevelled hippie manipulator in his mid-thirties with a harem of hot young cuties in tow would not have stood out especially in rock-and-roll Babylon at that time. Manson and his entourage would have been just another bunch of acid-scrambled longhairs participating in the stoned bacchanal. Hence Joan Didion and her circle's reaction to the slayings: alarmed, yes; shocked, no. Manson was Didion's entitlement poster-boy made flesh. He fitted her pen portrait to the letter, right down to the recidivist tendencies and the growing up absurd. He held up grocery stores and gas stations (albeit without ever having bothered to work in them first) and pimped and robbed his way across several county lines. As a result he'd spent half of his first thirty-two years in confinement. Charlie's biggest sense of entitlement and resentment was reserved for the music industry. Aggrieved that he couldn't secure a record contract, he exacted retribution in the most savage way imaginable. The recordings that have surfaced of Manson the singer-songwriter are not significantly better or worse than hundreds of other busker poets with limited talent who tried their luck in the second half of the 1960s. Once you get past the rambling campfire jams, the prison-cell polemic and the grating sense of infallibility (and the realisation that the people you are listening to committed acts of unspeakable atrocity), songs like 'Look at Your Game, Girl', 'Cease to Exist' (aka 'Never Learn Not to Love') and 'Eyes of a Dreamer' are the kind of half-OK efforts that wouldn't have disgraced many a bedenimed troubadour in the late 1960s.

Like Hitler being turned down by the Vienna Academy of Fine Arts in 1908, it's perhaps a touch fanciful to suggest that cataclysmic consequences might have been averted had someone just let Manson sign on the dotted line of a five-year contract, with a royalty rate sufficient to keep him in acid and autos. There's always the possibility that the second album would have been a concept work about dune buggies, race war and encrypted messages in Beatles records, but given the calamity that ensued, not to mention the legions of second-rate singer-songwriters who did manage to secure record deals, that might have been a chance worth taking.

Then again, if it hadn't been Charlie Manson, it would have been somebody else.

Mr. and Mrs. America – you are wrong. I am not the King of the Jews nor am I a hippie cult leader. I am what you have made me and the mad dog devil killer fiend leper is a reflection of your society. Whatever the outcome of this madness that you call a fair trial or Christian justice, you can know this: In my mind's eye my thoughts light fires in your cities.

CHARLES MANSON'S
STATEMENT AFTER HIS
CONVICTION FOR THE TATE
AND LABIANCA MURDERS

PSYCHEDELIA UK

9

YOU GET A TAN FROM STANDING
IN THE ENGLISH RAIN

I was seven when 'Love Me Do' made the Top Ten. There's a certain age below which you're not interested in music. I vaguely remember stuff before that. The only thing that really grabbed me was 'Telstar' by the Tornadoes, because I heard someone say it was the music of the future and I really liked that. But there's something which very few people write about or understand – but it's probably one of the most important processes of popular culture – a generation recognising itself in music.

And that often happens when a generation latch onto music which is designed for people much older than them. The Beatles weren't making music for seven year olds, they were making it for teenagers, I guess, but kids loved it. If you were older at the time The Beatles were a bit uncool. You were a beatnik or something like that, whereas for me it was one of the first things that spoke to me and kids of my age.

COLIN NEWMAN, April 2003[1]

'When I Was a Boy'

Like Wire guitarist Colin Newman, I was seven years old when 'Love Me Do' was released in October 1962 – one month shy of my eighth birthday, in fact – and everything he says is correct. To have just turned eight when 'Love Me Do' entered the charts means that I witnessed the birth and development of sixties pop culture through an attentive child's eye, and it partly explains the fabric of this book from here on in. For the corollary of being seven when 'Love Me Do' came out is that I was twelve when 'Penny Lane' was released and in my sixteenth year when the Beatles split. They are ever present throughout my childhood and adolescence. I can remember just – only just – what the world sounded like the day before the Beatles arrived. As I get older and this proportion of my life grows smaller, inevitably a sepia tint creeps in here and there, certain memories grow hazy round the edges, but mere distance alone cannot diminish the effect that first year of the Beatles had on my pop consciousness. What did the Beatles sound like to an eight-year-old? They sounded like a scream. Not the scream of the girls who were screaming at them. And certainly not the anguished yelp of inner primal pain that Arthur Janov later added to John Lennon's crippled insides. I mean the scream the Beatles made, the scream of their own voices. Girls (and some boys) learned to scream back at them as a matter of course, as a tribal rite, but they were only screaming because the Beatles screamed first. They started it.

The process by which the Beatles came to dominate my pop landscape was closer to osmosis than fandom, and the way it sustained itself can be measured out in incidentals and ephemera as much as in hysteria and passion. One minute there was a world before the Beatles, the next they were everywhere, permeating every aspect of a child's life. The records were just part of it. Colin Newman's comment about a generation 'latching onto' music suggests that we were forever playing catch up, and it's true, we were, assimilating ideas and images we barely understood but at the same time instinctively understanding that this was ours. And, moreover, it was ours first. Everyone was playing catch-up in one form or another once the Beatles got into their stride; they rarely stood still long enough for it to be otherwise. Out of all that grows a culture and all it entails. And as a child, assuming you are pliant and willing, as I was, you instinctively mould yourself to the contours of that culture as it gestates and assumes its shape. Philip Larkin ends his poem 'An Arundel Tomb' with the line 'What will survive of us is love.' And that is ultimately how I feel about the Beatles. Long after the last biographical detail has been laid to rest, long after the last surviving great-grandchild has gazed at the faded magazine photos and asked, 'Which one was Beaky?' what will remain of the Beatles will be the songs. That's not to say the songs are timeless. Many of them – the majority, in fact, from their covers of 'Besame Mucho' and 'My Bonnie Lies Over the Ocean' to 'Baby, You're a Rich Man' and 'Because' – are quite clearly of their time. That's precisely what is good about them.

Some groups sustained what might otherwise have been very short careers by cherry-picking the best Beatle songs to cover. From *With the Beatles* onwards groups waited to see which LP tracks weren't going to be released as singles and then plundered the Northern Songs catalogue for all it was worth, barely able to believe their good fortune. From the Overlanders, with 'Michelle', to Marmalade and 'Ob-La-Di, Ob-La-Da' a multitude of artists exploited the embarrassment of commercial riches that flowed from the Beatles' prolific pens. Even when the catalogue wasn't plundered directly the Fab Four's influence was evident in what was borrowed: a chord sequence here, a harmony there, each reflecting nuances the Beatles themselves had instigated as each new album improved upon the previous one. George Harrison's 'Taxman' riff runs like an unbroken thread through the development of English psychedelia; it's there as a trace element in many a mod-pop mutation.

The Beatles got the riff by emulating their R&B heroes, but the groups who subsequently appropriated it didn't. They got it from copying the Beatles. Likewise the string arrangements and lyrics about lonely people that came after 'Eleanor Rigby'. Or the codas and false endings that followed in the wake of 'Strawberry Fields Forever'. Ditto the trills, frills, fanfares and peals of piccolo trumpet that came after 'Penny Lane'. Ditto the calliopes and steam organs that crop up in almost every psychedelic song about a fairground or circus. And ditto other details far too numerous to mention. The Beatles are the benchmark by which everything else in the 1960s has to be measured. They are the foundation stone and the building blocks of sixties pop, and everything that came after is a reaction to them. Groups either copied them directly or deliberately set themselves against everything they supposed the Beatles represented. Either way, it was still about the Beatles. Even when you think it isn't about them, it probably is.

The American film-maker John Waters once claimed that the main reason he hated the Beatles was that they killed the girl-group era. As well as offering a refreshingly plausible take on why anyone could possibly hate the Beatles, Waters offers a rare instance of someone contextualising the group in terms of what they displaced rather than what they represented. It's essentially an American perspective, of course. By the time the Beatles hit America at the start of 1964 the girl-group era had already peaked, but in November 1962, when 'Love Me Do' charted in the UK, it had barely begun. Motown might have been the sound of young America, but in England it was still the sound of the underground. And because he adheres to an American timeline Waters overlooks one crucial detail: the Beatles didn't replace the girl groups. They became the girl groups, by surrogacy and supplantation.

In Hamburg the Beatles were testosterone-fuelled shag lads, pilled-up, wide-eyed wild boys agog on the Reeperbahn, their antics akin to those of any other group of working-class males doing their overseas apprenticeship while living on basic wages in shit digs. It was there that Astrid Kirchherr prettified them with bowl haircuts and cute fringes. Thus, with one forward sweep of a comb, she toppled the lacquered pompadours and bequiffed crowns of a generation. As a fashion stance this was hardly unique. Parisian youth and English art students who were hip to Jean Cocteau's *Le Testament d'Orphée* had been wearing the look since 1959.

Californian surfers wore a similar bowl cut long before the English invasion. But the look was new to rock and roll. When Brian Epstein came along he tried his best to reinvent the group in his own image, smartening their tailoring with collarless suits and buffing them up with a light-entertainment outlook, but the rest – the prettification, the feminisation – the Beatles took care of themselves. It took little coercion.

In a single day in February 1963 the Beatles recorded ten of the songs that would feature on their debut LP *Please Please Me*. Three of them – the Shirelles' 'Boys' and 'Baby It's You' and the Cookies' 'Chains' – were covers of girl-group songs. 'I Want to Hold Your Hand', the record that broke them in America, replicated the snuggle-up sentiments and hand claps of the girl-group songs, as did 'Hold Me Tight' on their second LP, *With the Beatles*. That album also contains covers of the Marvelletes' 'Please Mister Postman' and the Donays' 'Devil in Her Heart'. Many of Lennon and McCartney's earliest compositions adopted the billet-doux format of the girl-group love song. 'Love Me Do', its B-side 'P.S. I Love You', 'From Me to You' and 'All My Loving' are all feminised love letters, audio lipstick scrawls on a perfumed envelope. From the sha-la-las of 'Baby It's You' to the coyness of 'I'm Happy Just to Dance with You', from the way they deported themselves on stage – lead singer separate and stock still, backing singers cheek to cheek at the mic – to the way they arranged their music, the Beatles were immersed in girl-group vocabulary, girl-group identity, girl-group choreography, girl-group iconography.

What is most noticeable about the early songs is just how many of them make more sense when sung by a female. 'There's a Place', 'It Won't Be Long', 'Do You Want to Know a Secret?' and, but for one solitary mention of a man, 'I Want to Hold Your Hand' all situate themselves firmly within the emotional terrain of the best girl-group songs. The heartbreak, the longing and the flirtatiousness are all borrowed from the lingua franca of girl pop. These are girl-group songs that just happen to be sung by men.

Those who like to portray the history of popular music as a series of distinct linear epochs claim that the period between 1958 and 1963, specifically the period between Elvis joining the army and the arrival of Beatlemania, was some sort of cultural void, populated entirely by plastic, white-bread pop stars – all those Troys, Fabians and Bobbies – and manufactured showtune schmaltz. It's a marketing and merchandising view of the world, and one that a surprising number of music historians willingly and uncritically adhere to. And yet even a cursory glimpse at the UK and American pop charts in the period immediately prior to the arrival of the Beatles will show it to be utterly fallacious. In the UK the pop charts reverberated to the sound of Del Shannon, Duane Eddy, Ray Charles, Floyd Kramer, Johnny Kidd and the Pirates, surf instrumentals, the Shadows and all their imitators, the twist, the Hully Gully and countless other dance crazes. In the US 'Ya Ya' by Lee Dorsey, 'Green Onions' by Booker T. and the MGs, 'Hit the Road Jack' by Ray Charles, 'Shop Around' by the Miracles, 'Tossin' and Turnin'' by Bobby Lewis and 'The Mountain's High' by Dick and Dee Dee were all Top 10 records that directly shaped the Beatles' sound and made them who they were. In the *Cashbox* or *Billboard* Hot 100s during any one week there was abundant evidence of raw, energised alternatives to the milksop sound so commonly associated with the era. The idea that youth music had lost its spark and vibrancy during the period immediately prior to Beatlemania is a complete myth.

So too is the theory that the Beatles exploded in America when they did because they helped revive the morale of a nation still in mourning for its recently assassinated president, John F. Kennedy. Even Ian MacDonald, in his rigorous and authoritative account of the Beatles songbook, *Revolution in the Head*, subscribes to this view. Referring specifically to the success of 'I Want to Hold Your Hand', he states: 'In the USA release came too late for the festive season, which in any case had been dampened by the recent assassination of President Kennedy. When Capitol finally capitulated to Epstein's pressure and issued "I Want to Hold Your Hand", the record's joyous energy and invention lifted America out of its gloom.'[2] In fact, American youth seemed to have been lifting itself out of its gloom pretty nicely without the intervention of the Beatles. The record that 'I Want to Hold Your Hand' replaced at number one on 25 January 1964 was none other than 'Louie Louie' by the Kingsmen, the three-chord classic that launched the garage-band sound and was arguably the prototype for punk rock. 'Louie Louie' spent two weeks at the top of the *Cashbox* and *Billboard* Hot 100. American youth had also been coming to terms with its grief by buying 'Surfin' Bird' by the Trashmen in sufficient quantities to send it as high as number four in the charts, when 'Louie Louie' was number one. Also in the US Top 30 the week 'I Want to Hold Your Hand' went to number one were 'You Don't Own Me' by Lesley Gore (number 6), 'Anyone Who Had a Heart' by Dionne Warwick (10), 'The Nitty Gritty' by Shirley Ellis (13), 'When the Lovelight Starts Shining Through His Eyes' by the Supremes (23), 'Quicksand' by Martha and the Vandellas (24), 'Can I Get a Witness' by Marvin Gaye (25) and 'Baby, I Love You' by the Ronettes (26). Yes, Bobby Vinton and Bobby Rydell were there too, but so were Jerry Butler and Major Lance. That's a fabulous Top 30 by any standards. This was the teenage landscape that the Beatles encountered when they went to America and assumed their surrogacy.

The term that the American writer Michael Hicks coined to summarise the repository of influences and inputs that help shape an artist was 'the congregation of the voice'. He originally applied it to Elvis Presley's vocal style in order to critique the idea that Presley was unique. Hicks shows this not to be the case and cites astute comments made by the country singer Charlie Hodge, who detected that Presley's very audible influences ranged from Billy Eckstine to Hank Snow. Hicks modestly admits

that 'the congregation of the voice' was his 'off-the-cuff term for the collection of personalities implied by a rock singer's delivery',[3] but as a working model it has much to commend it. The Beatles too were the sum of their learned and inherited parts – which partly explains why to a seven-year-old they sounded like they were screaming, and to plenty of seventeen-year-olds too. And to composer Luciano Berio too, as it happens. 'One of the most attractive vocal characteristics is the naturalness, the spontaneity and the multitude of sounds,' said Berio of their singing. 'It's true that most of the time the singing is on the level of a scream, but everyone screams in his own fashion without affectation.'[4] Screaming had never entirely gone out of fashion. Girls had screamed at Sinatra, Presley and Johnny Ray. Little Richard and Screamin' Jay Hawkins screamed a fair bit too. The Beatles undoubtedly screamed in their own fashion, although the extent to which it was without affectation is disputable. Lennon and McCartney were astute enough to notice from very early on that when they shook their moptops and hit the higher register, the audience responded in kind. And so an age-old ritual, passed down from previous generations of bobbysoxers and teenyboppers, was buoyed (and girled) by the aggregation of the Beatles' own influences, the mass congregation of their voices.

The scream is there in the orgasmic call and response of 'Please Please Me' and in the climaxing falsetto of its chorus. It's in the octave leap of 'Is there anything I can do?' on 'From Me to You'. It's there at the end of every verse on 'I Want to Hold Your Hand'. It's there in the final 'you should be glad' on 'She Loves You' (a love song sung in the third person so no one feels left out). It's there in the backing vocals on 'Twist and Shout'. It's there in every ascending melody line and high harmony. It's everywhere, in fact, and it comes from all kinds of places. It's a distillation of all the Beatles' competing influences, all melded together and overlaid and underlaid in two- or three-part harmony, until it became a sound that was utterly their own. It comes from copying the girl groups, but it also comes from copying doo-wop, Little Richard, Larry Williams, Buddy Holly, Roy Orbison, Smokey Robinson, Del Shannon, the Isley Brothers and the Everly Brothers – especially the Everly Brothers, who more than any of their contemporaries built the bridge which spanned that early-sixties void that critics adhere to but nobody else does. It's detectable in 'Cathy's Clown'

and 'Lucille'. It's there in the thrilling and willing of 'Temptation', and it was still there when the Everlys went beat-group electric in 1964. It's why 'The Price of Love' and 'Love Is Strange' sounded so utterly modern when they were released, rather than the tired and desperate efforts of tired and desperate leftovers from a bygone era.

William Mann, who famously endorsed the Beatles in *The Times* in 1963 and talked of the 'chains of pandiatonic clusters' in 'This Boy' and 'the Aeolian cadence at the end of "Not a Second Time"', was also astute enough to surmise that the scream would soon become idiomatic, or, as he put it in his own inimitable fashion, 'Those submediant switches from C major into A flat major, and to a lesser extent mediant ones (eg the octave ascent in the famous "I Want to Hold Your Hand") are a trademark of Lennon–McCartney songs – they do not figure much in other pop repertories, or in the Beatles' arrangements of borrowed material – and show signs of becoming a mannerism.'[5] And he was right. They did become mannered, and as soon as the group recognised them as such they moved on. The muting of that scream marks the end of the Beatles' girl-group stage. The trouble was, no one told the fans. After a while the screaming got so loud that the Beatles could no longer hear themselves think, let alone play. On those rare occasions when the hysteria did relent, the group were shocked at just how ramshackle they sounded. John Lennon always maintained that the Beatles stopped progressing as a live act after 1963. One listen to any of the available concert recordings from 1966, their final year of touring, would bear this out. Between 1964 and 1966 any real progress the Beatles made happened away from the glare of the spotlight. They began to develop for the first time as a studio ensemble. Public exuberance gave way to private introspection. There was more than one reason for that, but the main one was pot.

'I Saw the Light'

Marijuana made the Beatles dreamy and contemplative, but it also made them duplicitous. Already enthralled by Bob Dylan's facility with words, enthralled to the point of self-conscious emulation in Lennon's case, they began writing songs that reflected their new experiences. Marijuana helped insulate the group from the constant hysteria that followed them everywhere. It cocooned them from Beatlemania, and it exerted a two-way pull on their creativity. On the one hand the subterfuge necessary to keep their vices secret gave their lyrics a fresh repertoire of disguises and double bluffs, new ways of encoding their emotions in euphemism, in jokes and third-person detachment. At the same time an explicit masculinity and more than a hint of chauvinism began to emerge in their writing. Many of the Beatles' early love songs were trite and candy-coated. Relationships were cosy and harmonious, or at least strived to be. From 1964 onwards all that changes. There is a shift away from the generalised and the non-gendered, as lyrics begin to deal more specifically with male ego and pain. Lennon and McCartney start writing hard-bitten tales about wounded pride, jealousy and betrayal. Love requited is replaced by love thwarted, love spurned, love hidden away.

The subterfuge and deception of Lennon's unfaithfulness to his wife Cynthia reveals itself, or rather cloaks its duplicitous intent, in 'You've Got to Hide Your Love Away' and 'Norwegian Wood (This Bird Has Flown)'. 'In My Life' reveals a sombre and reflective quality to his writing for the first time – although even here he shrouds his emotions in hazy evocations of unnamed places, lovers and friends. That same vagueness is there in the third-person meanderings of 'Nowhere Man', a song that Lennon later dismissed as mere word shapes but which anticipates the ennui that would settle on his muse as his drug intake increased. 'Nowhere Man' also introduces the inner dialogue that would inform some of his best psychedelic songs. Paul McCartney's compositions at this time range from the carefree ('I'll Follow the Sun') to the conciliatory ('We Can Work It Out') to the dismissive ('I'm Looking Through You'). He also wrote his fair share of full-blooded odes to fornication. 'She's a Woman', 'The Night Before', even the mockingly mournful 'Baby's in Black' all reek of a rich bachelor Beatle out on the pull.

During this period the Beatles developed into pop music's first chamber ensemble and began composing in a way that adhered more closely to the baroque sonata than to contemporary pop. In its traditional form the baroque sonata was a composition for four instruments, generally featuring two treble instruments, usually violas, and a bass instrument, with a keyboard instrument adding harmony. As the form evolved so too did the flexibility of these components. Pieces might be scored for a range of solo instruments or for duos, trios, quartets or sextets in various combinations. Two, three or four instruments might join a bass or melody line in unison, without any one component dominating. This is precisely what the Beatles were doing by 1965: utilising interchangeable instrumentation at will, doubling up bass lines on lead instruments, interweaving up to three separate guitar parts into a composite whole. The interplay of guitar sounds on 'I Feel Fine', 'Ticket to Ride' and 'Day Tripper' creates a tapestry of timbres that conceals each element's virtuosity. Such seemingly effortless fluidity was made easier by the fact that all three guitar players could take on each other's roles. Harrison was a perfectly adequate bass player, McCartney a more than decent lead guitarist. Lennon could play lead and rhythm. He and McCartney both played piano and organ, and from 1964 onwards increasingly began to compose songs at the keyboard as well as on the guitar.

On the Beatles' earliest recordings harmony was largely provided by the voices. Instruments stuck to their allocated roles, providing lead, rhythm, bass and percussion accompaniment strictly in accordance with the conventions of pop composition. Increasingly, though, from *A Hard Day's Night* and *Beatles for Sale* onwards, harmonic textures were created with guitars and keyboards, any further embellishment and augmentation normally being provided by George Martin. This ensemble approach to composition rapidly spread to every aspect of the recording process. Every new recording technique or piece of studio equipment was viewed as an aid to tonal colour, but the Beatles assiduously resisted the temptation to let any one sound or recording device dominate their output. Their use of flanging, phasing, fuzz boxes and wah-wah pedals was always subtle and never reduced to gimmickry. As with all great ensembles virtuosity was always subordinate to the group whole, and solos were kept brief and economical. It is extraordinary to consider that during this key period of their creative development no Beatles song broke the three-and-a-half-minute barrier.

The Beatles' evolution from pill band to pot group, and from surrogate girl group to boy band, took place over a period of two years and reached a conclusion on 11 November 1965 with the recording of 'Girl' for the *Rubber Soul* album. 'Girl' was another of Lennon's duplicitous identity songs, using generalised sentiments to disguise what is essentially a first-person confessional. It alludes to his troubled relationship with Cynthia, but also summarises past crushes and unrequited passions for existential poster girls Juliette Gréco and Brigitte Bardot. The lyric is an accumulation of regrets – regret at not leaving her, regret at ever meeting her, regret for treating her bad – but the dominant mood is one of detachment. The clumsy switch from first person to third for the final verse, suggested and partly penned by Paul McCartney, fails to universalise the sentiments; it simply makes them more oblique. 'Girl' is ultimately a love song about the idea of a love song, arranged with dry wit and a not so subtle nod to the prevailing narcotic influences. The title refrain, 'Aah, girl', was close-miked at Lennon's suggestion to give it intimacy, but the sharp intakes of breath at the end of each line also suggest a joint being inhaled. 'Girl''s two-step chorus features acoustic guitars strummed bouzouki-style in parodic homage to *Zorba the Greek*. The jape is intrusive and heavy-handed and suggests that the group can't decide when to be funny or serious any more. As Lennon sings, 'She's the kind of girl,' the backing singers, George and Paul, sing a backing refrain of 'Tit tit tit tit tit tit tit'. 'Girl' concludes with an unnaturally hasty fade-out that seems to be saying, 'That's enough loveable Scouse wit, lads. Joke's over, time to move on.'

'What's the New Mary Jane'

The Beatles first encountered LSD at the home of a well-connected Harley Street dentist, who injected the drug into a sugar cube and put it in the coffee of John Lennon, George Harrison and their respective partners. As Harrison later laconically noted, 'After that we started putting it in our own coffee.' That first night, singularly unprepared for the madness to come, Lennon and Harrison insisted on driving to a discotheque. When they arrived they got the full Christopher Mayhew 'extraordinary gradations of mauve' experience and thought the club was on fire, even though it was just the light cast from ordinary street lamps. Fire seemed to be a common motif throughout the trip. When they got into the lift to go up to the discotheque, they all assumed that was on fire as well because of the glowing effect of the red indicator light above the floor buttons. Later they went on to the Ad Lib club, from which they eventually emerged screaming into the night, before crawling back to George's house, with Harrison driving at a sedate 15 mph while doing his best not to be distracted by his cackling passengers. Lennon cracked manic jokes, while George's wife Pattie, seeing some goalposts in a field, insisted on getting out and playing football. Back chez Harrison everyone eventually went to bed, leaving Lennon alone. Having decided that the house was a submarine he spent all night navigating the building as it floated above the Harrisons' 18 ft garden wall. He also did some drawings, which he later gave to Ringo Starr, of four faces saying, 'We all agree with you.'

The effect all of this had on the Beatles' music announces itself with the multicoloured explosion of 'Tomorrow Never Knows' in April 1966 and concludes with the dreamy vapour trails of 'Across the Universe' in February 1968. And in between the two the Beatles reshaped pop as we know it.

'Tomorrow Never Knows' was the group's eureka moment. The song's imaginative use of tape loops and montage brought avant-garde techniques into the mainstream, liberating them from the increasingly arid and complacent world of the conservatoire, and its effect was long-lasting, particularly on the conservatoire world itself. 'I never go to classical concerts any more and I don't know anyone who does,' said composer and critic Ned Rorem in January 1968. 'I do often attend what used to be called avant-garde recitals, though seldom with delight, and inevitably I look around and wonder: What am I doing here? What am I learning? Where are the poets and painters and even composers who used to flock to these things? Meanwhile the absent artists are at home playing records; they are reacting again, finally, to something they no longer find at concerts. Reacting to what? To the Beatles, of course.'[6]

This reaction against academicism had been building for some time in the multimedia world. Dissatisfaction with avant-garde orthodoxy had been the primary impulse behind the Neon Rennaisance, the Acid Tests and all the other immersive environments, but it was the Beatles who took the popularisation of experimental techniques to another level. 'Tomorrow Never Knows' showed just what was possible when the pop world and the avant-garde found common ground.

The song's lyrics were partly inspired by Timothy Leary, Ralph Metzner and Richard Alpert's acid manual *The Psychedelic Experience*. Subtitled 'A Manual Based on the Tibetan Book of the Dead', it was a loose and somewhat tenuous translation of a 1927 theosophist interpretation of pages reputedly taken from an ancient Buddhist text. Only the opening lines of 'Tomorrow Never Knows' are lifted directly from Leary, Metzner and Alpert's book (the relevant

section reads, 'Whenever in doubt turn off your mind, relax, float downstream') but other key phrases are adapted from the sections entitled 'The First Bardo Instructions' and 'Vision Six: "The Retinal Circus"'. The First Bardo makes reference to 'game existence', while Vision Six refers to 'The Buddhas of the Realm of Game Existence'. Elsewhere in Vision Six the synaesthesia of 'Words become things, thoughts are music, music is smelled, sounds are touched' is echoed in Lennon's 'see the meaning of within' and 'listen to the colour of your dreams'. Lennon stated on more than one occasion that he had neither the patience nor the inclination to read the entire tome. Indeed, he later referred disparagingly to 'that stupid book of Leary's', but his characteristically acerbic dismissal couldn't entirely disguise his familiarity with key sections of *The Psychedelic Experience*. Throughout the song he shows distinctive evidence of having read and distilled the text to its essence. As, for instance, with these two extracts from the First Bardo:

The life process. Do not fear
it. Surrender to it. Join it. It is
part of you. You are part of it.
Remember also: Beyond the restless
flowing electricity of life is the
ultimate reality – The Void. Your

*own awareness, not formed into
anything possessing form or color, is
naturally void.*

*Unobstructed; shining, thrilling,
blissful. Diamond consciousness.
The All-Good Buddha. Your own
consciousness, not formed into
anything, No thought, no vision, no
color, is void. The intellect shining
and blissful and silent – This is
the state of perfect enlightenment.
Your own consciousness, shining,
void and inseparable from the great
body of radiance, has no birth, nor
death.[7]*

On one occasion Lennon made an offhand reference to what he described as 'Leary's pamphlet', which makes it likely that he adapted at least some of his source material from the *Psychedelic Review*. Issue 7 of the magazine, published early in 1966, contains Leary's 'Five Psychedelic Prayers Adapted from the Tao Te Ching', several of which utilise imagery not dissimilar to that contained in 'Tomorrow Never Knows'. The third prayer, for instance, contains the lines 'All things / all images / move slowly within' and 'All forms emerge from this second / back to the ancient beginning.'

'Tomorrow Never Knows' begins with an invitation and ends with a mantra to rebirth. En route Lennon acts as polysensory tour guide, taking us through the various stages of ego death and enlightenment. He stretches his vowel sounds on 'dyy-ing' and 'shiiiyning' to replicate the time distortions and warped perceptions of the acid trip. As with most of his psychedelic songs ('Rain', 'Strawberry Fields Forever', 'I Am the Walrus') he delivers the lyric in a somnambulistic drawl over a droning melody. George Harrison would become the Beatles' most enthusiastic exponent of Indian music, but it is Lennon who first references its sonority and harmonic stasis. Psychedelic drugs softened his rasp and his Dylan sneer, as well as compounding the stoned languidity already apparent in 'You've Got to Hide Your Love Away', 'Nowhere Man' and 'Girl'. On 'Tomorrow Never Knows' Lennon's delivery alternates between clarity and slur, surging and retreating as if by neurological impulse as it rises and falls in synch with the sound bed of audio concrète. At certain points his pronounciation becomes so blurred it is almost buried beneath the montage of loops. The accumulative effect of the interplay between the submerged textures of Lennon's larynx, the lyrical longing for transcendence and the sudden hallucinatory bursts of studio effects transform 'Tomorrow Never Knows' into the first truly convincing recreation of the psychedelic experience on record. In 1966 this was nothing less than a revelation.

The sources used for the tape loops were a seagull-squawk effect devised by Paul McCartney; two mellotron loops featuring the instrument's flute and string settings; a sustained orchestral chord of B flat major; a tambura drone played by George Harrison; and a reversed guitar line sampled from 'Taxman' and played by McCartney. Although they sound random and anarchic on first hearing, there was nothing random about the way in which they were utilised. The loops possess an internal logic of their own, offering abstract counterpoint as they respond to the lyric line. Each intricately crafted tape layer adds atonal orchestration to the overall piece. This was an incredible logistical achievement considering that they were mixed in live. EMI's engineers had to adopt an all-hands-to-the-pump approach to the sound desk, with all the tapes running simultaneously in real time. Bootleg recordings exist of a trial run-through of 'Tomorrow Never Knows', tape loops and all, which make its audacious intent even clearer. Lennon's vocal is low in the mix and the sound balance uneven.

Faders are opened and closed arbitrarily, allowing the listener to experience the extraordinary bricolage created by the loops as they thread in and out of the song.

Lennon's working title for the song was 'The Void', but he changed it in honour of one of Ringo's legendary non sequiturs ('A Hard Day's Night', 'Eight Days a Week', etc.). This one originated in 1964, when fervent fans tried to cut off the drummer's hair. In a BBC interview he is heard to say, 'I was just talking, having an interview. I looked round, and there were about 400 people just smiling. So, you know, what can you say?' 'What can you say?' asks John drily. 'Tomorrow never knows,' Ringo responds. It speaks volumes for the Beatles' democratic principles and their unceasing use of humour as a leveller that Lennon was prepared to sacrifice a title that embodied his thoughts on cosmic consciousness and replace it with Ringo's more earthbound contemplation of the unknown. Like most of Ringo's famous word jumbles, it was temporal in nature, but then Ringo always was the most grounded of the Beatles – grounded in time and place, grounded in circumstance, grounded in rhythm, grounded by nature. It was Ringo who, when asked how the newly minted pop millionaires spent their time off, responded, 'Well, sometimes I go round John's house and play with his toys and sometimes he comes round my house and plays with mine.' It was Ringo who returned home first from the visit to the Maharishi in India, comparing Rishikesh to Butlins. As well as possessing a barbed wit he is often the most undervalued member of the group, all too often cast as the willing fool. His drumming, the one compositional element, it is fair to say, that didn't have readers of William Mann or Wilfred Mellers rushing to consult their *New Grove Dictionaries*, really comes into its own on the Beatles' psychedelic songs. That lolloping hop-and-a-skip tape-treated beat, first heard on 'Ticket to Ride', dovetails perfectly with Lennon's disorientating drowsy delivery on many of the Beatles' psychedelic high points.

On 'Tomorrow Never Knows' Lennon locked himself into the drone world and stayed there for the best part of a year. His legendary instruction to George Martin was to ask the producer if he could make his vocals recreate the sound of thousands of Tibetan monks chanting from a mountain top. La Monte Young and the west-coast minimalists had been exploring the same territory for some time. Ramon Sender at the San Francisco Tape

Music Center had been experimenting with sustained low tones since the early 1960s. 'I had a very large Tibetan gong,' he said. 'I found that if I scraped it with a very stiff piece of plastic and then dropped the pitch about three or four times, going from high speed to low speed, I finally got this sound that sounded like a whole bunch of monks chanting.'[8] Sender and his fellow Tape Center collaborator Bill Maginnis worked with drone pieces constructed entirely out of stacked loops. His favourite was a tape piece he took from Maginnis, which he then slowed down umpteen times and overlaid with his own readings from *The Tibetan Book of the Dead*. He also mentioned that he liked to listen to the completed piece while on LSD. These explorations predate 'Tomorrow Never Knows' by two years. Film-maker Jordan Belson provides similar antecedents with *Allures* (1961), *Re-entry* (1964) and *Phenomena* (1965), a series of abstract cinematic paintings that made use of manipulated light projection and, in the case of *Phenomena*, influences drawn directly from *The Tibetan Book of the Dead*.

The Beatles had always been great embellishers and assimilators, but it was during their psychedelic period that these tendencies peaked. Their genius is often taken as a given but less attention is paid to the willingness and rapidity with which they absorbed new ideas. Paul McCartney's man-about-town affability and interest in the avant-garde during this period is well documented, whereas Lennon is usually portrayed as the stay-at-home hedonist, the drug-addled dad who could barely get off the sofa to give Julian his tea (or pass him his crayons). But it was Lennon who presided over the Beatles' psychedelic baptism, and it was Lennon who inspired George Martin to take the group's use of the studio as a compositional tool to a whole new level. Lennon was the initial enabler and conduit through which the Beatles' psychedelic output flowed.

'Rain', the B-side of McCartney's nifty, satirical 'Paperback Writer', introduced backward guitars and reversed vocals to the Beatles' sound palette, and to a large portion of the record-buying public. Again, the Beatles didn't invent the technique. Reversed tape had provided the rhythmic component of Ferrante and Teicher's version of 'The Lady Is a Tramp', which featured on their album *Dynamic Twin Pianos* in 1960. (Ferrante and Teicher probably deserve an entry in the pre-psychedelia hall of fame for the way in which they used echo as percussion and made undiscovered worlds audible simply by hammering at piano keys in a dementedly unclassifiable manner.) After they adopted the technique on 'Rain', reversed tape became part of the Beatles' textural landscape. So enthused was Lennon when he first heard the effect that in his acid pomp he asked for the entire song to be reversed before it was released. On 'Rain' sonic distortion was once again complemented by the hazy drawl of the vocal. The stretched vowel sounds that were such a feature of 'Tomorrow Never Knows' were elongated to the nth. The words 'rain' and 'shine' were stretched over thirteen beats, where previously there might have been a chorus or middle eight. Unlike the instructive treatise of 'Tomorrow Never Knows', 'Rain''s lyrical content verges on the bland. The rain, like everything else in Lennon's physical world at this point, is just a state of mind. 'Rain' gives the first real indication of the acid-compliant Lennon, the brain-zapped Lennon who would have nothing to say but 'It's OK' on 'Good Morning Good Morning'. Similar sentiments were apparent on 'I'm Only Sleeping' – which also features disorientating bursts of backward guitar. But that song is chiefly a by-product of Lennon's indolence. 'Rain' reduces a razor-sharp intellect to childlike awe. It's an acid convert's joy at seeing rain for the first time and marvelling at its essence.

'She Said She Said' reveals an altogether different side to Lennon's surrender to the void. On 'Tomorrow Never Knows' subjugation is unconditional; on 'She Said She Said' it comes with caveats. In the midst of bliss Lennon is in touch with his inner curmudgeon and having a bloody good moan. 'She Said She Said' is one of *Revolver*'s two great whinge tracks, 'Taxman' being the other. On the latter George Harrison lays down that great James Brown and Booker T. riff that became the prototype for mod psych. At the same time he has a gripe about the amount of income tax that the band is having to pay to the Exchequer. This very secular song emanates from a man on the verge of spiritual rebirth. 'She Said She Said' introduces us to that other acid perennial, the bum trip. Many LSD users have reported that after experiencing the life-altering multiverse opened up by that first revelatory venture into inner space, negotiating the second encounter is often a little more fraught. And so it transpired with the Beatles. In August 1965, in the idyllic setting of a ranch-house retreat in Benedict Canyon, Los Angeles, Lennon and Harrison took what was their second acid trip. They also reputedly

introduced Ringo Starr to the drug. Roger McGuinn, David Crosby and Joan Baez were at the ranch house too, as was actor Peter Fonda, who annoyed the arse off Lennon by repeatedly telling him he knew what it was like to be dead. Lennon's riposte, which he included in the original lyric, was 'Who put all that shit in your head?' Fonda has always maintained that he was trying to ease Lennon through his chemical turbulence by relating a near-death experience he'd had as a boy, when he accidentally shot himself. He thought he was being helpful by displaying the still-visible stomach scar from the original bullet wound, but this merely sent Lennon into a downward spiral, and in an attempt to ward off an impending bad trip he had Fonda ejected from the party. Viewed half a century later this oft-repeated tale seems faintly comical, but its central scenario will be familiar to any day tripper whose best-laid plans for a little recreational space travel have been ruined by the presence of that acid perennial, the vibe killer. When people talk about the Beatles' common touch they probably don't have 'She Said She Said' in mind, but in its own mind-altered way the song is as much of a reminder of mortality and mundanity as 'When I'm Sixty-Four'.

'She Said She Said' is essentially

an inner dialogue that Lennon has in order to keep himself anchored to sanity. Where 'Tomorrow Never Knows' is both expansive and inviting 'She Said She Said' is an incantatory spell cast upon a divided self. It is constantly warding off and waving away, forever refuting, permanently sidestepping pitfalls and dangers. The only mantra it offers is 'No, no, no, you're wrong.' One of the most rhythmically irregular songs that Lennon ever wrote, 'She Said She Said' marks out the disturbed psychological terrain that Syd Barrett would later make his own, all lurches and leaps, the sound of irrationality and reason criss-crossing and colliding. 'Tomorrow Never Knows' welcomes ego death. 'She Said She Said' fears it.

'Tomorrow Never Knows' was presented by Lennon to his colleagues in the spring of 1966 not so much as a fait accompli but as a blueprint for further explorations, a route map for soul and psyche. 'She Said She Said' was recorded in June 1966, almost a year after it was conceived. The two songs effectively bookend the *Revolver* sessions, the first and last tracks to be recorded. Had 'She Said She Said' not been so hastily completed in order to sign off the album, who knows what might have been achieved had it been given the tape-loop treatment. They

are in the end, though, two very different songs and they illustrate the schismatic nature of Lennon's acid encounters. 'Tomorrow Never Knows' resolves itself by ending at the beginning, by acknowledging karma; 'She Said She Said' simply wants to go back to the imagined security of childhood. This regressive aspect is most evident in the way the line 'When I was a boy' leaps out of the song, initiating a sudden change of tempo and an equally abrupt mood swing. The wording is significant: not 'Everything was fine', as in the weather, as in complacent hippie platitudes, but 'Everything was right'. In the midst of chemically induced turmoil Lennon clings to childhood certainties. In the middle of the Beatles' most revolutionary musical period it's not the Hacienda that must be built but an infant Arcadia. 'It was just an "acidy" song, I suppose,' he later mused. '"When I was a little boy," you see. A lot of early childhood was coming out.'[9] It's a throwaway reflection delivered with typical Lennon insouciance, but its implications informed the next eighteen months of the Beatles' output and, indeed, the next eighteen months of UK psychedelia. Childhood and nostalgia would become the leitmotifs of some of their finest psychedelic work. The group's publicist, Derek Taylor, suggested that when the Beatles took acid, it was a case of 'four Scousers exploring inner space and just finding more and more Scouser down there'. This search for the inner Scouser would have its finest flowering in the double A-sided single 'Strawberry Fields Forever'/'Penny Lane', but the tendency towards reflection and nostalgia would also dominate the mood of *Sgt Pepper's Lonely Hearts Club Band* and the *Magical Mystery Tour* film and EP.

The working method used to construct 'Tomorrow Never Knows' – building an elaborately layered sound montage in the studio from Lennon's basic sketch – was repeated on 'Strawberry Fields Forever'. If anything, the execution is even more remarkable second time around, given that the finished recording is a composite of two seemingly ill-matched components. Various studio snippets have come to light in recent years – some officially released in the *Beatles Anthology* series, others still only available as bootlegs – which allow the listener to eavesdrop on the song during its various stages of development. Lennon's original Weybridge demo shows him struggling with the irregular scansion of his lyrics. 'I cannae do it,' he says softly to himself. Initially he sings 'Let me take you back' rather than 'down'. Early studio versions are sparsely arranged, with Lennon finger-picking the folksy melody on the nylon strings of a classical guitar, while simple augmentations are tentatively suggested by his colleagues – Harrison's slide guitar, a burst of *Pet Sounds* harmonising, McCartney trying out textures and chord progressions on the mellotron. (Even at this early stage he underpins Lennon's childhood evocation with great sensitivity.) Those early unadorned takes allow the listener to hear Lennon's high-register vocal in all its fragile splendour. Already it carries the plangent quality of the song and its underlying sense of yearning. Unburdened by embellishment it reveals some surprising similarities in cadence to McCartney's 'Here, There and Everywhere'.

George Martin provided a punchy arrangement for four trumpets and three cellos, and it is his score that gives the track its rhythmic momentum, adding sparkling Tin Pan Alley brass and meaty strings to Lennon's disjointed perceptions, and lending coherence and continuity to what was possibly the most multi-focused and non-linear lyric he had ever written. The restless narrative, the pitch shifts, the swirling textures, none of these would have been possible without the catalyst of LSD, while the clanging outro, false ending and disturbing dream-loop coda create a sound world quite unlike any that had been heard on an English pop record up to that point.

'Strawberry Fields Forever' and 'Penny Lane' are the Beatles' crowning achievement as a psychedelic unit, perhaps the crowning achievements of psychedelia itself. Each song conveys key aspects of its creator's world view under chemical reconditioning. 'Strawberry Fields Forever' emphasises that nothing is real, each verse ending with a qualifier or disclaimer; 'Penny Lane' is hyperreal and wedded to routine and certainty. Lennon mystifies with each stuttering utterance; McCartney magnifies with matter-of-fact description. And yet when you attempt to trace the topography of 'Penny Lane' you discover that its perspective is as awry as that of 'Strawberry Fields Forever' and that it undermines its certainties with the same dreamlike propulsion. Everything is happening simultaneously in 'Penny Lane' – daytime, nighttime, summer, winter. The song offers a visual paradox similar to that seen in a Magritte painting such as *L'Empire des lumières II* or *La Revolution*. McCartney had begun collecting works by the Belgian surrealist by this time and 'Penny Lane''s conundrums possess a similarly unsettling air of heightened

normality. All the banker lacks is a bowler hat to go with his mac and the affinity with the Magrittean suburban landscape would be complete (and the rhyming scheme would certainly have allowed for it). The real acid giveaway is the line about the pretty nurse thinking she's in a play . . . and she is anyway. Lennon conveys the sense that nothing is real by gently leading the unsuspecting listener into the dream haze of his unsettled psyche; McCartney conveys that 'nothing is real' by casting a glazed gaze upon everyday banality.

Paul McCartney's experience of LSD was very different to John Lennon's and George Harrison's. The last of the four Beatles to take the drug but the first to admit it (as he would later be the last member to leave the group but the first one to do so publicly and thus end it), McCartney feared that LSD might bring on the very things that Lennon and Harrison relished: ego death and the dissolution of personality. Always the most driven member of the Beatles, he initially suspected that LSD might have a detrimental, even fatal effect on his productivity. In spite of his initial reservations, McCartney's acid songs, though few in number, are exquisite. They provide a perceptual counterpoint to Lennon's efforts that throws fresh light on their working relationship, while simultaneously illuminating the best of what was already there. The American religious teacher G. Ray Jordan, speaking of his first LSD session in 1956, described it as being 'more of the same only more so – by which I meant that it was much like my experience before taking LSD, except that there was an entirely new intensity or new dimension to everything'.[10] That perfectly describes Lennon and McCartney on acid: they were just the same as before, only more so.

Always an enthusiastic pot smoker during the Beatles' heyday (and, indeed, for long after the band split), McCartney only finally took LSD in late 1966 (some sources suggest the date was even later). When he made his public admission in June 1967, he claimed that he had only taken the drug four times. For a long time marijuana was mind-altering enough for McCartney. It fuelled some of his best songs on *Help!*, *Rubber Soul* and *Revolver*, without ever becoming intrusive or sappy. The only exception was the clunky surrealism of the face in a jar by the door in 'Eleanor Rigby', which as an image always seemed a tad too self-conscious and out of synch with the mood and narrative momentum of the song. 'Got to Get You into My Life', which Lennon incorrectly ascribed to

McCartney's belated discovery of LSD, was, as McCartney later admitted, an ode to pot. The line 'every single day of my life' ought to have been evidence enough that it was about smoking marijuana rather than taking psychedelics, although of course it could just as easily have been about a girl. The same 'girl and gear' infusion informs McCartney's 'Good Day Sunshine'. His continued preference for hash rather than acid partly explains why he persisted with dreamy melodic love songs like 'Here, There and Everywhere' and third-person ruminations on heartbreak and loneliness like 'For No One' and 'Eleanor Rigby' during the recording of *Revolver*, while Lennon was embarking upon his no-holds-barred voyage to the beyond.

The introduction of LSD into McCartney's writing added fresh perspective to an already rich writing partnership, without noticeably upsetting the equilibrium of that relationship. McCartney could no more have created a word jumble like 'I Am the Walrus' than Lennon could have written 'When I'm Sixty-Four', and although he could be satirical, biting, even mildly vindictive (as 'Drive My Car', 'I'm Looking Through You', 'You Won't See Me' and 'Paperback Writer' amply illustrate), McCartney had the least corrosive wit of all the Beatles. He would never have written anything as sarcastic as 'Taxman' or 'Only a Northern Song', or as ethereal as 'Tomorrow Never Knows'. Being alone and taking a ride and not knowing 'what I would find there' is not the same as unconditionally surrendering to the void.

McCartney's acid songs – 'Penny Lane', 'The Fool on the Hill', 'Magical Mystery Tour' – come clanging with bells on. They are full to the brim with clarity and vigour. Their tone is sprightly, their arrangements buoyant and breezy. Lennon's are conceived and executed as tone poems; McCartney's arrive fully formed. McCartney sounds like he has spring-cleaned his brain, whereas Lennon sometimes sounds like he has flame-throwered his. McCartney's acid songs are painted with bright primary colours; Lennon's are ethereally glazed and hazy of hue. McCartney's acid voice is purposeful and rarely gives way to doubt or indecision; Lennon's has an undertow of malcontentedness which rears up at the most unexpected moments. McCartney would never have envisaged elementary penguins chanting Hare Krishna while giving Edgar Allan Poe a good kicking. Although he lacked Lennon's intuition as a lyricist, McCartney was far more purposeful as an arranger.

Rarely incapable of bringing his musical ideas to fruition, he could usually convey precisely what he wanted in the studio; the piccolo trumpet on 'Penny Lane', which he hummed to George Martin after being inspired by a performance of Bach's second Brandenburg Concerto, is just one fruitful example from the vast repository of melodic inspiration that McCartney possessed at his peak. Lennon, on the other hand, would come to the studio with remnants of visionary impulses, which the band and production staff would then painstakingly attempt to reconstruct, as if reassembling a dream from instructions rendered in some long-forgotten language. The finished products were always magnificent but ultimately Lennon could never reconcile these simulations with the acid utopias summoned by his imagination. He is on record as saying he would still have preferred actual monks chanting on 'Tomorrow Never Knows', but what he really meant was the monks he heard in his own body temple at the height of his trip. Lennon also wanted to re-record 'Strawberry Fields Forever', and remained dissatisfied with the record's masterful synchronisation of incongruent elements. He expressed a similar wish to re-record 'Lucy in the Sky with Diamonds', which he considered, on reflection, lyrically contrived; the arrangement he thought too literal. He loved the cut-up of calliopes and steam organs on 'Being for the Benefit of Mr Kite' but thought the song itself trite. Compare all this with McCartney's initial disbelief that he had written the melody of 'Yesterday' and that it must have come from somewhere else, from some talent greater than his own. McCartney could craft standards out of commonplace aspirations and modest expectations (particularly when it came to lyric writing). Lennon, the overreacher, frequently aspired to the immortal, but always had to settle for less.

Between them Lennon and McCartney pretty much encompassed the creative possibilities of the LSD experience: Lennon internalising, McCartney externalising; Lennon painting messy mindscapes, McCartney painting domestic murals; Lennon working with large-scale canvases, McCartney crafting immaculate miniatures; Lennon channelling the unconscious, McCartney reportaging the actual; Lennon seeking truth in essentials, McCartney finding it in the incidentals. What they share, what all the best psychedelic Beatles songs share, in fact, is a penchant for images and ideas that are rooted in the quotidian and conveyed in familiar vernacular. There is an absence of simile and analogy in their acid songs, no tortuous metaphor, no poetry concrète, no cut-ups, nothing designed to alienate. Even the acrostic in 'Lucy in the Sky with Diamonds' was arrived at accidentally. Musically the Beatles embraced modernism at every turn. Lyrically they remained traditionalists, even when they were exploring the frontiers of inner and outer space. When it came to the cleansing wash of the English Tizer-Aid acid test, their powers of clear-eyed perception remained undiminished. Even on LSD they are acid everymen as often as they are seers and sages.

There's another narrative voice in all this that is never remarked upon. It partly springs from the Beatles' inner Scouser, but it carries echoes of their girl-group surrogacy too. It's a woman's voice, a working-class woman at that, gossipy, domestic, matter-of-fact when it wants to be but prone to wandering off the subject and making a short story long when circumstances permit. It tugs maternally at your sleeve and says, 'Do you remember that old children's home at Strawberry Fields we used to go and explore? And you'll never guess who I saw down Penny Lane the other day. That fireman – the one who's always acting strange. Did you read in the paper, about all them holes in Blackburn? Something should be done, it really should. Things are looking up, though, aren't they? That's what I think anyway. Well, it can't get much worse, can it? Stands to reason. Oh, didn't you know? She ran off with that fancy man. You know the one. The man from the motor trade. Her poor parents. What must they think? Isle of Wight is it again this year? Don't forget to send us a postcard. Must dash.'

LSD put people in touch with their feminine side in all kinds of unforeseen ways. It prettified mod groups and softened their blues hollers and howls, but with the Beatles it infiltrated their common touch too. 'Penny Lane', 'Strawberry Fields Forever', 'She's Leaving Home', 'When I'm Sixty-Four', 'Getting Better' and 'A Day in the Life' are as gender neutral as some of their best girl-group songs. Even when moments of male pain and misogynist confessional emerge, as they do unpleasantly on 'Getting Better', there's always Lennon and McCartney's reassuring call and response, like two women chatting across adjacent backyards as they peg out the washing.

If acid Paul is thesis and acid John is antithesis, acid George is synthesis. The youngest member of the Beatles, he was arguably the most accomplished musician, but indisputably the slowest developer of the three songwriters. Prior to *Revolver* his only convincing group compositions had been 'I Need You' on *Help!* and the Byrds-influenced 'If I Needed Someone' on *Rubber Soul*. Unlike Lennon and McCartney, who were both at the height of their creative powers by the time they encountered LSD, Harrison discovered psychedelics at the exact moment he was beginning to blossom as a songwriter. 'Love You To', one of the stand-out tracks on *Revolver*, was an astounding and unprecedented excursion into Indian music, yet it was only the sixth of Harrison's songs to have been recorded by the Beatles. His LSD experiences proved to be more tumultuous and life-changing than Lennon and McCartney's. More importantly, they irrevocably shifted the personality dynamics within the group. Until the arrival of LSD Harrison had been the junior partner. Acid changed all that. It was John and George, remember, not John and Paul who first set sail for Pepperland.

Bonded by their mutual experience, Lennon and Harrison became the best of acid buddies. Subsequently they embarked upon a multitude of trips, simultaneously surrendering to the void in their search for the meaning of beyond and within. Their initial encounters with LSD were remarkably similar and elicited similarly evangelical responses in song. The crucial difference was that Harrison ultimately found LSD life-affirming, and it put him on a spiritual quest that he pursued for the rest of his life. Lennon, after taking heroic doses of the stuff, ultimately found LSD disabling and subsequently had to go through a long, painful process of reconnection in order to restore his battered ego and scrambled sense of self. Although he recognised its limitations, Harrison never renounced LSD, and his later recollections contrasted sharply with Lennon's more acerbic dismissals. Speaking to Jann Wenner in 1970, during his famously therapeutic exorcism of Beatle John, Lennon recalled that 'I got a message on acid that you should destroy your ego, and I did, you know. I was reading that stupid book of Leary's and all that shit . . . and I destroyed myself.'[11] Speaking to *Rolling Stone* magazine for its twentieth-anniversary issue in 1987, Harrison claimed that LSD 'was like opening the door really, and before you didn't even know there was a door there. It just opened up this whole other consciousness, even if it was down to, like Aldous Huxley said, the wonderful folds in his grey flannel trousers.' Lennon looks back in anger and cites Leary with malice and misgiving. Harrison unwittingly perpetuates the mythology of those grey flannel trousers but acknowledges the life-enhancing joy of the encounter.

Personality-wise Harrison was every bit as complex as Lennon. His songs could veer from the transcendental to the secular in the blink of a third eye. 'Love You To' yin and yangs between earthly desire and eternal love. 'Taxman' is full of nouveau-riche resentment. The two songs were recorded within seven days of each other! Harrison was also one of the least flamboyant lead guitarists in the history of rock and roll, and the way in which he incorporated the timbres and techniques of Indian music into his repertoire was similarly unshowy. The first evidence of his interest in Indian music was his sitar-playing on 'Norwegian Wood', recorded in December 1965. On the Lennon composition he simply replicated the melody line of the lead guitar, but his subsequent forays into Indian music were considerably more accomplished. The tambura drone which introduces 'Tomorrow Never Knows' and underpins the second half of the song, the reversed guitar part on 'I'm Only Sleeping', transposed so that it resembles a sitar, the subtle swarmandal-playing on 'Strawberry

Fields Forever' and the tambura reprise on the fourth verse of 'Getting Better' all provide integral compositional elements rather than mere decorative effect and reveal just how rapidly Harrison acquired a feel for Eastern modalities and textures.

Harrison first encountered Indian music in less than auspicious circumstances while the Beatles filmed *Help!* in 1965. The film has little of the wit and charm of its predecessor, *A Hard Day's Night*. Its plot is trite, and to modern eyes and sensibilities parts of it now appear unpleasantly racist. *Help!* stars a 'browned-up' Leo McKern as a Hindi high priest called Clang who is trying to retrieve a sacred ring from Ringo Starr. Dialogue and plot lines resound with Asian and oriental stereotypes and 'oh dear dear dear' mannerisms. There are jokes about the Black Hole of Calcutta and lots of Gunga Din-style humour which wouldn't have looked out of place in a *Carry On* film. To complete the caricatures there's a Turkish belly dancer, a loincloth-wearing man who meditates while standing on his head and another who sleeps on a bed of nails. Human sacrifice to the goddess Kali is an integral part of the plot. Apart from the excellent song sequences the only real pleasure to be had is trying to spot the scenes in

which the group are clearly off their heads – by now they had discovered pot-smoking in a big way and Lennon and Harrison had already received their acid initiation. It was during the Indian restaurant scene in *Help!* that Harrison first picked up the sitar that was being played by a member of the resident house band. Soon afterwards he went out and bought one for himself.

There was nothing faddish about Harrison's motives for exploring Eastern music; the depth and sincerity of his interest was indisputable. Indeed, so sincere was he that he abandoned plans to immerse himself entirely in the study of Indian music when, after consultation with Ravi Shankar, he came to the realisation that such an all-consuming apprenticeship could not realistically be embarked upon at the ripe old age of twenty-three. Even though this was only five years older than Shankar had been when he began his musical studies, it represented a lifetime in terms of the two men's cultural differences. Harrison didn't wish to dabble, musically or philosophically. His incorporation of his spiritual leanings into his music was embarked upon with the same ascetic zeal that Lou Harrison, John Cage and Gary Snyder possessed when they began applying Zen teachings into their work. Nor did

Harrison wish to adopt the play-in-a-day approach to the sitar that was so popular (and much ridiculed) among his pop contemporaries. He diligently avoided the temptation to reduce the richness of Hindustani music to cliché. His enthusiasm and the body of work that emerged while he was under the influence of Shankar was unique to English pop at the time. It was more akin to devotional music than exotica, and could sometimes seem dour even to the most open-minded Beatles fan. 'Within You Without You', his sole writing credit on *Sgt Pepper*, is not only completely out of step with the rest of the album, it is philosophically judgemental at a time when the moral compass of the counter-culture favoured benign tolerance.

After the group's last live concert performance at Candlestick Park, San Francisco, on 29 August 1966 Harrison announced, 'That's it. I'm no longer a Beatle.' Brian Epstein had to talk him out of leaving the group. Harrison had been the first Beatle to want to stop touring, and had recoiled even more than Lennon at the sheer hysterical onslaught of Beatlemania. In September 1966, while Lennon went off and filmed *How I Won the War*, McCartney played with his tape loops and Ringo played with his toys, George and Pattie

Harrison visited India as guests of Ravi Shankar. The guitarist was immediately struck by the central role that spirituality played in people's everyday lives and how even the secular seemed religious, and even though he initially over-romanticised his experiences, as so many others, from Carl Jung to Allen Ginsberg, had done before him, his visit was to prove both life-affirming and life-changing.

Ginsberg and Peter Orlovsky had made a similar journey in 1962, visiting Swami Shivananda in the foothills of the Himalayas. As Barry Miles's biography of Ginsberg recalls, 'It was at Shivananda's ashram that Allen learned the Hare Krishna mantra in which the various names of Vishnu are repeated. Ginsberg was the first to introduce this to the United States.' Ginsberg and Orlovsky, along with poet Gary Snyder, also visited the heavily guarded compound of the Dalai Lama, who had been living in exile since fleeing the Chinese invasion of Tibet in 1959. Ginsberg asked him about the relationship between meditation and drug-induced states. 'The Dalai Lama gave the same answer everyone else did,' Snyder later recalled in his journal: 'drug states are real psychic states, but they aren't ultimately useful to you because you didn't get them on your own will and effort.

For a few glimpses into the unconscious mind and other realms they may be of use in loosening you up. After that you can too easily rely on them rather than undertaking such a discipline as will actually alter the structure of the personality in line with these insights. It isn't much help just to glimpse them with no ultimate basic alteration of the ego that is the source of lots of the psychic-spiritual ignorance that troubles one.'[12]

Harrison eventually came to similar conclusions himself, but in the short term his concerns were more pragmatic: how to reconcile his new-found world view with the day job. Asked in 1987 if religiosity had helped him cope with the rigours of Beatlemania, he replied, 'All the panic and pressure? Yeah, absolutely. Although up until LSD I never realized that there was anything beyond this state of consciousness . . . The first time I took it, it just blew everything away. I had such an overwhelming feeling of well-being, that there was a God, and I could see him in every blade of glass. It was like gaining hundreds of years of experience within 12 hours. It changed me and there was no way back to what I was before. It wasn't all good because it left a lot of questions as well. And we still had to continue being fab, you know?'[13]

During this period Harrison's music continued to oscillate between the earthly and the elevated. 'It's All Too Much', his most unrepentant acid song, was as much an exercise in levity as levitation and it contains the best evocation of the transience of the LSD trip that anyone ever wrote: 'Show me that I'm everywhere and get me home for tea.' In the midst of her first physical contortions Lewis Carroll's Alice worries if Dinah, her cat, will be getting her teatime saucer of milk. At the end of her adventures, just after the playing cards have risen up against her only to turn harmlessly into fluttering leaves, Alice awakes by the river bank. She relates her adventure to her sister, and the first thing her sister says is: 'It *was* a curious dream dear, certainly, but now run in to your tea. It's getting late.' It was ever thus, it seems. Thrust skywards by lysergics but grounded by pragmatism, George offers the same route home, the Grantchester clock at ten to three and buttered scones for tea. As a treatise on temporary enlightenment it has much to recommend it, and those sentiments, see-sawing between the thrill of space travel and the happy touchdown on terra firma, were enthusiastically endorsed by many a day tripper who, like Harrison, had perceived that while acid afforded a temporary glimpse of heaven, you wouldn't want to pin an entire philosophy to its kite tails. 'It's All Too Much' was Harrison's honest rejoinder to 'Day Tripper'. 'We are all day trippers,' he seems to be saying. 'That's the only ticket that LSD will allow you to buy, the ultimate acknowledgement that acid apportions its insights and discoveries in bright, spectacular starbursts, but the rest, my friend, is up to you.' Harrison, like many others, soon came to realise that LSD might show you heaven in a grain of sand, but it is still just a grain of sand. Philosopher Alan Watts said in 1972, 'My retrospective attitude to LSD is that when one has received the message one hangs up the phone. I think I have learned from it as much as I can'.[14] Watts mentioned that many people he knew who had enjoyed constructive experiences with LSD had then turned to spiritual disciplines, 'abandoning their water wings and learning to swim', as he put it. 'Without the catalytic experience of the drug they might never have come to this point, and thus my feeling about psychedelic chemicals as about most other drugs . . . is that they should serve as medicine rather than diet.'[15] George Harrison also learned not to confuse dietary supplement with supplicant. Like Watts, he also hung up the phone once he had got the message,

abandoned his water wings and learned to swim.

'It's All Too Much' combines physical love, ego loss and spiritual oneness as well as any song the Beatles recorded during their psychedelic phase. 'The more I learn the less I know' was the clearest signpost yet to where Harrison was heading. It was also the closest the Beatles ever came to jamming on record. A wild squall of feedback commences the song, and as Harrison sings of his encounter with the shining love light his awestruck utterances are punctuated by the most vitriolic screeds of rhythm guitar that John Lennon would commit to vinyl, until he made 'Cold Turkey'. Ringo Starr's drumming alternates between tape-slowed proto-trip hop and stoned stumble and clatter. At times he loses the beat completely and by the end has reduced proceedings to an undignified Dave Clark Five stomp, with the band reciting the song title like it's a football-terrace chant. (Anyone who has heard the unabridged fourteen-minute version of 'It's All Too Much' will know why it was faded on record when it was.) In the dying moments of the song, with pop sensibilities to the fore, Harrison playfully quotes the opening lines of the Merseys' 1966 hit 'Sorrow' (which are themselves reprised at the end of the Merseys' version in raga style) and follows this with an eerie modal scat. It's the sound of Harrison the pop fan and Harrison the truth-seeker in perfect harmony.

Unlike Lennon, who proved capable of rousing himself from his drug-induced sabbatical to knock out a couple of masterpieces for the new album, Harrison wrote virtually nothing during this period, or nothing he presented to the Beatles at any rate. His contribution to *Sgt Pepper* is minimal compared with his input on *Revolver*, and yet his sole writing credit is unforgettable. 'Within You Without You' reflects a growing disenchantment with shallow materialism, as well as doubts about the direction of the group itself. The opening words of each verse – 'We were talking' – mimic the instructional style of a guru or Zen master. Gently cajoling at first but increasingly dogmatic as it proceeds, 'Within You Without You' seems to be aimed as much at his band members as at the wider world. It also confirms the degree to which Harrison the scholar had familiarised himself with a range of Indian musical styles. The song features uncredited musicians playing dilruba, swarmandal, tabla and tambura in a concoction that owes nothing to Western pop. George Martin's additional orchestral

colourations seem a tad superfluous and tread a fine line between sympathetic embellishment and sophisticated pastiche. Indeed, sophisticated pastiche may well have been Martin's greatest contribution as an arranger. He could more than adequately pastiche the exotic motifs of the Beatles' music, as his score for the *Yellow Submarine* film amply illustrates. 'Theme One', the specially commissioned piece that Martin wrote to launch the BBC's first pop network, Radio 1, in 1967, stands as an inspired composition in its own right. Drenched in phasing, it is an audio fanfare to the spirit of the age, an affirmation of a mindset. The fact that Radio 1 was launched with a psychedelic instrumental speaks volumes about the times.

Although frequently disparaged, 'Within You Without You' is the most radical piece of music on *Sgt Pepper*. You only have to contrast its moral certainties with the blasé air and breezy indifference that Paul McCartney adopts in 'Fixing a Hole' to see how far and how fast Harrison had flown from the collective nest. McCartney's casual ruminations on the nature of right or wrong (answer: it really doesn't matter) owe more to his hash haze than the transformative powers of LSD. Had Harrison sang those lines they would have been elevated from the circum-stantial into the spiritual and taken on a completely different hue.

McCartney's solution to the increas-ingly burdensome baggage that came with being a Beatle was to devise a persona that the group could get play-ful with, an alter ego they could hide behind. Shrewdly perceiving that the emphasis might be just a little too much on the ego and not enough on the alter, Harrison saw *Sgt Pepper* as another wall of illusion. Like John Lennon, he remained unconvinced by the concept; he also detected, rightly or wrongly, that something was adrift in the ensemble itself, bemoaning the lack of genuine collaboration and the degree of fait accompli with which McCartney imposed his own creative directives. These were astute judgements, made during a period when eminent critics and musicologists were falling over each other to claim that *Sgt Pepper's Lonely Hearts Club Band* represented the pinnacle of pop's evolution. Ken-neth Tynan called the album 'a decisive moment in the history of Western civi-lisation'. Wilfred Mellers, in *Twilight of the Gods*, claimed that the songs were now to be listened to rather than danced to. Adopting McLuhanesque terminol-ogy, he declared *Sgt Pepper* to be 'a ritual involving the young – through its

electronic extension of musical sounds into the environment of the external world – in a ceremonial togetherness without the prop of church or state'.[16] Harrison's misgivings were probably nearer the mark. As a concept *Sgt Pep-per* is flawed; as a collection of songs it is inferior to *Revolver*. On musical merit it probably does not rank among the Beatles' top five LPs; *Revolver*, the 'White Album', *Abbey Road*, *Rubber Soul*, *A Hard Day's Night* and perhaps even *Help!* have more cohesion. Con-ceptual continuity, such as it is, evapo-rates after the first two songs – the title track and the gratingly chummy 'With a Little Help from My Friends', sung by the dispensable Billy Shears, who once he has tried and failed not to sing out of key is never heard from again. There might have been mileage in building an entire album around the plain-man sentiments of Shears and giving Ringo Starr as prominent a cameo role as he enjoys in *A Hard Day's Night* and *Help!*, but as with the concept as a whole, this potential remains undevel-oped. As John Lennon subsequently pointed out, continuity on *Sgt Pepper* simply consists of the tracks segueing into each other.

Paul McCartney's desire to cre-ate an alternative group persona was understandable. Tired of labouring under a punning group name that now seemed anachronistic (although no more anachronistic perhaps than the Rolling Stones, the Beach Boys or the Kinks), McCartney had been much taken with the exotic names of the west-coast groups. He also drew upon another west-coast legacy, one that had been a crucial component of the Acid Tests and the Mime Troupe: the idea of masque play and masquerade. Unfortunately, the weakest thing about the *Sgt Pepper* album is Sgt Pepper himself. The situation could have been resolved simply by making 'A Day in the Life' the title track. The Beatles didn't really need the contrivance of an alter ego. What they really needed was a poetic conceit that would have tapped into the trivial made sublime and revealed the conceptual unity that was there all the time: the acid everyman (and woman), the inner Scouser – that was their one consistently unwavering voice. 'A Day in the Life', with its juxtapositions of the profound and the mundane, carries the conceptual weight and the emotional burden that an imagined band and an end-of-the-pier Billy Shears show could never remotely hope to convey.

Sgt Pepper is actually the great English album that got away, and all because of a simple marketing decision. The group originally intended 'Strawberry Fields Forever' and 'Penny Lane' to be the first two tracks on their new LP, and it is their absence that handicaps *Sgt Pepper* from the outset. The themes they incorporate – transcendental reflection, hazy and crystalline evocations of time and place – are motifs that reoccur throughout *Sgt Pepper*, but without their pivotal role the album never truly adds up to the sum of its parts. Opening each side of *Sgt Pepper* with 'Penny Lane' and 'Strawberry Fields Forever' would have provided a clear statement of intent, and would have given shape and purpose to an uneven and underdeveloped narrative.

George Harrison's 'Only a Northern Song' was also rejected from *Sgt Pepper*, although for qualitative reasons rather than marketing ones. Had it been included its snarky sentiments would have provided a much-needed secular counterpart to the devotional 'Within You Without You'. It would have counterbalanced Harrison's dourness and the forced jauntiness that afflicts the album's weaker tracks. 'Only a Northern Song' is one of the most misunderstood and maligned works in the entire Beatles canon. Conceived in the same curmudgeonly mood that inspired 'Taxman', a superficial reading of the song would suggest that it was merely Harrison's resentful response to not owning the publishing rights to his material. Ian MacDonald subscribes to this reading and dismisses the song in less than seven lines in *Revolution in the Head*, calling it a self-indulgent dirge. As well as raising the question of when exactly a drone becomes a dirge, MacDonald's curt analysis overlooks vital nuances. It's only in the song's chorus that Harrison actually comments on his material circumstances, and even that comes with the caveat that it doesn't matter because ultimately nothing does – a very George Harrison thing to say in 1967. Dig beneath the grouchy surface and 'Only a Northern Song' is as much a comment on Harrison's spiritual quest as it is on the small print of his publishing contract. It is also utterly in keeping with the themes of disembodiment, disengagement and transcendence that inform most of his songs during this period. 'Only a Northern Song' says as much about the illusory nature of existence as 'Tomorrow Never Knows'. It also confronts something none of the Beatles' other psychedelic songs ever fully grapple with: the effect of listening to music on drugs. The chords are going wrong. The band are not quite right. The harmony is out of key. Except they aren't. And it's not. It's you listening late at night, blissed out of your brain.

All four of John Lennon's contributions to *Sgt Pepper* – 'Lucy in the Sky with Diamonds', 'Being for the Benefit of Mr Kite', 'Good Morning Good Morning' and 'A Day in the Life' – draw inspiration from found material: respectively a child's drawing, a circus poster, television and a seemingly random selection of newspaper stories. The use of *objets trouvés* refreshed Lennon's lyric-writing, snapping him out of acid ennui and liberating him from his debt to Bob Dylan and the entrapment of self-expression. These compositional methods dominated Lennon's creativity during the back end of 1966 and the early part of 1967, and it's worth documenting the timeline and the sequence of events in order to illustrate how these found processes impacted upon his writing.

12 December 1966: Lennon watches an episode of the BBC comedy series Meet the Wife *entitled 'This Christmas, Shop Early', starring Thora Hird and Freddie Frinton.*

December 1966: TV ad for Kellogg's Corn Flakes. Jingle goes:

Good morning, good morning,
the best to you each morning.

*Sunshine breakfast, Kellogg's
Corn Flakes,
best for everyone.*

*Late 1966: Julian Lennon brings
home a drawing from his nursery
in Weybridge. He tells his dad that
it's his friend Lucy. In the sky. With
some diamonds.*

*18 December 1966: Heir to the
Guinness fortune, Hon. Tara
Browne, killed in a car crash in
Earl's Court, London. He hadn't
noticed that the lights had changed.*

17 January 1967: The Daily Mail
*publishes on successive pages
coverage of the inquest into Tara
Browne's death and a news-in-brief
item from the now discontinued
'Far and Near' column about a
council survey that has estimated
the number of potholes in need of
repair in Blackburn, Lancashire.*

*19–20 January: Recording session
for 'A Day in the Life'.*

*30–31 January: The Beatles film
a promo for 'Strawberry Fields
Forever' in Knole Park, Sevenoaks,
Kent. On the second day of filming
Lennon buys an original 1843*

*poster advertising Pablo Fanque's
Circus Royal in an antique shop.*

*8 and 16 February: Recording
session for 'Good Morning Good
Morning'.*

*17 and 20 February: Recording
session for 'Being for the Benefit of
Mr Kite'.*

*28 February: Recording session for
'Lucy in the Sky with Diamonds'.*

'Lucy in the Sky with Diamonds' is
the most pastiched psychedelic lyric
of all time. Its florid imagery launched
an entire tradition of marshmallow
munchkins and lemonade-lollipop
lyrics and its legacy can be heard in
countless psychedelic pop songs. It
would be tempting to call 'Lucy' itself
psychedelia-by-numbers had Lennon not built the multicoloured aba-
cus in the first place. Unlike his other
psychedelic-era material, 'Lucy in the
Sky with Diamonds' contains no hint
of menace or abandonment to the void.
Instead its half-waking, half-sleeping
narrator's voice relates an inner travelogue, a child's-eye contemplation of
phantasmagoria that is clearly inspired
as much by *Alice in Wonderland* as it
is by Julian Lennon's nursery scrawl. In

'Lucy in the Sky with Diamonds' Carroll's 'rocking-horse fly' and 'looking-glass insects' become 'rocking-horse people' and 'looking-glass ties'. Claims that the song was actually about LSD can be easily dismissed. The Beatles were rarely coy about their sources and by the time they recorded *Sgt Pepper* their lyrics were liberally scattered with drug references. There is no reason why they would arbitrarily deny a song's origins in 1967. Lyrically 'Lucy' is clearly informed by Lennon's acid saturation but its adult perceptions are framed within a child's-eye view of the world. As with 'Rain' and 'Across the Universe' it's Lennon getting in touch with his inner innocent. The Julian Lennon drawing that gave the song its name evokes the same sense of awe and wonder that inspired some of Juan Miró's best surrealist titles: the 1968 painting *Bird Awakened by the Shrill Cry of the Azure Taking Flight over the Breathing Plain,* for instance; or, better still (and from 1967, no less), *The Lark's Wing, Encircled with Golden Blue, Rejoins the Heart of the Poppy Sleeping on a Diamond-Studded Meadow.* Then again, 'Lucy in the Sky with Diamonds' might just as easily have been inspired by Lennon's love of Burl Ives's 'Big Rock Candy Mountain', with its 'bees in the cigarette trees',

'soda-water fountains' and 'lemonade springs'.

The origins of 'Being for the Benefit of Mr Kite' are also well documented. The original 1843 poster advertising Pablo Fanque's Circus Royal that Lennon found in an antique shop in Sevenoaks while filming the 'Strawberry Fields Forever' promo provided him with his best 'found' lyric. The arcane phrasing of the circus billing reacquainted him with a relish for mimicry that had lain dormant since the publication of *In His Own Write* (1964) and *A Spaniard in the Works* (1965). Those two literary ventures made great play of punning wordplay, parody and grotesque characterisation. Pablo Fanque's celebrated roll call of bizarre acts offered Lennon fresh opportunities to indulge these reawakened pleasures. Only three phrases were lifted verbatim from the original circus poster: the song title itself and the phrases 'having been some days in preparation' and 'lastly through a Hogshead of real fire'. Others – 'over men and horses, through hoops, over garters' and 'Messrs Kite and Henderson', for instance – were adapted or elided in order to fit metre and scansion. Where he doesn't lift the wording directly Lennon provides his own approximations of the posters, Victorian-prose style. A nip here

– twenty-one summersets is changed to ten, the circus location Rochdale becomes the more palette-pleasing Bishopsgate – a tuck there – 'In this branch of the profession Mr H challenges the World' trips off the tongue better in Lennon's version – and, hey presto, the chance retrieval of a discarded item of Victorian ephemera is transformed into something magical and inspired.

'A Day in the Life' is *Sgt Pepper*'s magnum opus and has a sense of the epic that is missing from Lennon's other psychedelic songs. On one level it is a sombre meditation on the intangible nature of unrelated events, on a world where a senseless sudden road death due to a split second of carelessness is accorded equal significance with a council survey about road repairs. On another level it gives added cohesion to an understated narrative thread that runs throughout the entire album. Lennon often complained that several of his songs, from 'Help!' onwards, were either taken at too fast a tempo or ruined with insensitive or over-literal arrangements, but he remained inordinately proud of 'A Day in the Life'. The song proceeds at a stately pace, its sparse verses underscored with simple arrangements – voice, acoustic guitar, piano and minimal percussion

– interspersed with brief orchestral passages that seem to burst in through the paper-thin walls of an adjacent dream. Lennon's lamentation sways between pathos and pessimism, between blithe acceptance and quiet despair. So all-consuming is the battered grandeur that the desire to 'turn you on', intended, and usually interpreted, as a bold, unabashed clarion call, ends up sounding more like a desperate urging for elevation from drab circumstance, by whatever means necessary.

'A Day in the Life' is one of the last songs that Lennon and McCartney collaborated on with any degree of empathy. McCartney's 'Woke up, fell out of bed' interjects urgency and adherence to everyday routine into Lennon's more world-weary and detached contemplation of the humdrum. On an out-take McCartney can be heard overdramatising his cameo role, giving unnecessary rising intonation to 'made the bus in seconds flat' before obviously thinking better of it. On the finished track he delivers his lines with just the right degree of distraction. The contrast between the two narrative voices is embedded sublimely in the details. Lennon is sedentary and reflective; McCartney is bustling and on the move. He has to be somewhere, and he's late. Time only stands still when he has a smoke and goes into his own reverie. Lennon commences and concludes the song in silence and stasis, the idle turning of a page, a brief exhaled 'oh boy', and on to the next mind-numbing snapshot of mundanity.

Some critics made comparisons between 'A Day in the Life''s world-weary ruminations and T. S. Eliot's *The Waste Land*, but its espousals are far more modest. Its piecemeal fragments don't so much reveal fear in a handful of dust as the gradual accumulation of actions and inactions that give meaning and purpose to ordinary lives. It's a theme that runs through the entire LP, and it's *Sgt Pepper*'s great unspoken. There is no grand narrative, just unrelated and unconnected moments frozen in time. Rather than looking to the early-twentieth-century modernism of *The Waste Land*, a more appropriate parallel might be found in the unassuming 1950s provincialism of Philip Larkin's 'The Whitsun Weddings'. Larkin's poem, published in 1964, takes a train journey from Hull to London as its central metaphor for the journey through life. Vignettes of transitory moments are glimpsed fleetingly from the carriage window as the train moves south. The succession of Saturday-afternoon weddings that give the poem its title, each different yet somehow the same, are depicted in all their gaudy and grand display. Meanwhile, the world drifts by, rendered in prose as flat as the Lincolnshire landscape: farms, fields, glinting hothouses, Odeons, cooling towers, breakers' yards – and that perennial summer sight, the cricketer running in to bowl who you never quite manage to see at the moment of delivery. Then suddenly, in the midst of his own quiet ruminations, Larkin utters the lines that bond all these separate events together and show us our own humanity:

> . . . *and none*
> *thought of the others they would*
> *never meet*
> *or how their lives would all*
> *contain this hour.*

And that, ultimately, is the soulful affirmation and *raison d'être* of *Sgt Pepper* too. Not the sketchy unformulated fiction of an Edwardian brass band, but the chance intersections of circumstance and dispassionate depictions of unrelated figures in an unremarkable landscape – some of whom might just think they are in a play and are anyway. Rita, the meter maid. The girl slipping away at dawn to meet a man from the motor trade. And all the others who come and go and come and say hello. Life flows on within them and without them. Even Vera, Chuck and Dave.

For all its flaws there are moments on *Sgt Pepper* where the Beatles truly make the trivial world sublime, but this tendency peaked not with that much-lauded LP, but in the oft-derided charabanc adventure that followed. The received critical wisdom is that *Magical Mystery Tour* is too similar a concept to *Sgt Pepper*, and that by replacing the bandstand with a bus ride Paul McCartney was merely recycling worn-out ideas and old party invitations, but while the initial idea may once again have been patchily thought out and ill executed, it is *Magical Mystery Tour*, not *Sgt Pepper*, that most fully embraces the Beatles' Englishness. The five songs and one instrumental that appear in the film – 'Magical Mystery Tour', 'Fool on the Hill', 'Flying', 'I am the Walrus', 'Blue Jay Way' and 'Your Mother Should Know' – are the best that they ever wrote to order. Each represents a distinct facet of the group's psychedelic vision (celebration, innocence, bliss, absurdity, dislocation and nostalgia respectively). However, the hostility that greeted their grand folly when it was premiered at peak time on the BBC on Boxing Day evening in

December 1967 proved to be a watershed moment.

The late BBC radio producer John Walters once said of Bob Dylan's *Renaldo and Clara* that while it didn't convince him that Dylan was a good movie-maker, it did convince him that Dylan had probably seen a lot of good movies. There is something of this in the *Mystery Tour* too, and it is hard to argue with Ian MacDonald's assessment in *Revolution in the Head* that the Beatles 'wandered drug dozy into the medium of film, assuming that anyone with a few ideas could turn out something watchable'.[17] The least domesticated and only unattached Beatle during 1967, McCartney was always out on the town, assimilating, ears keenly attuned to avant-garde activities. As he's never grown tired of telling us, it was he, not Lennon, who first experimented with tape loops. It was he who checked out AMM and Karlheinz Stockhausen. It was he who devised the as yet still unreleased 'Carnival of Light', the fourteen-minute 'bit of random' that he provided for a mixed-media event at the Roundhouse in January 1967. And it was he who experimented with home-movie-making, citing Expanded Cinema pioneer Bruce Conner as a prime catalyst. A particular influence on McCartney was Conner's 1964 three-minute 16 mm short *Vivian*, which featured his friend Vivian Kurz cavorting playfully while swathed in mummy bandages and demurely smoothing her dress to the accompaniment of Conway Twitty's version of 'Mona Lisa'. Under Conner's spell McCartney sat in a Paris hotel room pointing his movie camera at the gendarmerie outside and then synching the footage up to Albert Ayler's frenetic free-jazz interpretation of 'The Marseillaise', which featured on his 1965 ESP-Disk LP *Spirits Rejoice*. McCartney filtered all of these avant-garde impulses into a homespun version of Ken Kesey's magic bus ride. But whereas Kesey and his intrepid travellers went off in search of America, the Beatles headed for the rolling hills and sandy beaches of the English West Country. Kesey had his friends and colleagues from the Perry writing class for company. The Beatles assembled a rich cast of extras by leafing through the situations-wanted pages of *The Stage*. Here they found Shirley Evans (who plays 'Shirley's wild accordion' in the film) and variety comic actor Nat Jackley ('Happy Nat the Rubber Man'). The Acid Tests had Hugh Romney and Del Close. The *Magical Mystery Tour* had Ivor Cutler, the stern Glaswegian laureate of childlike verse and admonishing

haiku, playing Buster Bloodvessel the tour guide, and Victor Spinetti – who had previously appeared in *A Hard Day's Night* and *Help!* – pantomiming it up as that perennial swinging sixties boo-hiss figure, the army recruiting sergeant. Kesey's house band was the Grateful Dead, who explored blues, folk and mind jazz while high on Owsley Stanley's acid. The Beatles had art-school absurdists the Bonzo Dog Band, who performed a 1950s spoof called 'Death Cab for Cutie', accompanied by a lusty stripper from a Soho revue bar.

George Harrison described *Magical Mystery Tour* as an elaborate home movie. Others were less charitable. Such was the storm that greeted its TV premiere that Paul McCartney felt obliged to appear on *The Frost Report* the following evening to defend it. The problem, as perceived by many viewers, was its lack of plot and disjointed (some might say complete absence of) narrative. Another problem was that it was made in colour at a time when most British households still only had black-and-white TV sets. Because of this crucial set pieces – the photo-chemical tinting of landscape and sky in the 'Flying' sequence, the multi-layered Expanded Cinema effects on 'Blue Jay Way' – were completely lost on the audience. Some suspected that something much deeper was lost too: that previously unbreakable bond between the Beatles and their audience. This was the defining moment, detractors say, when shit hit the fans and the Beatles finally failed to carry the mainstream audience with them. 'Come and see what we've found,' they were saying. 'Come and share our visions.' 'No thanks,' said those who only saw indulgence and incoherence, and especially 'No thanks' said a large portion of the press, who had been waiting for an opportunity to give the Beatles a good kicking for some time and now seized their moment with relish. '"I Am the Walrus," says John. "No, you're not," cries Nicola,' read one of the exchanges in the illustrated storybook that accompanied the *Magical Mystery Tour* EP. If the press was to be believed, little Nicola spoke for a significant section of the audience. Not since Kenneth Tynan had uttered the first 'fuck' on the late-night magazine programme *BBC-3* in November 1965 had a TV show caused such apoplectic headlines and savage reviews. And yet stripped of its accompanying hysteria and viewed with impartiality half a century later *Magical Mystery Tour* comes across as a sweet, good-natured little film, full of humour and brimming with British eccentricity.

As McCartney remarked, it was no worse than most of the TV fare that was served up that Christmas. And it was certainly no worse than most English pop films of the time. Like many a swinging sixties Brit flick, it has its longueurs. In its overlong chase sequences there is more than a hint that the Beatles hadn't shaken off as much of the Dick Lester influence as they might have hoped. What redeems *Magical Mystery Tour* is its irrepressible portrayal of the English at play, its village fete and carnival frolics – the midget wrestlers, the tug of war – and the unmistakable presence of a very British brand of surrealism that is always more daft than Dalí-esque, always closer to Bernard Bresslaw than Luis Buñuel. The scene where Wizard McCartney alerts Wizard Starr as to the whereabouts of the bus – 'ten miles north on the Dewsbury road' – would have been as incomprehensible to an American audience as the concept of a mystery tour itself, but when Ivor Cutler's tour guide Buster Bloodvessel utters his terse instruction to the bus passengers to enjoy themselves 'within the limits of British decency', many of the home audience would have instinctively recognised the stentorian portrayal of the pinched and repressed keep off the grass, playgrounds locked on Sundays, last orders half past ten little England they were living in.

Buster Bloodvessel's stern injunction precedes the most irrepressibly English sequence in the entire film. The shot on a shoestring surrealism of 'I Am the Walrus', nuns, policemen, animal skins and all, is the best bit of footage the Beatles ever conceived. Like the 'Strawberry Fields Forever' promo shot earlier in the year, it resonates with images of the English at our most bonkers. It also irrefutably represents the key moment when elements of the older audience, and some of the younger one too, must have been convinced that John Lennon had finally lost his marbles.

Lennon, as so often, conceived 'I Am the Walrus' as a mood piece and tone poem, and gave little thought initially to its melodic content. In its raw, un-embellished demo state it sounds like a dirge. Its paranoia-inducing two-note motif was reputedly inspired by a passing police siren, and by August 1967, when Lennon wrote the song, there was plenty to be paranoid about. Drug exposés of the pop aristocracy were beginning to appear under the guise of investigative journalism in Sunday newspapers such as the *News of the World* and the *People* as Scotland Yard and the Metropolitan Police

force started to get conspicuously hands-on in their approach to musicians who they thought needed taking down a peg or two. Brian Jones, Keith Richards, Mick Jagger and Donovan had already been busted, and it was widely assumed that 'Pilcher of the Yard' was setting his sights on even bigger prizes; indeed, both Lennon and George Harrison would get their visits soon enough. Panic and paranoia rather than harmony and inner peace were, therefore, fast becoming self-fulfilling aspects of the tripping experience by the time Lennon wrote 'I Am the Walrus'. The lyrics, declaimed savagely and nailed relentlessly to the on-beat for almost the entire song, are delivered in a strangulated bark that contrasts sharply with the airy melancholy of 'Strawberry Fields', the hazy drawl of 'Rain', the mantric drone of 'Tomorrow Never Knows' and the see-saw cadences of 'She Said She Said'. Its opening line only serves to lull the listener into a false sense of security, and once the illusory I Am He oneness has been dispensed with there is little sense of we-are-all-togetherness anywhere else in the song. From the 'Three Blind Mice' refrain of 'See how they run' onwards, 'I Am the Walrus' is a yellow-matter dog spew of word disassociation and random fragments, many of them, Lennon belligerently declared, designed to confuse the lit-crit crowd. Tossed like so many contemptuous bones to the hungry 'expert textperts' for them to chew on, some of these images are clearly anti-authoritarian (the corporation T-shirt, the city police-man, 'Semolina Pilchard' of the Yard), while others are the product of an acid-wracked sensuality (the crabalocker fishwife sounds like Lennon's elliptical response to the fish and finger pie of 'Penny Lane'). The song springs and uncoils with spatial distortions, *Alice in Wonderland* allusions and mucky schoolboy rhymes. There is an awful lot of mucous and messy goo, and enough mild blasphemy to keep 'Disgusted of Tunbridge Wells' in Basildon Bond for weeks. 'I Am the Walrus' surrenders sense and rationale completely to a chemically driven muse. It may have been written as a teasing riposte to the myth-makers and clue-seekers but, paradoxically, it is also the closest Lennon ever came to reproducing the incessant mind babble of the LSD trip without completely spilling over into dribbling incoherence. The song lunges and lurches along like Lewis Carroll's Walrus and Carpenter as they enact their own semantic paso doble while musing on cabbages and kings and whether pigs have wings. Like

Carroll's nonsensical duet, 'I Am the Walrus' gathers crazed momentum as it goes, scattering random word blurts before it, content to reassemble them wherever they settle. The comparison is frequently overused and abused but 'I Am the Walrus' is probably the nearest pop music ever came to painting a genuinely Joycean landscape.

There is something of an acid exorcism going on too: John the joker, laughing himself hoarse, laughing everything into what Richard Meltzer called 'cool semantic oblivion'. 'The key is surrender at every stage. Let the ego go. Let it die,' said Alcoholics Anonymous pioneer Tom Powers in a letter to Betty Eisner in January 1957, as he clarified his own thoughts on the LSD experience. 'The ego is an awful ham,' Powers claimed. 'It always tries to make a tragedy out of its own death. But this, as everything egotistical, is also false. At the death of the ego the real self laughs. Actually the real self laughs well before the ego death and this brings on the happy event as nothing else can. The ego cannot stand to be laughed at; it will go to any lengths to avoid it.'[18] Look at Lennon's expression as he performs 'I Am the Walrus' in the *Magical Mystery Tour* film. Too acid-mangled to gurn and do spazz faces any more, he has the demeanour of a purposeful simpleton; not the fool on the hill, but the fool who would persist in his folly and become wise. The joker who taunts himself as well as laughing at you.

The relentless mania of 'I Am the Walrus' only lets up when the introductory theme is reprised halfway through and Lennon delivers an elegant soliloquy to the English Acid-Test experience. Paul McCartney wills the pretty nurse in 'Penny Lane' to dream her play dreams as she offers poppies from a tray. Pragmatic George wanted to whizz round the universe but still be back by teatime. John Lennon in the not so sunny Summer of Love gazes out at an overcast Weybridge day, thinks of all those drizzly summer fetes and 'Indoors If Wet' signs and imagines everyone getting their tan in the rain. It is an effortlessly evocative image, sublimely surreal and rheumatically English to the marrow.

Any resentment or hostility that the watching audience might have felt towards the Boxing Day broadcast of *Magical Mystery Tour* was more than amply counterbalanced by the fact that for three weeks over the Christmas and new year period the 'Hello, Goodbye' single and the *Magical Mystery Tour* EP were numbers one and two in the UK singles chart. You heard them everywhere and all the time, resplendent in tandem. The title track from the *Magical Mystery Tour* commenced with an innuendo-driven, double-edged invitation to 'Roll up, roll up'. It sallied forth with a fanfare blaze of 'Penny Lane' trumpets and a woozy, slurred 'Mystery Trip' interjected into the bridge, just at the moment when the whole charabanc ride slows to half speed. Strangest of all, and unremarked upon by any critic that I have ever read, is that D to D minor Jazz Sebastian Bach outro, where McCartney doodles the prettiest of piano melodies, and as the song fades we hear a couple of bars of Swingle Singers vocalising. It's the oddest of trip teases, coldly ethereal and yet warmly inviting at the same time. It's as if the group are saying, 'The song was just the fanfare – the real trip begins here, on the other side of this fade.' The compulsively inane chatter of most radio DJs would have obscured it to all but the most eager ears, but that beckoning coda hinted at the promise of what further riches lie beyond and slightly out of reach.

'Hello, Goodbye' remained at number one for seven weeks, the longest run the Beatles had enjoyed at the top of the charts since 'She Loves You'. It was only appropriate that 1967 should have ended like this. All that snowflaky

December the airwaves sparkled to the echo of Paul McCartney's deceptively childlike ditty about a divided self, a self that simultaneously said 'stay' and 'go'. The dualism was significant. Who knew at the time what we were saying hello and goodbye-bye-bye-bye-bye to?

'Jai Guru Deva Om'

'Across the Universe', the last acid song the Beatles recorded, commences with the flutter of a dove and the phrase 'Words are flowing out'. With that utterance John Lennon brought the Beatles' psychedelic phase full circle. A life-changing period of experimentation that had begun just a little under two years earlier with an invitation to 'turn off your mind' came to rest with another meditative treatise on the fluidity of existence. The conclusion Lennon reached was the conclusion the Beatles always seemed to reach: no matter how elusive and ungraspable existence might appear, ultimately everything leads back to love. Coming so soon after the snarls, scoffs and snides of 'I Am the Walrus', 'Across the Universe' is a comfortingly harmonious finale to John Lennon's psychedelic voyage. It is driven by the same restless questing that informed all his psychedelic songs, but 'Across the Universe' offers

a more settled appraisal of the infinite. The thousand chanting monks he once heard in his head have dwindled down to a simple solo mantra: 'Jai Guru Deva Om' – 'Victory to the guru god'. The victory was illusory, of course, but if LSD had taught Lennon anything, he probably knew that already.

The Beatles always acknowledged with honesty and utter candour the direct and very audible effect that psychedelic drugs had on their music. It is hard to think of any other group or artist in a similar position of public prominence in modern times that has spoken so openly on the subject. The fulsome account that George Harrison gives in the *Beatles Anthology* book is one of the most erudite and considered that exists in the vast literature about LSD usage. He acknowledges the initial light-bulb moment of recognition when he first took the drug ('In ten minutes I lived a thousand years') and offers sober reflections that hark back to Huxley ('We didn't conjure up heaven and hell . . . all acid does is shoot you into space, where everything is so much greater. The hell is more hell . . . the heaven is more heaven'). He talks soberly about the drug's limitations ('Although the tablecloth might keep moving or the chairs get small, the basic thing that I first experienced was the thought: 'You shouldn't need this, because it's a state of awareness') and his disillusion with the drug culture ('I presumed mistakenly that everybody who took LSD was a most illuminated being and then I started finding that there were people who were just as stupid as they'd been before'). Ultimately, he comes to the realisation that 'It's the ego identity that fools us into thinking "I am this body". LSD gave me the experience of: "I am not this body. I am pure energy soaring about everywhere that happens to be in a body for a temporary period of time."'[19]

These viewpoints, rationally arrived at and pragmatically articulated, speak for the Beatles' experience of LSD as a whole. 'I didn't know what I would find there' and 'taking the easy way out' led each of them into deeper contemplation of 'the meaning of within' and 'the walls of illusion', and ultimately to a better understanding of themselves and each other, even if that understanding was that ultimately they no longer needed LSD to reach that understanding. LSD for the Beatles was a door that opened, a pathway to be trod, an acknowledgement, as Huxley had acknowledged, that the person who returns from those experiences is not the same as the one that embarked upon the journey. LSD didn't turn the Beatles into saints or seers, although there were those who would have quite happily beatified or crucified them for undertaking the journey in the first place. They became neither acid acolytes nor acid casualties. In the spirit of the times they simply submitted themselves to its sensory onslaught, immersed themselves in its possibilities, marvelled at its pretty twinkling colours and its glimpses of the infinite, and then moved on. Whatever trials or tribulations any of them faced later in life, none can be attributed to their LSD use, which was almost wholly positive and beneficial – beneficial to their music, beneficial to them as human beings, beneficial to the culture their music fed into.

In India, during February 1968, in the tranquillity of the Maharishi's Rishikesh compound, the Beatles wrote the majority of the thirty songs that would appear on an album simply called *The Beatles*. This body of new work contained only the barest of hints that they had ever been a psychedelic pop group. They commissioned pop art pioneer Richard Hamilton to design the sleeve for the LP, which was a shrewd conceptual move. Hamilton's all-white blankscape conveyed both a sense of blinding light and of a slate being wiped clean. 'I did them as an experiment to see how much you could pull away from an image and still have an image,' said Robert Rauschenberg of his own 1951 white-on-white canvases,[20] as he paid homage to a legacy that stretched back to the white-on-white paintings that Russian Suprematist Kasimir Malevich exhibited in 1918. As Hamilton recognised only too well, a multiplicity of ideas and interpretations could be projected onto an all-white canvas. Neutrality, paradoxically enough, was not an option. John Cage's notorious '4' 33"' was directly inspired by Rauschenberg, and his famous assertion that 'There is no such thing as silence' was, as Brandon W. Joseph noted, echoed in Rauschenberg's equally provocative 'A canvas is never empty.' Hamilton achieved the same effect with his Beatles cover. By utilising white on white he similarly drew attention to the image by the very act of being unable to eradicate the image. It was the most apposite and astute LP design the Beatles ever commissioned.

Peter Blake's assemblage of iconic figures for the *Sgt Pepper* cover has been endlessly eulogised, but Hamilton's deceptively illusory gesture of emptiness and absence carries far more conceptual weight. Blake's cover was the culmination of thirty years of post-war English art-school thinking.

It honours pop art's reciprocal relationship with pop music, even though the techniques it utilised were starting to look a little tired and formulaic by 1967. By using cardboard cut-outs Blake made his work intentionally one-dimensional. It is Hamilton's flat surface that has the greater depth. The *Sgt Pepper* sleeve is as cluttered as the typography on an old Victorian circus poster. It is self-consciously populist and anti-hierarchical in the way it frames its gathering, but its assemblage was also eminently open to parody, as Frank Zappa and the Mothers proved the following year with the mocking pastiche displayed on the cover of *We're Only in It for the Money*. With Peter Blake's sleeve we are invited to gaze at a gallery of heroes and icons. With the 'White Album' we are invited to take a look at ourselves. It's the latter sleeve that is somehow busier, more inclusive, more reflective.

On 8 February, the same day that the Beatles finished recording 'Across the Universe' and one week before they set off for Rishikesh to join the Maharishi, they completed work on George Harrison's 'The Inner Light', the third in a trilogy of songs – after 'Love You To' and 'Within You Without You' – that owed little to their composer's Western pop apprenticeship and everything to his LSD-inspired spiritual journey. On 'The Inner Light' Harrison adopted John Lennon's compositional methods, adapting found material taken from the *Tao Te Ching* and turning it into a three-minute song. In the Ursula K. Le Guin version of the *Tao Te Ching*, the opening of Chapter 47 reads:

> You don't have to go out the door
> to know what goes on in the
>   world.
> You don't have to look out the
>   window
> to see the way of heaven.
> The farther you go
> the less you know.

As Lennon had done with 'Mr Kite', Harrison minimally tweaks scansion and metre without fundamentally altering the meaning of the source material. Syd Barrett used the same approach on Pink Floyd's 'Chapter 24', and 'The Inner Light' shares that song's understanding of the transitory nature of action and the immutability of the soul. Its instructions ('arrive without travelling', 'see all without looking') bear comparison to those first explored on 'Tomorrow Never Knows' ('lay down all thoughts', 'see the meaning of within'). Listened to in sequence they read like an it's-all-one-song epiphany

to everything the Beatles had absorbed along the way. His own absorption complete, Harrison rarely felt the need to reference psychedelic motifs in Beatles songs again.

Once he had delved deeply enough into his inner Scouse child, Paul McCartney returned to his inner trad dad, borrowing the intro to Humphrey Lyttelton's 'Bad Penny Blues' and pounding out Fats Domino piano riffs on 'Lady Madonna'. Within a year he was telling us to get back to where we all belonged. As so often with the Beatles, the detours, diversions, inversions and reversions can't quite hide the continuity and consistency in that congregation of voices. Those Fats Domino chords were there all along, underpinning the sing-song lilt of 'Hello, Goodbye', just waiting to burst out again.

John Lennon went back to acid just the once in an attempt to put his fragile eggshell mind back together again. In her autobiography Cynthia Lennon castigated the irresponsibility of the unnamed person who gave John LSD at a time when his psyche was at its most vulnerable. Derek Taylor, who admits in *As Time Goes By* that he was the one who administered the acid, says that this was precisely why he did it. As they tripped together one last time Taylor therapeutically reminded John of all the great songs he had written while on acid and gently nudged him towards a pathway out of the mind maze as he slowly regained his psychological bearings. Somewhere along that pathway Lennon found Yoko, rediscovered his inner pain, resurrected his messiah complex and attempted to rebuild the ego that had been so severely battered by 'that stupid book of Leary's'. He savagely satirised the Maharishi in 'Sexy Sadie', poked gentle fun at the Beatles myth on 'Glass Onion' (a process of self-referencing that had begun with the nod to 'Lucy in the Sky' in 'I Am the Walrus') and shared a joke at his own expense in 'The Ballad of John and Yoko'. When he wasn't sounding peeved or exasperated in the latter he was happy to send himself up. Amid the Bagism, Dragism and Neo-Dadaism the two gurus in drag continued to seek out the truth, whether cocooned in heroin, ambushed by expectation or grief stricken by miscarriages. Lennon even found time to slip a line into 'The Ballad of John and Yoko' that suggested that despite that 'bloody Leary book', his LSD experience had not entirely been without purpose. 'You don't take nothing with you but your soul. Think!' he sang. The fact that he later attributes the line to 'the wife' somehow makes it all the more meaningful.

And, in the end, there is the impassive, bespectacled visage of the bard of Hull University library, speaking words of wisdom once again. In a touching eulogy, written for the *Observer* in 1983, Philip Larkin pointed out that the Beatles were far greater than the sum of their individual parts. In the immediate years after the break-up, with their talents still basking in the afterglow of their collective creations, it wasn't always easy to see that, even less so to say it. Several solo albums down the line, though, few would have disputed Larkin's assessment. But he was wrong about one thing. He said that when they went psychedelic, 'they lost the typists in the Cavern'.[21] They lost some of the Cavern typists the moment they decamped to London, actually. Some, but not all. For every provincial catcaller full of pent-up aggression and bottle-blonde resentment there was a woman who was prepared to lift up her skirts and fly. Larkin's lapse into caricature seems unworthy of him, although from reading his memoirs and diaries – everything but his elegiac poetry, in fact – perhaps it's not unworthy of him at all. In his dismissal Larkin lost sight of what those Cavern typists became instead. What we all became, in fact. Sure, some stayed at home, rooted to roots, typing pool, Liverpool, nursery rhyme, *Sunday Times* and thank you very much for the Aintree iron, etc. etc. But a fair few, who were no better than they ought to be (and no worse either), slipped away in a variety of guises. Some made their metaphorical appointment with the man from the motor trade, and some signed up for the magical mystery tour too. They didn't all go the full mystical nine miles, but then neither did three-quarters of the Beatles. Always remember that those Cavern typists were there first, before you, before me, before Epstein, before everyone. And some of them were there at the end too, the last to leave the cellar full of noise. They are the ones who have the longest memories and the best stories to tell. And anyway, we're all Cavern typists now.

10

THE SOFT MACHINE

Unfunky Cerebral Caterwauling, the Romilar Army and All the Wood that Doesn't Look Like Fish

My older brother Mark had a small but very hip record collection, and my roots lie with that generation before pop kicked in when jazz was the hip thing. People didn't buy so many records then. If you bought something and liked it, you'd play the same one over and over again for a very long time. You couldn't say, 'What's out this week?' because nobody knew. There wasn't the media coverage. It was more like a series of interlocked secret societies. You didn't expect to see your peer-group concerns reflected back at you.

ROBERT WYATT

'All I remember was the sound of change hitting the floor as I passed out. These centimes had fallen out of my pocket as I fell flat on my back. I saw a map of a dark island but it was lit from underneath by luminous colours. I'd never seen anything like it.'

These are not the words of some errant flower child describing his psychedelic rite of passage in 1967, or the testimony of a tourist who'd stumbled inadvertently into the UFO Club on Tottenham Court Road and had his drink spiked. This was guitarist Daevid Allen describing the summer of 1963, when he was living in Paris and happily acting as guinea pig for one of William Burroughs and Brion Gysin's mind-altering experiments. 'They'd tested the dream machine on me, you see. It was a light bulb suspended in the middle of a piece of cardboard. Tiny holes had been punched in the card, because it had been calculated that if you closed your eyes, these perforations turning at the exact circumference of a 78 rpm record would match your brain rhythms. When they coincided, you went into incredible colour hallucinations.'

Daevid Allen provides one of the crucial links between the activities of the older beats and the newer generation of hippies. The band he co-founded, the Soft Machine, named after a Burroughs novel, was the underground before there *was* an underground. In 1963, when the dream-machine experiments were taking place, Frank Ifield was at number one in the UK singles charts. When Allen first arrived in Paris in the early 1960s, the Beatles were still bawling out 'My Bonnie Lies Over the Ocean' in Hamburg. In

Paris, Allen resided at the Beat Hotel, a six-storey block on the Left Bank run by the redoubtable Madame Rachou, a former employee of French intelligence who was skilled at diplomatically keeping the gendarmes at bay while her clientele of exiled poets, painters and dope dealers pursued their pleasures. That clientele included Jack Kerouac, Brion Gysin, Peter Orlovsky and Allen Ginsberg. 'A scene in every room,' as Allen puts it. His first collaboration with Burroughs came in 1962, when he provided the music for a dramatisation of *The Ticket That Exploded.* 'I was the friendly straight with those guys. Acid used to arrive direct from the Sandoz factory in those days. You took about eighteen of these little tablets. There was another one called Romilar that we took in Ibiza, which had some unknown psychedelic agent in it and put you in the weirdest states. The locals in Ibiza used to call us the Romilar army.'

Allen had left Australia in 1960, vowing never to return. 'They were still killing Aborigines like kangaroos. Those redneck dudes from the deep north could hardly tell the difference. It was a horrific atmosphere and it's still not much spoken about. I arrive in Paris and next thing I'm sitting at the end of the piano with Bud Powell playing.' After seeing all of his jazz idols

in the flesh – Mingus, Monk, Dolphy, Rollins – Allen hitched to England and ended up lodging at Wellington House near Dover, a haven of creativity owned by broadcaster Honor Wyatt and her second husband, psychologist George Ellidge. Bohemians of the old school, they had connections with poet Robert Graves and his artistic colony in Deya, Majorca. Allen immediately bonded with their fifteen-year-old son, Robert. 'We had the same record collection, so instantaneously we were speaking the same language,' Allen says of the future Soft Machine drummer. 'He was a prodigy then, with his painting, piano-playing and everything. Robert was the same intellectual age as me – which doesn't say much for me, of course – but he was in a very advanced headspace for his years.'

While others formed skiffle groups, Wyatt and his school friends, brothers Hugh and Brian Hopper and Mike Ratledge, lived in full experimental mode. Hugh Hopper learned Charlie Haden bass lines from Ornette Coleman records, and recalls Wyatt's household being full of eclectic noise, ranging from Bartók to bebop, Stravinsky to Varèse. The Hopper brothers and Ratledge spent the early 1960s making rudimentary tape loops and surfing the ether for obscure jazz on

American Forces Network and the BBC Third Programme. 'It carried a much more avant-garde output than Radio 3 does today,' says Ratledge. 'But jazz was made much more accessible by the arrival of Daevid Allen, who turned up with about five hundred significant records – Monk, Mingus, Miles, Cecil Taylor, etc. – which then circulated to everyone's houses.'

Although they were no cultural slouches themselves, all his future co-collaborators cite Allen as *the* galvanising force. Allen had made tape loops with the loop guru himself, Terry Riley. 'They were all sixteen, seventeen,' he says. 'I was already the seasoned traveller, their big-brother beatnik.' Nights of atonal excess at Wellington House and at the Hoppers' equally tolerant parents' place eventually blossomed into a distinctive local sound. A whole mythology has subsequently sprung up around the fact that future Soft Machine and Caravan members once shared the same postal district, but the participants themselves are dismissive of such contrivances. 'An accident of geography,' says Ratledge. 'I get journalists asking me about the "Canterbury music school",' says Hugh Hopper, 'and with hindsight I'm sure it sounds like a great place. In fact, it was a small, quite conservative market town where nothing happened. There wasn't even a university until the late sixties.'

It was this unremarkable backwater habitat that allowed the future members of Soft Machine to pursue their musical agenda with impunity. Isolated without being isolationist, indulgent without being insular, eclecticism was the natural order of things. 'It's like that Tom Wolfe remark,' Ratledge says. 'In seeking a personal style you plagiarise so widely from everybody that you end up with an individual style.' During this period, Allen, Hugh Hopper, Wyatt and Ratledge had a go at being a jazz group. They secured a residency at Peter Cook's Establishment Club in Soho but were soon rumbled as imposters and were slung out after four nights. They also played an ICA gig with Burroughs and Gysin, and a jazz and poetry night at the Marquee, the largely unflattering results of which, complete with Allen's self-deprecating sleeve notes, were later released on CD as *Live 1963*. Figuring that, despite his hipster credentials, he wasn't going to be the next Charlie Christian or Wes Montgomery, Allen decided to become a full-time poet and headed for Robert Graves's artistic commune in Deya. He fondly recalls nights spent busking and reciting under the stars, plus the free accommodation courtesy of Graves. It was on one of these frequent sojourns in the islands that some unlikely pop dreams began to formulate. 'Kevin Ayers had some Beatles records and "Still I'm Sad" by the Yardbirds. We did an acid trip and I thought, "Bugger it, maybe I can make a living out of what I was doing before and call it pop." But first I had to adapt my guitar-playing to the language of rock and roll.' One slight inconvenience was that Allen hated rock and roll. 'Buddy Holly, "Rock Around the Clock", all that stuff – I loathed it,' he says. Ratledge shared this sentiment. 'We began to get interested in pop as a cultural excitement rather than a musical one,' he notes. 'Forming a band was a licence to do whatever you wanted to do and call it something saleable – pop music. Kevin was the only one with a real perspective on pop music when we started.'

Brought up in the Far East, the seventeen-year-old Ayers had moved to Canterbury in 1961. 'I'd been sent from London after a drugs bust. A policeman put his hand in my pocket and pulled out a lump of hash which I could never have afforded and said, "'Ello 'ello, what's this then?" I was sent to Ashford Remand Centre for two weeks. When the case came to court, they threw it out for lack of evidence, and the magistrate

said I should leave London because it was obviously a bad influence.' Instead the teenage pot fiend fell in with the Canterbury avant-garde. 'I was a musical ignoramus,' he says. 'All I'd ever heard was *The Sound of Music* and Chinese pop in Malaya. I was drawn to Daevid and Robert and Mike Ratledge and the Hoppers because they had wider interests than anyone else around. Daevid was a complete shock to the system. He had what were for that time outrageous alternative views. He was one of the originals. At that time, though, he was more into poetry readings than songs, and I hated poetry readings.'

Ayers's first serious musical collaboration in Canterbury involved playing bass and guitar with the Wilde Flowers. The name was originally going to be Wild Flowers, but Ayers suggested adding the 'e' in honour of Oscar Wilde. There was no grand design and the band line-up remained fluid. Future Caravan and Soft Machine members came and went on a whim. Ayers, Wyatt and Hugh Hopper would go off and join Allen in Paris or Majorca or Morocco at the drop of a busker's hat. Ratledge went to Oxford University to get his BA. The recorded evidence of these early incarnations reveals a mixed bag of soul, jazz and pop influences, played with varying degrees of competence and commitment, the sound of several bands in search of an identity. But early Soft Machine motifs were evident even then: the Hopper brothers' esoteric lyrics and angular arrangements; Ayers's clarity of vision and uncluttered imagery; Wyatt's idiosyncratically soulful vocals. There was a high quota of R&B covers in the early Wilde Flowers repertoire, with Wyatt providing vocals on everything from 'Get Out of My Life, Woman' to 'Nowhere to Run'. 'Seeing Otis Redding live was a wonderful shock to the system,' he recalls. 'There's a tendency when you learn music from records to underestimate the sheer physical impact. That lot would walk on stage at the Ram Jam Club in Brixton, 1–2–3–4 and in, and the overwhelming speed and power of it, the tightness. I just thought, "Blimey, this is as good as it can get." The first number started at the intensity that most people would reserve for their encore.'

'When I listen to those Wilde Flowers tracks now I can hear the Zombies' influence,' says Hugh Hopper. 'And the English Birds too, Ron Wood's Birds, not the American one: three raucous guitars, lots of shifting chords. They were one of the great forgotten bands of all time.' From Daevid Allen's perspective, though, it was all a bit too proper. 'The Wilde Flowers suffered from fraternal-approval syndrome – it was de rigueur for any band at that time, in order to be taken seriously, to be able to play "Papa's Got a Brand New Bag" with the right guitar sound and the right feel – but they could never get it right.'

By the summer of 1966 Allen's own plans for a beat combo, honed in the Romilar haze of the Balearics, were turning into something tangible. Three days of acid-fuelled anarchy with a nightclub owner from Tulsa called Wes Brunson led to Brunson pledging a considerable portion of his worldly goods to Ayers and Allen in return for them spreading the Aquarian love vibe. 'Sure,' they said. 'We'll need musical instruments, amplifiers and somewhere to rehearse.' The result was a four-piece called Mr Head, consisting of Ayers, Allen, Wyatt and guitarist Larry Nowlin. The most appropriately named group since the Small Faces entered beat competitions organised by *Melody Maker* and the pirate station Radio London, and got the music-biz agents buzzing. Mr Head toyed with the idea of changing their name to Nova Express, before settling for a slightly better known Burroughs novel. Larry Nowlin disappeared, Mike Ratledge came down from Oxford, and Soft Machine was born.

Signed to Chas Chandler's management company on the strength of Kevin Ayers's songs, the Soft Machine spent the latter half of 1966 making demos. Along with Pink Floyd, they played seminal London underground gigs at Notting Hill Free School, UFO and the *International Times* launch at the Roundhouse. Like the Floyd, the Soft Machine based their live performances around free-form innovation. Unlike the Floyd, they lacked a quirky little song about a transvestite to propel them into the pop charts. 'On the first Soft Machine single, "Love Makes Sweet Music", you could hear all the peer pressures of the time,' Daevid Allen says of a debut that could have passed itself off as Simon Dupree and the Big Sound if it hadn't been for Wyatt's imploring high-register voice. 'I wrote it in a squalid little hotel in Hamburg,' remembers Ayers. 'It was after we'd been fired from the Star Club – I think we lasted a day. I liked, and still do like, really good pop songs, and I thought I'd hit on that with "Love Makes Sweet Music". Had we had a good producer, and brought in a backing band, and got somebody else to sing it too . . . it might have been a hit.

'The Pink Floyd were our rivals at that time,' he admits, 'and when "Arnold Layne" came out, I thought,

"Fuck, that's so good," and although I was quite partisan and competitive with our record, I thought there was a lot more fairy dust on theirs. There was a mania with their early stuff, and we were never manic, apart from brief bursts when we played live. I think we were all too logical and clever. We could never be spontaneous enough and abandon ourselves.' The Soft Machine managed to be both studious and vicarious, depending on who was writing the songs. Their early recordings sound like a genre-defying amalgam of Dadaist absurdity, cerebral soul and jazz boplicity. This was a whole different apprenticeship to the blues scholars and R&B emulators who had found their way into mainstream pop. This was the sound of the Romilar army meeting the avant-garde academy.

'Everyone in the media was so surprised at how intelligent we were,' says Allen. 'There was this interview with a BBC guy who was astonished that Mike would come down from Oxford to play in a "pop group".' 'It was like a game at first,' admits Ratledge. 'It was something tangential to my life. It certainly wasn't a consuming passion.' When he first encountered the London underground scene he remained unfazed. 'It all seemed incredibly normal,' he says. 'I certainly didn't feel any disruption or change. I felt I'd been around people like that for most of my teens.'

The Softs were soon introduced to another of Chandler's management protégés, Jimi Hendrix. 'Kevin came back from Mike Jeffrey's office in Wardour Street,' remembers Allen, 'and said, "Hey, come and catch this amazing guitar player. He's better than Jeff Beck." Now Jeff Beck was my favourite guitarist, the most unpredictable, the most exciting, and when it really happened he could fly, but at least half the time he fucked up. When we got there, Hendrix was playing with no amp, yet the room was full of music. Really strong hands. Although actually Jeff Beck was still more exciting than Hendrix precisely because Hendrix didn't fuck up.'

By the spring of 1967 the Soft Machine had a mid-week residency at London's Speakeasy club. Allen recalls fond memories of unlimited drinking on Giorgio Gomelsky's expense account and Hendrix dropping in to jam the night away. 'I heard "Purple Haze" for the first time down there,' he marvels, 'and it sounded like classical music to me, but I couldn't see it being in the charts. I mean, how would the charts accommodate something like this?' While the Top 10 would indeed prove itself capable of accommodating

Hendrix, the UK took less of a shine to the Soft Machine. Like Pink Floyd, they found that when they ventured outside London or the university circuit their experimentation didn't go down so well. Particularly irksome was the Kevin Ayers-penned 'We Did It Again', with its two-note bass figure nestling somewhere between the Kinks' 'You Really Got Me' and Coltrane's 'A Love Supreme'. 'I had got into Sufism,' Ayers explains, 'and I liked the whirling dervish thing, the repetition. I always wanted to do it as a pure drone, but the band always got bored with that and kept adding things. We tried doing it like that at Chelmsford and people threw things. In fact, people threw things all the time when we did that number.'

'It only happened in England,' confirms Ratledge. 'If you appeared with, say, the equivalent of Status Quo in England, you would get booed off the stage. The expectation was that you would be a pop band and perform chart material.' 'We were pelted with stuff by Move fans at the Cambridge Corn Exchange,' remembers Allen. 'There was certainly an uneasy truce a lot of the time.' Always impeccably well connected, whether jamming at Robert Graves's place or getting acid-fuelled Okies to buy them equipment, Soft

Machine now fell in with the Riviera jet set. In the summer of 1967 they played a series of Happenings in the south of France, culminating in a gig in St Tropez town square organised by Eddie Barclay of Barclay Records and attended by the Parisian glitterati – Bardot, Delon, Godard, etc. Soft Machine's entire set consisted of an hour-long performance of 'We Did It Again'. 'It was the moment that elevated Soft Machine to the heights in the Parisians' view, and put us next to the Beatles and Rolling Stones for the next couple of years,' says Allen. For Ayers the St Tropez gig was an unrepeatable moment of musical satori. 'That was the only time "We Did It Again" really worked,' he says. 'Your best ideas happen when you're naive. There was something magical about that early band and I would challenge Robert or Mike to disagree with that. Later on, you become more sophisticated and competent but the content is rarely better.' The euphoria of the St Tropez gig was short-lived. On returning to England, Allen was refused re-entry at Dover. The official reason was an expired visa, but this was during a period when everyone from Lenny Bruce to Eldridge Cleaver was being denied entry to Britain for being undesirable aliens. Allen was red-stamped

and sent back to France. Suspicions still linger in the guitarist's mind as to whether he fell or was pushed out of the band. Always more assured as a cultural catalyst than as a musician, he was in those days a tad self-conscious about his technical limitations. Allen recalls in his book *Gong Dreaming* that after a particularly fraught gig Wyatt told him that he was ashamed to be on stage with him. 'When somebody tells you something that you already feel, it doubles the effect,' he says, and although he claims that 'being thrown out of the country was exhilarating, liberating, the best thing that could have happened to me', and talks excitedly of being in Paris during May 1968, he remains in no doubt that the Customs incident was highly convenient for the rest of the band.

Mike Ratledge saw things differently. 'I was quite shocked to hear that Daevid had indicated that we had kicked him out of the band, which is not my recollection at all. He was deported and was therefore no longer available to us. I don't remember any feeling of "Daevid must go" at the time.' He does concede, though, that saying goodbye to their big-brother beatnik marked the end of Soft Machine phase one. 'I only really started taking it seriously when Daevid left and we were down to a trio. It was then that I started writing for the band.'

Still lagging behind Pink Floyd in terms of UK popularity, Soft Machine found audiences more receptive in Europe and America. Live, the three-piece was a *tour de force*. Wyatt's vocals, all Eastern modality and bebop scat, merged with Ayers's Sufi drone over the layers of fuzz emitting from Ratledge's keyboard. 'We couldn't afford a Hammond, which was the authentic article,' Ratledge says, 'so I was playing this weedy Lowrey and I wanted to approximate the power that Hendrix had. I got sick of guitarists having all the balls.'

In April 1968, during a break from their first major US tour, the three-piece Soft Machine finally got to record their first album. Producer Tom Wilson had worked with Dylan and the Velvet Underground – 'Which is presumably why he was hired,' says Ayers. Despite Wilson's pedigree, and some great material, the resulting album lacked the power of their live shows. 'We started out with some very good ideas,' contends Ayers, 'but that album was amateurish, sloppy, badly produced – a nightmare, now I look back on it. All he did was phone his girlfriends. I think he thought we were a bunch of little white shits playing this unfunky cere-bral caterwauling.'

The album, with its distinctive 'pin-wheel' cover that pre-dates *Led Zep-pelin III* by two years, finally came out in November 1968 on Probe. Sleeve notes, written in period 'Hey, cats, dig their scene' style, were provided by Arnold Shaw, better known for his showbiz hagiographies. Two tracks on the album – Brian Hopper's 'Hope for Happiness' and Wyatt's 'Save Yourself' – were adaptations of material from the Wellington House days. The 'head is a nightclub' line on Ayers's George Gurd-jieff-inspired 'Why Are We Sleeping?' was taken from a Daevid Allen jazz poem. Gurdjieff was Ayers's Meher Baba, his flash bulb of inner wisdom. 'Gurdjieff's teachings were the lightning bolts that formulated my later ideas,' says Ayers. 'In my late teens and early twenties I embarked upon a personal odyssey through the world's philos-ophies. I wrote to Japan for all these books on Zen Buddhism. I read greed-ily and all the time. A bit later I took acid and expanded my mind – irretriev-ably. But Gurdjieff taught me that most philosophy is padding. That changed my attitude towards all these rather grave books I was reading. When most people start they don't want one-liners like "The truth of life is . . ." They want to hear how you came to that and a lot of mumbo-jumbo to make it colourful.

Gurdjieff's instruction for reading his *All and Everything*, this massively boring and arduous tome, was that you had to read it five or six times. I doubt if anyone ever read it all through once. For me it all clicked fairly early. I never believed in underlining things in songs, saying, "This is the important bit.' The Gurdjieff influence in "Why Are We Sleeping?" was about slipping things into normal situations which challenge your normality, but they don't come with trumpets or like express trains. Just slip them in without drama, so you think, "What was that?" You develop a fairly comfortable little storyline and then slip in something startling, as if nothing had happened. And that's what Gurdjieff was doing.'

One of the most graceful moments on the album was Ayers's instrumental 'Joy of a Toy', a title that was taken from an Ornette Coleman track and later reactivated for Ayers's first solo LP. 'I used a Gibson bass with nylon strings on that,' he remembers. 'Good for playing lead lines but not so good for a traditional bass sound. It sounds so elastic-bandy and plunky on that first album.' The album was recorded in one four-day session while the Softs toured with the Jimi Hendrix Experience. In contrast, Hendrix recorded *Electric Ladyland* over a leisurely six-month

period during the same marathon stint. 'On the first part of that tour with Hendrix there were moments of sheer magic,' says Ayers. 'I found Hendrix a very gentle, very sad guy. He was being ripped off emotionally, financially, and he had to strap on an enormous amount of chemical armour before he could become Jimi Hendrix on stage.' The tour took up most of 1968 and almost split the Soft Machine for good. 'I got heavily into macrobiotics on the second part of the tour,' remembers Ayers. 'I stopped drinking, stopped smoking, which was totally incompatible with the routine of touring. My energy level went right down and I was falling about all over the place. You can't do a two-hour gig on a green apple, a glass of water and a bowl of rice.' Future bass player Hugh Hopper was a roadie with the band at this point. 'When I look back now I think, "Great, I was on tour with Hendrix," but I never got to see much of the music, and even when I did I couldn't appreciate it because I was so knackered,' says Hopper. 'It wasn't sixteen articulated lorries like you have now. It was me and Hendrix's roadie with one van, praying that we would get to the venue on time. Hendrix was becoming really big during that period, so as soon as there was a gap in the schedule it got filled, and we ended up touring for months without a break. It did Hendrix's roadie's head in completely. He abandoned the van in the streets of New York at the end of it.'

It did Ayers's head in too, and he fled to Ibiza to regain equilibrium. 'Mike and Robert were far more musically literate than I was, and I think my simplicity bored them,' he said of his departure. 'I met Terry Riley and Gil Evans in New York, and I liked all those jazz people Daevid and Robert introduced me to, but it was all way beyond my musical comprehension, and I didn't have the interest in playing things in 19/7 just for the sake of it. I never really liked "fusion music". I much preferred the jazz as it was to start with, and rock as it was to start with. Fusion all seemed more fun for the players than the listener, people with virtuoso techniques blasting at each other to see how difficult they could be.' He dissolves into mirthful disdain. 'So I took my simplicity elsewhere, and lost this family. Being in a pure spiritual state at that time, clean of body and mind, I wasn't terribly worried. It only hit me later on that I was no longer close to these people.' Ayers gave his bass to Mitch Mitchell and took his simplicity to Ibiza, where he wrote most of the songs that eventually appeared on his first solo LP.

In his absence Soft Machine effectively disbanded. Ratledge, like Ayers, was burned out by the American tour. Wyatt hung out with Hendrix in LA and nurtured vague plans to pursue a solo career. Forced to record a second album as a contractual obligation to Probe, and with Ayers disinclined to budge from his sunny retreat, Ratledge and Wyatt brought in Hugh Hopper as a permanent replacement. The result, *Soft Machine Volume 2*, is an English underground classic. Much more of a piece than its predecessor, it kicks off with Wyatt's introduction to 'the official orchestra of the college of pataphysics' and a scholarly rendition of the British alphabet. The LP is full of wry self-referential nods. Ratledge and Wyatt's 'As Long as He Lies Perfectly Still' fondly recalls Kevin Ayers's macrobiotics regime. More caustically, 'Have You Ever Bean Green?' seizes on manager Mike Jeffries' comment that the band were just riding on Hendrix's coat-tails; Wyatt slips in an acerbic 'Thank you for his coat-tails, Mike, you did us proud' among the warm regards to Jimi, Noel and Mitch. The album's homage to Alfred Jarry came about when the band was invited to write the music for a performance of Jarry's *Ubu Enchanted* at the Edinburgh Festival, although Wyatt's own acquaintance with him went back to his teens, when his father had introduced him to Jarry's work. Daevid Allen describes the pataphysics project as 'creating a spiritual manifesto in an absurd form, casting a serious topic into an absurdist structure', something he turned into a fine art with his post-Soft Machine band, Gong. Ayers also applied the principle to his post-Soft Machine output, throwing a banana into the works whenever things threatened to get too serious. When asked to elaborate on the mechanics of pataphysics, Ratledge talks vaguely of 'the science of the impossible' and 'perverting the premises of scientific certainties'. I ask him how he applied that to the music. 'We didn't. Not in the least. Are you kidding?' He rocks with suitably absurdist laughter. '*Soft Machine 2* was people celebrating enthusiasms for things outside the music, be it French literature or whatever. Often song titles were just adverts for things we liked: "Read this, listen to that."' The album abounds with such references. 'As Long as He Lies Perfectly Still' contains the lines 'He's Lucky or Pozzo, Estragon and Vladimir / waiting for something that's already there.' And, like many people of my age, I first picked up Burroughs's book *The Soft Machine* in 1971 assuming it was a biography of the band. 'See,

it worked,' says Ratledge, with evident satisfaction.

Aside from referencing Beckett, Schoenberg, Dada and Jarry, the other distinctive component of *Soft Machine Volume 2* was the highly idiosyncratic compositional flare of Hugh Hopper. Hopper was a bookish-looking man with curly receding hair, horn-rimmed glasses and a moustache. He looked like he would have been more suitably employed in a professorial capacity at the college of advanced pataphysics rather than playing his debut Softs gig with Hendrix at the Albert Hall. Like Wyatt and Ayers, he wrote exquisitely English songs packed with abstruse imagery. One of the most magnificent moments on *Soft Machine Volume 2* is when Wyatt sings Hopper's 'Dedicated to You but You Weren't Listening'. 'Don't use magnets, geophysics / carry you back / Wholesome health food, home pride, satisfied,' Wyatt sings with impeccable pataphysical conviction. 'I had a terrible migraine when I wrote that,' Hopper offered a tad obliquely when I pressed him for an explanation.

Most of the tracks on *Soft Machine Volume 2* segue into each other, a common enough jazz device at the time, although Wyatt later justified the continuity as a defence mechanism against hostile audiences – it is, after all, harder to boo when there aren't any pauses. By 1970 such defensiveness was becoming increasingly unnecessary. In the summer of that year, while arguably at the height of their popularity, Soft Machine were invited to perform at the Albert Hall Proms. Ratledge was characteristically blasé: 'We'd played the Albert Hall twice before. It was just another gig. One was never surprised by anything during that period.' Despite its prestige value, the Proms performance masked growing internal divisions within the group. The release of their double album *Third*, just prior to the Albert Hall event, revealed a more jazz-influenced direction than before. The group was augmented by stalwarts of the English jazz-rock scene, such as Elton Dean, Lyn Dobson and Nick Evans, and the album was largely instrumental, apart from Wyatt's classic montage of life as seen from a New York hotel room, 'Moon in June', which the other members declined to have anything other than minimal involvement with. The evident hurt this caused Wyatt was a major factor in his eventual departure from the band. Always their most extrovert member – on stage his flailing long hair and exuberant drumming contrasted sharply with Hopper and Ratledge sitting hunched over their instruments – Wyatt found himself increasingly cut adrift in a sea of cerebral noodling. I reminded Hugh Hopper of a story where a purist progressive rock fan went backstage in 1970 to congratulate the Softs on a great gig and to sneer that they'd had to endure Geno Washington and the Ram Jam Band a week earlier. 'We'd play like that if we could,' Wyatt had commented. 'Oh absolutely,' confirms Hopper. 'I remember Robert meeting Phil Chen, the bass player with Jimmy James and the Vagabonds, and being knocked out by all these Temptations bass lines he was playing'.

Speaking of his earliest forays into rock and pop, Wyatt told me: 'I initially found it difficult to listen to words and music at the same time. I just thought words were a vehicle for making certain noises with your mouth, although I did learn to like Dylan later on. If anyone alerted me to that kind of thing, it was probably Hendrix. He took Dylan very seriously. It was Hendrix that put me onto white music. Before that I was getting my information from two sources: the jazz that I listened to at school plus the records that we listened to, to get clues as to how to play in amplified bands – Stax Records, Don Covay, James Brown.'

Shortly after the Proms gig Wyatt recorded his own solo album, *End of an Ear.* According to the liner notes he penned for the record's 1992 CD reissue, the venture hastened Wyatt's departure from the Softs. 'Perhaps – I was never told why – I was expelled soon afterwards from my original group by the very people I had invited to join it,' he observed ungrammatically but, it would appear, accurately. 'It was much more tricky than Kevin's departure, which was entirely amicable,' Ratledge acknowledges. Indeed, all of the Softs subsequently reconvened to play on Ayers's *Joy of a Toy* album in 1969. 'But after that tour with Hendrix things had polarised between Robert and everybody else,' says Ratledge. 'Hugh, myself and Elton were pursuing a vaguely jazz-related direction. Robert was violently opposed to this, which is strange, looking back on it, because he was passionate about jazz. But he had defined ideas about what pop music was and what jazz was. I think, like Kevin, he'd made conceptual decisions that pop should remain pop and jazz should remain jazz. And although the so-called conspiracy between Hugh, myself and Elton covered a lot of actual differences between us, we had sufficient similarity to define ourselves against Robert. The whole situation in the USA got very complicated. Robert used to walk off the stand because he didn't like what

we were playing or writing; you can't sustain a situation where your drummer is walking off the stand maybe one in four nights.' 'There were nights when we would make fun of him behind his back,' admits Hopper. 'It really had got that bad. Mike and I couldn't stand Robert, and he couldn't stand us. We were very cool and calculated, whereas Robert was very open and impulsive. During one evening of drunkenness at Ronnie Scott's he said to someone, "I wish I could find another band." The rest of us leapt on it and said, "Right, go on then." Robert was definitely pushed out of what he felt was his own group. He'd been one of the instigators, after all. And he seems as bitter about that now as he ever has been.'

This much was brought home to me when I contacted Wyatt in 1996 for an interview about his days with the Soft Machine. Back came a message written on a cereal box in that familiar child-like scrawl and skewed diction. 'I still have nightmares or rather daymares,' it read. 'I dream my rejection was a temporary blip and I'm welcomed back into the fold. Then I wake up. How bad was I affected by my being deported from SM? Well breaking my back was easier to deal with. That's how bad.' 'We handled it clumsily,' concedes Ratledge, with considerable understatement.

'Nobody in the band was trying to do the same thing at all, which is why it was quite original and why, after a couple of years, it fell apart,' Wyatt recalled in 1988 in a rare comment on his Soft Machine days. 'It was a constant process of disintegration really, getting in new people to fill the gaps. Which in the '60s was rare, because most bands were quite stable. But it kept changing, we kept on tinkering with it and tinkering with it and throwing each other out of it and leaving it until eventually all the kinks were ironed out, and in the end it became a standard British jazz-rock band. I don't know what happened in the end. I stopped listening after a while – I stopped listening before I even left.'[1]

'The very reason why the band was so good – with everyone pulling in different directions – became unsustainable,' says Ratledge. 'It reached a point where everyone wanted to do what they wanted to do so strongly that you couldn't have any sort of compromise. Nobody in that band was going to do anyone else's thing any more. It's the price you pay for being committed. You can sustain a band on compromise for years if there's no passion there.'

Between 1968 and 1970, both in Britain and the US, there was a significant gear shift in musical direction as former psych groups became progressive-rock groups or jazz-rock outfits, but the Soft Machine's jazz-rock allegiance was, it would appear, something of a misnomer. 'I never felt part of that English jazz scene,' says Ratledge, 'and the more we included those kind of players in the band, the more difference I felt between me and them, mainly because writing was very important to me and jazz at the time was very improvised and anti-writing. Hugh was much more at ease with that kind of departure than I was.' Hopper, though, maintains that he had equal misgivings about the jazz-prog detour taken by the band in the early 1970s. 'I was very influenced by *Uncle Meat* and *Hot Rats*-period Zappa, but that whole jazz-rock territory subsequently became very devalued. For me the best stuff was a mixture of real weirdness and good writing. Zappa was a great writer. But what you ended up with was lots of good technical players who didn't have that weirdness that could lift it.'

'In a curious sort of way, everybody discovered their individuality by being in the band,' Ratledge concludes. 'We all tried to do something cohesive to work out what we had in common, but everyone was acting out some idea of what they thought pop music was, and the longer it existed, everybody wanted to pull in different directions. That was both the reason for its success and the reason for it falling apart.'

The Soft Machine was perhaps the ultimate British manifestation of a band that constantly experimented in public. An ever-changing trio, quartet or quintet of wildly diffuse individuals of equally differing character and temperament, they were thrown together initially by happenstance, and were eventually separated by the very thing that had first united them – music. A mass of irresolvable contradictions, shared intelligence and counter-intuitions, they were the English underground's most prominent experiment in social engineering. The fact that the experiment failed made the undertaking no less thrilling.

All of the original members of the band had astute things to say about each other when I interviewed them. Of Ayers Daevid Allen perceptively noted that 'the thing about Kevin is that he is outwardly quite shy ['a sociophobe', was Ayers's own assessment], and when he isn't supplanting that with hedonism he goes away and reads all these books and gets very involved. There is this secret side to Kevin which he tends not to talk about. He prefers to let that social person be one of expanded extravagance.'

When I saw Ayers shortly after my original Soft Machine profile was published in *Mojo* magazine, he commented not on the content but on the photo spread from the band's early days. 'When we were young and beautiful,' said Ayers wistfully. Wyatt made a similar comment to me after a piece I'd written on him. 'That's just what Kevin said,' I responded. 'Ah, Kevin,' he exclaimed. 'We fucking ruined him. He should have been Ray Davies, but he fell in with a bunch of grammar-school wankers like us and we made him play all this difficult music.'

Ayers remained sanguine about this all his life. Towards the end of my interview with him he offered a typically tangential analogy, for creativity, for the journey through life, for everything. 'I was watching this local news programme the other night and they were interviewing this old guy who carved beautiful fish-head handles for umbrellas and walking sticks,' he ruminated. 'The interviewer asked him how he goes about his work. "Well," he said, "first of all I carves off all the wood that doesn't look like fish."'

11

PINK FLOYD

The Art-School Dance and the Hexagram Shuffle

You have a tendency, when things are going well for you, to interrupt the flow of events and to turn away from it negatively. When you have slipped back far enough you again reverse yourself and attempt to regain what you purposefully let go. This line is the line of self-defeatism – not in extremis, but the defeatism of constant backsliding, the defeatism of fear of climax, fear of contemplation, fear of attainment. You remain guiltless because the impulse does not stem from inhumane ideals and harms no one but yourself.
I CHING, Hexagram 24, 'Returning'

It begins appropriately enough with a song about leaving. Long before they signed a contract with EMI, Pink Floyd recorded one of Syd Barrett's earliest compositions, 'Lucy Leave'. Its melody and chord sequence are firmly in the tradition of the spasmodically paced R&B that produced the Pretty Things' 'Midnight to Six Man' and 'Buzz the Jerk', the Who's 'The Good's Gone' and countless other mod songs that now genuflect to another beat. 'The Good's Gone' is sung by Roger Daltrey in a flat, artless sneer that doesn't sit comfortably within his range. Like Daltrey, Barrett sings 'Lucy Leave' as if he's in an inappropriate register, as if he's approximating the requirements of a beatgroup vocalist, as if he hasn't found his voice yet – which, of course, he hasn't. To anyone hearing this unreleased item from the Pink Floyd's juvenilia days it will be clear why no one wanted to sign the band, or even offer them gigs on a regular basis. The changes are ramshackle and tentative. The whole thing lacks proficiency and polish. And those lyrics – 'Fall away from me, Lucy' – have a faintly hallucinatory edge that is completely out of synch with the standard pop vernacular of the time. When he sings, 'Mean, treat me and done me harm, Lucy,' Barrett sounds like he's parodying R&B. Which in a way he is. The madcap laughed even then.

Like Pete Townshend, Syd Barrett was landed with the role of providing lead and rhythm guitar for his group and frequently fluctuated between the two, fluctuation being the name of the game by 1966. Barrett was also fluctuating between his studies at Camberwell School of Art and the occasional gig with his band mates in the Pink

Floyd Sound, as they still sometimes called themselves. Art remained his first love and most people who knew him at this time regarded him as a painter who dabbled in music. Barrett had been a diligent and committed artist since his school days in Cambridge, where he used to attend extra Saturday-morning classes and frequently bunked off school lessons and cross-country runs so that he could go home and paint. Pink Floyd only made the great conceptual leap from R&B also-rans to improvisatory doyens of the English psychedelic underground once Barrett started to apply painterly techniques and philosophies to his guitar-playing. Again, like Townshend, Barrett was one of the few art students willing to put these principles into practice, and arguably he was the only one who articulated a fully realised conceptual connection between art-school methodology and pop appliqué. The cutting up and collaging of found materials (predominantly fairy tales and Mother Goose rhymes) was his greatest gift to pop music and would become part of the very fabric of the English psychedelic sound.

You sense new ideas in the air, a new atmosphere, a new excitement. You are almost at the point of accepting them and enjoying them. You have been won over gradually as this creative force has slowly permeated society and gradually has touched and influenced people you know.

HEXAGRAM 24

The Cambridge social milieu that Syd Barrett grew up in was not dissimilar to the one in Canterbury at around the same time. These were the children of parents whose politics ranged from progressive liberal to communist, the offspring of doctors, biochemists, university lecturers, artists, sculptors. Striving to find their own creative voices Barrett and his friends staged Happenings, read beat poetry and listened to free jazz. They went to see French, Italian and Polish new wave films. They dug Bo Diddley, the Stones and the Beatles, and they smoked pot. And at some point during 1964/5 they all started taking acid. Like Canterbury, Cambridge was a musical backwater. For all its intellectual wealth nobody expected a famous pop group to emerge from such cloistered confines. That's what London was there for, and London was only a train ride away – the centre of everything and yet a world apart.

What Cambridge did have was

comedy. Culturally, the first manifestation of the swinging sixties wasn't rock and roll; it wasn't even Beatlemania and the beat-group boom. It was the satire movement, and the origins of that were emerging courtesy of the Cambridge Footlights Club, in the shape of Peter Cook, Jonathan Miller, Eleanor Bron, John Wells, John Bird. Barrett already had a keen sense of the absurd, which was galvanised by his discovery of Cook, Dudley Moore, Miller and Alan Bennett. 'He adored Peter Cook very early on, and that's when we were fifteen,' remembers Barrett's former girlfriend, Libby Gausden, 'but he adored the Goons too, and he would not go out until they had been on. We all used to meet at the Mill pub on Sundays, and he wouldn't leave the house until the Goons had finished.'

This embracing of the absurd was fully formed by the time Barrett left school in 1962. In his final year he played the part of Mrs Martin in a dramatic-society production of Eugene Ionesco's *The Bald Prima Donna*. Being an all-boys school the two female parts in the production were played by males, who were distinguished from the real male characters by wearing pinafores – 'Although Syd indicated that he would have been more than happy to drag up for the part,' the production's producer

Peter Baker informed me. Described by Ionesco as an anti-play, *The Bald Prima Donna* was a satire on the English comedy of manners. Its sustained semantic attack on bourgeois convention sat well with Barrett's own finely honed disregard for social niceties. Ionesco's stage instruction required Mrs Martin to speak 'in a drawling monotonous voice, rather sing song without light or shade'. Not dissimilar, then, to the distinctively flattened timbre that Barrett would adopt once he became a pop performer. He settled on this singing style fairly rapidly and never bothered to develop it; sometimes slightly startled, sometimes hovering on the edge of a sneer, always well-mannered, it served him well from 'Lucy Leave' to his own eventual leaving. Mrs Martin's speeches were full of meaningless exclamations that displayed the futility of language. For a sixteen-year-old boy busy soaking up every last morsel of life's absurdities this was rich source material indeed.

As part of the questing spirit that typified Barrett's wider circle in the early 1960s, his school friends Andrew Rawlinson and Paul Charrier started to hitch down to London on Friday nights after school. They had little money and nowhere to sleep, so they stayed up all weekend on a diet of coffee, pills and sugar. 'What we came across was the outskirts of normal life,' remembers Rawlinson. 'One of the places we found was a cafe in Cromwell Road that was frequented by transvestites. They used to emerge at about eleven at night. It was a place for outcasts really. We weren't outcasts like them; we were schoolboys trying to find where the big time was. I liked those people. Most of them were pretty damaged, I have to say, because there wasn't the supportive culture for them.'

Regaled with tales of nocturnal trannies and outcasts, Barrett and his friends created their own bohemian clique. They still felt green and provincial in terms of what was happening (or what they assumed was happening) elsewhere, but in their own little enclave of stoned gatherings, gigs, parties, readings, screenings and Happenings a group consciousness began to develop which forged an identity very different to what was going on in any other town or city at the time. Gradually pretty much everyone from Barrett's wider social circle drifted down to London. His school friend Roger Waters commenced his architectural degree at the Regent Street Poly and told Barrett that if he ever moved down to town, they should think about getting a band together. Waters went

ahead and started without him anyway, forming embryonic bands with embryonic names: Sigma 6, the Megadeaths, the Screaming Abdabs, the Abdabs, the Tea Set.

In many ways Barrett's rechristening of the band remains his greatest legacy. All those earlier self-conscious efforts aligned themselves to specific tendencies that were emerging from the British counter-culture. Sigma 6 was derived from Alexander Trocchi's manifesto for 'the spontaneous university'. Megadeath evoked the H-bomb and the ever-present fear of obliteration. The Abdabs was a peculiarly English onomatopoeic term variously used to describe delirium tremens and shellshock. By 1964 its usage was more likely to suggest a college cabaret band who weren't in the habit of taking themselves too seriously, which was pretty much the case. Almost all of these early band names were Waters's suggestions; they sprung from the same verbal facility that gave us 'Flapdoodle Dealing', 'Take Up Thy Stethoscope and Walk', 'Pow R. Toc H.' and 'Corporal Clegg had a wooden leg'. The one exception was the Tea Set, which was jazz slang for smoking pot, an activity that was distinctly infra dig as far as Waters was concerned. The Tea Set was both a knowing nudge to the hip life – Louis Armstrong referred to 'tea' all his life – and an appropriation of an advertising slogan from the time – 'Join the Tea Set'. If you look at the cover of *Time* magazine's famous 'London: The Swinging City' edition from 15 April 1966, the red bus in the centre of the picture, right next to Big Ben, carries the slogan on its side.

For a while the group used the names Tea Set and Pink Floyd interchangeably. Barrett's former art-school contemporaries remember them playing college gigs under both billings. Cambridge friend Nigel Lesmoir-Gordon advised them to drop the Tea Set if they wanted to be taken seriously. 'Steve Stollman [ESP label co-founder] was talking of having these Happenings at the Marquee on Sunday afternoons. I said, "Yeah, poetry and jazz." It occurred to me that there was this band in Cambridge called the Tea Set who might be well suited. At that stage they were just beginning to be adventurous. Still doing the R&B stuff but starting to cut loose. I can't remember if I phoned Syd Barrett or Roger Waters. I said, "Don't call yourself the Tea Set. Call yourself by that other name, the Pink Floyd. It will sit much better." Tea Set sounds like such a joke. I didn't like it, too crass.'

As a name, Pink Floyd has endured far better than many of the other options available at the time. The Beatles' monumental creativity rapidly outgrew a name that was based on a feeble pun, derived from Buddy Holly and the Crickets. Equally time-bound is the Rolling Stones, taken from a Muddy Waters number, and chosen in haste by Brian Jones when required to come up for a name for an imminent gig. The Beach Boys, the Kinks and the Yardbirds are also unmistakably of their era, even if their music transcends it. Pink Floyd, though, has a certain subtle neutrality about it, suggestive and meaningless at the same time. Barrett had found references to two South Carolina bluesmen – Pink Anderson and Floyd Council – on a record sleeve and had combined the two forenames. Devastatingly simple in one respect, it belies deeper, more complex thought processes. 'Pink' variously connotes Caucasian, femininity, nakedness. 'Floyd' suggests black, rootsy, earthy. Floyd was not an uncommon name among blues and R&B musicians – Floyd Dixon, Floyd Jones, etc.; Woody Guthrie had immortalised bank robber Pretty Boy Floyd in song; and the recently deposed heavyweight boxing champion of the world was called Floyd Patterson. You can hear Barrett, the pop-art aesthete, cogitating over the options, sifting them laterally. Pink Floyd. Pretty Blues. Blushing Purity. Feminised Authenticity. Naked Outlaws. White Blackness. It's a name crafted out of intuitive juxtapositions. On one level it's an oblique play on the 'Can white men sing the blues?' syndrome that would preoccupy an entire generation of pop musicians during the 1960s. On another it's an indicator of Barrett's art-school sensibilities, a blank-canvas name, a looks-good-on-a-poster name.

For most of 1965 and well into 1966 Pink Floyd played the same rudimentary R&B as everybody else, just another average white band on an overcrowded circuit. They rehearsed up at Hornsey Art College, where their landlord, Mike Leonard, ran his light-and-sound workshop. It was here that the group first got a taste of the possibilities of mixed media. In Leonard's rehearsal space, performing in the flickering beam of his light and sound boxes, the group began to extemporise. They still performed their standard R&B repertoire when they played gigs, but in the light show they could stretch out into infinity. Barrett adapted his guitar style accordingly, sculpting with atonality, weaving new possibilities into old language. He stopped worrying about musical competence and technique

and began applying painterly textures and colouration. Within a matter of months he had pretty much abandoned his fine-art apprenticeship and started painting with sound instead.

You contemplate taking a course that is contrary to your deepest principles. Your thoughts have not yet been transformed into action. Banish unprincipled ideas immediately before they obsess you to the point of forcing you to act on them. There is no need to feel guilty – yet.

HEXAGRAM 24

Everyone threw the I Ching. Life became a game of chance and coincidence as adherents placed their faith in a recently revived oracle based on the Taoist wisdom of ancient China. The I Ching, the so-called Book of Changes, submitted action and interpretation to the casting of yarrow sticks or the throwing of coins. Meaningless actions were transformed into meaningful ritual. The I Ching became the stoner's parlour game *du jour*. While the political wing of hippiedom subscribed to the rhetoric of revolution, the mystical wing aligned itself to old-time theosophists and Rosicrucians and all the other esotericists who preferred palm readings, séances and yarrow sticks to throwing bricks through embassy windows or hurling marbles under police horses.

During that fruitful period in the late summer and autumn of 1966, when the words just seemed to pour out of him in a torrent, Syd Barrett wrote most of the songs that would appear on the Pink Floyd's debut LP, *The Piper at the Gates of Dawn*. Among them was a composition based on the I Ching called 'Chapter 24'. Barrett lifted the words pretty much verbatim from the Fu Hexagram ('The receptive earth above; the arousing thunder below'), which was chiefly concerned with the theme of 'Return – The Turning Point'. The song appeared on *Piper* embellished with harmonium, bells and mellotron, and Barrett sang it in a choirboy voice that now seemed to owe far more to folk music and the English hymnal tradition than it did to R&B. The song's ellipses were seamless. The Fu Hexagram's 'Return. Success. Going out and coming in without error' became 'Change. Return. Success. Going and coming without error.' As Lennon had done with 'Tomorrow Never Knows', Barrett borrowed specific phrases word for word and collapsed others to suit the metre. But he didn't get the technique from Lennon; he got it from

an art-school apprenticeship, which by the time he wrote 'Chapter 24' he had all but aborted. 'Action brings good fortune,' he sings. He sounds full of belief.

Early in 1967, during what should have been the final year of his studies, Barrett went to see Robert Medley, the head of Camberwell art school, and told him that he was earning £200 a week from gigs with the Pink Floyd. Medley generously offered him a sabbatical, but Barrett never did go back. According to those who knew him well, the wrench was apparently enormous. His close friend Anna Murray, who had appeared along with Susie Gawler-Wright in the original 1966 *24 Hours* programme about LSD, had no doubt about where his true talents lay. 'He was very carried away by the music and he liked performing, but at the time I thought he'd be better off as a painter,' she told John Cavanagh. 'His temperament suited it better. I was really surprised when he took off into the music so hugely. I felt he was swept up and it wasn't necessarily his intention or his driving force. It wasn't apparent to me that it was the most important thing in his life at all.'[1]

A month after Syd Barrett officially left art school Pink Floyd turned professional and signed a contract with EMI records for an advance of £5,000.

Along with other people you are experiencing a change of fortune – a turn for the better that is occurring without anyone having willed it, planned it or arranged for it. It occurs completely on its own, in its own slow time, in its own quiet way. Very gradually you will find your life becoming more eventful.

HEXAGRAM 24

It became eventful very quickly. There was nothing gradual about it at all. One minute the Pink Floyd were playing gigs at the Notting Hill Free School to a coterie of the devoted, the next they were the darlings of the London underground, headlining full-scale freak-outs at the UFO club and extemporising the blues into vapour in the swirling maelstrom of Mark Boyle and John Marsh's light shows. In January 1967 a German film crew from Bavarian Rundfunk filmed a one-hour documentary entitled *Die Jungen Nachtwandler* ('The Young Nightcrawler') inside UFO. Directed by Edmund Wolf, it featured a lengthy sequence that showed Pink Floyd performing an incredibly unshackled version of 'Interstellar Overdrive'. With the band immersed in John Marsh's light projections (Marsh is briefly glimpsed during the footage), Wolf intones, in German: 'These

people in their confusion try to experience a real community. Even here sometimes you can find a common pleasure – without any aggression. Something of a new quality of being together as people, that's what all the young ones are searching for. Much more kindness, much less aggression, that's what they are searching for. In all this confusion something really new will be born. That's what I believe.' Judging by the beatific looks on their faces, so do the blissed-out clubbers. They all seem to do what everyone did in the light show at that time: they choreograph themselves to its patterns, forming chemically enhanced dance shapes that merge with the pulsating blobs and drips of the light-show oils. The euphoria and oblivion on display as the camera plays across half-lit faces are testimony to the tidal wave that LSD was unleashing upon the London underground at the onset of 1967.

'And yet it does not matter that he's all in bits,' says Aldous Huxley in *The Doors of Perception*, as he listens to madrigals by the late-Renaissance composer Carlo Gesualdo while high on mescaline and perhaps not fully perceiving that it is he, the listener, that is in bits. 'The whole is disorganized. But each individual fragment is in order, is a representative of a Higher Order. The

Higher Order prevails even in the disintegration. The totality is present even
in the broken pieces.'[2]

That was Barrett in the early part of
1967. That was everyone.

You have sensed a change, a
regeneration, a turn for the better
in your situation. Your friends and
colleagues have not felt it yet. Move
with it freely and naturally, even
though this will alienate you from
others.

HEXAGRAM 24

Barrett went gung-ho for acid, and his
intake was prodigious. Unlike his band
mates, unlike the majority of musicians
on the scene, in fact, whose tastes for
stimulants rarely went beyond alcohol
and the odd puff on a joint, Barrett
enthusiastically endorsed the systematic disassembling of sense and psyche.
Cambridge compatriot and Hipgnosis's
LP-sleeve designer Storm Thorgerson
told me in 2012 about the time he and
Barrett ingested some hideous chemical compound cut with plastic deriv-
atives. As Thorgerson felt his entire
system undergo creeping paralysis,
'beginning with the legs and working
its way upwards', all he could remember was Barrett cackling with laughter
as he embraced the void.

In such circumstances fame tended
to be a hindrance, a bothersome intrusion into the more important business
of trepanning your soul. When the
Pink Floyd came to record their first
LP, producer Norman Smith felt the
full brunt of Barrett's truculence and
refusal. 'Syd was pretty difficult,' he
conceded in a 2007 interview with *Gui-*
tar World magazine. 'What I mean by
difficult is, they would be in the studio
recording a particular number. I would
bring them into the control room to listen to the playback. Syd was doing the
singing, of course. And I would suggest
perhaps a little phrasing alteration. Syd
was nodding. Didn't say anything, but
he was nodding, like a "yes" nod. He
seemed to be paying attention. I said,
"OK, go back into the studio and we'll
do another take." So they go back in
the studio and Syd did exactly the same
as he had done the previous take. So I
thought, "I think I'm wasting my time
here." But I realized as time went on
that Syd really and truly, in my opinion,
didn't get any pleasure out of recording.
Syd's thing was he would write these
songs, he would go to an underground
club or something of that nature and
perform in front of these fans. And that
really was his big thing.'

Smith was a product of the old
school, versed in the EMI way of doing

things. Barrett, equally methodical in his way, was versed in the spontaneous techniques of automatic writing and painterly abstraction. He baulked at the brain-sapping procedures of four-track recording, at the necessity of repetition. At school, performing in *The Bald Prima Donna*, he had tremendous sport with repetition, tilting at the absurdity of language until it surrendered its logic. In the college canteen, in stoned reverie with his friend, no two conversations were the same. In painting no two brush strokes were the same. Now he was being asked to play the same notes in the same order. Again and again and again.

'I'm an old jazz man,' said Smith. 'I played in jazz groups before joining EMI. So that was my kind of music. I walked into UFO and the group came on. Well, their music didn't mean very much to me at all. But they had this light show, which was very impressive. And I remember thinking to myself, "How can I get a light show onto disc?" I could see the following they had there and that they were extremely popular. So I thought, "Well, it looks as though we can sell some records here."' As well as nailing his commercial priorities to the mast, the Floyd's producer was astute enough to realise that Barrett's problem was insurmountable. How could he translate the thrill of immersion he felt at UFO into the clinical setting of Abbey Road studios? The more Barrett thought about it, the less he thought of it.

Down at UFO Mark Boyle provided the best of the light shows. He too had a fine-art practitioner's sense of perfectionism and a disdain for those who sold themselves short. By the end of the decade Boyle had forsaken painting with light and had become a fully fledged conceptualist and installationist. In May 1970, in collaboration with his partner Joan Hills, he put together an exhibition called *Journey to the Surface of the Earth*, a 'multi-sensual presentation of 1000 sites selected at random from the surface of the earth'. The exhibition was shown at the Gemeentemuseum Den Haag in Holland between 16 May and 12 July 1970, and in the programme catalogue Boyle wrote an extended polemic against the futility of 'explanation'. Its similarity to Syd Barrett's creative dilemma is startling. It anticipates and counterpoints Barrett's own withdrawal from the centre of his quest.

The head is drenched with thoughts and images that supercede one another with such rapidity that writing and even speaking become intolerable except as a sort of recreational activity, or as a social constitutional of a kind that appals you more and more.

MARK BOYLE

At his creative peak Barrett revealed a seemingly effortless capacity for scrambling meaning and logic. It's a rare lyrical gift, an instinctive freestyling approach to language that few songwriters possess. When he submitted himself to the obligations of the music industry – to pop-press interviews, for instance – he always sounded reined in and stilted by comparison. At the height of his fame he invariably came across either as polite, gauche or politely gauche. His formal and mannered responses reveal little of consequence about his art or himself. In Waters and Barrett's famous TV encounter with the music critic Hans Keller, both men appear composed, but they exchange frequent quizzical and amused glances as Keller fires off another of his 'Why precisely do you exist? Please explain' enquiries. Of the two, Waters looks slightly less ill at ease, the more willing spokesman, a role he would rapidly grow into in direct proportion to his colleague's withdrawal.

Barrett's strangest interview encounter during this period was with American journalist Meatball Fulton, just after the release of *The Piper at the Gates of Dawn* in August 1967. In 2008 Fulton unearthed a rare and previously unheard tape of his meeting with Barrett and posted the full unedited audio on the Internet.[3] Listening to it now is like eavesdropping on a conversation between two incapacitated stoners. Essentially it is an exercise in non-communication, but it speaks volumes about the times, and is revealing on several levels. Barrett is softly spoken to the point of inaudibility, and is as fluent as narcotic circumstances will allow. A minimally edited extract from his disjointed, rambling response to Fulton's first question runs as follows:

'Well, I'll say, for example, painting at an art school. Or painting, say, in infant school. The initial desire to paint or initial first successes at painting arose, I think, out of a very genuine basic drive . . . and because family and social set-ups are channelled into success or otherwise and, through schools and suchlike, one gets different things . . . one comes across teachers and people like that, teaching and instruction . . . and I feel now that having left art school that there are a lot of things that I could do. A lot of things I see now, a lot of things went into me, into my head . . . changing and altering things.

For instance, I made a painting the other day . . . and I could see and hear very clearly different instructions and different criticisms going into the picture, which were in fact criticisms that I could relate back to art school and teachers . . . So maybe this would be very valuable, this break. I don't know, to try painting again after a break of going into pop music.'

Even in this slightly tidied-up form the hash haze of the room is palpable. Although, as any music journalist who has ever been faced with the task of contriving quotable utterances out of the rambling inconsequentialities of stoned rock stars will tell you, the extract is no more inarticulate than many that writers encounter on a regular basis. Pick your way through the hesitant and halting delivery, the repetition, the cul-de-sacs and convoluted thought processes, and moments of clarity do emerge. The entire rambling discourse can be boiled down to this: Barrett has been thinking about his art-school training and is now wondering how he can best apply that conceptual grounding to the next stage of his creative development. At the time of the interview, August 1967, the Pink Floyd are taking a short break from touring, citing Barrett's 'nervous exhaustion' as the reason. Perhaps the most revealing

aspect of this conversational fragment is that Barrett is clearly thinking about resuming painting again, 'after a break of going into pop music'. He is still pondering the implications of having dropped his fine-art studies at Camberwell in favour of a pop career. What is not clear from the response is whether he is attempting to apply his theorising to painting alone or trying to facilitate further ways of making connections between his fine-art studies and his music. Either way, the fact that he is theorising at all, and attempting to articulate these thoughts from the depths of his stoned stupor to an equally stoned stranger, speaks volumes.

During the interview Barrett talks, albeit obliquely, about assimilating ideas and channelling thought processes. Unfortunately, his inquisitor reduces these potentially fruitful areas of enquiry to hippie shibboleths: conditioned response, thought control, the system, the man. Barrett is unfailingly polite and responds to all questions with a surface diplomacy, but he becomes increasingly guarded and non-committal as the tape rolls on. After the initial exchanges he perceptibly begins to withdraw from the whole charade that is unfurling like so much hash smoke before him. When Fulton attempts to press his interviewee further on the issue of freeing one-self from 'the system', Barrett tries to bring the question back to the specifics of painting. 'I finished a picture. I got through a lot of things. It's quite enjoyable, you know, and . . . I would like to get hold of that and be able to assimilate the system as it comes in, rather than as it goes out.' Again, gnomic though it seems, this is just a convoluted way of saying that he would like to be more methodical in his approach rather than simply relying on instincts. None of this registers with his interviewer, who changes tact and asks, 'Do you ever feel when you see people that you could tell them something about themselves that they don't already know? Or do you look at people that way? I feel you do, that you really sort of observe people. Do you?' Barrett initially tries to distance himself from the thrust of the question. His disjointed, contradictory reply hints both at a reluctance to deal with the enquiry and a degree of embarrassment at being put on the spot in this way. His response also contains a revealing nugget or two about the limits of journalistic encounters like this one:

'Nah. I think it's something about . . . I certainly do get a feeling of what people are like and, really, the complication comes out in talking, but this only comes out at certain times because of a feeling that talking is, in fact, a far less valuable thing than . . . it's almost superfluous to everything else, you know. But the same time, it's a contradiction that the words and talking to people should be difficult in any way. One is hesitant to say, "No, I can't say anything," you know. And I know as well this is something that occurs only at times, other times it doesn't . . . and it's cool.'

Again, choice phrases leap out of the brain fug – 'the complication comes out in talking', talking 'is superfluous to everything else'. And so it goes on. Inconsequentiality chases its own tail until all that can be heard is the tape machine whirring and the inhalation of ennui on an airless August day somewhere in London in the middle of the Summer of Love.

'There's so many different things that on different levels that I could say . . . maybe the most strange thing is . . . meeting you, very strange to meet you, well, it isn't really strange, it's not many people that . . . one can . . . interviewers and such like, and you come into that class. I mean generally it's just sort of say hello and to get to say the questions and go again . . . I don't know . . . I don't know.'

'I see you're holding back,' says Fulton.

'No. Not at all! I understand. I think

I learn a lot from you,' says Barrett, trying to put his interrogator at ease. As he struggles to extricate himself from this Ionesco-esque theatre of absurdity he merely binds himself in more semantic knots. 'I know I feel from you that . . . really, that I could say anything and do anything and you would still . . . I mean, you are recording it and that's cool and . . . I know that applies to you, to me and you, 'cos really I assure you, you can do anything you want, but . . . if . . . I want to . . . if I wanted to say nothing or if I want to act in an extra-extraordinary way . . . then I feel that that too is justified.'

The voice trails away. Click. Someone pushes an off button. In more ways than one.

You are the pivot of the changes
taking place. As you move in
the new direction – contrary
to accepted traditional ideas –
everyone and everything will fall in
behind you.
HEXAGRAM 24

Except they won't. 'Increasingly erratic' is the phrase that writers love to use about this particular phase of Barrett's disintegration: 'His behaviour became increasingly erratic.' It's a tired, hackneyed expression right up there with

'He let his imagination run riot,' and it's just as meaningless, or rather it's so true it's tautological. That's what the imagination does, it runs riot. That's what imagination is, a running riot. Oh, the futility of words. Barrett's imagination had always run riot. It had been running riot since he was two. 'You only have to read the lines / of scribbly black / and everything shines,' as he sings in 'Matilda Mother'. Ironically, the only time his imagination didn't run riot was when he knuckled down to the disciplined procedures of his art and his writing. When he wrote pop songs and painted he adhered to the conventions of pop songs and painting. It was when he wasn't being purposefully creative that his imagination ran riot. That's when he became 'increasingly erratic'. 'Increasingly erratic' was a loaded term. In context it meant too erratic to observe the procedures and obligations of the pop life (or, for that matter, the art life). Too erratic to toe the line. Touring. TV. Press. Promotion. Obligation. Be here now. Be there tomorrow. At some point during the summer of 1967 Syd Barrett crossed an invisible line. Improvisation in the context of a UFO performance was cherished and revered. Pete Townshend brings his mate Eric Clapton down just to check out what you are doing. Improvisation in the context of fucking up the career path and the well-rehearsed life your fellow band mates are carving out for themselves is irresponsible. Where are the boundaries? Where is the cliff edge and precipice? When you are self-medicating as often as Syd it becomes increasingly difficult to tell. And who is going to tell you anyway? 'Do you ever feel when you see people that you could tell them something about themselves that they don't already know?' asked Meatball Fulton, dropping verbal pebbles down a deep well and waiting for an echo that never comes. And how can you possibly answer that question when you hardly know your own self, when you no longer even want a sense of self?

You don't want any image, you want to be transparent, a projection almost seen on a cloud of cigarette smoke. And you know as you say it that all you're doing is to make another kind of image, perhaps more suited to your circumstances than any other. You're saying I am what I produce. I am a circuit of no importance. My anonymity is valuable to me.
MARK BOYLE

Barrett thrived in the light show. It appealed to his sense of anonymity.

Immersed in the multicoloured displays of the liquid lenses and the celluloid wheels, adorned in dappled refractions, backlit by flickering shadows and silhouettes, reduced to a shape, an outline Barrett could shed his obligation to stagecraft and ego projection. Performing in the light show was like merging with your own canvas. The troubles began when there wasn't a light show to hide in. When the Pink Floyd toured the ballrooms, they encountered another world. Barrett visibly wilted in the spotlight. Suddenly Hexagram 24 – earth above, thunder below – took on more ominous connotations.

Do not plunge into a new course – you will only find yourself thrashing helplessly about. What will happen has begun to happen. You sense it starting; as it proceeds you will sense its progress. Meanwhile, remain yourself. Practise only what you fully understand.
HEXAGRAM 24

The Pink Floyd go to America, and have to abandon the tour after only a handful of gigs. In November 1967 they embark upon one of the last of the old-school package tours around the UK with the Jimi Hendrix Experience, the Move, the Nice, Amen Corner, Eire Apparent and Outer Limits. Fifteen-minute sets for each band and thirty minutes for Hendrix, the headline act. Syd Barrett starts to go missing, sometimes while still on stage. On a couple of occasions Nice guitarist David O'List is drafted in as a replacement. No one really notices. No one really cares. It's a package tour. Fifteen minutes of fame. Shove 'em on and shove 'em off again.

> *You would like to have a bitter*
> *image of yourself. But you're not*
> *even bitter any longer. You have*
> *no ambitions. You've seen it all*
> *and you knew before you saw it*
> *that their Hilton Hotels and their*
> *Cadillacs were going to add up to*
> *precisely nothing. You're an onion,*
> *and to find the inner, essential onion*
> *you strip away the layers protecting*
> *the centre, to discover that at the*
> *centre there are only more layers*
> *and beyond them a smell and a blur*
> *of tears.*
>
> HEXAGRAM 24

The English beat poet Spike Hawkins tells Barrett that he has unlocked so many doors. 'Yes,' replies Barrett. 'But with cheap keys.' Disillusion hardens like quick-setting cement. Required to come up with a new single Barrett writes 'Vegetable Man', a sardonic sneer

at the whole process of pop fame. He delivers it in that flat, artless sneer, the one he reserves for all the songs that aren't about gnomes and Emily and Puck and Pan. The lyrics will be mis-read for years as a lacerating treatise on his crumbling state of mind. He also writes 'Scream Thy Last Scream', a tale as dark and menacing as any Grimms' fairy tale. Both songs are rejected as 'uncommercial'.

> *A turn for the better has come and*
> *gone. You have let it pass you by . . .*
> *you believe you display backbone*
> *by resisting change, you mistake*
> *your fear for stubbornness. This*
> *attitude is disastrous. It denies*
> *the inevitable flow of change in*
> *the universe – a flow which will*
> *carry you along, if not buoyant and*
> *upright then tumbled headlong and*
> *willy-nilly. But the moment has*
> *passed. You can do nothing about*
> *it now. You must patiently wait for*
> *things again to resolve themselves.*
>
> HEXAGRAM 24

'If not buoyant and upright then tumbled headlong and willy-nilly' would be the shape of it for some time to come. On BBC Radio 1, on 31 December 1967, John Peel and Tommy Vance presented a three-hour end-of-year edition of *Top*

Gear. It was a stupendously rich celebration of all that was great and good about 1967. As well as featuring Syd Barrett's last session with Pink Floyd there were live sessions by the Moody Blues, the Herd, the Alan Bown! and Eric Burdon and the Animals, all of whom performed four numbers apiece. The best of the year on vinyl was featured too. There were bulletins from the American underground like 'I Can Take You to the Sun' by the Misunderstood, 'Porpoise Mouth' by Country Joe and the Fish, 'Castles Made of Sand' by the Jimi Hendrix Experience, 'Dropout Boogie' by Captain Beefheart, 'Pandora's Golden Heebie Jeebies' by the Association, 'A Child's Claim to Fame' by Buffalo Springfield, 'Fall on You' by Moby Grape. There were all those English singles and LP tracks that had gone into making the great psychedelic spring, summer, autumn and winter of love: 'Blue Jay Way' by the Beatles, 'Coloured Rain' by Traffic, 'Armenia City in the Sky' by the Who, 'Time Seller' by the Spencer Davis Group, 'Supernatural Fairy Tale' by Art, 'Fredereek Hernando' by One in a Million. And in the midst of all these riches Syd Barrett's absence hovers like light-show spectral shadows. He's there on tape but his spirit is somewhere else. He sings 'Scream the Last Scream',

'Vegetable Man' and 'Jugband Blues'; the latter would be the last of his compositions the Pink Floyd recorded. The last word he sings on a Pink Floyd LP is 'joke'.

In his final months with the band there was an undoing of everything and a sense of unravelling. In need of reinforcements they brought in Barrett's old Cambridge pal David Gilmour to bolster the sound and maybe, who knows, reignite a flagging spirit. Syd's mate Dave, with whom he had swapped riffs in the tech college canteen, with whom he had busked in the south of France. The five-piece line-up did rejuvenate him briefly. He perked up for a gig or two, but then lapsed back into incommunicado. 'His head did no thinking / his arms didn't move,' as he sang on 'Scarecrow'. And then one day – hooray! – the band didn't pick him up any more, reasoning that there was no one there any more to pick up anyway.

While Syd Barrett embarked upon a decade-long quest to impale himself upon ennui and indecision, Pink Floyd furnished his absence and his unfinished canvases with their own architectural ab-dabs and abstractions. Groups are often at their best when they don't know what it is that they are doing, when the boundary markers are ill defined, when the goal is still beyond, when the dreams (or, in the Floyd's case, the dystopias) are only half formed. It is also during this period, paradoxically enough, when they are at their most influential. The spacey imprecision that Pink Floyd hazily sketched out between 1968 and 1970 – impulses in progress, fleetingly captured and episodically rendered on *A Saucerful of Secrets*, *Ummagumma*, *More* and *La Vallée* and on their numerous radio sessions – influenced everything from the German space rock of Tangerine Dream to the ambient dance fusions of the Orb and beyond, influenced everything but Pink Floyd, in fact. Their best music during this transitional period is tentative, ethereal and unsullied. Its hauntingly wistful beauty encapsulates both where its founding spirits came from and what they were never entirely able to leave behind.

'I really think that the architecture has a lot to do with it,' reasons Barry Miles. 'That's why the Pink Floyd's music is so slow and English and environmental. It's the sound of Grantchester Meadows. It's a very English upper-middle-class environment that is required to produce that. Canterbury is the only other place like that. Even Oxford has a metal-box factory and a ring of industry around

it. It seemed to me that that was a very important element in the Pink Floyd – the fact that the three different leaders all came out of that same background, incredibly privileged, not just middle-class but very privileged in the sense of what they had access to. And the visual aspect too. I'm a great believer in the situationist idea that the actual geography and buildings and the built environment is of tremendous importance. Just growing up there and walking around those streets, going to the meadows and always being in the presence of medieval architecture. And the very slow pace of life in the sense that everything just continues. There's the keeper of the fabric, and when he dies there's another keeper of the fabric. These are just offices that get renewed.'

While the Pink Floyd assembled monuments of sound that reflected their architectural heritage, their original guiding spirit remained in Cambridge, abstract and listless, occasionally regathering thoughts that would never quite assemble themselves in the same way again. As in light show as in life.

You remember fragments of 50,000 experiences, and you suspect them, and you suspect the conscious

*and unconscious forces that keep
dredging them up. They're all
part of the proper snobberies, the
prejudices and preferences built
in by your heredity and your
upbringing. Most of all you suspect
the way you formulate. And so
finally you say there is this, there is
this, there is this.*

MARK BOYLE

Until in the end there isn't even that.

12

SMASHED BLOCKED

Art-Pop Renegades and the R&B Mutations

Remember how Pop-art and Op-art influenced fashion and fabrics? Well stand by for the next craze. It's not easy to say. It's 'psychedelic art'. And if you haven't got your tongue around that one how about hallucinogenic?

Both these words are being used to describe the weird and wonderful coloured patterns that manifest themselves to takers of the new mind drugs like LSD (fashion goes to some strange places for its inspiration these days).

According to Home Furnishing Daily, *an American trade journal, these 'psychedelic prints seem to move, come in and out of focus, blur. They reach the unconscious. They bring to mind Outer Space . . . a dream . . . A trip.'*

Colours are 'waves of emotion', 'kinetic' . . . 'dots of movement'.

For American fashion designers to get the psychedelic idea they don't happily have to take the drugs and get the visions. It's all being specially set up with coloured lights at museums and art exhibitions in New York.

Already available in London 'psychedelic' goggles at 30 shillings. They have built-in glass prisms which make everything look multi-coloured and mixed up. Pauline Fordham, who makes them, says 'they're a good visual trip'.

DAILY MIRROR fashion feature, January 1967

Watch any of the surviving film footage from the early days of UK psychedelia, at UFO, say, or the Roundhouse, and you can see a similar scenario being played out. Something of the changing times can be glimpsed in the way the girls are dancing. Ostensibly, most of them are still mod-stepping, or at least trying to. But something else has taken hold, some weird gravity-denying push and pull. Everything's gone a bit loose-limbed and gangly. Physically everyone is still genuflecting to familiar dance-floor habits and rituals. There's a hint of the mashed potato here, an absently executed shuffle, shake or slide there, but everything is starting to get a little uncoordinated, a little what you might call 'interpretive'. But then it must be pretty hard to shoop-shoop when your cheekbones are radiating ultraviolet light and your elbows are turning to cellophane.

The same shape-shifting process can be detected in the music too. Between 1965 and 1967 British R&B rapidly mutates into something altogether more supple, and you can trace those mutations in the output of almost every famous group of the period, and quite a few non-famous ones too. If the multitude of changes that occurred in UK pop between 1965 and 1967 can be boiled down to one essential characteristic, it is that audible shift between taut, jerky R&B and the more flaccid and fluid manoeuvres of psychedelic pop. The head buzz and hot-wired heart palpitations of speed are giving way to the nirvana rush and brain mash of acid, and can't you just tell. You can see it in the dancing and you can see it in the way musicians move, or no longer move, on stage. The wide-boy swagger and barrow-boy braggadocio of mod is replaced by dreamy-eyed, mush-mouthed immobility. It's the difference between Steve Marriott singing 'Whatcha Gonna Do About It' and Ronnie Lane singing 'Green Circles'. It's the difference between the Pretty Things singing, 'Oh Rosalyn / tell me where ya bin,' to a Bo Diddley shuffle beat in 1964 and the Pretty Things dribbling, 'Sitting alone on a bench with you / mirrowed [*sic*] above in the sky,' three years later.

The way clothes were cut during the mod era made people pose in a certain way, turning everyone into mini-Modigliani sculptures or cubist photo images, dandies descending a staircase. For purposes of decorum the miniskirt dictated the way a female sat. Knees together pointed inwards, legs splayed at right angles, feet apart. A generation subsequently adopted the pose regardless of what they were wearing and that angular look dominated fashion photography for the next five years, and rock-star posturing for long after that. George Melly noticed the all-encompassing effect on poise and deportment in 1965, when he observed a gathering of art students: 'Heads craned forward, shoulders slightly raised, trunks off centre, but leaning either forward or to one side, never

straight or backwards. Arms and legs were pushed out at angles so that there seemed no flow either singularly or as a group. When they moved, which was infrequently, everything seemed to jerk into new awkward angular shapes.'[1] As new pharmaceutical imperatives took hold, that lop-sided stance was increasingly choreographed by lop-sided beats in the music. Soon enough there was lop-sided thinking in the lyrics and the outlook too.

Mod, in all its manifold permutations, rampages through the entire story of English psychedelia. The mod's peacock parade was a complex amalgam of dandyism and brutism, a constant clash between heightened aesthetic sensibilities and base instincts. The friction between these two tendencies colours every shade and variation of psychedelic pop, and the mod aesthetic informs every last gesture, utterance and emasculated strut of what follows here. By 1967 traditional male swagger was under chemical bombardment; from the androgyny of the mod boy–girl look to the hazy drone and drawl of the music everything went melty-headed and soft-centred. Callow, lilywhite singers of unconvincing larynx who only months before might have been trying to convince you that they were your back-door man were now arriving metaphorically doused in cheap after-shave and dressed in a whole new set of poncey threads, with a bouquet of graveyard-grabbed daffodils in hand, trying to convince you that their motor wasn't nicked and their wallet was over-flowing. It was all a front, of course, but in song at least the nervous machismo it produced briefly usurped the blues boasters of yore. Sometime around the latter half of 1966 and the early part of 1967 the momentum of those who had been influenced by post-war R&B was derailed, and the mannish boy gener-ation began to explore other options. There always was another male 1960s, of course – the 1960s of boys cry when no one can see them and similar secret fragilities – but this was something else. Psychedelic drugs presented fresh new guises and disguises to explore. Every-body stopped flexing to the pill rush and submitted themselves to the new pharmaceutical circumstances. The effects on the music and the culture were audible, visible and everywhere.

The dance moves, the musical trans-formations, the vocal inflections, the lyrical matter of the songs, they all betray the difference between being blocked in and tripped out, receptors closed or receptors open. 'Blocked' was a great mod slang term for being pilled-up and, like all the great forgotten jazz words – 'reefer', 'wigged-out', etc. – it deserves to be revived and kept alive. 'Blocked' perfectly conveyed the accumulative effect that all those mother's little helpers could have on a night's leaping and lack of sleeping. There's a certain incriminating doe-eyed stare and facial impedance that you see all the time in archive footage of 1960s models. When they speak, you can hear it in the inanimate dry-mouthed drawl and the way they take in tiny little gulps of air between utter-ances. Blocked. Every one of them.

John's Children made an anthem out of such impulses. 'Smashed Blocked' was the A-side of their first single, released in late 1966. 'Smashed' was another great 'buzz' word, temporarily appropriated by potheads from juice heads in the mid-sixties. Put the two words together and – *voilà!* – twice the obliteration. 'Everything's spinning. My eyes are tired,' sings Andy Elli-son, during the song's opening dream sequence. 'Blocked, blocked, blocked. My way of getting through.' 'Smashed Blocked' was originally released with the title 'The Love I Thought I'd Found' in order to get airplay, but it's that hook line that endures. After the opening disorientation drama it settles down into a waltzy serenade delivered with as much piss-take insolence as a smashed blocked mod could muster in 1966. By 1967, with Marc Bolan briefly on board, John's Children were singing songs with titles like 'Midsummer Night's Scene', 'Jagged Time Lapse' and 'Sara, Crazy Child'. And on a single shunned by the BBC they invited Desdemona to lift up her skirt and fly. Those track titles tell you all you need to know about the difference – the jagged time lapse indeed – between 1966 and 1967. Last year's blocked mod was this year's crazy child, dressed in allusions and apparel to match. Desdemona taking flight, pleading to Othello 'kill me tomorrow, let me live tonight'.

Marc Bolan was there before the beginning. An eleven-year-old Face. The original working-class dandy in the underworld. The boy who invented himself, over and over again. He softened his East End vowels, affected a lisp and sought out that amoral netherworld that readily embraced all those barrow boys who might be mistaken for rent boys, that 42nd Street of the mind 'where the underworld meet the elite' that constituted the less publicised side of swinging London, that decadent meritocracy where deb culture on the way down met prole culture on the way up, as *Queen* magazine put it. 'Everyone else wanted to sound like cockneys. We all wanted to sound better than our

backgrounds,' noted Bolan's close friend and fellow individualist Jeff Dexter. Producer Tony Visconti calls Bolan 'the most focused artist I've ever worked with'; his detractors called him a pushy little hustler on the make, a scheming wannabe, ready to hitch a ride on any bandwagon in order to achieve the fame he so clearly craved. Born Mark Feld to a market-trader mum and a lorry-driving dad in Hackney, east London, in 1947, he had little formal education and left school at fourteen. Analysis of his illegible scribble suggests that he may have been dyslexic, but they didn't have dyslexia in the 1950s. You just sat at the back of class and either buggered about or dreamed and doodled. An entire generation of 11-plus rejects did that, and it was here, in the going-nowhere zone of the 1950s secondary modern school, that Bolan's imagination took wing – his and a few thousand others. 'All those lads from that kind of background were into getting out of what they were surrounded by,' notes Jeff Dexter, who first met Bolan at Connick's, a tailor's on Kingsland Road. 'It had a great boys' department. I became a model for their 1961 show at Earl's Court. So did Marc. We just used to glare at each other, check each other's clothes out.'

Initially, the teenage Feld flirted with the stage name Toby Tyler before allegedly francophiling the harsh K of his forename and collapsing Bo(b Dy) lan into Bolan. The story may be apocryphal. It hardly matters. Bolan was dream-weaving from the off, and if anyone can lay claim to the first English underground single, it's probably him. Released in November 1965 on Decca, 'The Wizard' was an astonishing piece of work for its time, a truly extraordinary two-minute slice of orchestrated pop sorcery that doesn't sound remotely like anything else from that period. It tells of Bolan's almost certainly fabricated meeting with a magic man and gave birth to one of its creator's most enduring myths. 'He came back from France, where he claimed he'd met this wizard in the woods and lived with him for three months and learned his magic spells,' remembers Simon Napier-Bell, Bolan's early mentor and manager of John's Children. 'In fact, he'd been for a weekend package tour and met some gay guy. But Marc was a great fantasist and in the end he believed he'd met a wizard. But the great thing about him was that if he knew you knew the truth, he'd have a laugh. I said, "It's just some bloke you met in a gay club, isn't it?" Marc said, "Yeah, but he could do conjuring tricks." Marc got this reputation for being precious, but he wasn't really. He was always funny with his friends.'

'He could spout a lot of bullshit but give you the wink while he was saying it,' confirms Dexter. 'He was always totally sussed to what was going on around him.' This combination of adaptability and ambition meant that Bolan was tailor made (literally) for the pop-mod mutations that were going on around him. His time with John's Children was brief, brash and opportunist, just another rung on a career ladder that led upwards, but the collaboration produced some great art-pop moments.

Bolan's follow-up to 'The Wizard', 'The Third Degree', released in June 1966, was played extensively by the offshore pirate stations. Again, its raw, spiky, demo-like quality sounded completely out of kilter with everything else around. When his third and arguably most inventive solo single, 'Hippy Gumbo', made zero impression at the tail end of 1966, Simon Napier-Bell co-opted his young protégé into John's Children. 'I said to him, "Go and write a song where Andy (Ellison) can sing the verse but you can come in with the chorus." We'd decided that this funny quivering voice was too much for the public to take in a full song.' The result of that first collaboration was 'Desdemona'. On the follow-up, 'Midsummer Night's Scene', the contrast between Bolan's and Ellison's vocals is pronounced. Bolan is only let loose at the very end, screaming the chorus line like he has no previous acquaintance with the lyrics or indeed the key he's supposed to be singing in. He sounds unhinged. Although he responded enthusiastically enough to Napier-Bell's penchant for instrument smashing and riot incitement, Bolan was clearly never going to be a team player and he departed John's Children in June 1967. That month the following ad appeared in the one-shilling-a-word 'Musicians Wanted' section of *Melody Maker*: 'Freaky lead guitarist, bass guitarist and drummer wanted for Marc Bolan's new group. Also any other astral flyers like with cars, amplification and that which never grew in window boxes.' New dawn. New argot. Same sharp eye for the main chance.

Another group that rode the changes pretty well was the Creation. The Creation had started out life as Mark Four, playing patented British R&B, but, encouraged by producer Shel Talmy to indulge their experimental tendencies, they adopted Pete Townshend's feedback squeaks and squalls and began making great art pop. Guitarist Eddie Phillips played his instrument with a violin bow, a technique that was emulated to equally good effect by Jimmy Page a year or so later, and on tracks like 'Life's Just Beginning' and 'Through My Eyes' the Creation showed that they were more than accomplished Yardbirds copyists. In their finest song, 'Painter Man', they created an antidote to the myth that has grown up around the fact that a few prominent pop stars attended art school. It's a myth that fails to take into account the tenuous, at times non-existent link between several of these stars and their art-school training (e.g. Keith Richards, Eric Clapton, Ray Davies), or the fact that many of the most conceptually astute musicians of the 1960s (e.g. Marc Bolan, Paul McCartney, Robert Wyatt, Roger Waters) didn't attend art school. In claiming that art schools were a repository for bohemianism and hanging out, the myth fails to take into account the fact that the majority of people who attended these institutions did so to become artists, and that the vast majority of those who had the same disenchanting experience of art school as John Lennon, Keith Richards and Ray Davies didn't go on to become John Lennon, Keith Richards and Ray Davies. 'Painter Man' conveys a more typical art-school experience. The song's central character spends his days designing cartoons, comic books, dirty postcards, soap boxes, tea packets, TV ads and tin-can labels. He isn't the next Andy Warhol or Jasper Johns; he's a hired pair of hands in a commercial world. 'Classic art has had its day,' sneers singer Kenny Pickett, who four years later went on to co-write Clive Dunn's 'Grandad' and clearly knew what he was talking about.

The Creation were full of moody-boy bluffing and attitude and had great tailor-made songs to match. 'Biff Bang Pow' incorporated comic-book iconography into its my g-g-g-generation tribulations about a mod boy affronted by a former girlfriend's continued looming presence in his life. As singles go, it's all pop-art hook and little more, but a pop-art hook is all it needs to be. 'How Does It Feel to Feel' was a smashed blocked anthem. Released in February 1968, it conveyed a jittery generation's comedown but was alleviated by a tell-tale last-verse line about sliding down a sunbeam and bursting clouds on the way, a sure sign that things had changed a little since the days when they went out as the Mark Four and that many groups were now getting their lyrical pick-me-ups from other sources.

The music of the Pretty Things also went through some radical changes during this period. They had started off as a raw, raucous R&B outfit; guitarist Dick Taylor had been a member of an early line-up of the Stones, playing bass alongside Mick Jagger, Keith Richards and Brian Jones before teaming up with art-school colleague Phil May to form his own band. The Pretty Things had Top 40 hits with their first four singles – 'Rosalyn', 'Don't Bring Me Down', 'Honey, I Need' and 'Cry to Me'. On songs like 'Midnight to Six Man' and 'Buzz the Jerk' they pioneered the jerky and angular complexity that mod pop was built on. Phil May's snarling vocals on their first two LPs sound like the prototype for countless garage bands that came out of America in the mid-sixties. By the time the Pretty Things recorded their third LP, *Emotions*, in 1966 the sound had softened and become more folksy and whimsical. Swinging London vignettes like 'Death of a Socialite' and 'Photographer' were knowingly arch and satirical, while Reg Tilsley's florid orchestration on tracks like 'The Sun' and 'House of Ten' is the prototype for the kind of pop-psych arrangements that would become ubiquitous in the late sixties. But one track on *Emotions* more than any other signposts the future. On first listen 'Trippin'' sounds like an innocuous satirical throwaway. Set to a rural blues ramble, with a melody that references the Stones' 'Play with Fire', the song's three verses address, in turn, a painter, a writer and a record-maker. They just happen to be called Mr L, Mr S and Mr D. 'Mr L, they love your paintings / is it something that you use?' the lyric enquires. Mr S's books 'have more perception with every one you complete'. The records Mr D makes 'are strange / some folks even find them confusing / they say it's the sunshine that lights you up'. The Mr D verse mentions Methedrine, the second pop song to do so following Donovan's 'The Trip'. In addition to the hefty 'Sunshine Superman' nudge in the lyric, Phil May appears to slur Donovan's name in the final chorus. Just in case we haven't got the message yet, the chorus goes, 'I won't ask you more than twice / are you trippin, mister? / Whatever it is, it's nice.'

Following a move from Fontana to EMI the Pretty Things issued a brace of singles that announced their arrival as fully fledged psychedelicists. 'Defecting Grey'/'Mr Evasion', released in November 1967, and 'Talkin' About the Good Times'/'Walking Through My Dreams', which followed in February 1968, are a million miles from the Bo Diddley-inspired singles that got them on *Top of the Pops* in 1964. 'Defecting Grey' sounds like a collage of four separate songs. Beginning with the ominous low rumble of a tone generator and a whoozy nursery-rhyme melody

seemingly played by a drunken pub pianist, it suddenly lurches into a 'Merry-Go-Round' waltz and a lyric about two lovers on a park bench who appear to be astral-travelling their tits off. These fey ruminations are abruptly curtailed by a snatch of tape-reversed sitar, followed by a raucous R&B section that reverts to the band's early style, before heading back into a waltz-time verse. A middle eight replete with spacey high harmonies is followed by another waltz-time verse, a reprise of the reversed-sitar section, a Yardbirds-style rave-up, a further verse, four bars of cockney knees-up and a finale that fades out on a one-word chant: 'Sky–sky–sky–sky'.

'Defecting Grey''s follow-up 'Talkin' About the Good Times' takes the coda of 'Strawberry Fields Forever' and the two-note oscillations of 'I Am the Walrus' as its inspiration and builds an entire song out of them. Like its predecessor, it is dominated by lurching see-saw tempi and echo-drenched, high-register harmonies that manage to sound both exhilarating and eerie. It also features the subtle use of a mellotron, clanging rhythm guitars, some decidedly Ringo-esque drumming and that slowed-down 'Taxman' riff that pretty much every psychedelically inclined outfit borrowed at some point during 1967.

The Pretty Things' move into new pharmaceutical terrain was gradual and accumulative, taking place over a period of two years. Others were transformed overnight into awestruck (sometimes dumbstruck) converts. Zoot Money had been a stalwart of the London R&B scene since the early sixties. He was briefly a member of Alexis Korner's Blues Incorporated, but made his name as the extrovert front man of Zoot Money's Big Roll Band. It's a familiar résumé: a residency at the Flamingo Club, a reputation and a tight-ass band to match, a flamboyant stage act heavy on the Hammond, all topped off with Zoot's likeable loon persona. The Big Roll Band made singles with poppy A-sides and serious workouts on the flip for the club connoisseurs. On their LPs they paid homage to their heroes: Jimmy Smith, James Brown, Jimmy Reed et al. In September 1966 they had a minor UK hit with the Tony Colton/Ray Smith composition 'Big Time Operator', a brassy mod anthem to aspiration, lightened by Zoot's genial rasp and mock boastfulness. 'I'm going to be so big you won't even be able to look at me,' he jokes Muhammad Ali-style on the fade-out. In the spring of 1967 the Big Roll Band released a single called 'Nick Knack', a gimmicky number that riffs a little tiredly on the old give-a-dog-a-bone refrain. It rhymes 'bone' with 'stoned' but alcohol is still clearly the drug of choice, even though the song slips in a sly reference to getting spiked ('he drunk mickey finns / anything') and getting high; admittedly it's on pink champagne, but Zoot waves a flower in the promo film and the inference is obvious. Everything is about to change.

A few weeks later Zoot Money formed a band called Dantalian's Chariot and, as he succinctly put it on their first record, 'I was OK / and then one day / pow!' Dantalian's Chariot was basically the Big Roll Band with a new name borrowed from a 1904 translation of a seventeenth-century compendium of demonology known variously as *The Lesser Keys of Solomon, Clavicula Salomonis Regis* or *The Lemegeton*. The 71st spirit of Solomon, according to the book, was Duke Dantalian. Dantalian's Chariot (the band, not the demonic evocation) played their debut gig in front of 15,000 people at the Seventh National Jazz and Blues Festival at Windsor race course, the forerunner to the Reading Festival. On 12 August, just four months after the release of 'Nick Knack', and on the same Saturday-night bill as the Nice, Paul Jones, the Crazy World of Arthur Brown and Ten Years After, Dantalian's Chariot appeared resplendent in white robes and played an R&B set doused liberally in fairy dust. Their reception, both from the crowd and pop journalists, varied from polite bemusement to outright ridicule. The following week the Chariot played the opening night of the Middle Earth club, but fared a little less well when they took the show on the road. 'We are too far ahead of the audience outside of London: East Grinstead is not Haight-Ashbury,' noted Zoot, not unreasonably. Dantalian's Chariot released one manically inspired single, 'Madman (Running Through the Fields)', and gigged solidly for six months before the bookings dwindled and the money ran out. They recorded several tracks for a proposed album for the Direction label, which the company then decided not to release. The working title for the LP was *The Elephants They Are Dance*, which probably tells you all you need to know about the prevailing influences. The eventual emergence of these recordings on a Wooden Hill CD released in 1996 reveals not so much a lost classic as a compendium of mismatched curios and inspired moments of high lunacy.

What Zoot Money lacked as a new-age prophet he more than made up for in zonked-out charm. On 'World War Three' he managed to make the impending Armageddon sound like an after-hours jam session at the Speakeasy. 'This Island' was a dreamy instrumental featuring Andy Summers on sitar, accompanied by crashing waves and a female chorale that ventures boldly into Yma Sumac territory. On 'Suma' Summers's sitar and Nick Newall's flute explore the Indo jazz-fusion territory popularised by John Mayer and Joe Harriott. The unreleased album's high points (in every sense) are 'Fourpenny Bus Ride' and 'Four Firemen'. The former takes the little-man theme that runs through mid-sixties pop and tells of Charlie, a humdrum employee with a humdrum job and a drudge-filled life (and wife). 'From Tooting to Chiswick his mind is free to roam far from his home,' Zoot huskily intones, with more than a suggestion that the bus ride might be a metaphor. 'Four Firemen' relates the tale of a fire crew who are called out on a job, only to get there and find that it's nothing more than an army sergeant major wishing them to mop up some water he has spilled on the bathroom floor of his barracks. The subsequent stand-off, as the firemen refuse to comply, is relayed with all the narrative tension and philosophical rumination of a major spiritual conflict. Lines like 'They still had to do their jobs' are delivered with all the wigged-out conviction of the terminally wasted. Firemen Henry and William reason that having fought in two world wars they shouldn't have to do this sort of thing. The story doesn't so much unfold as congeal. It's an epic tale of nothing-muchness, Sam Beckett's *Endgame* for the acid crowd. You are left with the feeling that this was a great lost opportunity and that they should probably have turned the whole thing into a concept double album, with each of the four firemen being given a whole side on which to relate the puddle-mopping episode from his own perspective. It could have been *Quadrophenia* meets Fireman Sam. Instead Zoot Money, and eventually Andy Summers too, joined Eric Burdon's psychedelic Animals.

Of all the stars who played with Laughing Sam's Dice Eric Burdon made perhaps the most radical transformation of them all. In 1964 he was a Geordie blues brat with a stage stance and persona to match, staring down the barrel of a television camera on *Top of the Pops* as he sang a borrowed song about a bordello in New Orleans with a sneer on his lips and insolence in his eyes. In their earliest incarnation the Animals stood on the shoulders of giants: John Lee Hooker, Ray Charles,

Chuck Berry, Jimmy Reed. They were at the forefront of the first English invasion of America, and Burdon wore his WMCA Good Guys sweatshirt with pride, thrilled to be part of it all. Their Trad. Arr. version of 'House of the Rising Sun' inspired Dylan to go electric. Burdon took one of the finest songs ever to come out of the Brill Building, Mann and Weil's 'We Gotta Get Out of This Place', and made it sound like it was about his own father. When the Animals covered 'Please Don't Let Me Be Misunderstood', a song written for Nina Simone, Burdon handled its tricky phrasing as expertly as she did. In an age when even the best English pop singers – McCartney in Little Richard mode, Jagger as James Brown mannequin – offered fan-boy pastiches of their heroes, Burdon just dared you to snigger at his sincerity. He meant it, man. His band mates, Chas Chandler in particular, found it amusing that this diminutive, greasy-haired gnome should adopt the mantle of the seen-it-all bluesman, but Burdon just hunched himself against the brickbats and carried on regardless. Between 1964 and 1966 the hits just kept on coming – 'I'm Crying', 'Bring It on Home to Me', 'It's My Life', 'Don't Bring Me Down' – but apart from the occasional mischievous twinkle that stare never let up. While his fellow musicians mugged and grinned behind him, Burdon continued to look down the barrel of that light-entertainment lens like the Brit-punk prototype that he was.

There was a brief transition period between beat-group Burdon and psychedelic-band Burdon, and it was marked by an album called *Eric Is Here*, recorded with the Horace Ott Orchestra in late 1966, when the singer first relocated to America. *Eric Is Here* showcased what might have been had Burdon gone down the pop route. He sang arrangements of twelve numbers straight off the LA and New York publishing-house production line, including Randy Newman's 'Mama Told Me Not to Come' and 'I Think It's Gonna Rain Today', Mann and Weil's 'It's Not Easy' and English and Weiss's 'Help Me, Girl'. The latter, a Top 20 hit in the US and UK, was billed as Eric Burdon and the Animals, even though drummer Barry Jenkins was the only band member featured. By the time *Eric Is Here* was released in March 1967 Burdon had relocated permanently to the west coast, with a new band in tow and an evangelical glint in his eyes.

The new musical direction immediately became apparent with the single 'When I Was Young'/'A Girl Named Sandoz'. Released in April 1967, the A-side is a blues-rock confessional that pays lip service to Burdon's earlier earthy style. In it he smokes his first cigarette at ten and loses his virginity at thirteen, incorporating Dylan's 'I was so much older then' into the storyline. If 'When I was Young' hints at rebirth, 'A Girl Named Sandoz' confirms the reason. The musical style is still hard-rock and riffy but the woman now teaching him ('good things / very, very sweet things) speaks of more cerebral initiations ('strange things / very strange things / my mind has wings'). To hear Burdon coo 'Sandoz, you taught me love' in such a limp-lunged simper is to be alerted to the fact that something very significant has happened to the man who used to sing John Lee Hooker's 'Boom Boom'.

By the spring of 1967 Burdon had become a fully fledged convert and unpaid spokesman for the cause. He stopped imitating bluesmen and started preaching live and direct from Sandoz Mission Hall. In interviews he was a wide-eyed advocate. 'Freaking out is connected with the effects produced by the drug LSD in the States,' he explained helpfully to Keith Altham of *NME*. 'All the groups who play it will tell you that they never touch the stuff – which is rubbish!' The next two years were prolific ones for Burdon. Between

October 1967 and December 1968 the new Animals released four albums: *Winds of Change, The Twain Shall Meet, Every One of Us* and *Love Is*, the last of which was a double. Unlike some of his contemporaries Burdon retained his pop sensibilities and throughout 1967 the Animals continued to enjoy a run of hit singles, both in Britain and America: 'When I Was Young', 'Good Times', 'San Franciscan Nights', 'Sky Pilot' and 'Ring of Fire' all went Top 40. Up to this point in his career Burdon had had only four songwriting credits to his name, and three of those had been co-written, but now the lyrics came in a lysergic torrent: lessons in hip musical history ('Winds of Change'), ringing the cultural changes ('San Franciscan Nights', 'Monterey'), self-evaluating confessionals about too many nights down the speakeasy ('Good Times'), cod-spaghetti-western space drivel ('Black Plague'), tender lyricism ('Poem by the Sea'), anti-war sentiments ('Sky Pilot') – all of it tweaked and treated by Tom Wilson's production, which bathed everything in a hallucinatory glow. Although he experienced frequent hostility towards his change of direction, Burdon never seemed to have any trouble reconciling the former blues brat with the new psychedelic warrior. 'It's all meat from the same bone,' he sang on the closing track on *Winds of Change*, as he namechecked Ray Charles, Ravi Shankar, Muhammad Ali and Eric Clapton. He referenced Hendrix in 'Yes, I Am Experienced', the SF scene in 'Gratefully Dead', Donovan and Jefferson Airplane on 'San Franciscan Nights' and the Byrds' 'Renaissance Fair' on 'Monterey'. When he lays claim to his heritage on *Winds of Change*, the family tree that begins with King Oliver and Duke Ellington is made to sound like everything was leading up to the present moment in history. 'Frank Zappa zapped / Mamas and Papas knew where it was at,' he sings unequivocally on 'Winds of Change', eschewing false demarcation and hip snobberies. Behind the born-again platitudes of 'San Franciscan Nights' lies a sincere attempt to reach out beyond the stoned faithful. The song was one long plea for tolerance and understanding addressed as much to the 'old cop/young cop' who breaks heads on Love Street as it was to the denizens of the Haight. Similar open-heartedness informs 'Sky Pilot', a comment on the Vietnam war that addresses the young conscript and his conscience rather than the already converted draft-dodger and anti-war marcher.

Burdon's generosity of spirit was also displayed in the plethora of cover versions his band performed, both live and on record. The old Animals borrowed from the blues. The psychedelic Animals embraced modernity. Their thirty-minute set at Monterey included versions of Donovan's 'Hey Gyp', Nina Simone's 'Gin House Blues' and the Rolling Stones' 'Paint It Black'. Three-quarters of the *Love Is* album was devoted to cover versions, including interpretations of Ike and Tina Turner's 'River Deep – Mountain High', Sly Stone's 'I'm an Animal', June Carter's 'Ring of Fire', Traffic's 'Coloured Rain', the Bee Gees' 'To Love Somebody' and, with Andy Summers and Zoot Money now in tow, an extended version of Dantalian's Chariot's 'Madman (Running Through the Fields)'.

By June 1968, though, Burdon indicated that he was reverting to earlier role models. 'The Maharishi never sung like Ray Charles,' he told Chris Welch of *Melody Maker*. He seemed to have reached an impasse with the girl from Sandoz too. 'LSD is temporary insanity,' he said. 'It's beautiful but you can't stay there all your life.' On the subject of his new band mates he claimed, 'Zoot Money has changed a lot, and I'm trying to get him to change back.' 'What changed him?' asks Welch. 'LSD,' states Burdon simply. 'It changed me too. I don't regret having

used it. Now I've done a complete circle. I've just got to the point where, well . . . a human being can think too much and become insane.'

Someone else who was always more inclined towards Ray Charles than the Maharishi was Steve Winwood. At the beginning of 1967 Winwood was still belting out a plausible impression of his hero with the Spencer Davis Group. Their latest hit, 'I'm a Man', dominated by Winwood's beefy Hammond chords and hoarse blues holler, was in the Top 10. In March it was officially announced that Winwood was quitting the group, although behind the scenes he had been planning his next venture for some time, with a trio of musicians from the Brum beat scene: guitarist Dave Mason, flautist and saxophone player Chris Wood and drummer Jim Capaldi. By June that new outfit, Traffic, was in the Top Ten with 'Paper Sun', a single that provided more compelling evidence that yet another gang of R&B disciples had succumbed to the mind-expanding joys of acid. Introduced by Jim Capaldi's tabla and Dave Mason's sitar, and driven by Winwood's soulfully wasted vocal and Chris Wood's skittering flute, 'Paper Sun' possesses an enigmatic sense of bleary-eyed disengagement. Penned by Capaldi its lyric switches dreamily between an amorous encounter on the beach and the dimly lit realities of a dingy bedsit life. It's a strangely shimmering single, pathos-ridden and yet passive and non-judgemental, that manages to sound intimate and out of reach at the same time. And in images like 'the icicles you're crying' its defining influences are unmistakable.

Traffic followed up the success of 'Paper Sun' with the Dave Mason composition 'Hole in My Shoe', an ultra-commercial childlike ditty that, like 'Paper Sun', featured a sitar and lyrical references to awaking from a dreamy slumber, the difference being that when the girl awakes in the final verse of 'Paper Sun' a seagull is stealing the ring from her hand. In 'Hole in My Shoe' the dew has merely soaked through his coat. Where 'Paper Sun' is disoriented, dry-mouthed and heat-scorched 'Hole in My Shoe' is gently bedraggled. To compound its innocence 'Hole in My Shoe' has a spoken middle section recited in an impressively awestruck manner over a sustained wave of mellotron by Francine Heimann, the six-year-old step-daughter of Island Records boss Chris Blackwell. In later years Mason came to regard many of his Traffic lyrics as trite, but no amount of disassociation can disguise how thrilling it was to see

'Hole in My Shoe' sitting in the Top 10 for seven weeks during the autumn of 1967, nestling next to the Engelbert Humperdincks and Tom Jones's of this world and giving clear indication of just how easily psychedelia's childlike charms might be assimilated into the mainstream.

The ethereal heat haze of 'Paper Sun' and dew-soaked ambience of 'Hole in My Shoe' combine to equally good effect in Traffic's third successive Top 10 hit, 'Here We Go Round the Mulberry Bush'. The blithe optimism of the song's nursery-rhyme verse is undermined by Winwood's ghostly interjections, the spookiest of which – 'Will you shelter me when I am naked and cold?' – sounds like it has escaped in the dead of night from a seventeenth-century murder ballad and stumbled through the undergrowth until it has reached the safe haven of an isolated cottage. Written as the theme for Clive Donner's film adaptation of Hunter Davies's coming-of-age novel of the same name, 'Here We Go Round the Mulberry Bush' was one of the first things that Traffic recorded and its mix of dream swirl and shadowy menace would become a key characteristic of their early work. Sadly, nothing of this atmosphere was captured in the film, which reduces Davies's subtle rite-of-passage observations to an adolescent farce. A monument to miscasting, it tramples all over the book's nuances and understated poignancy and turns it into a facile swinging-sixties sex romp. Every time the swirling organ intro of the theme tune swells up it promises other-dimensional journeys to far-off lands, but the action remains resolutely rooted in a celluloid landscape that hasn't bothered to update its reference points since *Summer Holiday* and *Carry On Constable*.

Soon after they formed Traffic initiated what would become a late-sixties rock cliché when they announced that they were 'getting it together in the country'. Renting a remote cottage near the village of Aston Tirrold at the foot of the Berkshire Downs, they got rip-roaringly stoned and composed most of the music that would appear on their debut album, *Mr Fantasy*. There were impromptu performances in the garden, jam sessions with the likes of Eric Burdon, Pete Townshend and the Small Faces, and lots of strange, dark acid trips, including one where a roadie spooked the band into thinking that they were being drafted to Vietnam, forcing them to go out and buy a newspaper in order to convince themselves that the story wasn't true.[2] Traffic's rural retreat was subsequently much

imitated as others headed for the hills in search of drug-fuelled creativity free from the attentions of the inner-city fuzz; usually they ended up with little to show for their endeavours other than a few campfire jams and unusable demos. Against all odds, certainly against all prevailing narcotic tendencies, the album that emerged from Traffic's Berkshire escapade has a cohesion that justifies the entire venture. Released in December 1967 *Mr Fantasy* is an inspired hybrid of spectral soul, Summer of Love wistfulness, impromptu frivolity and lyrics that occasionally get tangled in the brambles or stumble off the crumbling chalk cliff of their own profundity. The album's cover photo is shot through a red-and-yellow-filtered glow, with what looks like dawn's early light breaking through the window. It captures the record's mood of wood smoke and wasted intimacy perfectly.

The Spencer Davis Group, the outfit that Steve Winwood left, promptly reinvented themselves as a psychedelic outfit and released a couple of stunning singles that could just as easily have been made by Traffic, so similar were they in texture and so seamless was the transition from soul pop to psych pop. Eddie Hardin replaced Winwood on keyboards, and while he lacked his predecessor's vocal dexterity, the band more than made up for it with the quality of their singles. On 'Time Seller', a Top 30 hit in the summer of 1967, sawing cellos cut a swathe through acres of phasing in a style that anticipated the terrain that another Birmingham-based unit, ELO, would exploit in the 1970s. 'Time Seller''s portentous sound is charmingly undermined by some decidedly Lucyesque lyrics (lemonade rain, money made of chocolate, etc.), while leaning heavily on 'Strawberry Fields Forever' for its disorientating dynamics. Ringo's percussive flourishes (sudden flurries of hi-hat on the chorus, for example) are all over the song. 'Time Seller' also contains one of the clunkiest edits ever heard on a pop record, when the cello fade thirty seconds from the end is hastily overdubbed with a perfunctory burst of tympani, which seems to serve no purpose whatsoever other than to cover up a mistake.

The group's next single, 'Mr Second Class', was another terrific slab of psych pop. Released in January 1968 its slow-fuse intro was out of the same epic mould as the Small Faces' 'Tin Soldier', which had been released just a few weeks earlier. Both songs are the sound of mod soul gone psych but retain just enough of their Booker T. roots to keep the ravers happy. Lyrically 'Mr Second

Class' was straight out of the drudge and begrudge school of English pen portraits that Ray Davies perfected. The late sixties abound with songs that sneer at straights, full of accusatory, finger-pointing, 'Hey, Mr Three-Piece Suit, look at you leading your pathetic buttoned-up life' lyrics. Hindsight can be cruel, and back then it would never have occurred to any of these musicians that half a lifetime later, with the pop success of their youth now just a dwindling memory, they would be leading an existence every bit as humdrum and prospect-deprived as the office-work conformists they sneered at when they were in their paisley-shirted prime. 'Make your money fast / It had better last for you,' sings Eddie Hardin without discernible pathos or irony. Musically 'Mr Second Class' is punchy and anthemic. Lyrically it falls down where so many Ray Davies emulators fall down – too much energy expended on the put-down, not enough on any sense that 'Mr Second Class' might be redeemable.

Of all the groups whose style was transformed between 1964 and 1967 Procol Harum's evolution was perhaps the most rapid and radical of all. In January 1964, in their pre-Procol incarnation the Paramounts, they had a minor Top 40 hit with a cover of Leiber and

Stoller's 'Poison Ivy'. A little over three years later 'A Whiter Shade of Pale' went to number one in the UK singles chart within a fortnight of its release and stayed there for the next six weeks. If there is one single epochal moment when the English Summer of Love was officially declared open, it was the sight of R&B stalwarts who seemed to have reinvented themselves overnight and were now sporting kaftans, capes and cowls on *Top of the Pops*, while singing a song about vestal virgins, set to a slow, sonorous baroque-and-roll melody.

As the Paramounts they had played a mixture of rock-and-roll and R&B covers, and were contemporaries of the Rolling Stones (who also covered 'Poison Ivy'). When the Stones hit the big time, the Paramounts inherited their discarded club residencies and shared bills with the Who when they were still the High Numbers, but by late 1965, while Pete Townshend was penning mini-pop operas by day and engaging in auto-destruction by night, the Paramounts were backing Sandie Shaw on the cabaret circuit. 'A purely financial decision,' recalled keyboard player Gary Brooker when I interviewed him in 1996. 'When you're looking at the month or two ahead and you've only got five gigs and someone says, "Back Sandie Shaw and we'll give you fifty

quid a week," you do it.' On the eve of a similarly expedient tour, this time backing pop star Chris Andrews, guitarist Robin Trower chose to quit rather than have to play Andrews's jaunty pop hit 'Yesterday Man' every night. Brooker also decided he'd driven up a musical cul-de-sac. 'I didn't want to play R&B covers any more because the people who made the originals had started coming over. Booker T. was actually onstage in Walthamstow if you wanted to see him.' In this simple pragmatic rationalisation lies the single most plausible reason why so many British R&B bands began to forge a new musical direction in the mid-sixties: the black R&B combos who had been revered, exoticised and mythologised were now touring the UK on a regular basis. Enterprising agents often secured guest spots for UK acts on these tours, but even though such bookings made good sense from a business point of view, they made little sense creatively. Why risk humiliation when the visiting soul stars had the original chops and were far more accomplished musicians and, indeed, entertainers?

It was while considering what he wanted to do next that Brooker met his Mile End Milton, lyricist Keith Reid. Reid had known Marc Bolan when he was still Mark Feld. 'Long before the

Mod movement – when they were still being referred to as modernists – there were two teams, one in the East End, one in the Stamford Hill area, which was where Marc lived. Everybody used to go and hang out at a Wimpy Bar near Whitechapel Art Gallery on a Sunday morning. I was twelve and I thought I was the youngest kid on the scene, but he was even younger. First time I met him he was very proudly wearing a pair of Levi's which he'd pinched from this shop in Leman Street. We just got talking 'cos we were the youngest in this scene of people who totally lived for clothes. We were two precocious snot-nosed kids.'

When he first started writing lyrics, Reid was heavily influenced by *Bringing It All Back Home*-period Bob Dylan. With typical mod precocity he asked Chris Blackwell, head of the newly formed Island Records, if he would give him the money to go to America in return for the publishing rights to his songs. 'He wasn't prepared to do that, of course, and he shuffled me off to DJ Guy Stevens instead, who by then was working as A&R man for Island. Guy originally tried to put me with Steve Winwood, who at the time was secretly working with Jim Capaldi, though he was still officially with Spencer Davis.' Indeed, Reid confirms that

half the lyrics that turned up on the first Procol Harum album were originally offered to the embryonic Traffic. He remained in thrall to the influence of Bob Dylan, and his lyrics, full of obtuse symbolism and often a little too wordy for the melodies that carried them, became one of Procol Harum's defining features.

In May 1967 the Reid-penned 'A Whiter Shade of Pale' was released. The *NME* gave it a tentative short review in its 'Potted Pops' round-up of unknown bands. 'A gripping blues-tinged ballad warbled in heartfelt style,' it said. 'Hummable. Thoroughly impressive.' 'We'd recorded it live in the studio,' recalls Brooker. 'And we thought the cymbals were really clashy. We wanted to hear what it would sound like on the radio, so Tony Hall [Decca A&R man] arranged to get it played on the pirate Radio London.' A nation immediately turned cartwheels 'cross the floor for a four-and-a-half-minute organ melody inspired in equal measure by Bach's 'Air on the G String' and 'When a Man Loves a Woman' by Percy Sledge. The record went on to sell two and a half million copies in the UK alone and its influence was felt everywhere as many a keyboard player ditched the Jimmy Smith and Brother Jack McDuff sermonising and began to indulge their inner baroque. Over the next couple of years the soulful mutations of 'Whiter Shade of Pale' could be heard in an abundance of organ-led dirges that similarly pitched themselves somewhere between Percy Sledge and J. S. Bach. Felius Andromeda recorded the Procol-inspired 'Meditations' in a Cricklewood church, supposedly for that essential ecclesiastical authenticity, but mostly, one suspects, for the publicity. Felius Andromeda shamelessly dressed up in monks' robes to promote the song and the accompanying PR blurb spoke of séances and devil visitations. 'Reputation' by Shy Limbs featured a pre-King Crimson/ELP Greg Lake on bass and vocals and had heavily phased 'Whiter Shade of Pale' keyboards. 'Mr Armageddon' by Locomotive featured a jazz-rock line-up augmented by Dick Heckstall-Smith, Chris Mercer and Henry Lowther, and commenced with a portentous swoosh of Hammond block chords and the unforgettable opening line, 'I am everything you see and what is more.' Locomotive's previous record, the blue beat-inspired 'Rudi's in Love', had been a minor Top 30 hit in October 1968, but Tony Blackburn made the apocalyptic 'Mr Armageddon' his record of the week on his Radio 1 breakfast show. The past was indeed a foreign country.

They did things different there.

In America stylistic evolution tended to follow a similar pattern: folk rock, psychedelic rock, country rock. In the UK the more common trajectory was R&B group, psych group, progressive rock band. In this respect Procol Harum's development was typical: R&B covers gave way to a brief and florid flirtation with the trappings of psych rococo, before the band began to pursue a more grandiose orchestrated path in the 1970s. Some of the most iconic records of the psychedelic era featured musicians who had learned their craft on the R&B club circuit before donning paisley in the name of the cause and then plying their new-found virtuosity in some of the most high-profile progressive acts in the UK. 'My White Bicycle' by Tomorrow and '14 Hour Technicolour Dream' by the Syn featured Steve Howe and Chris Squire of Yes respectively, without betraying a hint of how those two might sound a couple of years later. The Action became Mighty Baby. Art became Spooky Tooth. Simon Dupree and the Big Sound became Gentle Giant. The Nice evolved into ELP. Less feted than most were Blossom Toes, who eventually became the progressive-rock group BB Blunder, two of whose members also contributed to Keith

Tippett's grand fifty-piece jazz-rock project Centipede. In 1967 Blossom Toes released one of the Summer of Love's most overlooked LPs, *We Are Ever So Clean*. Guitarist Brian Godding remembers the group performing at a Labour Club venue in 1967, when an aggrieved punter stepped forward to pass judgement on their free-form extemporising. 'A RIGHT bucket of LSD if ever I heard one,' he said. It's a commonly aired reminiscence among musicians of a certain vintage. A provincial promoter phones a London agency and asks them to send up one of these new-fangled psychedelic groups he's read about. Said group spend most of the gig hoping they aren't going to get physically pummelled by the audience. In another pop universe Brian Godding could have taken the Graham Gouldman route. A publishing-house writer of finely crafted pop songs, Godding also played R&B in the Ingoes with fellow Blossom Toes members guitarist Jim Cregan and bass player Brian Belshaw. The eventual Blossom Toes line-up was completed by drummer Kevin Westlake, who had previously backed Little Richard in a Sounds Incorporated-style outfit called Johnny B. Great and the Quotations. The Yardbirds' manager Giorgio Gomelsky signed the group to his Marmalade

label, put them up in a King's Road communal pad and encouraged them to 'experiment'. 'Gomelsky brought us an acetate of *Sgt Pepper*,' remembers Westlake, 'and he made us listen to Olivier Messaien for ideas.' The results can be heard in *We Are Ever So Clean*'s opening track, 'Look at Me I'm You', which was an attempt to incorporate Messaienic tonality into traditional pop structures. David Whittaker orchestrated the album with strings and brass, but the unsung star of the project was engineer John Timperley, who spent painstaking hours bouncing down endless layers of sound onto four-track. 'What on Earth', which lent the album its title, contains the winning psychedelic couplet 'We are ever so clean / Cleaner than the tub on your washing machine.' While others were heading east to contemplate the great wheel of karma, the Blossom Toes explored the cyclical possibilities of the Hotpoint domestic appliance. Kevin Westlake's 'The Remarkable Saga of the Frozen Dog' was a delightful acid cameo of winter walks with a mangy mutt that 'fell in love with a lady who sings folk music'. 'People of the Royal Parks', another Westlake composition, was a lysergic knees-up in the Marriott–Lane tradition, its Summer of Love topicality evident in lines like 'They've closed the pop stations and locked the parks on Sunday afternoons.' 'We lived in the King's Road, but we never felt like pop stars,' says Westlake. 'You'd meet other people in bands who were starting to act the part and believe it, but the Blossom Toes never did. 'Actually, Jim Cregan [who went on to be part of Family, Cockney Rebel and Rod Stewart's backing band] always had it in him to be a star and he would find that extra bit of cash to buy a velvet jacket when we were down to our last pint of Guinness, but you have to believe in the act, right down to the way you respond when someone calls your name, and we never did, being a bit modest and normal.' And cleaner than the tub on your washing machine.

Family, the group Jim Cregan subsequently joined, had started life in Leicester as the Farinas, playing the usual mixture of R&B, blues and soul covers before decamping to London, where they were immediately adopted by the UFO crowd as clued-in provincials. Immortalised as 'Relation' in Jenny Fabian's autobiographical novel *Groupie*, and critically endorsed by John Lennon, Family brought something entirely original to the late-sixties psychedelic scene. The band's debut single, 'Scene Through the Eye of a Lens', released on Liberty in October 1967,

was one of the great acid revelations of the era. 'Suddenly everything blends / raindrops that sparkle like gems,' sings Roger Chapman on a song that sounds like it could have been beamed in from the Incredible String Band's *5000 Spirits or the Layers of the Onion*. Several group members were multi-instrumentalists, including violin, cello and bass player Ric Grech, who later decamped to supergroup Blind Faith. Grech's adornments weave in and out of the group's debut LP, *Music in a Doll's House*, which was released on Reprise in the summer of 1968 and had been the working title for the Beatles' follow-up to *Sgt Pepper* before they generously gave way. The overtly psychedelic elements on *Doll's House* were as much down to producer Dave Mason as to the band themselves, who, although clearly immersed in the hazy spirit of the age, retained distinct aspects of their R&B clubland apprenticeship, not to mention more jazz-orientated leanings than most UK underground acts. Mason played sitar on *Doll's House* and applied judicious phasing and echo to give it that necessary spacey flavour, but for all its period trappings it is Roger Chapman and John Whitney's songs that stand out. Chapman possessed a blast furnace of a voice that ranged from a bleating vibrato to a distressed howl. It was sometimes hard to reconcile the powerhouse on-stage presence of Family's lead singer, all malevolent prowl and recidivist grin, with the man who could write folk pastorals like 'Mellowing Grey', 'Winter' and 'The Weaver's Answer'.

Family wore their fluency lightly. They could incorporate tricky time changes without it all seeming like a pointless exercise in musical proficiency, and they weaved their charm well into the next decade, during which they enjoyed a run of hit albums and, unlike a lot of their progressive contemporaries, a clutch of Top 30 singles too.

The Nice started life as P. P. Arnold's backing group, with musicians drawn from R&B club acts like Gary Farr and the T-Bones (keyboard player Keith Emerson, bassist Lee Jackson and original drummer Ian Hague), the Mark Leeman Five (replacement drummer Brian Davison) and pop group the Attack (guitarist David O'List). They swiftly evolved into a cracking good psychedelic outfit capable of producing bright and brittle three-minute gems like 'Flower King of Flies', 'The Thoughts of Emerlist Davjack', 'The Diamond Hard Blue Apples of the Moon' and 'Happy Freuds', songs that were full of splintery shards of sharp-edged sound and understated classical

flourishes and had a refreshing absence of pomposity. That didn't last long.

The Nice's mad gallop through 'Rondo' on their 1968 debut album *The Thoughts of Emerlist Davjack* was a raver's version of Dave Brubeck's 'Blue Rondo à la Turk' and became an Idiot Dancers anthem, but even at this early stage Keith Emerson was relying on showmanship rather than technique and dropping more than a hint that he would like to spend less time on the pianissimo in order to devote more of his energies to plunging knives into his instrument. Even at their most druggy no one could have ever have accused the Nice of being subtle, but in the ham-fisted schlock classicism that gradually imposes itself on their material progressive rock can clearly be heard bubbling in the amniotic fluid of its first trimester. While David O'List was in the band this wasn't an issue. The interplay between his abrasive guitar and Emerson's churchy interludes on 'Rondo' and on their audacious adaptation of Leonard Bernstein's 'America' are reminiscent of Syd Barrett and Rick Wright at their most exploratory in the early Pink Floyd. Emerson was clearly never cut out to be a droney minimalist, but once O'List was edged out of the band – Syd Barrett-style – for his erratic behaviour, egomania rapidly came to the fore. To trace the group's output through their five studio albums is to witness the humour and quirkiness of psychedelia gradually bloating into the gargantuan beast that was prog.

On their first session for John Peel's *Top Gear*, recorded in October 1967, the Nice approach cover versions of Charles Lloyd's 'Sombrero Sam' and The Byrds' 'Get to You' with a freshness that infuses and invigorates both compositions. In their August 1968 *Top Gear* session they are equally playful and inventive, with an interpretation of the main theme from Frank Zappa's *Lumpy Gravy* and their take on 'Aries', one of the tracks from *The Zodiac: Cosmic Sounds*, an Elektra Moog album featuring Mort Garson, Paul Beaver, Emil Richards and members of the LA Wrecking Crew. In more recent years *The Zodiac: Cosmic Sounds* has been appropriated by the kitsch crowd and accorded cult appeal, but it was much played on the pirate radio stations during the summer of 1967, not just on John Peel's *Perfumed Garden* but on more mainstream daytime shows too, where its exotic flavours were not at all out of place next to the Procol Harums and the 'Paper Sun's. The Moody Blues later credited the album as being one of the chief inspirations that helped them shape *Days of Future Passed*.

In December 1968, when the Nice returned for their fifth *Top Gear* appearance, they recorded adapted versions of 'The Karelia Suite' by Sibelius and Bach's Brandenburg Concerto. John Peel later observed that they left him in no doubt that they felt they were improving on the originals. To indicate just how integral the Nice were to Peel's programme they were accorded the honour of writing a new theme tune, which was unveiled with great ceremony on *Top Gear* in April 1969. With its low growling bass and Hammond fuzz it was utterly in keeping with the underground vibe of the show and replaced its previous theme, a bright bouncy number by Sounds Incorporated that had survived intact since *Top Gear*'s bright bouncy origins on the BBC Light Programme.

Like many a proto-prog outfit that didn't have a resident Ray Charles or Mose Allison imitator, the Nice audibly lacked a convincing lead vocalist. The short straw was generally drawn by bass player Lee Jackson, and his gruff, growling impression of an animal that has had its thorax stamped on made tracks like 'The Cry of Eugene' and 'Azrael' particularly hard going. Their Dylan interpretations 'She Belongs to Me' and 'Country Pie' are singularly gruesome listening for this reason alone. The heavy-handed delivery also tips 'Little Arabella''s notional ambiguity into what sounds suspiciously like snide misogyny. During a period when fey daintiness was being deified in psychedelic pop song the Nice's charmless putdown of the empty-headed hanger-on, complete with cautionary pay-off line – 'She's sitting right next to you' – was a chauvinist throwback. 'Happy Freuds' could easily have gone down the same misanthropic road had it not been for the Zappa-inspired production – the speeded-up vocals are straight out of *We're Only in It for the Money* – and Emerson's uncharacteristically light-hearted delivery of some clever elisions and the killer pay-off line – 'Only really shallow people know themselves.' Listeners were still left to ponder what 'your Capricorn is showing and the edge is getting frayed' might mean, but then lyrics were never really the point of the Nice once David O'List left. The ubiquity of shallow dolly birds in their music was a mere trifle compared with the untapped potential of the classical tradition, which Emerson regarded as his natural stamping ground. By their fourth album, *Five Bridges*, released in 1970, they were taking on classical commissions with confidence, and ELP was just a cannon's roar away.

When the original power trio, Cream, formed in the summer of 1966, their reputations went before them. Bass player Jack Bruce and drummer Ginger Baker had played together in the Graham Bond Organisation; guitarist Eric Clapton had been a member of the Yardbirds and John Mayall's Bluesbreakers. The band's name, suggested by Clapton, was a knowing and confident nod to their collective pedigree. Essentially there were two Creams: the live Leviathan with unrestrainable ego that played bludgeoning blues jams of interminable duration at tinnitus-inducing volume to packed stadiums on endless American tours; and an altogether odder and less presumptuous beast, a thoughtful studio ensemble augmented by cellos, bells and trumpets. This version of Cream recorded three-minute songs crammed full of imagist poetry that was declaimed in operatic libretto over thunderous and polydextrous beats. The live version of Cream, critically lauded at the time but hardly listened to now, became a byword for excess and decibel-driven dynamics. The studio version, undervalued at the time, was more reflective and possessed lyricism, humour and melancholy in abundance.

Cream announced themselves with a Dadaist joke. The critics were expecting rock gods to descend from Mount Olympus. What they got instead was a softly crooned cabaret shuffle called 'Wrapping Paper', which only reached number 34 in the singles chart when it was released in October 1966. Singles weren't really what Cream were about, even though the half dozen they did put out all made the Top 40. Their debut album, *Fresh Cream*, released in December 1966, was a polite and underwhelming affair. Only the poly-rhythmic rumble of Ginger Baker suggests the maelstrom to come. It was Baker's ability to marry jazz pyrotechnics to sheer primal savagery that drove the band's sound in its early days. The moment he ceases clicking his sticks twenty-eight seconds into 'I Feel Free' is the moment the heavy-rock sixties begin in earnest. Bruce later quipped that as far as he was concerned the band was a jazz trio, it's just that he hadn't bothered to tell the others, but it was Baker who unleashed the spirit of Elvin Jones and Max Roach. What Bruce did have, though, was lyricist Pete Brown. Brown brought to Cream an English beat poet's sensibilities and screeds of idiosyncratic imagery hitherto unheard in British rock music. The Bruce and Brown writing team would forge some of the most distinctive rock songs of the 1960s, and it was Brown's

obtuse elliptical lyrics, as much as Cream's consummate musicianship, that elevated them above all the other since-my-baby-left-me merchants.

Cream's second album was entitled *Disraeli Gears*, a punning play on words based on derailleur gears, an in-joke that every bicycling school kid in Britain would have immediately recognised. The LP, recorded in New York and released in November 1967, transformed a cut-above blues band into nailed-to-the-mast psychedelicists. Producer Felix Pappalardi gave one listen to their Trad. Arr. blues arrangement of 'Lawdy Mama' and shape-shifted it into a piece of lysergic voodoo called 'Strange Brew', complete with new lyrics co-written with his wife Gail. The pair also penned 'World of Pain' on the same album, and over the next couple of years Felix Pappalardi's input would prove to be as distinctive as Pete Brown's as he quickly became an integral part of the studio set-up, embellishing the group's sound with an array of instrumentation, including viola, organ, trumpet, tonette, hand bells, piano and mellotron.

Apart from 'Strange Brew', the most overtly psychedelic moments on *Disraeli Gears* were 'Dance the Night Away' and 'Tales of Brave Ulysses'. The former was Pete Brown's wistful farewell to the visceral thrills of his own nightly ego obliteration at UFO. The spirit of Anna Halprin and the Acid Tests looms large in the lyrics. 'Dance myself to nothing / vanish from this place,' intones Jack Bruce in an elongated croon over a nimble arrangement that could only have been executed by musicians with a tonnage of hard graft behind them. Clapton throws in a perfectly weighted psyche-delic solo, paying homage in his soaring crescendos to the Byrds' 'Eight Miles High'. 'Tales of Brave Ulysses' was the result of a collaboration between Clapton and *Oz* magazine illustrator Martin Sharp. Written on the island of Formentera in trochee form (the same metrical style that Longfellow used for *The Song of Hiawatha*), it was a sen-sual Homerian epic filtered through a prism of pure liquid Sandoz and forged in the blinding Balearic light. Clapton had recently acquired his first wah-wah pedal and daubs the song in its cry-baby tears. He doesn't show off his new toy but uses it sparingly as ensemble texture. He repeats the trick to equally good effect on 'World of Pain'.

In concert Clapton could be as showy and indulgent as his colleagues, but on the best of his studio work with Cream he sounds reined-in and disci-plined. On *Disraeli Gears* his seething,

understated intensity is the lynchpin of Bruce's 'We're Going Wrong', a song which constantly threatens to go off like a bomb. It rumbles along, all bottom end and prowling intent. Brooding bass and fidgety toms mark time as if they are about to explode at any moment. Clapton, clearly not daring to upset the uneasy calm by doing anything too showy, interjects with only the briefest and most tentative of blues runs, while Bruce gives it his best gothic aria. Only at the end, with an apologetic nod to Spoonful, do they attempt a traditional twelve-bar resolution. It's a remarkable piece of work, simmering with danger and malevolence.

By 1968 live Cream and studio Cream had become irreconcilable. While the live unit played to vast sold-out amphitheatres and extemporised on blues patterns ad infinitum, the stu-dio ensemble grew ever more sophisti-cated. The group's third album, *Wheels of Fire*, was a double: one live, one stu-dio. The live portion is redeemed only by Clapton's four-minute burn-up of Robert Johnson's 'Crossroads', while the studio set serves as a reminder of what Cream might have been, had the rails not carried off the train, as Pete Brown allegorically put it on 'As You Said'. The most rhythmically complex song that Cream ever attempted, 'As

You Said' featured Bruce playing cello and acoustic guitar with open tunings, as taught to him by Richie Havens. Brown's bittersweet remembrance of things past is delivered in drone tones that complement the music's Eastern modality. 'Deserted Cities of the Heart', another of Brown's lost lovescapes, has verses bridged by weaving cello phrases, until Clapton plays a psychedelic solo that for disciplined intensity rivals the one he performed on 'Dance the Night Away'.

Aside from Felix Pappalardi's increasingly ornate arrangements, *Wheels of Fire* also saw the sudden blossoming of the songwriting partnership of Ginger Baker and jazz pianist Mike Taylor. The relationship yields three great songs: 'Passing the Time', 'Those Were the Days' and 'Pressed Rat and Warthog', all of which give Pete Brown a run for his money in their use of oblique imagery. 'Passing the Time' was a mood piece scored for cello, pedal organ and glockenspiel, with two sombre lullaby verses about wintertime solitude divided by a tape-spliced passage of rock improvisation. 'Those Were the Days' features Pappalardi on Swiss hand bells, and with its mythical evocations of Atlantis and wild Medusa's serpents it offers a lyrical counterpoint to 'Tales of Brave Ulysses'. Baker's drumming on

the choruses, playing across the beat with short clipped phrases of piston-like precision, is phenomenal. 'Those Were the Days' clocks in at two minutes and fifty-three seconds – a monument to pared-down intensity amid all the bloated excess. 'Pressed Rat and Warthog', croakily declaimed by Baker, tells the eccentric tale of two unlikely grotesques of dubious vintage who sound like cast-offs from some time-warp Dickension netherworld, where they ply their trade 'selling atonal apples and amplified heat' and other surreal wares. The bedraggled pathos of the lyric is beautifully offset by Pappalardi's pastoral arrangement, which features an elegiac fanfare of trumpet and tonette.

The band's final album, *Goodbye Cream*, was, like its predecessor, half live, half studio. The trio of studio songs – 'Doing that Scrapyard Thing', 'Badge' and 'What a Bringdown' – form a suite in all but name, three gloriously enigmatic pieces, individually composed yet delivered in a collectively skewed lingua franca. 'Doing that Scrapyard Thing' and 'What a Bringdown' in particular provide an all too belated reminder that at the death the Bruce–Brown and Taylor–Baker writing teams were beginning to compose songs cut from identical cloth. There was always a wintry side to Cream's lyrics, deep shudders of foreboding forged in storm-tossed turmoil and prematurely darkened days. It announces itself on 'We're Going Wrong' and 'World of Pain'; it's there in 'Those Were the Days' and 'Passing the Time'. Even 'Tales of Brave Ulysses' begins with a retreat from leaden winter. Wintertime's icy waltz figure-skates all over *Goodbye Cream*, as the group offer cryptic commentary on the culture that spawned them and all too rapidly swallowed them up.

Eric Clapton's 'Badge' is the most majestic and stately of the three studio compositions. It features a guitar solo played incognito by George Harrison, a man who, like Clapton, knew a thing or two by 1968 about trying to cling to individual identity within a group context. The lyric speaks entirely in the past tense and is clouded by caution, regret and musings on what might have been. Bruce and Brown's 'Doing that Scrapyard Thing' is a Dylanesque eulogy set to a rollicking piano boogie. Positively skittish and demob-happy in their final days, 'Scrapyard' is Cream's autobiography rendered in scrambled fragments. The studio side of the album closes with Ginger Baker's astounding 'What a Bringdown', a frenetic eulogy in 5/4, and a last-gasp testimony to the demise of a dream. Sung by Bruce, it offers warped cockney doggerel ('Take

a butcher's at the dodgy mincers on old bill') and an inkling of sanity being spat out in resentful ellipses. A despairing 'Don't you know when a head's dead?' mutates into a taunting 'Don't you want to make more bread?' Bruce emits a pained background yelp as if to say 'no more', and the song finally runs aground on a cascade of unheeded warning bells before dashing itself to death on the rocks. A final funereal organ rises from the inky depths, only to be cut dead by an abrupt tape edit. Goodbye, Cream.

An abundance of lesser-known material released between 1965 and 1969 faithfully followed the same line of musical development. Records that were ostensibly mod soul were liberally doused in fuzz, reverb and other distortion techniques to give them that essential psychedelic desensibility. Received wisdom would have it that maverick record producer Joe Meek was washed up by the mid-sixties and had failed to keep pace with public taste. In fact, the manic energy and compulsively eccentric studio trickery he brought to records like 'Watcha Gonna Do, Baby' by Jason Eddie and the Centremen, a Parlophone release in 1965, and 'Too Far Out' by the Impacs, which came out on CBS in 1966, were totally in keeping with the emerging new sound, and who knows what he might have achieved with the smorgasbord of psychedelic delights had he not blown his brains out in February 1967, just when things were really starting to get interesting.

The Craig's 'I Must Be Mad' and the Answers' 'Just a Fear', both released in 1966, were pulsating, pill-fuelled R&B, with frantic lyrics that see-sawed between lust and neurosis. From the same year 'Searching for My Love', by the splendidly named Allen Pound's Get Rich, was another frantic brainstomper, an English approximation of the garage sound. But whereas the legacy line of US garage invariably led back to surf, 'Searching for My Love' evoked the Shadows' 'Apache'. 'When the Night Falls' by the Eyes was released in 1965 and sounds two years ahead of its time. It kicks off with a menacing Pete Townshend hanging chord that can barely wait for the regulation she-done-me-wrong platitudes to end before it spills into unruly feedback. The leakage is overlaid by a high, wailing harmonica, more influenced by Morricone than Walter Shakey Horton, and adds ominous intent to a song that already sounds like psychosis. 'Red Sky at Night' by the Accent cooks up some similarly spooky atmospherics by reciting the old shepherd's delight/

shepherd's warning folklore over a salvo of fuzz. It doesn't evoke a farmer greeting his flock at dawn so much as a bunch of twitchy mods who have been up all night after sampling the proceeds of their latest chemist's raid. Spectral shimmer also infuses 'Vacuum Cleaner' by Tintern Abbey, which is all guitar distortion, splashy cymbals, stretched syllables, numbed delivery and pinned eyeballs. 'Buffalo Billy Can' by Apple is set to a McCartneyesque boogie piano and a mutated 'Taxman' shuffle, and it allows just the occasional tantalising snatch of lucidity to peep through the purple haze. The song announces itself with a force field of wah-wah and a trebly guitar diminuendo before plunging headlong into screeds of unintelligibility worthy of Syd Barrett at his most out there. The words are gabbled in lurching staccato wheezes, as if the singer is taking regular hits on an airbag full of nitrate. 'His head thrown back as though to aim some stammered utterance, howitzer-like, at the blue dome of heaven,' said Aldous Huxley as he recalled a snapshot of Arnold Bennett in the midst of his mescaline reverie.[3] Many a similar stammered utterance was heard in the late sixties, as the blue dome of heaven came under constant attack.

Winston's Fumbs featured Small

Faces founder member Jimmy Winston and future Yes keyboard player Tony Kaye. On their single 'Real Crazy Apartment' the backing vocalists sing 'Fur-nit-ure – whooooah' in helium-high voices, while the wigged-out chorus goes, 'I like the paper on the wall / it is so kind / plays on my mind / it is so warm.' It's not exactly 'Kubla Khan' but it wears its influences with pride. The B-side, 'Snow White', is similarly diverted by the new style of interior decor and implores the listener to 'look at the pretty posters hanging on the wall'. Musically it's another trademark example of late-1960s R&B in transition: jagged guitars and chunky Hammond organ juxtaposed with floaty vocals that do their best to sound effete but can't quite conceal their soul-boy roots. In Winston's Fumbs' take on the traditional fairy tale the innocent princess is transformed into a voracious and scheming club girl. 'Thinks she's mighty / thinks she's a queen / thinks she's the greatest thing ever seen,' taunts the singer as R&B machismo refuses to go gently into that good night.

By the end of the decade everything had slowed to a hazy drawl of fuzz tones. Emasculated former soul boys staggered around in the ultraviolet night, searching for their last remaining brain cells and wailing into the void. The kind of sentiments formerly reserved for dance-floor braggadocio or a knee-trembler in a back alley had been usurped in the name of more cerebral ruminations. Future Foreigner guitarist Mick Jones started life in early-1960s instrumental beat combo Nero and the Gladiators. In 1965 he teamed up with Tommy Brown to form the J&B, and in 1966 they released 'There She Goes', a stately shuffle doused in echo, ghostly strings and wistful sentiments aimed at a passing It Girl 'all dressed up in the latest clothes'. Like so many songs of the period it typifies the style mutations par excellence, a beat ballad made eerie by the simple expediency of an unearthly production. In 1967 the J&B changed their name to the State of Micky and Tommy and started making state-of-the-art psych pop. They slur their words in the time-accustomed mush-mouthed manner on the tabla- and sitar-driven 'Nobody Knows Where You've Been', while drowning in a whirlpool of phasing. And they sound as keen as choirboys when they sing of 'clockwork oranges without any springs' on the lavishly orchestrated 'Love from One to Five'. By 1969 they had been born yet again, this time as Nimrod, under which name they recorded 'The Bird', a Small Faces-inspired epistle to mind elevation and psychic immersion.

'Hold my hand so they won't drag me under,' pleads Jones, already sounding like he's already way too far into his trip to be considering survival strategies. Only two years earlier the group had been doing cover versions of 'Get Out of My Life, Woman' and 'The In Crowd'; here they sound like they would still be quite partial to a rave-up if only they had the wherewithal and their limbs weren't made of treacle.

'The sounds of love are in my head,' sing the Factory in 'Try a Little Sunshine', released on CBS in 1969. Previously such idle contemplations would have been crowded out by speed buzz, but times have changed. 'Try a little sunshine and you'll be right there,' they gently urge, while soaring on a feather-bed of falsetto. The song feigns a fade-out at the two minutes and twenty seconds mark, a perfectly acceptable departure point for a mod-pop single only three years earlier, but three years is a stylistic lifetime in the second half of the 1960s. The false ending leaves the listener momentarily suspended in limbo before 'Try a Little Sunshine' comes crashing back in on a wave of rumbling percussion, cymbal wash and a cascading coda of blissed-out love chords. And somewhere in a suburban discotheque an abdicating Face regains the use of his legs, rises unsteadily to his feet, checks his crumpled threads and smooths his barnet back into shape. Moving into the centre of the crowded dance floor, bathed in celestial light, he raises his hands to the heavens and feels the warm inviting embrace of the vibrating air around him. A mod supreme.

13

'HE'S BEEN TRAVELLING EVERYWHERE'

Innuendo, Euphemism and the Lucy Effect

These references are often obscure and couched in language and jargon not readily understood by ordinary people.
FRANK GILLARD, BBC director of sound broadcasting, 1967[1]

The release of the Beatles' *Sgt Pepper's Lonely Hearts Club Band* in May 1967 was greeted as a landmark event across the world. In San Francisco members of the Grateful Dead, Jefferson Airplane and many other Bay Area residents all remember a common scenario during the days following its release, in which you could walk or drive around the Haight-Ashbury district and hear the album blaring out of every other window you passed. In the UK *Sgt Pepper* arrived at the offshore pirate station Radio London during DJ Ed Stewart's lunchtime show. He immediately put the album on the turntable. After a few moments he noticed that John Peel was standing behind him and had been reduced to tears by the music he was hearing. 'This obviously means more to you than it does to me,' said Stewart and handed the rest of the show over to Peel, who proceeded to play the LP in its entirety.

Meanwhile, the BBC celebrated the release of *Sgt Pepper* by banning 'A Day in the Life' on the grounds that it appeared to advocate drug use. 'The BBC takes a pretty liberal attitude towards the products of the gramophone industry,' said assistant head of publicity Roland Fox in a memo to BBC press officers on Friday 19 May 1967. 'However, we have listened to this particular song over and over again and we have decided that as far as we are concerned it goes a little too far and can encourage a permissive attitude to drug-taking. Therefore we have exercised our editorial discretion in deciding not to broadcast this particular song.'[2]

The purpose of Fox's memo was to alert BBC press officers to the possibility of a major news story breaking over the weekend. Hopeful of averting a crisis at this stage, the memo added: 'This information is on no account to be volunteered but it may break from other sources, in which case you may talk as follows.'[3] No press statement was issued on the Friday but, as Fox rightly suspected, the news did break from other sources – that very Friday evening, in fact, at the official launch party for the album, and the Corporation faced a steady barrage of calls from the newspapers all weekend.

The BBC had first been alerted to the controversial content of 'A Day in the Life' by a news story that *Disc and Music Echo* carried in its 6 May edition, which reported that some Los Angeles radio stations had already banned the song. Taking its moral lead from the US stations the BBC's objection to 'A Day in the Life' centred on the phrase 'I'd love to turn you on'. Clarifying matters in a memo to the head of EMI, Sir Joseph Lockwood, on 25 May, Frank Gillard, the BBC's director of sound broadcasting, explained that 'We are increasingly concerned over the allegation that some pop records contain references to drug taking and can be construed as giving encouragement to unfortunate habits and perhaps even to vice.'[4] Such terminology spoke

volumes about the way in which BBC senior managers approached the thorny area of youth culture in the 1960s. The Corporation's objection wasn't to *Sgt Pepper* per se, merely the wider connotations of 'A Day in the Life'. Indeed, the day after Roland Fox's cautionary memo it devoted an entire sixty-minute edition of the Light Programme's *Where It's At* show to a preview of the LP, presented by Kenny Everett but minus the offending track. The Beatles were also the centrepiece of the BBC's *Our World* live TV link-up on 25 June, in which they previewed 'All You Need Is Love' to a global audience. The glaring omission of 'A Day in the Life' from the BBC's airplay did, however, highlight the Corporation's troubled and sometimes inconsistent approach to censorship.

At the BBC the issue of censorship had traditionally centred on lewd or salacious lyrics, songs that were considered to be in bad taste, lyrics that offended religious sensibilities, records that contained direct product placement or brand names, and records that compromised the BBC's commitment to political impartiality. In this regard the Corporation was far more likely to prohibit a song that promoted Scottish or Irish nationalism than one that suggested the listener take a magic-carpet ride to the centre of their mind. Drug references, however, did not fit easily into any of the existing categories for banning records, nor were they common in pop lyrics before 1967. There was a rich history of risqué allusions in folk and blues music, but even these controversial items, deemed unsuitable for inclusion in general entertainment programming, could still be played in specialist slots that catered for those particular genres. Contemporary pop presented a whole new set of problems, and, as senior managers within the BBC conceded, nobody but the initiated understood the argot anyway.

Drug addiction, however, was another matter. In January 1967 EMI hastily withdrew 'The Addicted Man' by the Game after seven minutes of an episode of the BBC record-review show *Juke Box Jury* had to be cut, following a heated discussion between the guest panellists. Despite the controversy – the title phrase appears nowhere in the song itself – and the fact that the opening words are 'Take it, boy' and the chorus goes 'Reach there, man / and get there fast,' there is little in the song to distinguish it from any of the other Who-influenced R&B that was released during the period. The subject matter might have been abundantly clear to anyone in the know, but had the song just been called 'Reach There, Man', it's quite possible that the *Juke Box Jury* panellists would have remained oblivious to what the Game were really singing about. The lyrics, delivered in an insolent slur through a wall of feedback and fuzz, would have been as unintelligible to the unconverted as many rap lyrics are now. That's part of the reason why so many drug-inspired songs did slip by unnoticed and why a whole codified language of innuendo and euphemism developed in the way that it did during the late 1960s. Nobody sang, 'Right now I am experiencing piercing shards of ultraviolet light passing through my skull owing to the LSD tablet I swallowed a couple of hours ago,' not when there were so many other linguistic options available.

'He's been travelling everywhere,' sang the Smoke on the less than subtle 'My Friend Jack', released on Columbia just a month after the 'Addicted Man' controversy. The song had been recorded in the summer of 1966 and contained the first allusion on record to the ingesting of LSD via liquid droplets absorbed by a sugar cube. An early version included the lines 'Oh, what beautiful things he sees' and 'Lost in a wonderland of colour and of sound', but these were later replaced by the

less controversial 'He's been travelling everywhere' and the more self-
consciously florid 'He's seen the hawk
fly high to hail the setting sun.' On balance it's debatable which of the two sets
of lyrics is the more drug-influenced.
On the released version the dated argot
of 'He's the weirdest cat in town' is
replaced by 'On the west coast he's real
famous / kids all call him sugar man,'
a thinly veiled reference to Owsley
Stanley. And anyway 'My Friend Jack''s
most blatant drug signifier doesn't
appear in the lyric at all; it's evident
instead in the nerve-shredding, heavily
reverbed guitar sound that introduces
the song. Added at the insistence of
producer Monty Babson, that introductory dose of distortion is where 'My
Friend Jack''s true intentions are made
manifest. Without that it could just as
easily be a song about a horse that likes
sugar lumps.

'How do we know if it's a drug song?'
was the plaintive response from within
the BBC to the whole issue of censorship. In a memo issued on Monday 22
May 1967, Robin Scott, then controller
of the BBC Light Programme and about
to become head of the newly formed
Radio 1, readily conceded: 'We are
aware that some offending records will
get through and some innocent ones
will suffer, but there could be no doubt

about the rightness of our intentions.'[5]
So convinced was it of the rightness of
its intentions that the Corporation sent
a letter to the heads of all major record
companies outlining its policy. On 23
May Frank Gillard wrote personally
to Sir Joseph Lockwood explaining the
BBC's decision. 'I never thought the
day would come when we would have
to put a ban on an EMI record but
sadly that is what has happened over
this track,' he began, in hand-wringing
tones. 'We cannot avoid coming to the
conclusion that the words "I'd love to
turn you on" followed by that mounting
montage of sounds could have a rather
sinister meaning.'[6] Such reasoning
could easily have initiated a whole new
set of procedures whereby BBC producers might have had to start listening
out for further sinister intent in records
that contained 'mounting montages of
sound', but Gillard's letter made it clear
that the BBC was more concerned with
'A Day in the Life''s lyrical connotations than its ability to replicate hallucinatory experiences via sonic trickery.
'The record may have been made in
innocence and good faith,' he said, 'but
we must take account of the interpretation that many young people would
inevitably put upon it. "Turn on" is a
phrase which can be used in many different circumstances, but it is currently

much in vogue in the jargon of the drug addicts.'[7]

In his reply Lockwood assumed a posture of befuddlement. 'I read that some stations in America have taken the same line so I read through the words to see if I could find what is objected to, but frankly I did not understand a good deal of the lyrics – which is really rather the case on most pop songs. However I have heard from Americans that they do talk about "turned on" in connection with drug taking.'[8] Having apparently taken on board what he had 'heard from Americans', Lockwood assured the BBC of his full support.

'Sir Joseph Lockwood was a crafty old sod,' Pink Floyd's manager Peter Jenner told me when I interviewed him about EMI's signing of the band in January 1967 (actually the phrase he used was considerably more colourful and slanderous than that). 'They couldn't possibly have said, "Oh yes, they're a drug band and we're giving them money." He knew that we were playing on that psychedelic thing and the drug culture.' Although Lockwood was prepared to play the diplomacy game with the BBC (while his record labels issued 'My Friend Jack', 'My White Bicycle', *Sgt Pepper's Lonely Hearts Club Band*, *The Piper at the Gates of Dawn* and *S. F. Sorrow*), other major

record companies, at boardroom level at least, offered unqualified support for the Corporation's policy. There were a few dissenting voices, however. Andrew Loog Oldham's Immediate label refused to play the game at all, while Robert Reisdorff, managing director at Liberty Records, wrote: 'I must confess that very often only a few "hippy composers" are aware of the double meanings of the lyrics they write.'[9] CBS's managing director Kenneth Glancy responded with similar caveats. 'I am sure that you will agree that the problem becomes all the more vexing because of the "inside" character of much of the lexicon of contemporary pop writing,' he wrote. Just the faintest trace of sarcasm might have been detected in his conclusion: 'Nonetheless, we continue to wrestle with the problem, as does our American parent company [Columbia], but I am grateful that you have shared your feelings with us. We shall be guided accordingly.'[10]

Initially, the BBC even considered prohibiting the use of the word 'psychedelic'. The same May memo about the decision to ban 'A Day in the Life' mentioned that 'We also agreed that the word psychedelic could not be banned but that we should do everything possible to discourage its use.'[11] Discouragement rather than outright censorship turned out to be the BBC's strategy, and for all its initial bluster and apoplexy over 'I'd love to turn you on', the Corporation only banned one other record for drug references during 1967: 'Heroin' by the Velvet Underground. Several groups later claimed to have had records banned by the BBC (or rather their publicists did), and in some cases disapproval did lead to a record being ignored rather than censored (the aforementioned 'My Friend Jack' and the Purple Gang's 'Granny Takes a Trip', for instance), but after trawling extensively through the BBC written archive the only other reference I can find to a record even being reviewed for a questionable lyric with possible drug connotations in 1967 was 'Step Out of Your Mind' by the American Breed on CBS. A memo dated 3 August caustically noted: 'I had to use my intelligibility booster (no bass and peaked at 1100 c/s) to play the thing several times to decipher the crucial couplet ("you gotta be able to bend your brain if you want to get on in the world / you gotta be just a little insane if you want to get on in the world") which seems to me to be sceptic rather than psychedelic. The title line though is repeated insistently.' Describing the item as 'a discotheque sound', the memo concluded: 'not to be universally excluded'.[12] Apart from that

the only other psychedelic song that fell foul of BBC procedures was 'Streatham Hippodrome' by Cuppa T, a harmless vaudevillian ditty about a sexy girl who sells intermission ice creams at her local cinema, which was banned in March 1968 because of concerns that it might be seen to be giving free advertising to a leisure venue.[13] Despite its occasionally nannyish attitude, the BBC was, in fact, incredibly magnanimous when it came to drug controversies. At the height of the Jagger and Richards drug trial a memo was issued stating that the Rolling Stones were already being punished in a court of law and should not be further punished by the BBC. Programme-makers were told that they were free to continue playing the Stones' records.

'A Day in the Life', however, remained a cause célèbre, the trip that dare not speak its name. The Beatles' own representatives spent the rest of the 1960s trying to get the restrictions on airplay lifted. As late as April 1970, the month the band officially split up, Apple was still sending polite letters asking if the ban might be rescinded. 'I am not sure I would have originally imposed it,' conceded future director general Ian Trethowan. 'But I agree that this is certainly not the time to lift it. We don't want to appear to make any gestures towards permissiveness.'[14] By 1970 the BBC's own pop charts and playlists, not to mention the entire shape and sound of contemporary pop music, would suggest that Trethowan's unconciliatory response had come at least three years too late.

Those of a censorial disposition could have found hidden meanings in the most innocuous of pop songs, while simultaneously missing an abundance of references elsewhere. As Robin Scott admitted, some offending records would get through and some innocent ones would suffer. In the event few suffered at all because the BBC devolved all decision-making to its producers, and by the time Radio 1 started broadcasting in September 1967 several of these producers were young, sympathetic to the new sound and on the same cultural wavelength as the DJs they worked with. They were less likely than their Light Programme predecessors to agonise over whether the Herd's 'I Can Fly' or the Moody Blues' 'Fly Me High' were encouraging young people to experiment with narcotics. And what criteria could they utilise anyway? In an age when even Peter, Paul and Mary's 'Puff the Magic Dragon' came under suspicion almost anything could be read as a drug reference.

Was 'Magic Spectacles' by the Nerve a drug song? Issued on the Page One label in 1967 and produced by Reg Presley of the Troggs, the aforementioned spectacles allowed you to see 'magic everywhere'. A suspiciously drawled middle eight contains the phrase 'all these things and more I see'. In fact, the only thing even marginally psychedelic about the song was its title. Apart from that it was just a run-of-the-mill pop ballad given a little dayglo dressing. Ersatz drug references like this were everywhere in 1967 as mod and soul groups turned into psych groups and donned the appropriate semantic apparel. Studio Six were a Glaswegian septet who in April 1967 played on the legendary Stax-Volt Revue tour with Booker T. and the MGs, the Mar-Keys, Sam and Dave, and Otis Redding. Publicity photos from a year earlier show them wearing pinstriped suits and surly mod scowls; by the summer of 1967 they had forsaken the pinstripes for op-art gear, and by November they were in the studio recording a single called 'Strawberry Window' for Polydor, under the guidance of Robert Stigwood. The instruction appears to have been, 'OK, boys, we're going for the flower-power market with this one, so, Neil, if you could quote from Molly Malone and the Association's "Windy" in your "freaky" intro, then we'll bring in the "Strawberry Fields Forever" coda before hitting the Tremeloes' tra-la-las at full tilt. Oh, and don't forget the Ivy League harmonies. You never know, it could work.' It didn't, of course. It rarely ever did, but somehow 'Strawberry Window' still adds up to far more than its ridiculous parts. It's a wondrously mismatched mélange of incongruous influences all thrown into the mix in the hope that some of them would land hit side up. Utterly typical of the times, it's the sound of a record company second-guessing and the work of a group who would still rather be on that Stax tour. But by 1967 windows (strawberry or otherwise) were all the rage, as were views in general. Elevated perspectives were particularly fashionable. On the Clarke–Nash (but mostly Nash) composition 'Wings' the Hollies made light of Arthur Koestler's comments about cable-car rides to the summit when they sang, 'Why do they want us to walk when we can fly?' If someone was ascending in a balloon, flying a kite or descending by parachute, the chances are they were singing about something other than balloons, kites and parachutes. Mentions of the weather were also a sure sign that something analogous was afoot. Hazy skies might not carry a hidden message, but paisley skies definitely did. And when the

Easybeats sang about a 'Peculiar Hole in the Sky' on a 1967 Parlophone single, it was clear that we were now a world away from the mod-fuelled anti-work ethics of 'Monday, I have Friday on my mind'. The seemingly innocuous act of walking in the sunshine could also be construed as suspicious. Sunshine per se became suspect once Owsley Stanley began to manufacture his 'orange sunshine' acid (to go with his other popular brands, purple haze and blue cheer). References to 'clouds lifting' and 'walking on a cloud' might not be all that they seemed and things getting 'brighter' could also be viewed through a whole new pair of magic spectacles. The Escher-like architecture of the acid trip also inspired a marked increase in rooms without doors, and spiral staircases – particularly ones that reached the sky. The 'elevator to the brain hotel' that appears in Donovan's 'Epistle to Dippy' was just asking for it, as indeed was most of Donovan's material. Mirrors, paintings and portraits were no longer mere fixtures and fittings but indicators of distorted perspective and deeper intent. 'House of Many Windows' by Motherlight, released on Morgan Blue Town in 1969, was another of those great Monty Babson productions created entirely by session musicians. Commencing with a cavernous rumble of piano strings and a John Barry zither, it explodes into life with an everything-but-the-kitchen-sink cavalcade of keyboard pyrotechnics, tricksy phrasing and the kind of portentous lyrics ('black fire escapes against the dawn sky') that signify that progressive rock is merely a matter of months away.

As the BBC's wary surveillance of the American Breed record had shown, the mind could be construed as the most suspect mechanism of all, particularly if you showed an inclination to step outside of it, as the Breed did, or take a giant step inside it, as the Monkees were occasionally wont to do. This had clearly not been an issue when the Easybeats had Friday on their mind, even though that song overtly celebrated the Monday-morning countdown to another smashed blocked weekend. The phrase 'within your mind' now connoted a whole new way of thinking. In fact, almost any song could take on a startling new aspect just by inserting the word 'mind' at an appropriate juncture. The language of questing and soul-searching also called upon a whole new set of criteria, while the simple acts of 'knowing' and 'showing' were cast in illuminating light, particularly if they were stretched over four bars and sung raga-style. References to 'change' were also worthy of close scrutiny.

Prior to 1967 the only colours to appear consistently in pop songs were black to denote misery, blue to denote dejection and the occasional dash of red to signify anger. Psychedelia opened up a whole new paintbox and splashed the contents gleefully all over the playroom walls. Sometimes the resulting mess made pretty patterns – 'Shades of Orange' by the End, 'Technicolor Dreams' by Status Quo – but at other times it created something as toxic as 'Pink, Purple, Yellow and Red' by the Sorrows. Released on Piccadilly in 1967, the song is ostensibly just another transition marker between mod and psych but its content indicates that some deeper turmoil has been triggered by the switch from purple hearts to purple haze. Two years earlier the Sorrows had been in the UK Top 10 with 'Take a Heart', a moody beat-era snarl of a song brimming with masculine anger and resentment. 'Pink, Purple, Yellow and Red' is pretty much the same song only in multicolour rather than monochrome. It has a similar throbbing bass line, albeit taken at a more jittery lick, and the bitterness and rancour is still wrapped in fuzz and distortion as before. Its reference points are a throwback to the beat era too. His whisky bottle is almost drained and he's in his cups. His woman has left him.

His friends all wish him dead. The sea change from mod to psych sensibilities comes in one derisive sneer as the mind-numbed narrator muses on what his so-called friends might think of him if he was dead. 'Maybe then they'll agree that the flowers improve me,' he sings, with spittle-flecked irony. Despite its pretty pastel title, 'Pink, Purple, Yellow and Red' is an incendiary slab of pill-fuelled hate pop; not so much a eulogy to a born-again flower child, more the irrationale of a man who, realising his drink has been spiked, has lurched reeling out of the nightclub and just about made it back to the sanctuary of his spinning bed before the furies take flight. 'Something's gonna blow / inside my head,' he sings like a Brum-beat Travis Bickle as the walls contract and expand around him.

Aside from psychedelia's techni-colour expansion of the colour field, 'visions' and 'patterns' came in for close attention too. Not when Cliff Richard sang 'visions of you', obviously, but when the Bystanders trilled, 'We're the pattern people,' on their cover of the Jim Webb composition, they were revealing subcultural affinities that lay far beyond interior design in the tradi-tional sense. And if you were so bereft of lyrical inspiration that you couldn't think of a colour, you could always just say the word 'colour'; better still if you could combine it with 'mind', as the Attack did on their mod-psych B-side 'Colours of My Mind'. Failing that, the tautological fail-safe 'Dream on My Mind', as sung by Rupert's People, was always a good bet.

Exaggerated distance, spatial dis-tortion, warped perception – many were the ways of analogising the vola-tile propulsion of the acid experience as psychedelia opened up whole new terminological vistas to describe the quantifiable infinite. 'Eight Miles High' started it, and even though Roger McGuinn remained teasingly ambigu-ous about whether that was eight phar-maceutical miles or aeronautical ones, it was undoubtedly the Byrds' 1966 star log that set the trend for applying mileage rates to the road less travelled. According to reliable astronomical sources, Aldebaran, the intended des-tination of the Rolling Stones in '2,000 Light Years from Home', is actually sixty-five light years from Earth, which meant that Jagger and Richards had overshot their destination by some dis-tance, but accuracy was never really the issue during the relentless inter-galactic storm of 1967. 'There he goes on another voyage of his own delusion,' sang Twink Alder on '10,000 Words in a Cardboard Box' by the Aquarian Age, readily acknowledging that evocations of distance were only ever as plausible as the acid-raddled narrator who was doing the evoking.

By 1967 the distorted views (and, indeed, the see-through baby blues) that Syd Barrett sang about on Pink Floyd's 'Arnold Layne' were evident everywhere, and not just in the music. On album sleeves the standard group photo op was discarded and portraiture began to be fed through a fish-eye lens, draped in gauze and blurred beyond recognition. Cream sat tinted and apostle-like atop multicoloured phoenix wings on *Disraeli Gears*. Traffic looked toasted and aglow on *Mr Fantasy*. The Troggs peered pensively through cellophane, as perhaps the Troggs only could, on the album cover of the same name. From every irregular angle psychedelic graphics reconfigured linear images into abstraction. LSD's all-pervasive decentring of the self rapidly seeped into everything. It was there in the molecular rearrangement of the drug itself as persona willingly non grata floated in egoless limbo land and watched helplessly as endless astral projections of their subdivided souls bubble-popped into infinity. It was there in the St Elmo's arc of the light show as performers disappeared into the glycerine drips and

the celluloid wheels to be remoulded as spectral apparition and outline, as shadows and reflections. There was even a song called 'Shadows and Reflections', written by Tandyn Almer and covered in the UK by mod group the Action. 'Shadows and Reflections' heralded the new immersion. The song was about what a lot of great mid-sixties pop songs were about – absence. It concerns a guy who compulsively revisits the empty apartment where his ex used to live. All he's left with are memories and ghostly visitations. There are the shapes she used to make when her physical presence inhabited this room. In her place is a neon-lit nightscape as the past is recast in a dark empty room with no curtains and the electricity cut off.

The Action's previous singles had all been blue-eyed soul covers – 'Land of a Thousand Dances', 'In My Lonely Room', 'I'll Keep Holding On', 'Baby, You've Got It'; now they sang, 'Just these neon reflections / cast their frightening glow / Drifting patterns of shadows below.' 'Shadows and Reflections' pointed the way out of mod pop towards psych pop, a huge, luminous pop-art arrow that signposted other possibilities. Pretty soon all kinds of people would be singing about shadows and reflections, as they surrendered to the head-shredding flickerscape. That feeling of everything being slightly out of synch with itself was a feature of 'Baby Your Phrasing Is Bad' by Caleb Quaye, who sings the title line in a narcoleptic blur: each syllable is slowed down and stretched out in a brain-blitzed homage to bad diction and ill communication. Ringo-esque drums pound leadenly while the singer sounds like he can barely lift his head to utter the words. 'Night Is A'Comin' by Warm Sounds has the ubiquitous 'Taxman' riff, heavy guitars, unhinged helium vocals and a nudging lyric that namechecks the Grateful Dead, and asks what you're growing in your flower pot, as if we don't already know. It fades out with some of the most radical tape reversal heard on a sixties pop single. The archly named 'Bee Side' by Tintern Abbey – actually an A-side – features all manner of subtle embellishments: splashy phased cymbals, echo-treated unintelligible vocals, a soupçon of mellotron and a sparse horn arrangement. The verses are all hazy drawl but the chorus breaks down into churchy canticles. It's all topped and tailed with a two-finger piano exercise that doesn't feature anywhere else in the song.

The best English psych pop had a wonky momentum all of its own. The lurches and leaps of the trip, rendered in sudden tempo shifts and erratic clashes of timbre, were matched by the wonky momentum of the words. The Pink Floyd's 'Apples and Oranges' is a masterclass in zigzag meanderings and acid-splattered insights, but 'Smokey Pokey World' by Tickle runs it pretty close. The wigged-out call and response between the left-brain, right-brain vocal lines is blue-eyed gospel mutated to the nth. The duo of vocalists sound like disembodied glove puppets popping up from adjacent rabbit holes or moon craters as a ringmaster MC unsuccessfully tries to club them to death with a mallet made of calcified Jelly Tots. (That's the promo film I would have made, anyway.) When some future civilisation disinters the song from beneath the scorched rubble, it will discover the genetic coding of psychedelia itself: it can be located in the moment when the singers give free rein to their high harmonies on the words 'tootsie roll'. 'Smokey Pokey''s B-side, 'Good Evening', is cut from similar multicoloured cloth. With its time-warped contractions and its strident pub piano it's a psychedelic night down at the Old Bull and Bush. 'Good to see a friendly face once more,' they sing, only to be lured into a tap room full of acid pranksters who are all dressed like infrared skeletons shot full of radioactive dye, just so they can mess with your mind when the ultraviolet light show begins. The gradations are more gentle, the lurches less extreme in 'Gone Is the Sad Man' by Timebox, but the results are equally resplendent. The rhythm trampolines along on a springy bed of piano and tinkling vibes that sound like four bars from 'Strawberry Fields Forever''s coda looped to infinity, but the vocals pirouette to a momentum of their own design, criss-crossing the tempo, tumbling joyously over the root chords, bursting with high harmonies and soaring octave leaps.

Like a lot of the best codified psychedelic songs, 'Gone Is the Sad Man' delivers its message with a gentle nudge. Not every acid-inspired lyric announced itself with bells and whistles and self-conscious allusions plucked from the 'How to Converse in Fluent Psych' songbook. Often it took just one subtly delivered word or phrase to alert the knowing. Had it been written in 1966, 'Amy Peate' by Orange Bicycle would have been just another invitation to gaze at a pop-art poster girl, but it's 1967 and just look at her now. She's got 'smiling secret knowledge', 'she's not the same as other girls' and 'life has so much more'. If she ever takes off those big boutique sunglasses, you'll be able to see her deadly nightshade eyes.

'Secret' by Virgin Sleep comes adorned with an achingly exquisite arrangement for cello and mellotron, and has that bobbing-just-above-the-waterline rhythm that characterises a lot of the mod R&B that has swapped the appeal of the dance floor for drowning in drugs. The song is a miniature paisley pastorale, a teddy bear's picnic with spiked sugar lumps. The vocalist sings of hushed certainties and secrets that can't be spilled. The creatures in the forest know. Nature knows. The birds and the bees know. The spider spinning his web of silk, he definitely knows. Everybody in the song knows, but do you know? If we all keep perfectly still and nobody disturbs the spell, it will stay like this for ever. It's wasted and fey in a way that only a dosed-up ex-mod could be in 1968. The equally enigmatic 'It' by Excelsior Spring condenses acid bliss to one word, one strobe-flashed 'Wow' on a wall. Produced by Andrew Loog Oldham, 'It' comes and goes in one minute fifty-eight seconds, an all-enveloping vision of unreality that bows out just before it blows it with one too many attempts at summarising the unutterable.

'The Otherside' by Apple is announced by a thin trebly guitar line that plummets into the awaiting arms of a McCartneyesque piano. The lyric struggles to express its noble intent, burdened as it is with the inadequacies of the vernacular. The goal beyond is reduced to familiar phraseology: 'seeds are sown', 'my ship has sailed', 'life beyond eternity', 'visions far from reach'. And yet somehow the end result is magnificent. Thought and expression are irreconcilable, but we continue to yearn and search nonetheless. It's a universal sentiment grounded by the devil in the details. So majestic is the lysergic ebb and flow of the melody that you can almost forgive them for the dreadful couplet 'spirits fly / halfway to the sky'.

While the Beatles' 'Lucy in the Sky with Diamonds' and the Jimi Hendrix Experience's 'The Stars that Play with Laughing Sam's Dice' were getting all the acrostic attention, the smartest in-joke of all slipped quietly by on a poorly distributed LP that all but died a death when Andrew Loog Oldham's Immediate label went bust in 1968. Billy Nicholls's 'London Social Degree' was set to a typically sixties piano beat, but the song owes its shimmer to a whole new set of impulses. 'If you pass it and you see a new meaning, girl / You won't have to go to church and believe / you will see the love that makes you think better / it's a London Social Degree,' sings Nicholls in joyous homage to the new chemical religion. In his missionary fervour to spread the love he also urges 'that you tell your mum and dad', although there is substantial anecdotal evidence to suggest that this was not always advisable.

'All of a sudden there's a different world appearing in front of my eyes,' sang the Open Mind on 'Magic Potion' in 1969, a rumbling avalanche of proto-Stooges fuzz-rock issued at the frazzled end of the decade. The Open Mind began life as the Apaches. Then they became the Drag Set. Of course they did. It was the law. They were observing the thermodynamic principles of sixties pop: from Shadows copyists to foppish mods to deep-fried, pan-galactic pill wizards with wah-wah pedals instead of wands. It's debatable which offers the bigger clue: the name of the band, the name of the song or the Alice-inspired talk of 'taking a sip'. 'How do you feel?' enquires the singer. 'I feel fine,' comes the response. This is no longer the feeling fine that the Beatles were singing about in 1964. The currency has changed. Drug is the love.

Tangerine Dreams and Strawberry Windows

'A Day in the Life', despite the BBC's prim attitude, was hailed as a masterpiece and was indisputably the most talked about track on *Sgt Pepper*. 'She's Leaving Home', like 'Eleanor Rigby' before it, inspired a spate of domestic vignettes and kitchen-sink melodramas about small affairs and big circumstances. 'Being for the Benefit of Mr Kite' led to a junkyard full of calliopes and steam organs appearing on records. But by far the most influential track on the LP was 'Lucy in the Sky with Diamonds'. Its rococo lyricism had an immediate impact upon the lingua franca of psychedelic pop, and in the eighteen months following its release the airwaves were filled with florid imagery inspired entirely by John Lennon's enchanting childlike tale of the girl with kaleidoscope eyes.

The posters, the light shows, the fashions and the album graphics of psychedelia all owed a debt to the decorative arts of bygone times, so it was no surprise that pop lyrics would assume equally flowery and frivolous shapes. Suddenly every last workaday wordsmith was adopting the techniques of William Holman Hunt and John Everett Millais and coating their songs with a fine hallucinatory glaze, in the hope that they might replicate the glittery surface sparkle of the acid trip. The evidence could be heard everywhere as all kinds of groups began to inject a little dayglo luminosity into speed-blurred eyeballs. 'Lucy in the Sky with Diamonds' did more than any other song to hasten the metamorphosis of brutish, hard-edged R&B into prissy and effete pop rococo. Most copyists neglected 'Lucy''s seamless glideoscope and settled instead for an indiscriminate plundering of its more imitable components – the tangerine trees, the cellophane flowers, the marmalade skies. But good, bad or indifferent, it was impossible to avoid the 'Lucy' effect. It's there in 'and when it rains / it rains lemonade' in the Spencer Davis Group's 'Time Seller'. It's there in Dave Mason's 'House for Everyone', from Traffic's *Mr Fantasy* album, with its 'My bed is made of candy floss / the house is made of cheese', and it was everywhere during 1967 and 1968. You didn't even have to search for it in the lyrics. The titles often told you everything you needed to know.

'Turquoise Tandem Cycle' by Jason Crest offered 'houses of papier mâché' and 'scarlet ribbons hanging from the sky'. Angel Pavement's 'Green Mello Hill' has a 'purple alligator swimming in his cup of tea'. 'Send My Love to Lucy' by Toyshop came laden with evocations of 'sunset harmonies and rainbows made of glass', 'forests of oblivion' and 'golden swordfish'. Even a routine pop ballad like 'How Could You Say

You're Leaving Me?' by Piccadilly Line managed to slip in a reference to 'taffeta skies'. There was something delightfully, English-ly absurd in ex-mods and Denmark Street hacks attempting to match their commercial instincts to the new lysergic sensibility. Some used imagery that was so interchangeable and generic no one would really have noticed, or cared, if the songs had been called 'Marmalade Cycle', 'Hyacinth Popcorn' and 'Turquoise Threads' and been performed by Wimple Tandem, Orange Crest and Jason and the Scruggonauts. Had they been so inclined USCO could probably have made a fortune by customising Gerd Stern's three-dimensional 'mechanical poem' 'Contact Is the Only Love', feeding the new psychedelic argot into its kaleidoscopic word wheel and selling the random ready-mades to music publishers for a fee.

That, in the end (and in the very beginning too), was the heart of the matter. Some took a little sugared pill that made them mystics for a day; others just put on a paisley shirt and pretended. And that some of the best exponents of UK psych pop didn't touch drugs at all is a truth that should be universally acknowledged. Kaleidoscope made two LPs – *Tangerine Dream* (1967) and *Faintly Blowing* (1969) – that

were absolutely dripping in 'Lucy'-isms. At their best they sounded like the finest *Piper at the Gates of Dawn* tribute band in the world. 'Dive into Yesterday' accelerates and slows like a wonky clock. 'Flight from Ashiya' has all the necessary see-saw propulsion and a nudging get-the-message lyric that promises 'one minute high / the next minute low'. 'Nobody knows where we are,' they sing in their best Syd Barrett mind-blown whimper. They trippily tra-la-la'd in all the appropriate places. They sang about watch repairers, the seaside and sky children. They referenced 'the white clouds of no-time'. They used words like 'iridescent' with confidence. They pronounced 'nobody' and 'knows' with the requisite fluting vowels. And by their own admission Kaleidoscope never necked anything stronger than alcohol. 'Cigarettes burning faster and faster / everyone talking about the ever after,' they sang on 'Flight from Ashiya', and plain filter-tipped cigarettes is just what they were.

Another of psych pop's great rococo outfits was Status Quo. Between the period in early 1967 when they were forced to change their name from Traffic to the moment early in 1970 when they decided to spend the next decade rewriting the Doors' 'Roadhouse Blues', Status Quo made music to match their shirts: paisley-patterned pop that swirled and curled in plumes of phasing, all delivered in Francis Rossi's trebly nasal drone or Rick Parfitt's lovestruck pout. The moment on 'Technicolor Dreams' where Rossi sings, 'If I could escape through the windows of my mind I would fly to your magic mountain land,' and puts the necessary wavery raga emphasis on the stretched vowels of the word 'land' ('lay-ay-ay-and') is one of the truly great offerings of English psychedelia, but Status Quo delivered many others during their psych-pop prime. Due to a quirk of fate the only edition of *Top of the Pops* to survive from 1968 features them performing their Top 10 hit 'Pictures of Matchstick Men', allowing the viewer to glimpse them in all their frock-coated, neatly coiffured, slightly bashful black-and-white glory. On 'Ice in the Sun', their other chart hit from that year, they rampage through the Marty Wilde-penned cod-psychedelic verses with reckless abandon, crunching through the changes like the glorious one-chord wonders they were clearly destined to be. Their tinny psychedelic sound, all turquoise tandem wah-wah, girly-boy harmonies and pop-mod riffing, was a thing of beauty. Their song titles when laid end to end – 'Mr Mind Detector', 'When My Mind Is

Not Live', 'Black Veils of Melancholy', 'Elizabeth Dreams', 'Sunny Cellophane Skies' – spelled out the word 'ersatz'.

The most convincing 'Lucy' adopters were often groups whose underground credentials ranged from marginal to non-existent. The Troggs, the Bee Gees and the Move were all unashamedly pop at a time when rock was in its ascendancy. All three had old-school pop managers (Larry Page, Robert Stigwood and Tony Secunda respectively) who adhered to old-school management principles (another of pop's fabulous oxymorons) and were prone to instigating equally old-school publicity stunts. These groups did cabaret, not Monterey, and only with great reluctance did they adopt flower-power couture. Page initially put the Troggs in barbershop candy stripes. Secunda played on the Move's menacing image and cast them as 1920s gangsters. Robert Stigwood didn't bequeath the Bee Gees any sense of style at all. He initially thought the serious money would be in publishing and hawked the Gibb brothers' songs round Denmark Street and the Charing Cross Road in search of clients. All three groups found endless ways in which to fall foul of anti-provincial snobberies. The Troggs, despite being the first UK garage band, were seen as bumpkins from Wiltshire, with attitudes to match. The Bee Gees spent their formative years in Australia and were already geeky child stars with a track record in saccharine pop before arriving back in England. And in an age of dandified mods and mutated R&B the Move contained two unreconstructed rockers among their ranks, singer Carl Wayne and drummer Bev Bevan, who were as happy playing Eddie Cochran numbers as Tamla covers.

During an animated studio discussion on the legendary *Troggs Tapes*, a discussion that directly inspired a scene in *Spinal Tap*, an exasperated Reg Presley can be heard imploring engineer Clive Franks to 'put a little bit of fucking fairy dust over the bastard'. After a moment's reflection he amends his original request. 'I know that it needs strings,' he says quietly. 'That I do know.' And indeed there was a period in the mid- to late 1960s when that was all the music industry knew too: sprinkle some fairy dust over the bastard and add some strings. Giddy with Beatlemania, increasingly empowered by the growing belief that perhaps guitar groups weren't on the way out after all and devoted to a scale of overproduction that would have brought most other industries to their knees, record companies lavished generous budgets

and grandiose expectations on the most unlikely and unassuming of discs. Even the most mediocre of efforts (and their equally nondescript B-sides) could expect the full orchestral works, or a string section at the very least, all budgeted for at musicians' union scale rates in the vain hope of a hit. Reg Presley knew a thing or two about making hit records, and for the best part of a decade his logic was adhered to by record companies great and small.

The Troggs were hugely incorrigible and massively influential. Musically they were more accomplished than they are ever given credit for. They may have been progenitors of the garage sound but they were proto-bubblegum, proto-glam and proto-grunge too. In a parallel pop universe they contain the only Presley who really matters, the true savour of the English savant-garde. Reg Presley sang with a visible twinkle and a metaphorical wink that suggested he was in on the joke too. Adopting the louche manner of a bar-room balladeer, he was far more typical of the average English lothario than we like to admit. Beneath the cool veneer of every dandified Brian Jones or Stag-O-Lee bluesman lurked a bleary booze-goggled Reg Presley just dying to strut his stuff.

The Troggs (shortened from Troglodytes at Larry Page's insistence) initially made their name with cabalistic paeans to lust at first sight like 'Wild Thing', 'With a Girl Like You', 'I Can't Control Myself' and 'Give It to Me'; or, in the case of the Larry Page composition 'Cousin Jane', paeans to secret late-night liaisons with your blood relatives. When psychedelia arrived, they replaced the candy stripes with lilac and velvet and scrubbed up pretty well, without losing any of their leery (as opposed to Leary) charm. Their 1967 single 'Night of the Long Grass' was a gothic moorland tryst, with spooky Joe Meek wind-machine effects. An abundance of similar oddities were to be found on the band's B-sides and album tracks. The fairy dust they sprinkled on 'Jingle Jangle', on their 1966 LP *From Nowhere*, showed that they could spin a nice line in folky-baroquey. They could also dampen the ardour sufficiently to turn out tender hot-breathed ballads like 'Love Is All Around' and 'Any Way that You Want Me'. They were nothing if not adaptable. 'When Will the Rain Come', the B-side to 'Love Is All Around', and 'Head or Tails', from 1968's *Mixed Bag*, sound like prototypes for every garage band that has ever crawled out from underneath a rolling stone. 'It's Showing', from 1967's *Cellophane*, would have perfectly suited Eric Burdon in his late-1966

'between old and new Animals' period.

Like Ringo's drumming, Reg Presley's Wiltshire burr really came into its own when the Troggs went paisley. The 'Lucy'-isms of 'Butterflies and Bees' ('dandelion seeds to rainbow trees') showed that when they eased off on the lechery they could turn out lysergic balladry with the best of them. But it is with their specialised brand of acid gonzo that the Troggs really made their mark. The synthetic side of psych was summarised magisterially on 'Purple Shades', a track on *Mixed Bag*. 'Purple Shades' is full to the luminous brim with wondrous nonsense. Reg and the boys are dancing on cellophane moons by the third line. At one point Presley sings 'Bamboo butterflies, twice their normal size, flying around in my mind' with such disturbingly drawling West Country conviction that you want to travel back in time, reach for the Andover phone directory and call him up to explain that 'Well, Reg, a butterfly twice its normal size still isn't very large, you know.' I've rehearsed that observation into oblivion over the years. I used it as the opening line to the sleeve notes I wrote for a CD compilation called *Paisley Pop* in 1991. I reprised the anecdote for a home-taping feature for *Mojo* magazine in 1997 called 'Dozy Takes a Trip', an imaginary twenty-two-track compilation that highlighted the 'so wrong they got it right' aspect of daffy psych. And I was thrilled beyond words when a Channel 4 interviewer, obviously prompted by my observations, asked Reg Presley what had inspired his rococo flight of fancy. Presley revealed that it was nothing more potent than Rich Tea biscuits and a nice cup of tea, which is exactly as it should be.

Actually, the most telling observation on 'Purple Shades' is not the one about bamboo butterflies. It's the bit where Presley envisions giant teddy bears climbing up his stairs. 'What they symbolise / I don't realise,' he sings, with disarmingly convincing befuddlement, adding a superfluous 'something I don't understand' just to round off the magical mystery tour of his Rich Tea-saturated psyche. There, in essence, was the Troggs' take on psychedelia, and they sound no less illuminated and certainly no more philosophically impoverished for the non-experience than many of their supposedly more elevated acid-soaked peers. And while Chris Britton's 'Maybe the Madman', from the same LP, was hardly going to assist radical psychiatrists Ronnie Laing and David Cooper with their enquiries, it does contain some absolute nuggets. 'Building fairy castles in a hostile space of undiscovered skies' is

just one of the many lyrical gems that dribble out as Britton's brain thoughts run away from the colours of his mind. 'The sun travels on round the world and keeps shining while we sleep at night,' sings Presley during the chorus, in his finest *mondo profondo* accent. Little did we know it at the time, but in such Copernicus- and Kepler-denying insights seeds were being sown that would reap a rich cosmological harvest when Presley began his pioneering research into the origins of crop circles.

Had they not reinvented themselves in the mid-1970s as disco pioneers the Bee Gees might by now be more highly regarded as a pop act. The first four LPs they made for Polydor – *Bee Gees' 1st* (1967), *Horizontal* (1968), *Idea* (1968) and *Odessa* (1969) – contain immaculately crafted songs full of sumptuous melodies and beautiful orchestration, arranged and directed by their very own George Martin, Bill Shepherd. Apart from Lennon and McCartney, Barry, Robin and Maurice Gibb were probably the most melodically gifted English pop composers of the 1960s. In their early days they were accused of being Beatles copyists, a claim that led John Peel to comment on his *Perfumed Garden* programme, 'If you're going to copy anyone, it might as well be the Beatles,' but there clearly was credence in the accusation. Their debut UK hit, 'New York Mining Disaster', lifted its melody line from the Beatles' 'You Like Me Too Much'. 'In My Own Time,' from their debut LP, borrowed the 'Taxman' riff, while the pounding pianos at the beginning of *Horizontal*'s 'Harry Braff' leaned heavily on 'Good Day Sunshine'. The 'in my time' bridge on the same LP's 'Birdie Told Me' takes 'In My Life' as its inspiration. Like the Beatles, the Bee Gees were early adopters of the mellotron; its eerie textures were well suited to the equally eerie timbre of the Gibb brothers' vocalising. The Beatles were also a source of inspiration for quirky character vignettes like 'Craise Finton Kirk Royal Academy of Arts', a song about a billboard man who advertised the Royal Academy, and the aforementioned 'Harry Braff', a breathless manic rant about a racing driver. On 'The Earnest of Being George' the Bee Gees betray a Liverpudlian weakness for bad puns, but on 'World', a plaintive anthem for the uprooted and the anxious, they sound like John Lennon at his most disenchanted, and the song contains an ode to regret that Lennon himself could have written: 'If I remember all of the things I have done / I remember all of the times I've gone wrong.'

Despite the obvious debt to the Beatles in their harmony singing, there was a tremulous quavering quality to their voices that no one else had. On 'Holiday', a huge hit in America but never released as a single in the UK, Robin Gibb's haunting, desolate tones make the idea of a vacation sound like a lament. It's a quality that frequently undermines any sense of celebration in their songs, giving even their love songs a melancholy air and imposing a distancing that few others apart from the perennially semi-detached Ray Davies ever managed. But then again, it's worth reiterating that their debut UK hit was about a pit disaster.

The Bee Gees were never remotely hip, not even by association. Critically they were regarded as interlopers, arrivistes, an image that stayed with them throughout the 1960s and helped detract from the fact that they were superb tunesmiths and master craftsmen. Asked by *NME* in February 1973 to name ten favourite records for its regular 'Under the Influence' column, Robert Wyatt raised a few eyebrows (and highbrows) by placing the Bee Gees' *Horizontal* in among his favoured Charles Mingus, John Coltrane and Sonny Rollins albums. 'No one would have said anything if I'd put John Cage or Schoenberg,' he told me. 'I always thought they were very good – song-writers as skilled as Burt Bacharach but actually doing it themselves as rock groups are supposed to do. But people would ask them who their heroes were and they said Winston Churchill, which didn't resonate in the burgeoning alternative society.' 'I'll tell you how naive we were,' said Maurice Gibb. 'I went out drinking with Lennon once when he was on LSD and I never even noticed! He covered it very well, and he was much funnier. He wasn't sarcastic but he was very witty. He also got very creative. He kept running off into a room to draw or write things down.' On another occasion Gibb recalled being at a party when someone passed him a joint, 'and I got out my fags and said it's all right, I've got plenty. There's no need to share one!'[15]

The palpably nostalgic air, the eccentric music-hall twang of their character songs, the mellotrons, the hazy nasal drawl – all these qualities suggest that the Bee Gees were tailor-made, if not tailor-styled, for psychedelia. They were certainly masters of the elusive 'Lucy'-esque lyric: 'I can feel the speaking sky,' on 'Red Chair, Fade Away'; 'An apple is a fool but lemons never do forget,' on 'Lemons Never Forget'; 'Please don't make no hesitation / there will be no recreation,' on

'Jumbo'. The words mean nothing but suggest everything. They wriggle free of codification and cultural baggage. They are perfect psychedelic facsimiles, fashionable forgeries, impeccably rendered. 'There must be something there,' they sing on 'Barker of the UFO', a song which despite its title is more Foreign Office than Tottenham Court Road club. It was no good asking the Bee Gees themselves to shed further light. They were rarely forthcoming about the influences behind those early songs, and when they were they were less than insightful. The frenzied accelerations of 'Harry Braff' they put down to nothing more than a wild late-night drunken writing session.

When it worked, when lyric and sentiment were in tandem and they weren't just throwing word shapes, the Bee Gees sounded sublime. *Horizontal*'s title track was a tone poem equal to anything that Brian Wilson and Van Dyke Parks were attempting with *Smile*. It sounds like a requiem – 'This is the start of the end / goodbye' – but it's actually a song about writing a finale rather than the finale itself. The Gibb brothers explored similar self-referential territory on 'Gilbert Green', a song they gave to Gerry Marsden to record as a single in 1967 before realising they could have done a better job themselves. 'Gilbert Green' is a song about writing a song about a character who writes songs that no one ever hears. Gilbert mends carpets for a living and, in a denouement worthy of Pete Townshend, had he written *Teenage Opera* instead of Mark Wirtz, he perishes in a house fire. When Gilbert's undiscovered song is found in the basement, it's not a long-lost masterpiece; it simply 'tells the tale of laughing men and yellow beans'. It's a taunting rejoinder to Lennon's 'Don't you know the joker laughs at you?' and it summarises the Bee Gees' psych-pop endeavours perfectly. There's an obliqueness and insularity about many of those early songs that make you think they were having a quiet Lennonesque in-joke at everybody's expense. Not insincere, just weird.

The Barry Gibb song 'Kilburn Towers', from their third LP *Idea*, begins with a haunting mellotron slowly wheezing out the melody line before settling into a warm samba lilt, except when you listen closely it's a song about drifting and disengagement. And Barry Gibb isn't part of the action; he's sitting on a hillside, serenading his jug of wine like the Chinese poets of old in their solitude. 'I am a street / watching the people walk,' he sings, a line that Scott Walker would probably have given his

Jacques Brel songbook to have written. 'That could mean everything,' he shrugs in response to his own listlessness. It's a line that could serve as the perfect epitaph to the Bee Gees' fleeting, tantalising engagement with psychedelia.

By 1966 the five members of the Move were already veterans of the Birmingham beat scene. Still only in their teens and early twenties, they had been playing in one combo or another since the rock-and-roll days. As a result they were all accomplished musicians by the time they came together as a group. All five were competent vocalists: they could harmonise interchangeably and four of them sang lead. Everyone who saw them perform at the height of psychedelia paid testimony to their stage presence and prowess. In their live act they stomped their way through an art-prole variant on Pete Townshend's auto-destruction show that was not so much Metzger-inspired, more a gleeful smashing of stuff without a hint of intellectual pretension. Needless to say, they scared the shit out of some of the less hardened UFO regulars. It was hard to concentrate on your karmic realignment as shards of vandalised TV sets went whizzing past your face. The Move's most notorious stunt was to issue a set of photo-montaged postcards to promote 'Flowers in the Rain', one of which graphically suggested that Prime Minister Harold Wilson was having an affair with his private secretary, Marcia Williams. In 2006, when a BBC play, *The Lavender List*, contained a similar inference, Baroness Falkender, as she was by then, successfully sued. In 1967 the prank received the attentions of MI5 and an out-of-court settlement with the prime minister himself; as a result Roy Wood has never seen a penny of the royalties for 'Flowers in the Rain' to this day.

Musically the Move possessed a thuggish beauty all of their own. Their sound was built on a bedrock of rumbling bass and powerhouse drums, with guitars sawing away like cellos, all topped off with that Brum barbershop quartet of adenoidal vocalists. Its effect could be both seductive and alarming, especially when the anxiety-inducing register of Wood's piercing nasal whine leapt out of the mix. As a group they could be disarmingly nursery-rhymish one minute ('(Here We Go Round) The Lemon Tree', 'Flowers in the Rain'), folksy and pastoral the next ('The Girl Outside', 'Mist on a Monday Morning', 'Beautiful Daughter'), but they were rarely more than a groin thrust away from the lairy and the priapic ('Fire Brigade', 'Wild Tiger Woman'). 'Fire Brigade', a riotous

teenage rampage of a single, is about a girl so hot they need to send in the emergency services just to quell the ardour of her admirers. It begins with the screaming bells of a fire engine and ends with a few punked-up bars of Eddie Cochran's 'C'mon Everybody'. Roy Wood never took drugs but was happy to borrow his reference points from those members of his band who did. He was the Alan Lomax of psychedelia, the front-line psycho-anthropologist who made field recordings among the chemically charged natives and reported his findings in three-minute vox pops with great middle eights.

The Move's nervy, panic-driven debut single 'Night of Fear' quoted from Tchaikovsky's *1812 Overture* and contained a nagging, incessant chorus line guaranteed to get its intentions across: 'Just about to flip your mind / just about to trip your mind.' The synaesthesic follow-up 'I Can Hear the Grass Grow' ended each chorus with a joyous 'I see rainbows in the evening'. Like several of their contemporaries, including the Hollies and Traffic, the Move remained deeply divided about the extent to which they should embrace the new style, but they were rarely shy of adopting the necessary psychedelic mannerisms when it was expedient. Puckish opportunism is audibly evident in Carl Wayne's twee, arch delivery on 'Walk Upon the Water', all fluting vowel sounds and effete affectations. And it's there in spades on the shameless, unabashed cry of 'flower power in the rain' during the fade-out to 'Flowers in the Rain', the only time the phrase ever appeared on a Top 10 hit. With lessons learned from their crowd-pleasing apprenticeship, the Move performed credible cover versions of several west-coast classics, including the Byrds' 'So You Want to Be a Rock 'n' Roll Star', Love's 'Stephanie Knows Who' and Moby Grape's 'Hey Grandma'. On the latter, clearly unfamiliar with the codeine-based American cough syrup Robitussin, they sing the line as 'Robusals and elderberry wine'.

Their finest three minutes was 'Blackberry Way', Wood's haunting eulogy to lost love, a bleak counterpoint to 'Penny Lane' full of ghost whispers and taunting refrains. Its melody bore a passing resemblance to 'Flowers in the Rain' and its oow-aah bridge was borrowed from Harry Nilsson's 'Good Old Desk', but the rest of the song was planted firmly in the tradition of English melancholia. It's pouring with rain, the trees are bare, the boating lake is empty and abandoned, and love is a fleeting presence pain-stained by memory. It's a song that seeks reassurance in once-familiar settings but upon returning finds only regret. It also contains the finest lines that Roy Wood ever wrote: 'See the battlefield of careless sins / cast to the wind.'

All of the best Move songs sound dark and slightly sinister, especially their singles. I have a simple theory about this: it's because they were all hits in the early spring, late autumn or winter. With the sole exception of the chirpy, cheeky 'Curly', they never had a summer hit during the 1960s. You can hear the nights drawing in on all their best records.

Like the Velvet Underground, the Move's original members fell away one by one. Bass player Ace Kefford left after a 1967 package tour with Jimi Hendrix, Pink Floyd and the Nice, officially from nervous exhaustion, unofficially from too much tripping. Guitarist Trevor Burton hated 'Blackberry Way' and left shortly after its release, forming Balls with Denny Laine, Steve Gibbons and Alan White. They retired to get it together in the country and made one single: the magnificently ramshackle peacenik anthem 'Fight for My Country'. Move vocalist Carl Wayne had always entertained ideas of being a cabaret singer and used to serenade the band on the way home from gigs with his interpretations of Sinatra standards.

True to his word, he left after the 1970 *Shazam* LP to pursue his dream. He didn't make it to Las Vegas but did enjoy a lucrative living singing for his supper on adverts, jingles and daytime TV.

Four months after banning 'A Day in the Life' the BBC launched its new pop service, Radio 1. The first record played on the station was 'Flowers in the Rain' by the Move. It seems that despite all the initial fuss, the distance from 'somebody spoke and I went into a dream' to 'relieved to leave reality behind me' was not so far after all.

14

THE PSYCHEDELIC MUSIC HALL

That humanity at large will ever be able to dispense with Artificial Paradises seems very unlikely. Most men and women lead lives at the worst so painful, at the best so monotonous, poor and limited that the urge to escape, the longing to transcend themselves if only for a few moments, is and has always been one of the principal appetites of the soul.
ALDOUS HUXLEY, *The Doors of Perception*[1]

Are you all seated comfortybold, two-square on your botty? Then I'll begin . . .
STANLEY UNWIN

Cream chose to end their 1967 *Disraeli Gears* album not with one of Pete Brown's symbolist conundrums, or a blues master class, but with what may be the best Dadaist stunt they ever pulled: a group rendition of the old music-hall song 'Your Baby Has Gone Down the Plughole', renamed 'Mother's Lament' and credited 'Traditional. Arranged by Ginger Baker, Jack Bruce, Eric Clapton.' Counted in with an exaggerated 'a wun, a two-ah, a free, a four' and sung in impeccable mockney, it's one of the darkest tracks on the album, telling as it does the story of a mother of ten whose carelessness at bath time leads to the death of two of her children. In a denouement typical of the music hall, she vows never to wash her surviving children again, reasoning, 'It's the smell that keeps the angels away.'

'Dogs', the B-side of the Who's 1968 single 'Call Me Lightning', is a heart-warming evocation of the time Pete Townshend spent at the White City greyhound track with his dad when he was a kid. It's the tale of a couple who are united by their love of dog racing, that peculiarly British pastime that was once so popular that the annual Greyhound Derby used to be shown on prime-time television. The song's spoken interludes are full of dog-track vernacular and its chorus – 'There was nothing in my life bigger than beer' – would have raised the rafters in the music halls a century earlier. It also has one of the cheekiest fade-outs in English pop: 'Twenty-five knicker please on Yellow Printer . . . saw it run at White City just last week, broke the record . . . Nice dog, yes, lovely form, lovely buttocks.'

From the same year, 'Rene (The Dockers' Delight)' relates the ribald tale of the sailors' best friend found in every port. The song featured on the Small Faces' *Ogdens' Nut Gone Flake* and, like Cream's 'Mother's Lament', Steve Marriott delivers the song in exaggerated Jack the Lad vowels, suffixing every other word with '-ah', just as Kate Carney, the cockney Coster Comedienne, had done in the halls. Few psychedelic songs were ever as coarse as those in the original music-hall repertoire – all that acid seemed to make many a young mod go all twee and chaste – but 'Rene' was a shamelessly unreconstructed homage to sex with a prostitute of mature years. The song's arrangement was a pure throwback to Marriott's stage-school apprenticeship, and so comically conveyed was his raucous tale of 'groping with a stoker from the coast of Kuala Lumpur' that it was easy to overlook the fact that 'Rene' was based on a real-life dockside lady of the night, visited by the callow singer in his wide-eyed youth. 'Everything me mother hit me for she taught me,' Marriott later admitted.

'She's Bought a Hat Like Princess Marina', a track on the Kinks' 1969 LP *Arthur*, was one of those perfectly weighted vignettes to deference that Ray Davies excelled at. It tells the story of a dutiful 1950s wife who embellishes her otherwise drab life by aspiring to the exotic headwear of Princess Marina, the Duchess of Kent, who was well known in the post-war years for her decorative millinery. The woman's husband, meanwhile, buys a hat like the one worn by Conservative prime minister Anthony Eden. In truth neither of them have two pennies to rub together. He drives a second-hand Ford and there's no food in the larder, but they look the part and keeping up appearances is all that counts. It's a very British post-war premise – fur coat, no knickers, as the old saying goes – and once again it's a theme that goes all the way back to the music hall. Talking to *Rolling Stone* magazine in 1969, Ray Davies explicitly acknowledged his debt to the halls and the direct influence they had on the writing of 'She's Bought a Hat Like Princess Marina'. '[It] starts pretty sad,' he says, 'then it goes into the bit about what it's all about – "I haven't got any money." They're having a hard time.' Explaining the double time tempo in the second half of the song he says, 'Then they sing the way they did in the music hall, *because that's the way they used to express it* [emphasis mine].' Davies cites Harry Castling and James Walsh's 1926 song 'Don't Have Any More, Mrs Moore' as an example of the kind of composition he's thinking about. Popularised by the comedic singer Lily Morris, 'Don't Have Any More, Mrs Moore' was an ironic take on excess that tells the story of the hapless lady who in successive verses has too many children, strong alcoholic drinks and husbands, each catalogue of mounting calamity being answered with the title refrain. It's the melody as much as the lyrical content that Davies lifts from the original song, but once again it illustrates the extent to which the music hall influenced British pop music during the psychedelic era.

There had been vaudevillian novelty songs in pop's recent past but they were of a different character and hue. In 1965 Herman's Hermits sealed their fame in America with two such items: 'Mrs Brown, You've Got a Lovely Daughter' and 'I'm Henry VIII, I Am'. The former was originally sung by Tom Courtenay in a 1963 TV play called *The Lads*; the latter was made famous by music-hall singer and comedian Harry Champion during the Edwardian era. Champion was even better known for that other music-hall staple, 'Any Old Iron'. Herman's Hermits' versions were originally recorded as album fillers and neither was released as a single in the UK, but in America both went to number one, as did the New Vaudeville Band's

similarly vaudevillian 'Winchester Cathedral' in November 1966. In the year of 'We Can Work It Out', 'Paperback Writer', 'Yellow Submarine', 'Paint It Black', '19th Nervous Breakdown' and 'Sunshine Superman', 'Winchester Cathedral' was the biggest-selling British single in America, spawning a multitude of soundalikes both in the UK and the US. But before any of these there was Lonnie Donegan. Lauded for his role in the skiffle movement and his seminal influence on British rock and roll, Donegan was less critically acclaimed for his best-selling novelty numbers like 'Does Your Chewing Gum Lose Its Flavour', 'My Old Man's a Dustman' and 'Lively'. He was probably the first victim in the rock-and-roll era of that peculiarly English notion of 'selling out'. In the same way that Eric Burdon could be applauded for imitating John Lee Hooker but ridiculed for aspiring to be a cosmic sky pilot, Donegan was on assured ground while he was channelling Woody Guthrie but not, it seems, when he began performing numbers from his own indigenous novelty tradition. Presumably those who bought the novelty numbers in their millions didn't feel this way, but it's a particularly British critical snobbery to despise the potency of cheap music while somehow revering and exoticising the folk traditions of others. And yet it is the material Donegan performed when he gained wider mainstream appeal that more truly reflects his roots, which are to be found not in the Mississippi Delta or the Midwest dustbowl but in the music-hall and variety songs of the nineteenth and early twentieth centuries. There is an unbroken line of development in British popular entertainment that runs from Marie Lloyd, Harry Champion and Alice Leamar, through Gracie Fields, Wee George Wood and Max Miller to *Fings Ain't Wot They Used T'Be* and *Half a Sixpence*, and at some point in the late sixties it gathers some unlikely adherents and produces 'Mother's Lament', 'Dogs', 'Rene', 'She's Bought a Hat Like Princess Marina' and countless others.

Anthony Bennett describes the development of music-hall song in the nineteenth century as 'a radical break with earlier popular song – the first and arguably most important upheaval in an area where change had hitherto been gradual'.[2] The same might be said for the sudden stylistic lurches that pop music underwent a century later. As with the R&B mutations, the sheer oddball nature of these changes can be measured in time-lapse images. It's the difference between Roger Daltrey

talking "bout his g-g-g-generation' and singing 'We're a happy couple you and me / with a greyhound at either knee.' It's the difference between the Small Faces singing 'Picked her up on a Friday night / sha la la la lee' and 'Gor blimey, hello, Mrs Jones / how's your Bert's lumbago?' And in case you need reminding, the first of those lyrics is followed by a 'yeah', the second by 'Mustn't grumble.' A lot can be accounted for in the time it takes to get from Steve Marriott's soul-boy exhortation to a chirpy enquiry about his neighbour's lower-back ailment.

One of the less acknowledged innovations of British psychedelia was its revival of one of the mainstays of the music hall, the character song. Lennon and McCartney had made it an industry prerogative that groups and artists should write their own material, the vast majority of which was boy-meets-girl songs, while the success of Bob Dylan had made expression synonymous with self-expression. As a result observational songs, usually sung in the third person, had become a rarity in pop by the mid-sixties. In this respect Paul Simon's 'A Most Peculiar Man' was an anomaly. Written and recorded in England during the summer of 1965, the song first appeared on *The Paul Simon Songbook* and was re-recorded that December for inclusion on Simon and Garfunkel's *Sound of Silence*. Of all the material Simon wrote, or adapted, during his stay in England ('Homeward Bound', 'Scarborough Fair', etc.), least attention has been paid to this unassuming song about an unassuming man who lives alone, dies alone and leaves nothing but rumour and gossip among neighbours who didn't know him very well and didn't care much for him anyway. 'A Most Peculiar Man' proved to be the archetype for a particular kind of character song that would flourish in English pop from 1966 until the end of the decade: idiosyncratic vignettes chronicling the lives of eccentric characters, written from a non-judgemental or detached perspective. In the space of a few months came the Beatles' 'Eleanor Rigby' (August 1966), The Who's 'I'm a Boy' (August 1966) and 'Happy Jack' (December 1966), Cat Stevens's 'Matthew and Son' (December 1966) and Pink Floyd's 'Arnold Layne' (March 1967) – songs about loneliness, gender confusion, imbecility, drudgery and transvestism respectively. After that it was open season for the character song, and they came in every conceivable permutation. Variations on 'Simple Simon'. Songs about a teenage boy's infatuation with vintage erotica.

Songs about star-crossed lovers bonding over a mutual love of greyhound racing. Songs about a promising female singer whose big break is thwarted by personal-hygiene problems. And those were just the ones written by Pete Townshend. Elsewhere there were songs about tramps and buskers, watchmakers, toymakers, pawnbrokers, grocers, gravediggers, policemen, firemen, ice-cream men, gingerbread men, ton-up boys and shy boys, office girls and pin-up girls, weird uncles, lonely spinsters, jilted brides, sweet little old ladies. From 1966 onwards they all came pouring out in an unprecedented flurry of A-sides, B-sides and EP and album tracks. And by 1970 the phenomenon was all but over.

The three most influential groups in the evolution of the English psychedelic music hall – the Who, the Small Faces and the Kinks – had distinctly varying relationships with psychedelia. The Kinks were not in the least bit psychedelic, while the Small Faces utterly immersed themselves in pharmaceutical excess. With the Who, and particularly with Pete Townshend, the situation is more complex. The themes that Townshend dealt with in his songs – disengagement, dual identity, fractured personality, divided selves, multiple selves, warped perception – should have made him a prime candidate for the psychotherapeutic benefits of the acid experience. On the surface the influence of LSD on much of the material he wrote between 1966 and 1968 would appear to be a given. On 'I Can See for Miles' he sings of being able to see the Eiffel Tower and the Taj Mahal. On 'I Can't Reach You' he talks of distance in terms of a billion ages, a million years, a thousand miles. The *A Quick One* and *The Who Sell Out* LPs are liberally sprinkled with fairy dust. Tracks like 'Disguises', 'Armenia City in the Sky' and 'Mary Anne with the Shaky Hand' radiate with echo and distortion. However, in his 2012 autobiography *Who I Am* Townshend claimed to have taken LSD only four times and that his experiences, including one particularly turbulent encounter with STP after the Monterey Festival, were neither pleasant nor insightful. After these less than euphoric encounters Townshend came to the conclusion that he had enough neuroses to be going on with, without flooding the mental circuitry any further with volatile and unpredictable substances.

Townshend was the pop-art Brothers Grimm. Many of the songs that he wrote during this period crackle with malevolence and sinister intent. His characters – Bill the headcase, Happy

Jack, Mary Anne with the Shaky Hand, Sally Simpson, that deaf, dumb and blind kid – were quirks, oddballs, outcasts. 'I Can See for Miles', which many assumed was an epistle to LSD, was in fact driven by suspicion and a desire for retribution. It contains one of the most malicious 'you got a lot of nerve' opening lines outside of Bob Dylan: 'I know you've deceived me, now here's a surprise.' There may be magic in his eyes but the dilated pupils are of the deepest, darkest hue.

And yet when the Who donned their music-hall masks they revealed wit in abundance. On the cover of *The Who Sell Out* Pete Townshend has an outsized tube of Odorono wedged under his armpit. The LP track it references is about a girl who pongs a bit. There is a flippancy to Townshend's best psychedelic music-hall material that rapidly dissipates once he embarks upon his all-consuming quest to realise his *Lifehouse* project or work out what *Tommy* was really about. The levity is there in 'Happy Jack' and 'I'm a Boy'; it's there in 'Pictures of Lily', a song about finding a substitute for unrequited lust in Edwardian erotica; and it's especially there on 'Tattoo', on *The Who Sell Out*. 'Tattoo' is one of the most affecting songs that Townshend ever wrote. It takes a simple premise – two young brothers discussing 'what makes a man a man' – and reveals that even when identity is only skin deep, the repercussions of youthful impulses can last a lifetime. 'I expect I'll regret you,' sings Roger Daltrey, 'but you'll be there when I die.' With typical Townshend brutality, one brother gets beaten by his father for having a tattoo of his mother; the other gets beaten by his mother for having a tattoo of a naked lady. One brother eventually gets tattooed all over and marries a tattooed lady. The denouement is deliberately farcical. All the carefully constructed pathos that the verses so tenderly set up is undone by the absurdity of personal circumstances, exactly the same device that is used to deflate posturing and pomposity in countless music-hall songs.

A tattoo is an act of faith. The act once committed is fixed for ever and remains long after the original impulse has been forgotten. The best pop songs are like that too. They remind us in time both of what we were and what we have since become. Ultimately, they reveal how some things never truly die. The truth Daltrey doesn't expand upon is that the tattoo will outlive him. Memories, like tattoos, fade with time but can never be completely erased. Away from the glare of the spotlight and the soul-searching of 'I Can't Explain' and

'My Generation', sideshow attractions like 'Tattoo' and 'Dogs' will tell future generations as much about the 1960s as some of the old songs tell us about the 1860s. Like the best of the music-hall material, they resonate with pathos, sentimentality, stoicism and a robust vulgarity.

'Tattoo' ends with a quick burst of 'rooty tooty too'. The same phrase appears in the chorus of another great psychedelic music-hall song, the Small Faces' 'Lazy Sunday'. One of the most noticeable things about the Who's 'Dogs' was the close similarity between Roger Daltrey's exaggerated 'Laaarndon' pronunciation and Steve Marriott's barrow-boy delivery on several of the Small Faces' hits. John Entwistle later claimed that he thought the Who should have given the song to the Small Faces anyway, and he's probably right. The two bands may have been products of London's east/west divide but culturally they were blood brothers. Both were immersed in mod without actually being mods, both loved American R&B and both transcended their influences. The big difference was that the Small Faces took to acid like an Itchycoo Park duck to water.

There is a celluloid clip of the early Small Faces performing their second single, 'I've Got Mine', in the 1965 movie *Dateline Diamonds*. Original keyboard player and guitarist Jimmy Winston is still in the line-up. They are wearing suits and ties and impeccably tapered mod haircuts. Close up the unforgiving cameras reveal pimples and mottled skin. They look about fourteen. They strut on the spot, dancing from the shoulders upwards. There's lots of spasmodic head-jerking and rooster neck going on. Jimmy Winston looks blocked.

Trot along the skyways a couple of years to May 1967, to where the group, with Ian McLagan now on keyboards, are miming 'Green Circles' on the German TV show *Beat Club*. McLagan plays a pretty, jingly-jangly intro on a pub piano. Ronnie Lane, resplendent in flowery frock coat, steps up to the mike and dribbles out a cascading word slur that is both euphoric and bucolic. 'And with the rain / a stranger came,' he sings as the melody tumbles and plummets. Lane looks so feather-light that he seems in danger of being lifted aloft on the airstream of the song's sweet harmonies. His bass hangs limp by his side and he makes only cursory attempts to pretend he's playing it. 'And you and I and everywhere,' he drawls, marvelling at the oneness of everyone and everything.

The lyrics of 'I've Got Mine', like the movie they are featured in, are disposable and trite – baby this, baby that. 'Green Circles' hints at a Pan-like visitation. What's happened in the interim? You can probably guess.

Prior to joining the Small Faces Steve Marriott had been a promising child actor, a product of the prestigious Italia Conti school. He had played the Artful Dodger in Lionel Bart's *Oliver*, and appeared on the original soundtrack recording, singing 'Consider Yourself' and 'I'd Do Anything' in impeccable stage cockney. He played up that cheeky-scamp persona in early-sixties pop flicks like *Live It Up!* (1963) and *Be My Guest* (1965). In the latter he was cast as Ricky next to David Hemmings's David, performing in a fictitious beat group called the Smart Alecks. Marriott plays a drummer, with moves clearly copped from Keith Moon. Hemmings does a passable impression of a lead guitarist. A year later Hemmings would portray a thinly disguised David Bailey in Antonioni's *Blow-Up* and Marriott would be in the Top 10. Somewhere along the line the squeaky-voiced young scamp that can be heard on the *Oliver* soundtrack developed a great barrel-house rasp and transformed himself into a pint-sized Solomon Burke, a miniature Bobby Bland. Marriott could have gone the Tommy

Steele route and found himself *Half a Sixpencing* for the rest of his days. Had things not worked out with the pop career he might easily have found himself auditioning alongside another *Oliver* refugee, Davy Jones, for a role in *The Monkees*. Instead he artfully dodged his way out of a lifetime of character parts in British B movies and stage shows and incorporated his exuberant cockney cabaret turn into the greatest mod band of them all. Forever fidgety, always on, and by all accounts a bit of a pain to have to deal with on a daily basis, Marriott was the buzzing extrovert imp of the perverse in the Small Faces. In that 'Green Circles' clip he can be seen attempting to throw guitar shapes, even when the opportunities are non-existent. Whenever the camera lingers on him he executes a truncated Chuck Berry duckwalk, just to keep himself busy while Ronnie slurs away about 'you and I and everywhere'.

Ronnie Lane was the perfect foil for Marriott's restless urgency, providing beautiful harmonies, whimsical charm and a glimpse of the sublime. It was Lane who introduced a sense of spirituality to the group. He was also the first member of the band to take LSD – unwittingly, it seems, at a Brian Epstein party during the autumn of 1966, when he took one of the specially laced orange segments from a tray. 'Blew my bloody mind!' he told Allan Vorda. 'The lyrics for "Itchycoo Park" came from that experience where I wrote, "It's all too beautiful!" I couldn't believe it! Where had I been all my life? The whole thing is all laid out there. And it is all too beautiful! I went out into the street and people were coming past me with these long faces, and I cried! I couldn't believe all these people didn't realise what a fantastic gift they had. I burst into tears. That's when Glyn Johns came to my rescue. He took me out in his E-type Jaguar and drove me around to help straighten me out. It was a bit of a long drive. I had been scarred deeply by what I had seen where all these people were ignorant of their gift.'[3] Lane offered further clues to his transformation in an interview with Keith Altham for *NME* in September 1966. 'He is at present going through a disturbing emotional period when he feels that his whole character is altering through a new outlook on life,' notes Altham euphemistically. 'In the last six months I've completely changed my attitude,' Lane announces. 'I suddenly realised that I had achieved my ambition of playing in a big group and life must hold something more. I mean, we're not just this,' he says, indicating his skin. 'There are other things

424

that I'm finding out about – they're as old as time. It's just that I'm beginning to see them more clearly.' Pretty soon the rest of the band were beginning to see them more clearly too. Lane's spiritual search would lead him, on Pete Townshend's recommendation, to Meher Baba, but whereas Townshend always seemed to carry a heavy burden, Lane wore his love like heaven. The pop songs he wrote at the time manage to be both easy-going and awestruck, switching from one to the other in the blink of a third eye.

Two months after Lane's acid initiation the Small Faces released 'My Mind's Eye'. Taking its melody from a nineteenth-century carol, 'Angels from the Realms of Glory', the song's title signposted the future, merging the cerebral and the celestial in one joyous three-word refrain. It made number four in the UK singles chart the week before Christmas, heralding a sensory blizzard that would continue throughout the early months of 1967 as 'Sunshine Superman', 'Mellow Yellow', 'I Feel Free', 'Penny Lane/Strawberry Fields Forever', 'Purple Haze' and 'Arnold Layne' all heeded the call. It's worth pointing out that at number two in that same Yuletide chart was Val Doonican's 'What Would I Be'. Marriot and Lane spoke for those who suddenly

had a whole other metaphysical take on that question.

If 'My Mind's Eye' wore its influences subtly, its follow-up, 'Here Come the Nice', was brazen and overt. The song's title was partly inspired by the group's love of Lord Buckley – a variation on 'here come the Nazz', Buckley's nom de plume for Jesus – while 'nice to be nice' was one of the group's many in-house euphemisms for getting high, but nothing else about 'Here Come the Nice' was discreet or surreptitious. If there was ever any doubt what the song was about, they come straight out with it at the end of the first verse: 'He's always there if you need some speed.' The Small Faces were barely five minutes ahead of the game but they completely got away with it. The most overt drug song the group had released so far, a veritable anthem to the charge of the purple-heart brigade, was given unrestricted airplay on BBC TV and radio.

If LSD put the Beatles in touch with their 'inner Scouser', the Small Faces' acid escapades connected them with their inner cockney. Like the Beatles, many of their best acid songs remain rooted in the provincial, even when that province was the universe and beyond. In August 1967 they released the most heavily phased pop hit of the summer. 'Itchycoo Park' was named after a lovers' rendezvous in Manor Park, east London, where couples went to canoodle in the long grass. Ronnie Lane claimed that the idea for the song's 'under dreaming spires' intro came to him when he was leafing through a tourist guide to Oxford while sitting in a hotel room. In typical Lane fashion, 'Itchycoo Park' mixes euphoria ('It's all too beautiful') and the commonplace ('feed the ducks with a bun') in equal measure. Impeccably English, from its locale to its incidentals, the song's endorsement of truancy ('Why go to learn the words of fools?') resonated strongly with a generation of disaffected school kids in the late sixties. I should know – I was one of them. The fact that 'Itchycoo Park' can skip so effortlessly between evocations of Oxford's ancient seat of learning, skipping school and amorous gropings on a piece of east London scrubland speaks volumes about the breadth and vision of Ronnie Lane's acid muse. There is none of the fractured mindscape of a John Lennon or a Syd Barrett, no edgy mod neurosis, only harmony and transcendence. 'Itchycoo Park' blends the ethereal and the earthly as well as any pop song released during that golden summer. As with many of Lane's compositions, it's essentially an inner

dialogue, an acid meditation. Like 'My Mind's Eye', it borrows its tune from the English hymnal, in this case the sixteenth-century prayer for guidance 'God Be in My Head'. The hymn is only five lines long but its effect on Lane was seismic:

> *God be in my head and in my*
> *understanding;*
> *God be in my eyes and in my*
> *looking;*
> *God be in my mouth and in my*
> *speaking;*
> *God be in my heart and in my*
> *thinking;*
> *God be at my end and at my*
> *departing.*

'God be in my eyes' translates fairly obviously into 'Itchycoo Park''s 'to rest my eyes', but the fourth line is significant too. On an alternative, slower version of 'Green Circles', Lane amends the line 'He dreamt of circles in the air and you and I and everywhere' to 'in his heart and everywhere'. Heart was very important to Lane. Assailed by acid overload, many were reduced to babble. Few chroniclers of the LSD experience thought to mention heart, and the word crops up in remarkably few psychedelic songs. Most were content to merely marvel at the colour show and then move breathlessly on to the next sensory delight. Ronnie Lane was always ready to stop and reflect on the euphoria that he felt in his heart and soul. There was nothing preachy or earnest about his acid songs; they manage to be both reverent and conversational. The ascending/descending call and response of 'Itchycoo Park''s second verse ('I'll tell you what I'll do / What will you do?') carries echoes of the Small Faces' R&B roots: Sandoz soul via Bethnal and Bow. Nonetheless, Ian McLagan always found Steve Marriott's delivery of the song a little too jaunty. 'It was all too perky for me,' he said. 'Ronnie and me had really great acid trips, and what he's singing about isn't just about getting high. He's saying it's all too beautiful, not it's-all-too-boo-tifull.'

Lane was the band's full-time dreamer, and it was he who took the Small Faces into the English mystic. As with the Who, many of their best songs were to be found among the throwaways – the flip sides and LP tracks. 'Just Passing', the B-side of 'I Can't Make It', sounds like a companion piece to Traffic's 'Berkshire Poppies' (which Steve Marriott guested on). Its two-minute woozy waltz is preceded by an exaggerated old-codger count-in ('a wunna and a two-ah') from Marriott

the music-hall MC. In her book *The Victorian Music Hall* Dagmar Kift mentions that one of the chief vocal characteristics of a chairman introducing acts in the music halls was to offer a 'satirical exaggeration of middle-class and aristocratic speech patterns':[4] that's Marriott the showman and piss-taker to a tee. He's at it again on 'All Our Yesterdays', introducing his bass player with 'And now for your delight the darling of Wapping Wharf launderette, Mr Ronald Leafy Lane'. The song's title was borrowed from a popular ITV nostalgia show which ran from 1960 to 1973. In the days of three-channel TV the programme was massively popular and combined the showing of wartime newsreel footage with other topical reminiscences of the time.

Further evidence of Ronnie Lane's questing spirit comes in the hauntingly beautiful 'Show Me the Way'. Built on Ian McLagan's electric-piano melody, a reconfiguration of 'Here Come the Nice' as if transposed by J. S. Bach, Lane in two disarming short verses embarks on an inner dialogue with a wiser self ('There's an old man in me / who I talk to, you see'). He considers the fragility of wisdom ('All the truth that I've known had been scattered and blown') and the overridding sense that life's ego games are just that, games.

'Someone else's part I am playing,' sings the mod supreme as he continues his search for the beyond within.

The title of Ian McLagan's 'Up the Wooden Hills to Bedfordshire' had first been used in 1936 to showcase the talents of another east Londoner, an up-and-coming nineteen-year-old singer called Vera Lynn. Lynn's debut recording, on which she sounds much older than her teenage years, looks back to the happier days of childhood, when parents lulled her to sleep with nursery rhymes, when the stairs were hills and 'Bedfordshire a house where I knelt to say my prayers'. The song evokes 'the village school / the winding lane / the fields of waving corn', sentiments that were about to become immeasurably more poignant with the onset of the Second World War. McLagan's song conjures a more contemporary dreamscape, 'a time beyond time' where 'all the sounds around you seem to have a new meaning', but in mood the distance between Vera Lynn's adaptation of an old nursery rhyme and the Small Faces' reverie thirty years later is not so far. Lynn's song contains the line 'My childhood days in fancy I could see': that could just as easily sum up an entire school of reflective English pop songs that surfaced in the second half of the 1960s.

In May 1968 the Small Faces unveiled their psychedelic music-hall masterpiece, *Ogdens' Nut Gone Flake*. Having moved from Decca to Andrew Loog Oldham's recently founded Immediate label the band were allowed to luxuriate in a post-*Sgt Pepper* atmosphere of indulgence. Oldham gave them unlimited pre-production and studio time for the project. Recording commenced in the summer of 1967 but 'pre-production' involved a week-long, drug-fuelled barge holiday along the Thames, travelling inland from east to west, reverse seafarers going backwards into the narrowing tributaries, as Ken Kesey might have put it had he been inclined towards a cockney knees-up. Ian McLagan recalls a disgusted tug-boatman shouting 'scourge of London' at the band as they negotiated their way unsteadily along the water, crashing into riverbanks and moorings and generally outraging the blue-blazer brigade as they ventured into the heart of the Windsor and Eton Riverside darkness. It was during the boat trip that Ronnie Lane came up with the album's central concept. In best 'Fool on the Hill' mode he decided that the LP would address the burning philosophical question of why is there only half a moon in the sky, and who pinched the other half? Showing remarkable collective foresight for a bunch of seasoned stoners, the band had the good sense not to stretch the concept over a whole LP. (God forbid that somebody would one day want to make an entire concept album about one side of the moon!) Instead the story of Happiness Stan and his hapless search was confined to side two. Side one commences with the instrumental title track, a slowed-down, phased-up orchestral revamp of the band's second single, 'I've Got Mine'. Andrew Oldham was keen on this sort of thing. Taking a leaf out of Phil Spector's book, and with a keen eye on the publishing royalties, he occasionally peppered Immediate B-sides with his own instrumentals. The B-side of the Factotums' 'In My Lonely Room', for instance – which none of the Factotums played on – was the Oldham-penned 'A Run in the Green' and 'Tangerine Flaked Forest', which was an orchestrated rewrite of 'The Last Mile', the flip side of Nico's debut single 'I'm Not Saying'. The Small Faces' instrumental revamp gives the album a sense of hazy grandeur right from the off. It sounds epic, a little George Martinesque, very much in the mould of Martin's 'Theme One'. If side two of *Ogdens'* honours Ronnie Lane's wonky loonscape, side one belongs to Marriott. 'Afterglow (of Your Love)' perfectly encapsulates the period, roughly spanning 'My Way of Giving' to 'Tin Soldier', when Marriott was writing his most inspired love songs. Subsequently released as a single after the band had split up, 'Afterglow' was a perfect fusion of acid imagery and molten sentiment. 'Song of a Baker', Lane's sole songwriting contribution to side one, weds lyrics inspired by a Sufi parable to a thunderous hard-rock riff. Very Ronnie Lane. Very Small Faces.

Also included on side one is the hit single 'Lazy Sunday'. The band regarded it as a bit of a throwaway at the time, a chance for Marriott and Lane to indulge their inner vaudevillian, but it became one of their biggest-selling records. 'Lazy Sunday' was the song that introduced drug vernacular like 'doing me crust in' and 'suss out' to the pop repertoire. It was probably the first time the word 'khazi' had been heard outside of a *Steptoe and Son* episode or a *Carry On* film, and it was indisputably the only chart hit ever to mention lumbago. Entering the Top 30 in April 1968, a month before the album was released, 'Lazy Sunday' was only prevented from reaching number one by Louis Armstrong's 'Wonderful World'. The two songs spoke ostensibly to different generations but reflected the same world view. Both possessed a sense of pathos and irony that undermined their celebratory facade. The subtext to 'Wonderful World' was racial and evoked the civil-rights struggle. Marriott's song was set in a multicultural street and his gripe was a little more short-term, although no less pressing. Both were essentially pleas for tolerance and unity in an intolerant and disunited world. And both mentioned rainbows; one of them was just a little more conspicuously dayglo than the other. For all its diddly-dee diddly-dum mannerisms 'Lazy Sunday' is an unrepentant anthem to turning on. Marriott runs the gamut of his vocal repertoire, moving effortlessly from the cockney sparra' intro to vintage 'Watcha Gonna Do About It' blues belting by the end. Each verse is interspersed with sound effects: galloping horses, seagull cries, church bells, whistling. They are unassuming little interludes and yet they are among psychedelia's finest and most affecting, and when the second montage subsides Ronnie Lane launches into his best music-hall rooty-tooty-too, as he pays playful tribute to the Who's road manager, Bob Pridden, aka Ben Pump, who was given to singing in cockney scat. Meanwhile, Marriott cheekily references the riff to the Rolling Stones' 'Satisfaction' through what sounds like a paper and comb. And later, long after the sun has set on

the rainbow street, there's Stevie, still penning his song with no words and no tune as he sits in the outside lav, sussing out the moon.

Like 'Here Come the Nice', the album's title, *Ogdens' Nut Gone Flake*, was a nod to the band's in-house humour, 'Me nut's gone' being Small Faces speak for what an arresting officer would no doubt have called 'an advanced state of intoxication'. When they were stoned the group frequently fantasised about the legalisation of marijuana, and the possibility of the Ogden's tobacco company marketing a blend called Nut Gone Flake. This was not as far-fetched as it might have seemed, and it was strongly rumoured at the time that the major tobacco companies and brewers had already patented names like Panama Red and Acapulco Gold in case decriminalisation became a reality. In their pot-headed state the group mused on how wonderful it might be to get an actual Ogden's tobacco tin design for the LP cover. Instead of the blanket refusal they were expecting Ogden's were thrilled at the prospect. Not only did their own designers get involved with the project, they made available vintage tin designs, which provided the basis for the actual cover. The distinctive circular sleeve that resulted from the collaboration is rightly revered as a design classic, one which perfectly reflected British psychedelia's love affair with Victorian and Edwardian iconography.

The real masterstroke, though, was to get renowned South African doyen of 'double-talk' Stanley Unwin to narrate the storyline on side two. The band had first asked Spike Milligan, which was an inspired choice in itself. Milligan would have brought his own unique brand of illogic and disproportion to the venture, but he declined to participate. The fifty-six-year-old Unwin proved ultimately to be just what *Ogdens'* needed, the necessary skewed link between the half-baked tale and its potential audience. Unwin was a ubiquitous presence on BBC TV and radio during the 1960s and much in demand as a voice-over for adverts. His 1961 LP *Rotatey Diskers with Unwin* was a firm favourite with the band. On side one Unwin precised folk tales such as 'The Pidey Pipeload of Hamling' and 'Goldyloppers and the Three Bearloaders'. The track 'Hi-De-Fido' begins with a brief extract from Tchaikovsky's *1812 Overture*, before the needle suddenly scrapes across the record and Unwin exclaims, 'Oh, sacrilade! For the sliding needload or sapphire through the groobers of a disky right to the middling!' Side one concludes with 'Artycraft', and contains the following apposite musings on abstract expressionism: 'Today we just get a pot of paintloagers and grurp it on the floor, riding a bicycole through it, and so the interpret for the arters of this: ooh, no, no, no, no! Far better to get a pot of paintings, severaload bottles of inkit, scrurp it huffalo-dowder the wall and stand hupside-dowdle and play a skating march. Because in this it would express the idea in the viewer.'

Side two of *Rotatey Diskers* was a tour de force, featuring live questions from a specially invited audience of press reporters, with Unwin 'answery most questions on manifold subjy'. These included such topical issues as 'The Populode of the Musicolly', skiffle, Elvis Presley and the Tottenham Hotspur football team. Most astounding of all was an improvised lecture on 'Modern Trends in Music', in which Unwin unleashed a stream of consciousness worthy of *Finnegans Wake*:

> *We are musically in a state of flux. Let's take rhythm: you have 'one, two, trittly how, grurt this fort and snuffle in the bow'. Now that is just an ordinary sequence of rhythm which indicates a rhythmic trend of heppy or a form of self-expressy. But I do think we ought to swing it about a bit. I'll give you a little*

thyrcus on this if I may, in beating.
We start off: 'one, two, trittly in
the foe, grurtsort and urt and urt
tockly fiddly and howgah. Now that
sounds a bit abstruse to you, doesn't
it? But when you get several barlide
of this, all congregale together,
the manifest as a whole is a deep
rhythmic fundamould.

When Ronnie Lane was introduced to Unwin he congratulated him on his recent Gale's honey commercial, citing the Unwinisms 'sunnyglow' and 'purimost' as his favourite words. It became clear from the start that the two parties, the East End music-hall mods and the poet laureate of linguistic illogicality, were tailor-made for each other. Unwin was duly invited to sit in on a Small Faces recording session and his deft ear immediately picked up on the group's in-jokes and lingo. Ian McLagan recalls him diligently making notes and then turning up the next day 'talking more like us than we did'. It was Unwin's interjections – 'Where at, man?' 'Oh, what a mind blast' – and double-talk narration that helped transform *Ogdens'* from what could have been just another piece of acid whimsy into one of the great English pop albums of its day.

The actual storyline doesn't take itself too seriously, which is probably just as well given that it can be summarised thus: a dim, innocent man-child called Happiness Stan who lives deep inside a rainbow in a Victorian charabanc ponders the missing half of the moon, goes off in search of it and communes with a hungry fly, who magics himself into a huge person carrier, which promptly takes Stan to meet a tramp called Mad John, who spills the not-so-complicated secret of the missing moon, before the fly steps forward to sing the finale about life being just like a bowl of All-Bran. As with so many concept albums, the Small Faces suspected in hindsight that they sacrificed their musical strengths in order to maintain narrative flow, but they needn't have worried. It's Unwin's surreal MC who gives *Ogdens'* its *ars poetica*, with the emphasis decidedly on *ars*. Or, as Unwin himself so aptly put it at the beginning of 'Happiness Stan':

So, gathering all behind in the
hintermost, he ploddy ploddy
forward into the deep fundemould
of the complicade and forry to sort
this one out, matey. Where at, man,
he thoucus, where at, man?

Sgt Pepper's Lonely Hearts Club Band famously concludes with the world-weary profundity of 'Day in the Life'. *Ogdens' Nut Gone Flake* ends with a knees-up, 'Happy Days Toy Town', or ''Appy Daze Toy Taahn' to give it the correct Bow Bells phonetics. The Beatles' magnum opus ends with a rising orchestral glissando and a long, decaying E-major chord. *Ogdens'* ends with Stanley Unwin reciting, 'I hope you'll turn out as three-quarters half as lovely, won't you? Wouldn't half enjoy it. Stay cool, won't you?'

Ogdens' Nut Gone Flake was a resounding critical and commercial success, spending six weeks at number one in the UK album charts during the damp, drizzly summer of 1968. Members of the group later expressed regret that they didn't give a little more consideration to performing *Ogdens'* as a stage show and fleshing out its theatrical possibilities. Instead, rusty through lack of live performance, they embarked upon a tour with the Who, who promptly blew them off stage every night. The nearest the audience got to an actual performance of *Ogdens'* was a 1968 BBC2 *Colour Me Pop* special, in which the band, along with Stanley Unwin, resplendent in crown and ermine cloak, sang live to a pre-recorded backing track. On the closing number, 'Happy Days Toy Town', they appear to be having a ball. There

is a cheeky exchange of 'nice' between Marriot and Lane, who spark off each other hilariously, with frequent nods and glances. In the final verse Lane changes the words from 'and if you're very true to it / you can't go wrong' to 'and if you're very shrewd with it'. Just the way he screws up his face and pronounces the word 'shrewd' provokes a huge laugh from Marriott. It's a seemingly minor detail but it encapsulates the infectious camaraderie the Small Faces possessed at their peak. Being shrewd with it was an ideal summation of Ronnie Lane's purposeful and conscientious approach to LSD.

The Small Faces were only around for four years but in that time their trajectory (both musical and pharmaceutical) perfectly encapsulated the creative evolution of the period. They shifted gear (in more ways than one) through speed and soul into the warm universal embrace of acid, and emerged out the other side still playing epic soul pop, and with their marbles still intact. Steve Ellis, lead vocalist with 1960s contemporaries the Love Affair, recalled on Radio 2's *Sounds of the Sixties* in 1987 that when the Small Faces and guest vocalist P. P. Arnold finished a blistering run-through of 'Tin Soldier' at a *Top of the Pops* rehearsal in January 1968, the notoriously blasé seen-it-all-before floor crew and technicians broke into spontaneous applause.

Discontented with the direction the group was taking, Steve Marriott, much to the rest of the band's chagrin, drafted in Herd guitarist Peter Frampton for a few sessions. Immediate then released what was pretty much a Marriott solo effort, 'The Universal', as the Small Faces' last official single. Recorded mostly in Marriott's back garden, complete with audible open-air ambience and occasional interjections from his dog, Seamus, 'The Universal' was a gloriously raggle-taggle piece of busker psych, its come-what-may philosophy best summarised in the line 'I mind my own and my own minds me,' a simple utterance worthy of the Marriott–Lane songwriting partnership at its carefree best. The B-side, 'Donkey Rides, a Penny a Glass', was the band's last 'knees up Mother Brodie' music-hall hurrah, as they continued to evoke quintessentially English experiences, in this case a day out at the seaside, to the end of their days. By the time 'The Universal' entered the UK singles chart Marriott was already in the process of forming Humble Pie with Frampton, Jerry Shirley and Greg Ridley. The Small Faces' final group release, the posthumously issued *The Autumn Stone*, gathered up a few live tracks and unfinished recordings which offered tantalising hints of new musical pastures. The achingly beautiful title track signposted the post-psychedelia direction that many English bands would follow. 'I'm looking for an open door,' sings Marriott to a simple acoustic accompaniment, before a gentle flute interlude takes flight and leaves old haunts far behind. 'Yesterday is dead / but not my memory,' he sings one last time in requiem to his band, and to his past, not realising that he would never be this good again.

Critics of the music hall point to its inherent conservatism. 'Key social institutions are always presented on an unchanging backdrop,' says cultural commentator Dave Russell. 'The existence of a huge gap between rich and poor was accepted . . . The social order was immutable . . . Accompanying this social conservatism was a deep-rooted fatalism. Life simply happened to music-hall characters: they had no control over their destiny.'[5] He could just as easily have been talking about the songs of Raymond Douglas Davies. The most accurate chronicler of fatalism in the psychedelic music hall was the least psychedelically inclined songwriter of the lot. Next to Bob Dylan, Ray Davies was arguably the highest-profile rock musician on the planet who chose to ignore psychedelia completely. Dylan was in self-imposed exile during 1967, making moonshine Americana with the Band up at Woodstock. When he did finally re-emerge as a recording artist the following year, with the folk- and country-influenced *John Wesley Harding* LP, he helped fashion the direction of post-psychedelic music in America. Unlike Dylan, Ray Davies remained an active and prolific recording artist during 1967, but he was equally noncompliant in his choice of subject matter. The Kinks' biggest hits either side of the Summer of Love, 'Waterloo Sunset' and 'Autumn Almanac', were resolutely unburdened by the stylistic trappings of the day.

Even when he was belting out big, raucous pop hits during the Kinks' first flush of fame, Ray Davies only ever seemed a warble away from a music-hall singalong. 'Where Have All the Good Times Gone', the B-side of the Kinks' 1965 hit 'Till the End of the Day', was sung from the perspective of an older generation. It spoke of, and to, honest God-fearing folk who didn't have a lot and expected even less. Like the premature eulogising of the Who's 'The Good's Gone', these were remarkable sentiments to be expressing in the middle of the never-had-it-so-good sixties. 'Where Have All the Good Times

Gone' was the product of a rare sensitivity, stoical, fatalistic, not inclined to twist and shout. Davies never bought the swinging-sixties myth and was all too aware even at the time that two separate narratives were unfolding: the media version of the decade and the one that was lived by the overwhelming majority of people. Davies wrote about that other sixties, the Eng-er-land that didn't swing, the England that lacked investment, the England where the factory windows and the steam trains hadn't been cleaned in twenty years. And while many of his contemporaries were frazzled on acid or pretending to be frazzled on acid, he wrote English character sketches that sought refuge and salvation in the simple things.

Davies liked to write what he called 'plain Jane' songs. Unlike John Lennon, who railed against Paul McCartney's tendency to write about meter maids and spinsters, Davies positively revelled in the humdrum. 'Greyness is beauty in boredom,' he told *Rolling Stone* magazine in 1969. One of the hallmarks of the music-hall song was the travails and tribulations of the little man. Davies was directly in that tradition and he elevated the form to a fine art. Possibly the greatest of these little-man songs, possibly the greatest song he ever wrote, was 'Shangri-La', from the 1969 album *Arthur*. Shangri-La is the name of Arthur's house but it's also his state of mind. Like the illusory earthly paradise presented in James Hilton's novel *Lost Horizon*, the land where no one ages unless they leave, Arthur's Shangri-La springs from a similarly delusional state of mind. The song opens where most would aspire to end ('Now that you've found your paradise') and descends into drabness from there. 'Shangri-La' is Ray Davies's version of Dante's *Inferno*. Death by dreariness. His nine circles of hell are deferred gratification, social stratification, inertia, fear, blandness, gossip, obedience, small-mindedness and insecurity. Arthur has traded in his soul for a house in suburbia that looks like all the other houses in suburbia. When he finally pays off his big debts, he celebrates by taking on smaller ones. That's the nature of his pyrrhic victory, his idea of bliss. And at the end of the day this little man sinks contendedly into the comfort of his rocking chair and slippers. Like England in the 1950s, he's knackered.

Living in reduced circumstances was a theme common to both the music hall and psychedelic pop songs. The 'prosaic aspects of everyday life',[6] Dagmar Kift called them, 'the visits to the pawnbroker and secretly moving house at night because of the failure to keep up with the rent'.[7] The pawnbroker's sign and the 'moonlight flit' were as common during the affluent swinging sixties as they had been a century earlier. For many life was still a daily drudge of avoiding the rent man, the electricity man, the bailiff and all the others who came calling for their money. For all the sociological rhetoric about embourgeoisement and the affluent society most working-class people inhabited a world where cigarette coupons and Green Shield stamps were saved and traded in for goods, the football pools were the weekly lottery and hire-purchase payment plans were colloquially known as the 'never never', because items were rarely paid for in full and would frequently be repossessed. Debt-filled drudgery was commonplace in sixties pop. In 'Shangri-La' Arthur rents his TV and radio 'for seven shillings a week'. The downtrodden little man who slaves for 'Matthew and Son' in Cat Stevens's song is in arrears with his rent. Non-preachy, non-polemical pop songs that set the music hall's immutable social order to a catchy tune were everywhere during 1967. Jeff Beck followed up his Summer of Love Top 10 hit 'Hi Ho Silver Lining' with the Graham Gouldman-penned 'Tallyman'. 'Tallyman' was an English slang term for the smooth-talking door-to-door salesman who let you purchase goods (anything from kitchenware to carpets) on a weekly payment plan, which he would 'tally up' in his book and tick off each time a repayment was made, hence the euphemism 'living on tick'. It's a term that goes back to the seventeenth century, when a ticket was issued to the indebted as a written acknowledgement of the transaction. J. C. Hotten's 1859 *Slang Dictionary* speaks of 'weak-minded women who purchase in haste and repent at leisure' in relation to the term. A satirical folk song called 'Tally-man', in print by 1905, features two lenders called Mr Cheatem and Mr Swindle and tells of women hiding in neighbours' houses or in the coal hole when the men come calling for their money. The final verse of Jeff Beck's 'Tallyman' conveys the same fatalism: 'From cradle to grave / we're expected to save,' he sings. 'Here's tick to the end / so we've made him a friend.'

In the penultimate chapter of Nell Dunn's *Up the Junction*, the author accompanies a tallyman on his rounds. With her shrewd eye for artless detail Dunn conveys the exploitative nature of his work, the contempt he has for many of his customers, particularly the black ones, and the tricks of the trade as he sells them items that they don't really need and can barely afford. At the same time Dunn manages to convey a sense that the tallyman is just on the make like everybody else, just trying to make a living in this life. 'Moneylender' by Rhubarb Rhubarb trawls similar territory. Where the tone of Jeff Beck's 'Tallyman' is resigned and benign, 'Moneylender' is closer to Nell Dunn's Battersea shyster. 'Can't you see that if you trust in him / your future light is very dim?' may not be the most thought-provoking metaphor anyone has ever written but it serves its purpose. There is even a suggestion in the song's denouement that the money-lender might just get his day of reckoning if he wanders down one too many back alleys after dark, but ultimately it's just a pipe dream, as much of a fantasy as the idea of a fully paid-for carpet or washing machine.

In more recent times the idea of street performance has come to be associated with grant-assisted artists and regulated pitches, but in the 1960s the humble busker was synonymous with the one-man band, that cartoon caricature often to be seen working the theatre queues in television comedy sketches and usually synonymous with destitution or reduced circumstances. This resourceful character, with his elaborate mobile musical kit, bass drum fastened to his back, cymbals clasped between his knees, harmonica, whistles and wind instruments hung round his neck, was personified by Don Partridge, a real-life busker who enjoyed Top 20 hits during 1968–9 with 'Rosie', 'Blue Eyes' and 'Breakfast on Pluto'. Citing Henry Mayhew's classic nineteenth-century study *London Labour and the London Poor*, Geoffrey Fletcher quoted Mayhew's definition of the street performer:

These appear to possess many of the characteristics of the lower class of actor, viz., a strong desire to excite admiration, an indisposition to pursue any settled occupation, a love of the tap room, though more for the society and display than from the drink connected with it, a great fondness for finery and predilection for the performance of dexterous and dangerous feats . . .[8]

In Mayhew's world many of these people have stepped straight out of John Lennon's old circus poster to perform fire-eating and acrobatics for the unruly Victorian throng. Fletcher points out how commonplace these street entertainers still were in the 1960s; many were blind or physically disabled and, as Fletcher indicates,

their numbers had swelled considerably in the 1930s, when cinemas switched from silent movies to the talkies.[9] Many of these by now elderly musicians were still pounding the beat in the 1960s, and songs about them were plentiful.

'Gypsy Fred' by the Koobas casts the busker as a Romany seer/savant who flees the countryside due to the hostility of the locals. When he arrives in the city he finds that his simple homilies about the meaning of life are greeted as pearls of wisdom. Feeling uncomfortable with his new-found fame, he returns to the security of the hedgerows and his simple rustic ways. 'Spare a Shilling' by the Bunch was another fallen-on-hard-times tale about a young beggar who pleads that he would still be on the straight and narrow if only his girl hadn't left him. The song has a pop-soul sound typical of the period, pitching itself somewhere between the Alan Bown! and the Herd. It's only the unorthodox twist in the boy-loses-girl lyric – his descent into vagrancy – that reveals this is 1967, not 1966. No discerning mod would have been singing about being a down-and-out in 1966. Begging for love or forgiveness maybe, but not food. Such were the nuances that separated a year in British pop life.

'Chocolate Buster Dan' by Pandamonium cribs its title from an 1884 music-hall song called 'Railway Porter Dan', and offers another variant on the busker who has seen better days. Musically it has all the requisite vaudevillian touches: a barrel piano, 'Penny Lane' piccolo fanfares and a 'roll up, roll up' quick-time interlude straight out of the 'Magical Mystery Tour'. There's an additional nod to Ray Davies in the delivery, and the song tugs unashamedly on the audience's heartstrings as it solicits sympathy and respect for Dan's long-gone days of glory. 'Sycamore Sid' by Focal Point was about a different kind of outcast and was probably the first psychedelic record to eulogise one of its own. Although it wasn't written about Syd Barrett, who, as far as can be ascertained, didn't have grey hair and wasn't living in a tree in 1968, it uncannily presages the hermit-like existence that Barrett would eventually settle for and is full of suitably eccentric imagery ('in his tortoiseshell room / eating words with a spoon / writing songs with no tunes').

With a band name lifted from Dickens and subject matter rooted in the nineteenth-century travelling show, 'Joe, Organ & Co.' by Barnaby Rudge is delivered in baritone cockney by a Joe Brown soundalike. Produced by Monty Babson, it fades in on a dreamlike waltz-time barrel organ and owes its trippy, swirling dynamics to 'Being for the Benefit of Mr Kite'. Barrel organs were a common sight on the streets of Britain's cities up until the Great War but were in decline by the 1960s. They hadn't died out altogether, though, and, as Geoffrey Fletcher points out, as late as 1963 musical scores for theatre productions like *Half a Sixpence* were still being transposed into sheets of dots for use on these hand-turned instruments.[10] The barrel organ didn't require any musical skill; all the player had to do was turn the handle steadily in order to keep the pitch of the music constant. The instrument retained its popularity among the East End poor long after it had disappeared elsewhere and its arrival would be greeted with enthusiastic crowds and impromptu dancing. Fletcher cites Axel Munthe's *Memories and Vagaries* as 'the most finished expression of the melancholy character of the street organist's life'. In it Munthe observes: 'It is well known that the barrel-organ, like the violin, gets a fuller and more sympathetic tone the older it is.' He describes the organ at the centre of his story as being 'not of the modern noisy type which imitates a whole orchestra with flutes and bells and beats of drums, but a melancholy old-fashioned barrel-organ which knew how to lend a dreamy mystery to the gayest allegretto and in whose proudest tempo di Marcia [marching time] there sounded an unmistakable undertone of resignation. And in the tenderer pieces of the repertoire, where the melody, muffled and staggering like a cracked old human voice, groped its way among the rusty pipes of the treble, then there was a trembling in the bass like suppressed sobs.'[11] He could have been talking about the mellotron on 'Strawberry Fields Forever'. Something of Munthe's descriptive pathos is captured in 'Joe, Organ & Co.' too. There's lots of oompah brass, hallucinatory bursts of audience applause and plenty of psychedelic subtext in the lyrics. 'There they go on a cloud of magical notes' is a bit of a giveaway. It takes a couple of listens before the magnitude of lines like 'winding his wheel as the minutes pass' and 'Don't they know that you soon to have to go on your way where the sun doesn't shine?' fully sinks in and you realise that Joe is dying. The song fades out with the same barrel-organ swirl that introduced it; the notes carry the substance of Joe's life in their echo. For those living and dying on the dead-end streets of the East End the sound will have choreographed their lives from entrance to exit.

Love, in music-hall songs, was, as Dagmar Kift put it, 'either portrayed as a rose-tinted dream of bliss or a comic disaster'.[12] While comic disaster gently mutated into pathos over the course of a century, rose-tinted dreams of bliss adapted pretty well to the new psychedelic circumstances. Despite the media's portrayal of the 1960s' rampant permissiveness, the majority of the Tin Pan Alley pop songs kept faith with a world where earnest young men with good intentions asked a father for a daughter's hand in marriage, pledged their troth, vowed to be true and assumed that the object of their affections would do likewise. Beneath the stylistic trappings of fuzz guitars and phasing the traditional travails of the lovestruck endured, and many a chaste and old-fashioned courtship sentiment continued to be expressed. In the psychedelic music hall these traditional scenarios grew more dreamlike and detached. Boy meets girl was frequently counteracted by boy doesn't meet girl, boy imagines dream girl, boy falls in love with poster girl, boy falls in love with girl who doesn't exist. Desire evaporates into mirage evocations. Anomie replaces empathy.

'Office Girl' by Mike Leslie was released in 1966 but it anticipates the coming climate of distanced amour. It's a cool and curiously disengaging tale of crowded rush-hour streets, subway trains and unfulfilled yearning. The girl of the title is only briefly glimpsed before she disappears into the morning crowd. The song's anonymous narrator, who merely refers to himself as 'someone', imagines her glancing out of the window of her 'building of steel and stone', oblivious to the fact that 'someone' is out there among the anonymous throng, unrequited and equally alone. An air of melancholy hangs over the whole still-born affair. Every morning the same unresolved scenario is acted out. They seem as if they are in a play, and they are anyway. He sees her. She disappears into her concrete tower, swallowed up by the brutalist architecture of the city. In the fast-paced, unreciprocating sixties the narrator, brooding, silent and existential, can only stand and watch, like a character in a Truffaut movie.

A wittier pop-art take on the unobtainable is 'Advertising Girl' by Davey Sands and the Essex. The object of affection here is an inanimate poster girl, variously promoting soup, soap and cars, resplendent in purple miniskirt and manageable hair. She's the manufactured ideal, staring down from billboards and forever out of reach. 'She looks so real,' chants the singer over a 'She's About a Mover' organ riff. 'Where do I find a girl like that?' The

Attack's 'Created by Clive' is a more disparaging take on the It-girl song. The narrator agonises over the skinny pilled-up model who has traded in her past for deportment and elocution lessons, and swapped her personality for 'a plastic heart'. 'I've got feelings and I need love / like you need a mirror and a powder puff,' he denounces in petulant and preening tones over a pounding mod beat. His resentful disapprovals can't quite disguise the fact that she sounds like she's having the time of her life. 'Girl in a Bus Queue' by the Unauthorised Version is a curio even by psychedelic-pop standards. It was the B-side of the group's version of 'Hey Jude' (oh to have been a fly on the record-company wall when that was suggested as a money-making venture) and sounds like the kind of thing Dudley Moore might have attempted as a psychedelic pastiche, or written if he'd joined Caravan in 1969, or been fourth on the bill in an unknown varsity band at a Cambridge rag ball. Over a frantic 5/4 arrangement, replete with insistent 'doo-wah' backing vocals, complex three-part counter-melodies and echoey washes of trebly guitar played by ex-Tornado Alan Caddy, a well-bred young blade muses on the girl he spies 'all alone / not a love in her heart' at the bus stop. He makes repeated references to his 'incomprehensible dichotomy / what I dream and what I see', which confirms that this is not your average bunch of beat-music oiks talking. And so it proved. 'Girl in a Bus Queue' was actually the work of a group of choral singers from Magdalene College, Cambridge, which if nothing else reveals the sheer diversity of talent that was briefly whirlpooled into the psychedelic vortex and illustrates what could be achieved with a few well-placed Swingle Singers harmonies and the production values of a Joe Meek protégé.

Another common component of the original music-hall love song was the shy maiden and her counterpart, the naughty girl.[13] The psychedelic music hall added a fresh demasculinised variant: the coy boy. Written by Keith West and produced by Mark Wirtz, 'Shy Boy' by Kippington Lodge was about an acne-ridden misfit in ill-fitting clothes who is oblivious to the adoration of the mousy-haired, freckle-skinned girl who lives across the road. Instead, 'at the firm he works / among the small-time clerks', he coyly sneaks glances at the legs of the new typist. Full of snappy, tight rhymes that would have done Syd Barrett proud ('wears glasses / takes evening classes / never dances'), this cameo of inadequacy and imperfection ends with the gauche young office boy finally plucking up the courage to buy the new girl a ring, having not noticed that she is already wearing one. This was unrequited passion on a par with Dudley Moore's Stanley Moon in the 1967 movie *Bedazzled*, as he glances dolefully at Eleanor Bron's Margaret Spencer across the sizzling onions and ketchup bottles in the Wimpy Bar where they both work.

'Phoebe's Flower Shop' by the Cortinas evokes the Victorian street-corner flower-seller and relates the bittersweet tale of the boy who becomes smitten and buys roses from her every day. Inevitably, he discovers in the final verse that she has a husband and four kids at home. The fact that the chorus remains unchanged despite this bad news ('Phoebe, let your hair down / let it down for me') suggests that he's not going to be put off by the minor inconvenience of her marital status and is going to ask her out anyway. Misplaced lust of the 'Pictures of Lily' variety occurs in 'Shirley' by Cliff Wade, the tale of a young boy who falls in love with the glamour girl he spots on page sixteen of a magazine. He finds her name ('just a name', he acknowledges, knowing full well that Shirley is the pin-up's nom de plume) and decides to seek out more images of her. He peruses mucky magazines in the corner shop, which he can't afford to buy, and remains resigned to meeting her only in his dreams. There's no resolution and none of the hormonal frustration that drives 'Pictures of Lily', there's no understanding dad with a garden shed full of porn either, just unreachable 'Shirley' with her curly hair and girlish stare. It's the stare that's all important here. Like Davey Sands's 'Advertising Girl', the singer fleshes out a myth by locking eyes with a photo-shot gaze. A more comic variation on all this was 'Miss Pinkerton' by Cuppa T. Sung in stage-school cockney, complete with music-hall nudges and suggestive asides, it's a Bonzo-esque melange of trilling piccolos and rasping brass. Only the lilting Eastern intro and exotic bridge remind you that this is 1967, not 1867. Miss Pinkerton is the archetypal office spinster who, after constant rejection from her boss, decides to take her own life. Standing on a window ledge she is rescued by a hunky fireman ('who sets her heart on fire') and lives happily ever after. It's a song that, fire brigade, uncaring colleagues and all, could have been performed in the halls a hundred years earlier.

Jilted-at-the-altar songs were common in the nineteenth century, as were tales of sorry spinsters and old maids, and these stories of unrequited love underwent a sudden and unexpected revival in the psychedelic music hall. 'The Wedding of Ramona Blair' by Mirage, told in three short verses and clocking in at a little over two minutes, is an 'Eleanor Rigby'-inspired story of a young girl left at the altar on her wedding day. It could easily be a prequel to the McCartney song, offering an explanation as to what might have happened to Rigby earlier in her life. In the first verse Ramona 'dreams of the very next day'. On the morning of her wedding, with a nod to Eleanor Rigby's face in a jar by the door, she 'tried on her very best face', but disappointed that she doesn't look any different, she 'sighed / and carried on sewing her lace'. In the last verse she cries in her bridal gown 'on her very new bed'. The sorry tale is told from the viewpoint of the pitying congregation, who all agree it was nice to see Ramona in prayer as they 'give an occasional stare at the door' for the groom who never comes. A pretty accordion melody and ecclesiastical harmonies fail to offset the emptiness that lies at the heart of the song.

'Neville Thumbcatch' by the Attack is the story of an eccentric who happily grows vegetables and flowers on his allotment, while lonely Mrs Thumbcatch waits at home, alone and unfulfilled, with only her alabaster gnomes and a budgie called Mabel for company.

Eventually she runs off with that comic staple, the randy milkman, leaving Neville to cook, clean and sew for himself. The comic twist is that Neville hardly notices and remains resiliently happy. He has to give up his allotment, but he still has a window box.

The comic disaster element in the old music-hall love songs mutates into something altogether stranger during the psychedelic era. These songs don't exactly revel in the misfortune of others but neither do they elicit much sympathy; they just seem to stand aside and coldly observe, offering the same dispassionate gaze that John Steed and Emma Peel displayed in *The Avengers* whenever they arrived just a little too late at the scene of yet another unlikely and bizarre murder. It's rarely remarked upon, this emotional removal, this glazed and inanimate quality, but it's one of the most distinctive features of late-1960s English psychedelic pop song.

Perhaps the most under-acknowledged music-hall influence on psychedelia was the 'lion comique'. This nineteenth-century stage persona descended from the Regency dandy and the swaggering pastiche known as the 'swell'. It finds literary form in Dickens's haberdasher's apprentice Trabb's boy, who pricks Pip's social pretensions in *Great Expectations* with parodies of the aspiring Pip's posh posturing and affectation. Trabb's boy is a taunting, mocking grotesque, mirroring and mimicking a character who he in turn considers to be a grotesque. In music-hall song the *lion comique* was immortalised by George Leybourne's Champagne Charlie, and subsequently Americanised by Irving Berlin's 'A Couple of Swells'. Dagmar Kift defined the *lion comique* as 'lazy and hedonistic' and his songs as 'hymns of praise to the virtues of idleness, womanising and drinking'.[14] Cheap tailoring made much of this possible in the nineteenth century, says Kift, as it did a century later, when Italian and French fashions crossed the English Channel and young men began to don apparel that would have had the wearer identified, and more than likely beaten up, as a homosexual five or six years earlier. 'The counterfeit swell was especially attractive to upstart clerks and apprentices who were able to make use of cheaper mass-produced clothing to dress up in style if not in substance,' says Kift.[15] Once again, she was talking about the nineteenth century, but she could just as easily have been describing the legions of upstart clerks and apprentices who put style before substance (or rather put on style and took substances) in the 1960s.

The legacy of the *lion comique* survives in mod folklore with the legendary tale of the young offender who offered to pay his court fine by cheque after the Margate beach confrontations of 1964. This defiant act made the national newspapers at the time and the culprit in question was depicted as a symbol of all that was wrong with modern society. Less frequently reported was the fact that the young mod didn't even have a bank account, let alone a chequebook. Despite being comprehensively demythologised in Stanley Cohen's seminal study *Folk Devils and Moral Panics*, this empty gesture of bravado has trickled unchecked into numerous accounts of the mod era since, including Franc Roddam's 1979 film version of *Quadrophenia*.

In psychedelic pop these tendencies manifest themselves in a variety of postures. They have a certain cartoon mod insouciance about them that's simultaneously thrilling, incorrigible and tongue-in-cheek. 'It's Shocking What They Call Me' by the Game was discordant Who-influenced pop, full of 'who me?' audacity and barefaced lies. The protagonist puts on the charm and feigns outrage when his girl complains that he leads a life of degeneracy and comes home at all hours. In response he promises that he doesn't lie that often, never uses strong language and underneath it all is just deeply misunderstood. He sounds like he's rehearsed his excuses on his way home after another night of pilled-up excess. Equally barefaced was 'Father's Name Is Dad' by Fire. The song boasts a killer riff and a soaring chorus of 'My father's name was Dad / my mother's name was Mum.' It's the ultimate 'What are you rebelling against? What have you got?' anthem and depicts in perfect teenage semaphore a world of purposeful irresponsibility, where failure and lack of opportunity are working-class birthrights, and where adolescence, 'the awkward stage', is one long series of 'insane escapades'. The disenchanted world view is perfectly summarised in a derisory 'I laugh at it all', the only life strategy a boy in his mid- to late teens really needs.

Baudelaire called dandyism 'heroism in decay', vainglorious and misanthropic in its heyday but doomed to melancholy as youth fades. Obsessed with the external but 'spiritually opaque', as Cyril Connolly puts it, 'trifles are taken seriously and serious things made light of'.[16] Such inversions take on a particularly distinctive form in the pop music of the 1960s. They don't just signify themselves in teenage rebellion; they articulate their heroism in decay in idle boasts and empty threats, impulsive pledges and broken promises, nights on the town followed by dawn in the gutter. All manner of duplicitous double-crossing, deceitful showmanship and bad-boy behaviour get an airing, but underneath it all can be detected that same prevailing sense of threatened machismo, the faintest whiff of fear, recalcitrance and insecurity as tried and tested strategies no longer seem quite so fail-safe when defiant Jack the Lads fail to adapt to changing times. These are the men the girl groups warned you of.

'Matrimonial Fears' by Cymbaline could easily serve as an answer song to 'The Wedding of Ramona Blair', as sung by the heartless groom who jilted her. It commences with twenty-five seconds of swirling sound effects and a taunting nightmare voice-over reading the wedding vows ('Do you take this woman to be your lawful wedded wife? Do you? Do You? Do You?'). The narrator is jolted out of his bad dream by the sound of a telephone ringing and the reassurance of a soothing female voice giving him his early-morning alarm call. Set to a delicate piano melody we hear the story of the youthful lothario who has been enjoying the single life for several years and isn't ready to settle down. Except he doesn't sound

that youthful any more, just weary. And that early-morning call suggests he's no longer some young mod playing the field but a commercial traveller all alone in a hotel room. 'I'm just going to carry on carrying on,' he sings unconvincingly. This is prime 'What's it all about, Alfie?' territory, the character who hasn't yet realised that events have overtaken him and time has called his bluff. You wait in vain for the comeuppance that never comes, but there's only more bluster and bullshit. 'I'll leave you in the lurch,' he taunts. 'I'm using you, using you,' he repeats over the outro, seemingly unaware (or perhaps only too painfully aware) of the fate that awaits every unattached mod who, one day, is going to wake up aged thirty without a single clean pressed and ironed shirt in his wardrobe.

An altogether more charming counterpoint is depicted in 'You've Gotta Be with Me' by Onyx, a brisk and breezy slice of late-sixties psych pop boasting Beach Boys harmonies and sophisticated chord changes. Its middle eight hints at the synaesthesia of the drug trip – 'Your mind starts to reel / and you feel what you see / and you touch what you hear' – but it might just as easily be the heady rush of one too many complimentary Babychams in the VIP bar. 'I can get you into places / show you all the faces,' boasts the singer, with all the allure that a provincial town's night life can offer. It's a cheeky wink of a song; had they made a promo film to go with it it would have featured Barry Evans, the gauche, grinning star of *Here We Go Round the Mulberry Bush*. It's inclusive, smart but casual, and utterly typical of its time: daytime radio-friendly pop performed by a band who were themselves daytime-session regulars on Radio 1 in the late 1960s.

The great unsung hero of the psychedelic music hall was David Bowie. Although he has largely airbrushed this period out of his musical history, his debut LP, recorded for Decca in 1967, is a fascinating curio. The fourteen cuts on the album are completely out of synch with everything else that was going on around him. In the year of *Sgt Pepper*, *Disraeli Gears* and *The Piper at the Gates of Dawn* Bowie was channelling the spirit of Anthony Newley, specifically the Anthony Newley who in 1960 made the bizarre ITV sitcom *The Strange World of Gurney Slade*. *Gurney Slade* was to situation comedy what *The Prisoner* was to espionage, i.e. only tangentially related to its genre and guaranteed to frighten off sponsors and bemuse the majority of its viewing audience. In *Gurney Slade* Newley played the part of a perennial daydreamer and

fantasist. Back in suburban Bromley the teenage Bowie loved it. He was also hugely influenced by a 1962 single of Newley's called 'That Noise', which featured a rhythm section constructed out of sound effects. The scripted ad-libs and asides that Bowie dropped into his material at the height of his Newley fixation – on his self-inflicted bête noire 'The Laughing Gnome', for instance – were cribbed entirely from 'That Noise'.

Bowie's 1967 recordings sound like dress rehearsals and try-outs for the alter egos he would develop with such conceptual panache in the following decade. The settings are self-consciously stagey, the presentation theatrical. Indeed, Bowie made short promotional films for several of the songs and clearly envisaged them being presented in a wider theatrical context at some point. What he hadn't found yet was a consistent voice, so for a short time at least he adopted Anthony Newley's, while inhabiting *Gurney Slade's* off-kilter universe. By his own admission Bowie spent the 1960s trying to work out what it was that he wanted to do, and more importantly, what (and who) he wanted to present. He tried being a mod, he tried mime, he tried miming being a mod. He had a go at being a Buddhist, a man in a dress, a family man and a stranded astronaut who misses his family. These mannequins and masques would reach fruition with Ziggy Stardust, Aladdin Sane, the plastic soul boy and the Thin White Duke. But long before he was the cracked actor and the moon-age daydreamer he sang of mummy's boys, love-struck wimps, laughing gnomes, gender-bending soldiers, lonely war veterans, shopkeepers, gravediggers and psychopaths. And he sang of what it was like to be five, not from the perspective of prelapsarian lost innocence but from the viewpoint of a four-year-old. Had he never made another record his eponymous debut album would still merit a place in the psychedelic music hall of fame.

'Uncle Arthur' concerns a young man who works in the family shop, until at thirty-two he defiantly unties the apron strings and finds himself a girl. Alas, Sally can't cook, so Arthur flees back home to the family nest and mother's home cooking. For all the song's quirky charm, Arthur was in fact archetypal. There is an Arthur, or there certainly used to be, in every town. He could often be found working in the family baker's or butcher's or grocer's. The gossip about him would be handed down from generation to generation in conspiratorial nods and knowing whispers. 'He never married,' was always a favourite. Or, in Arthur's case, 'marriage didn't suit him'.

'Please Mr Gravedigger', the closing track on Bowie's debut album, is also its most macabre. The chirpy arrangements that characterise his other songs from this period are replaced with ominous tolling bells, thunderclaps and dripping rain. Hamming it up something rotten, Bowie affects a heavy cold and sneezes theatrically as he recites the story of a gravedigger who works in a bombed-out Lambeth churchyard, where he passes his time casually pocketing graveside mementos left by grieving mourners. The narrator, we eventually learn, is not the actual gravedigger but a psychopathic child murderer watching him at work. Each day he visits the graveside of Mary Ann, a girl he murdered when she was just ten. In the final verse he reveals that he is digging a grave himself – for the gravedigger. The song ends with the psychopathic narrator shovelling away in the relentless rain. It's *Gurney Slade* gone gothic.

Perhaps the most unlikely, certainly the least documented, link between the music hall and British pop music in the second half of the 1960s was the dramatised war tableau. Theatrical songs about war were regularly performed in the music halls during the second half of the nineteenth century. The Crimean and Boer conflicts were both given topical coverage, as was the broader theme of colonial expansion. The tone of these songs was, as Dagmar Kift points out, 'at the same time unequivocally patriotic and contradictory'.[17] Soldiers were portrayed both as cannon fodder and stoical good-hearted volunteers. Overtly jingoistic songs were often answered in kind by sardonic parodies. Indeed the word 'jingoism' owes its life to a music-hall song: G. W. Hunt's 1877 composition 'We Don't Want to Fight' (aka 'The Jingo Song'), which contained the rousing chorus:

> *We don't want to fight but by*
> *jingo if we do*
> *We've got the ships. We've got the*
> *men, and got the money too.*

These songs, says Kift, were simultaneously 'anti-heroic because they refused to glorify war, and heroic because they sang of the heroic deeds not of the generals, but of the little man'.[18] The music-hall audience, for whom the Crimean War was still fresh in the memory, empathised strongly with the plight of the common soldier, who, as Kift says, had been 'badly fed and quartered, suffered from the appalling tactical errors of their commanders and been miserably treated on their return home'.[19] The most effective way to get this message across was not by being overtly preachy but by adopting the form of the short dramatic tableau. Kift gives one example in which a lone soldier at Sebastopol is first shown on guard and then being wounded by an enemy bullet. The scene shifts to the exterior of an English village churchyard, where the same invalided ex-soldier, enfeebled by work and old age, makes a short, impassioned speech about the way he has been neglected by his country before collapsing onto the nearest gravestone. He dies to the accompaniment of softly falling snow and the sound of the church organ. Inside the church the congregation and choir can be heard observing God's word while ignoring the ex-soldier's plight.

These powerful tableau presentations were an art form in themselves and they were commonplace in the halls right up until the first decade of the twentieth century, but were eventually killed off by increased pressure from conservative political forces and, in London at least, the rise in respectable middle-class audiences. This led to self-censorship among the proprietors and a corresponding increase in overtly patriotic sentiments in the songs that were performed. By the time the halls began actively recruiting volunteers to fight in the 1914–18 war the tableau presentations had all but died out. However, they find their modern-day counterpart in the unlikely setting of psychedelia. Three of the major concept albums of the period – the Who's *Tommy*, the Kinks' *Arthur* and the Pretty Things' *S. F. Sorrow* – all feature the First World War in some capacity. On *Tommy*, an album that, as Pete Townshend acknowledged in his autobiography, was directly influenced by the music hall, the 1914–18 conflict features only in a brief introductory scenario, albeit the one that actually traumatises Tommy into becoming deaf, dumb and blind. On the Kinks' *Arthur* two songs specifically about the Great War are included: 'Yes Sir, No Sir' and 'Some Mother's Son'. The Pretty Things' album *S. F. Sorrow*, which preceded both *Tommy* and *Arthur*, was built around a short story singer Phil May had written about the life of a First World War conscript called Sebastian F. Sorrow. In addition to these the Zombies' *Odessey and Oracle* features bass player Alan White's 'Butcher's Tale Somme 1916' (erroneously printed on the LP's sleeve as 'Butcher's Tale (Western Front 1914)'), which was based in part on the experiences of his uncle, who died at Passchendaele, and his reading about the 60,000 who died on the first morning of the the Battle of the Somme. 'Butcher's Tale' also references the battles at Gommecourt, Thiepval, Mametz Wood and Verdun. Like a music-hall tableau it depicts the preacher in his pulpit urging soldiers to do God's work but turning his back on the consequences. Its simple and plaintive chorus says, 'I want to go home / please let me go home.' It's a refrain that echoes down through the twentieth century.

The Kinks' 'Yes Sir, No Sir' commences with a drum roll and tells of how the youthful Arthur, worker turned soldier, trades in one form of subservience, his labour, for another in the trenches of World War I. Life is a perpetual cycle of orders from above. Permission to breathe. Permission to think, eat and sleep. As the generals play war games with real lives, Ray Davies unleashes the most contemptuous polemical outburst he had written up to that point. 'Doesn't matter who you are / you're there and there you are,' he jaw-jaws in a mocking upper-class accent. 'Give the scum a gun and make the bugger fight / And be sure to have deserters shot on sight / If he dies, we'll send a medal to his wife.' The diatribe ends with a cackle of derisive upper-class laughter. If 'Yes Sir, No Sir' is driven by rage, 'Some Mother's Son' is a moving account of a parent's bereavement. The song was based in part on the brother of Davies's own brother-in-law Stuart, a fighter pilot killed in action during the Second World War, but the brother commemorated here is the universal soldier, buried in a foreign field, mourned in every town, every village, every household. There is one line in 'Some Mother's Son', so devastatingly simple, and at first glance mildly insensitive, that it may be one of the best that Ray Davies ever penned. 'Back home they put his picture in a frame,' he sings. 'But all dead soldiers look the same.' And he's right, they do. The same faded and sepia-tinted photos that sat on the mantelpiece of a million parlours, they did all look the same. Like the thousands of white crosses that dot the burial fields of Belgium and northern France, or the names on the Menin Gate, they blur into one universal Sanskrit of senseless slaughter and sacrifice. In another lyrical masterstroke Davies quietly juxtaposes grieving and loss with the dependable routines of normal life – children coming home from school, the world still turning on its axis.

Memory and loss are conjoined throughout the song. The soldier in the trench who 'dreams of games he played when he was young' just seconds before he is shot dead is a cinematic image straight out of *All Quiet on the Western Front*. It also recalls Siegfried Sassoon's own trench-bound Dreamers 'Dreaming of things they did with balls and bats' (dreaming also, incidentally, of some distinctly Ray Davies themes – 'firelit homes, clean beds and wives', 'Bank-holidays, and picture shows', 'going to the office in the train').

The tragic element of 'Some Mother's Son' is that each fallen young soldier is freeze-framed identically in his mother's eyes, never to grow old, forever looking the same as the day he went away. The loss is irretrievable. There is no body to commemorate. Memory is the only keepsake. The last line of the song is 'Some mother's memory remains': the mind lingers on the ambiguity of the word 'remains' long after the song has faded.

Had they never recorded again, the two singles the Pretty Things released either side of Christmas 1967, 'Defecting Grey' and 'Talkin' About the Good Times', would still have guaranteed the group a place among the pantheon of psychedelic pop. Like 'Penny Lane' and 'Strawberry Fields Forever', 'Talkin' About the Good Times' and its

B-side, 'Walking Through My Dreams', were originally conceived with a bigger project in mind, and as with the Beatles' songs, the album they were intended for is poorer for their absence. *S. F. Sorrow* has often been mooted as the first rock concept work, predating *Tommy* and *Arthur* by 18 months. Of the three the Pretty Things' album is lyrically the weakest, musically the most adventurous and sonically by far the most expansive. Producer Norman Smith endured a fractious time in the studio with Syd Barrett while making Pink Floyd's debut LP, but by the time he came to work on *S. F. Sorrow* six months later he had either learned to let go a little or had given up trying to curtail and contain. The album is a masterful engineering accomplishment, awash with echo-drenched high-register harmonies, clanging rhythm guitars, droning sitars and drowsy mellotrons. In terms of texture and timbre *S. F. Sorrow* is one of the finest ensemble works to come out of Abbey Road. Lyrically it only really makes sense when presented as a hallucinatory tableau. *S. F. Sorrow*'s main weakness, as with most concept albums, doesn't lie so much with the story as its execution. Narrative continuity is provided by the explanatory linking passages that Phil May adapted from

his original short story, and which are contained in an accompanying booklet along with the song lyrics. At certain points the explanations are longer than the lyrics. One of the golden rules of screenwriting is to convey plot development in the action, not in pointless extemporisation. Show, don't tell, as the adage goes. In cinematic terms *S. F. Sorrow* not only has too little show and too much tell, it spends too much time telling the listener what it is going to tell. The subject matter should always be at the service of the songs and not the other way around, but all too often on *S. F. Sorrow* the storyline becomes secondary, an adjunct to the explanations. This is why ultimately the album works best as a montage of blissed-out mood pieces, an inner tripscape. Had a few more rock concept works adopted the format of the music-hall tableau we might have been spared hours of creaky linkage, narrative contrivance and plot longueurs.

By the 1960s there had been a fundamental shift in British youth's perception of the military. Unencumbered by national service, bolstered by previously unimaginable spending power and, unlike their American counterparts, not unduly concerned by the prospect of fighting a war in far-off lands, young people developed a more flippant attitude towards the armed forces. Oxbridge satirists portrayed the military as bumbling figures of fun, whereas their 1920s predecessors had offered to drive the buses during the General Strike. By the mid-sixties military insignia were pop-art decoration. One of the leading London boutiques was called I Was Lord Kitchener's Valet and it co-opted Kitchener's original recruitment poster as an advertising slogan. From senseless slaughter and loss to commerce and logos in less than half a century. If a generation gap could be detected anywhere, it was here: not in the perceived slackening of morals and the unruly mods and rockers who rampaged across the bank holiday beaches, but in post-conscription attitudes towards the armed forces. When the Beatles were awarded their MBEs, not for their music but for services to the export trade, many who had fought in two world wars were outraged that bolstering the economy with the sale of pop records could be regarded in the same light as someone who had stormed an enemy sentry post at El Alamein or nursed a wounded colleague under gunfire until reinforcements arrived. In an age when gongs are routinely handed out to entertainers and sports personalities it might seem odd that the awarding of the Beatles' MBEs in 1965

caused so much fuss. But these were different times and there was a feeling that sacrosanct sensibilities were being trampled upon. This was the real source of the generational divide: not music, miniskirts and accusations that the kids of today had more money than sense, but in their perceived insensitivity towards the sacrifices that had made these privileges possible. The ironic wearing of medals and service stripes on a military tunic embellished with a velvet collar and gilt buttons did not always go down well with those who had forfeited so much, including their own carefree youth, so that Britain might be free from tyranny.

'What you won't find me doing, I promise you, is getting red in the face and furious because some of the boys enjoy dressing up,' said J. B. Priestley, an unlikely champion of the mods in 1966, as he reflected on his own dandy days. 'Who are we, far more responsible than they are for the idiotic world they are living in, to sneer and jeer because they want to be dandies for a few years? A lad who lives in a dingy back street and does a boring stupid job all day is surely entitled to change into some colour and do a little swaggering.'[20] But not everyone of Priestley's generation agreed with that assessment, particularly when it came to putting on a second-hand

RAF flying jacket or a row of antique-shop medals, and even though tinpot dictators the world over and members of the royal family who had never seen active combat were free to pin on ceremonial ribbons on formal occasions, it actually remained a criminal offence, punishable under the Uniforms Act of 1894, for any person not serving in the military forces to wear, 'without Her Majesty's permission', the uniform of any of those forces. A few unlucky customers of I Was Lord Kitchener's Valet were fined the princely sum of £1 for such sartorial transgressions, a sum which the shop's owners happily agreed to pay on their behalf.

There was a certain I Was Lord Kitchener's Valet levity to some of the late-sixties pop songs that dwelt on the theme of war. If they were the remnants of the music-hall tableau, they were mildly mocking ones, darkly comedic in a way that would have been unthinkable at the height of the music hall. Three of them appear on David Bowie's debut album. 'She's Got Medals' is the tale of a girl, Mary, who disguises herself as a boy called Tommy and joins the army, but just before the bomb drops she deserts and becomes a woman again, changes her name to Eileen and moves to London. It's tempting to view the song as a dress rehearsal (literally) for what was to come, but in his androgynous prime it's doubtful that Bowie would have explained the name change from Mary to Tommy with a Newleyesque aside like 'she's a one'. 'Little Bombardier' featured an inadequate, unskilled and psychologically damaged war veteran called Frankie Mear, who spends his lonely days in the local cinema until his good-hearted intentions towards the children who befriend him are mistaken for those of a pederast. He is threatened with imprisonment ('We've had blokes like you in the station before') and forced to leave town. 'Little Bombardier' is set to a charming waltz arrangement but the milieu it depicts is cruel and threatening, a world that has no place and little sympathy for outsiders or outcasts. 'Rubber Band' was also about a soldier who fought in the 1914–18 war. This one passes his time watching the brass band that plays 'in the library garden / Sunday afternoon'. As he watches he reminisces about when he used to listen to them in 1910 with the girl he was courting. In the final verse it's revealed that the girl he left behind is now married to the band leader. Five years before Bowie apocalyptically pronounced that we had five years left he ends 'Rubber Band' with a flouncing 'I hope you break your baton'.

'Colonel Brown' by Tomorrow tells of a retired soldier with an insufficient pension and no security of tenure. We learn that his wife departed last year, although whether she's deceased or just run off with a man from the motor trade we aren't told. He sits alone looking at photos of his army wedding: 'On his moustache hangs a tear / now all his life is souvenir.' The phrasing is cruelly apposite, an acknowledgement that all he fought for can now be purchased in a junk shop and worn as decorative insignia by foppish trendsetters. Only in the final verse do we learn that Colonel Brown is in a wheelchair. Like many a music-hall tableau the song ends with him praying in church, his faith undiminished to the end.

'Colour Sgt Lillywhite' by West Coast Consortium concerns a soldier home on leave. He has six daughters and has never lived anywhere but in married quarters. Meanwhile, his breaks between active service get ever shorter and he rarely sees his family. 'Gets his board and lodgings free / plus a taste of hell,' they sing as Lillywhite remains patriotic but apprehensive about the future. 'Signing for his pension / he'll still be standing to attention,' the song notes as it hammers home his lifelong subservience to orders. Posted overseas he wonders if he'll ever see his children again. By the end of the song he is beginning to wonder why he ever volunteered. The khaki and grey of the subject matter is offset by the bright tonal colours of pop psych. With its phasing, high harmonies and chiming trebly guitars it's a satirical poster-art reworking of Kitchener's original slogan: your country doesn't really need you.

The original music hall was killed off by a number of factors. In the first two decades of the twentieth century American imports like ragtime and the Charleston made the dance hall a more exciting proposition than the variety bill. The advent of cinema and radio in the 1920s all but sounded the death knell, as many of the star performers from the halls either made the transition to the big screen or decamped to sound broadcasting. By the late 1960s the prevailing circumstances were slightly different but the end result was the same. The arrival of the heavy-rock artillery and a corresponding rejection of frippery and dandyism was what did for the psychedelic music hall. Arch little songs about buskers and spinsters didn't stand a chance in the more austere and unforgiving climate of the early seventies.

The other factor that really did for the music hall was the standardisation of performance criteria. By the end of the nineteenth century eclecticism and an idiosyncratic approach to presentation were on the wane. The language of promotion became more formal and hierarchical. Factors that we now take for granted, like top and bottom billing, were introduced, and the kind of hard-nosed business imperatives that we think of as modern inventions were already in their ascendancy. In 1846 the performer R. J. Hayward was advertised in the *Bolton Free Press* as 'The great antipodean Wonder [who] will tie his Body in a complete knot and will also Sing a variety of Comic Songs while standing on his Head'.[21] The unruly capitalisation on the billing and the eccentricity of the act bear a marked similarity to the wording on the old circus poster that John Lennon discovered in a Sevenoaks junk shop in 1967. By the end of the nineteenth century all that had changed. 'The printed programmes of the variety theatres in the 1890s were much more sober in their descriptions,' says Dagmar Kift. 'They were generally restricted to numbering the order of appearance of the artistes in question with their names and a short summary of their particular speciality.'[22] John Lennon's 'found material', celebrated as a historical curio at the height of psychedelia, was, it turns out, already an anachronism by the end of the nineteenth century. All those calliope- and steam-powered songs inspired by 'Being for the Benefit of Mr Kite' sounded similarly anachronistic by the end of the 1960s.

15

THE PENNY ARCADIA

I remember being in my back garden
one day in the very hot summer of
1966 listening to Radio Caroline.
Every single record they were playing
was great. I just looked up at the
sky in a sort of ecstasy and thought,
'This is fantastic. This is the best it's
ever been.' I think everyone from my
generation agrees: 1965–67 were the
peak years in pop.
IAN MACDONALD[1]

On first hearing, 'At the Third Stroke' by Piccadilly Line sounds like typical Summer of Love fare. A dialling-tone sound effect is bolted onto the beginning and end of the record for no discernible reason – the title is never actually mentioned in the song – and the same goes for the disembodied voice of the speaking clock, which ends the track. It's a slightly desperate A&R department's idea of novelty. Something for the disc jockeys to latch on to. Something that might, just might conceivably distinguish 'At the Third Stroke' from all the other vaguely catchy pop singles released that week that didn't have a dialling tone on them. The arrangement is bright and breezy, the chorus tra-la-las, the circus has come to town and here's the obligatory trumpet fanfare to announce it. In contrast the verses are sung in hushed, understated tones and speak of something less celebratory, something more tentative and reflective: 'I remember rainy days'; 'Thinking back when I was six'; 'Bonfire night and Christmas Eve / kicking up the fallen leaves'. Even in its up moments bustling city nightscapes and the confidence of youth are contrasted with the hopes, fears and dreams of a less settled psyche.

'The Death of the Seaside' by Human Instinct is set to a rollicking pub-piano melody straight out of the music hall. It ba-ba-bas where Piccadilly Line trill and tra-la-la, and a husky Lennonesque vocalist sings about the summer that has just been and gone, recalling events so recent that you can smell the salty air and the suntan lotion. Children make sand pies. Lovers stroll along the prom ('in hats with "kiss me quick" on'). All this is contrasted with the sad afterscene. Kids are back at school now. Hotels are silent and empty. The sand is litter-strewn and deserted. The end of the holiday season is mourned explicitly in the song's title and summarised in war-zone imagery: 'Beaches now are no-man's-land.'

'Got to Get Away' by New York Public Library opens with a flourish of Rickenbacker twelve-string that in other circumstances might have been introducing a song about spiritual transcendence or a Byrdsian homage to a beguiling girl glimpsed from the window of a Greenwich Village coffee shop. But New York Public Library, despite their name, are a beat combo from Leeds formerly known as the Cherokees. They do a twenty-minute version of 'If I Were a Carpenter' in their live act. They know their Byrds from their Buffalo Springfield, and they have their own take on transcendence. It's not dissimilar to the Bay Area variety, as it happens, but it's delivered with fewer folky inflections and a tad more disillusion. 'The days come and go / summer sunshine, winter snow / before you know where you are / another year has gone,' sings a restless figure in an unchanging landscape bemoaning his lot. He longs to escape his loveless relationship. He mentions that he's living a lie (always a good indicator of a

feckless philanderer) and is a prisoner without bars (ditto, only with more self-pity), but there is something in the tone of the song that hints that his quest is more philosophical, and that his horoscope has told him the moon isn't in the seventh house, and that Jupiter isn't aligned with Mars. He's quietly going out of his mind in Nowhere Land with all the nobodies. The title line is sung at the end of each chorus with increasing urgency, a taunting self-reminder from a man counting out the passing of wasted days. Gotta get away. Gotta get away.

These are just three examples from a long list of late-sixties pop songs that speak of similar things: longing, leaving and evocation. Where does it come from, this yearning for yesterday, this burning desire to be somewhere, anywhere but in the here and now? It's not simply a product of teen frustration or commercial imperatives. It runs deeper than that. These melancholic longings and nostalgic reveries crop up frequently in English pop songs of a certain vintage.

Take the Mindbenders' 1966 single 'Can't Live with You, Can't Live without You'. The title conveys a trite Valentine card truism, but the song itself isn't trite. It's haunting and a little bit bleak. 'Can't Live with You, Can't Live without You' was the Mindbenders' third release after parting company with singer Wayne Fontana in 1965. It was co-written by Carole Bayer and Toni Wine, who were also responsible for the Mindbenders' debut single and Top 5 hit 'Groovy Kind of Love' and its moderately successful follow-up 'Ashes to Ashes'. Bayer later married Burt Bacharach and had solo hits of her own; she also wrote the title song to the movie *Arthur*. Wine was a child prodigy, a Juilliard graduate and Screen Gems writer who sang the solo female part on the Archies' 'Sugar, Sugar'. There you have high and low culture in one collective résumé, a songwriting lineage that encompasses the Conservatoire, classic-era Brill Building, bubblegum, and Oscar- and Grammy-winning soundtracks. But nothing else that Bayer and Wine ever wrote contains quite as much understated yearning as 'Can't Live with You, Can't Live without You', as interpreted by a mid-sixties beat group from rainy Manchester. Introduced by a nagging one-note guitar figure that resurfaces throughout the song, it's a slow-tempo love ballad, typical of late Mersey-era pop. It is simple and sparse in structure, just two short verses of concise lyrical couplets, each of which ends in repeats rather than rhymes (not all there/not

all there, walk away/walk away) and a three-line chorus that croons the title line followed by a desperate 'It's never gonna work out fine.' The song's coda simply reeks of desolation. 'Couldn't you try just a little bit harder to love me?' pleads the singer, transcribing girl-group sentiments into boy tears. 'Can't Live with You, Can't Live without You' was made for couples to dance close up to, cheek to cheek, as couples still did in 1966. A smoochy break from the rave-ups for the audience and a breather for the band. But really it sounds like it shouldn't be heard in a dance hall at all. It sounds like it should be listened to on a five-kilowatt pirate radio station in a dimly lit living room on a late winter's afternoon, through crappy little transistor-radio speakers that shake and vibrate with over-modulation, while encroaching medium-wave interference and static threaten to obliterate the signal.

It might be because I first experienced a lot of these records in precisely those circumstances, but I always felt like this about such songs, and in the period just before psychedelia arrived there were lots of them to feel like that about. Songs that even if they were released in the summer cast long shadows and spoke as much of the shade. Songs that on the surface were celebratory but were brimful of emptiness. Graham Gouldman was a master of such shadow play. The louder you played some of his compositions, the more hollow was their echo: 'Evil Hearted You' and 'Heart Full of Soul' by the Yardbirds; 'Cheryl's Going Home' recorded by Bob Lind, Cher and Adam Faith, with its opening line 'The thunder cracks against the night'. Even a song as anodyne as 'No Milk Today', sung by the relentlessly chirpy Herman's Hermits, makes empty milk bottles on a doorstep its forlorn focus of attention, rather than the spurned lover. Another Gouldman composition, 'I'm Gonna Take You There', recorded by Dave Berry and released at the end of 1965, is ostensibly a celebration of nightlife, out of the same mould as Dobie Gray's 'The "In" Crowd', Chubby Checker's 'At the Discotheque' and Petula Clark's 'Downtown'. Except when Dave Berry sings in those ghostly gossamer tones of his he makes the discotheque sound less a sociable habitat, more a secret meeting place populated by lonely outcasts. Things start optimistically enough with a trademark John Barry harpsichord pounding away on the on-beat, à la 'Heart Full of Soul'. It features a cracking session band and a strident arrangement, but the moment Berry starts singing he sounds like a disembodied spirit serenading a congregation of lost souls. His detachment offers stark counterpoint to the inclusivity of the song. 'There's a place / where we can go,' goes the opening line. OK. So far so purposeful. 'And no one cares / just what you know.' That sounds agreeably non-elitist. Leave your cares and burdens at the door, etc. 'Or what you wear / I'm gonna take you there.' Friendly door policy too. Excellent. But the ambivalence increases with each subsequent line. In the second verse it's 'And no one cares / just what you know / or who you are.' In the final verse, accompanied by the kind of ethereal female chorus that Joe Meek turned into a leitmotif, the checklist reads: 'or what you know / or who you are / or what you say'. Individuality diminishes with each taut four-syllable stab, until anonymity merges with the night. 'I'm Gonna Take You There' is great existential pop. Nothing matters. No one cares. And no one is listening anyway. It doesn't take too much of a stretch of the imagination to see how the onset of psychedelia would further pulverise such platitudes into vapour and nothingness, and how all that aching and melancholy could readily be reshaped to accommodate another kind of void. But where does all this dislocation come from in the first place? And why does it sit so well with English pop songs of a certain vintage?

'From Greek mnemonic art to Proust, memory has always been encoded through a trace, a detail, a suggestive synecdoche,' says Svetlana Boym in *The Future of Nostalgia*.[2] And in music too, she might have added. Pop is as well equipped to evoke these fleeting impulses as any other art form. To paraphrase Jim Webb, it is always running one step ahead as we follow in the dance. All notes are diminuendo if you listen closely enough. We are forever condemned to chase resonance in fading chords, in sentiments that die a little the moment they leave a lyricist's lips. Memory offers an approximation of what once existed, and we are forever genuflecting to its echo. Songwriters reflect all the time, of course, but they do so in a way that the music industry doesn't. The industry is constantly, as Ray Davies put it, 'eagerly pursuing all the latest fads and trends'. It exploits and reassembles the past whenever and wherever it detects a revivalist impulse. But revival isn't the same as reflection, and industry-led evocations are not the same as individual ones. There is a constant push and pull between personal reminiscence and the institutional construction of nostalgia. Both are prone to their distortions – 'only false memories can be totally recalled', says Svetlana Boym[3] – and heritage is sold back to us all the time, mostly in forms we barely recognise. But despite its marketed contrivances and its hard sell the music industry can never quite diminish the particularity of our dreams and the shapes they carve into our soul.

Nostalgia can be both tangible – a longing for what has been replaced – and abstract – an indefinable rootless yearning which inhabits the absence itself and stirs deeper emotional currents. Different people get nostalgic about different things at different times for different reasons. Nostalgia is a universal condition but it can be selective too. It's rarely all encompassing or absolute. It can be temporary and arbitrary and not simply a yearning for a time when everything was better. Love for certain aspects of the here and now can quite easily co-exist with an episodic wistfulness for the past. We are far more nostalgic about the resonances of old music than we are about piss-stained phone boxes, flea-pit cinemas, three-channel television or parks that used to lock their gates on Sundays, even if we might express a desire to go back to the time when such things existed – the time of our youth in most cases, a time where coincidentally enough most golden ages are located.

There's a familiar well-trodden path through the English idyll that many people have written about, but it's not one that I want to document here. I would like to propose a more esoteric lineage, one that conveys a less ortho-dox, although I hope no less persua-sive, account of that peculiarly British ability to be both celebratory and com-memorative at the same time, one that simultaneously embodies our ability to live both in the moment and yearn for yesterday. It's a legacy that contains an idiosyncratic mix of the commonplace and the eccentric, the humdrum and the elegiac, the disposable and the everlasting, the predictable and the daft, the tragic and the comic, the tra-ditional and the modern. The way that these contrasting tendencies learn to rub along and inhabit adjacent emo-tional terrain tells us something about ourselves and something about why our music sounded the way it did once upon a time.

The Cecil Sharp of Typographica

'Even when the guns had ceased fire, I could not come back to cricket for a season or two,' reflected poet Edmund Blunden on the devastation of the Great War in his 1943 memoir *Cricket Country*. 'And I think cricket itself did not come back all at once. It had been dismayed; it did not guess in the golden days at things like world wars, or that the score-books should be splashed with the blood of the quiet men.'[4] Noth-ing came back very quickly after the First World War, and many things did not come back at all. There certainly wasn't much enthusiasm in the 1920s for the spoils of empire and the deco-rative knick-knacks it produced. 'Dur-ing the 1920s everything Edwardian was sneered at,' noted Barbara Jones in a piece written for *Vogue* magazine in March 1947. Evelyn Waugh's bright young things, coked to the gills, might have partied like it was 1899, but dur-ing the otherwise not so roaring twen-ties everyone else was on the breadline, involved in the General Strike or watching their country estates fall into disrepair. Victorian and Edwardian iconography has always been subject to the whims of fashion and taste and went in and out of style, depending on the prevailing sensibilities, throughout the twentieth century. Psychedelia's appropriation of that iconography was part of a wider periodic cycle of cul-tural plunder and had stylistic ante-cedents that were established several decades before Sgt Pepper taught the band how to play, but that tendency was slow to take hold in the years after the Great War, with so much blood spilled on foreign fields, so many names etched into memorial stones and so many survivors, as Wilfred Owen put it, having crept back 'silent, to still village wells, up half-known roads'.[5]

The first real indication of a revival in pre-war culture came in the form of children's literature – Lewis Carroll, J. M. Barrie, etc. – but even that served as a form of escapism, an understandable desire to retreat to the prelapsarian. The re-evaluation of the everyday visual landscape, rather than the interior dreamlike one, was championed by two people. Poet John Betjeman's aim was to preserve Victorian architecture; Nicolete Gray's was to revive Victorian typefaces. Gray was the Cecil Sharp of typographica. She derived the same pleasure from an eight-line Tuscan reversed or a two-line Bourgeois ornamented that Sharp or Ralph Vaughan Williams gained from discovering an eighteenth-century Lincolnshire fishing ballad. Gray likened the dramatic stylistic shifts in Victorian ornamented letter design to Chinese and Japanese calligraphy and she marvelled at its contribution to nineteenth-century art. 'Suddenly without warning the insular English craftsman began to use a complicated and sophisticated artistic medium in a way totally foreign to his culture, and used it with verve and subtlety,' she said. 'It is a remarkable phenomenon.'[6] In his book *Pop Design: Modernism to Mod* Nigel Whiteley credits Gray's 1938 tome *XIXth Century Ornamented Types and Title Pages* as the catalyst for the twentieth-century revival in Victoriana. When Gray's book was republished in 1951, it had a massive influence on post-war graphic design. The new enlarged edition contained over 250 illustrations of nineteenth-century founts, as well as a further 450 examples sourced from the type founders' original specimen books.

'The typefaces were designed by the anonymous employees of commercial firms of founders, supplying commercial printers,' she stated. 'The aim of both the founders and printers was continuously to supply the public with novelties which would attract and please; *to succeed in this they had to keep in touch with the exact mood of the moment. Their business being purely commercial*, considerations of scholarship, individual personality or typographical principle do not blur the contact [emphasis mine]. The result is a communal art as pure as that of any primitive society.'[7] Gray describes an aesthetic that applies equally well to pop music, and like any discerning champion of the popular she confronts a paradox that applies to all popular cultural forms: the modern phenomenon of mass-marketed craftsmanship. Gray approached her task as a form of folk retrieval, but her methodology was democratic and non-hierarchical. In her book she frequently makes value judgements about good and bad signage but there is no privileging of artisan or auteur tendencies. She is as unapologetically utilitarian as any 1960s pop artist when considering the uses to which commercially produced typefaces could be put. They were found on handbills and children's books, street signs and hotel signs, coffee houses, auction houses, opera houses, zoological gardens, church memorials, railway timetables and theatre programmes. To Gray all visual displays were equal in the eyes of the lithographer.

XIXth Century Ornamented Types and Title Pages should be read as an erotic text. Its vocabulary satisfies Roland Barthes' definition of *jouissance* as outlined in his 1973 book *The Pleasure of the Text*. Gray lovingly pores over idiosyncrasies of proportion, barbed terminals, pointed spurs, jolly curves and curls in the same way that the author of a Victorian novella would lingeringly describe a well-appointed décolletage or glimpse of ankle. The curved leg of a lower-case 'r' in Caslon condensed and a shadowed Egyptian liaise on the page like indiscreet lovers. Gray imbues a sentence like 'the M may turn Runic and its diagonal lines cross one another'[8] with all the sensuality of splayed legs in a Parisian brothel. Her analysis is equally idiosyncratic. She sees the origins of surrealism in the mysticism and high romanticism of the 1840s, not a common view and certainly not a lineage you would recognise in most histories of art. She refers to Stuck and Mucha, now regarded as standard-bearers for nouveau poster design, as ranking among 'the less experimental continental artists'.[9] And she dispels the idea that there was ever one kind of Victoriana. The term has never been adequate when describing a time span of seventy years. Do people mean the age of scientific rationalism or romantic mysticism, utilitarianism or transcendentalism, benevolence or decadence, industrial modernity or wage-slave brutality, machine inventors or loom wreckers, childhood innocence or child prostitution? Are we referring to the Victoriana of clutter and kitsch or the Victoriana of strict adherence to form and function, the matriarchal age or the patriarchal one, nanny or mill owner, wet nurse or squire? Gray's answer, in typographical terms at least, is both, neither and all of them.

She also illustrates how the vogue for cultural retrieval was itself a nineteenth-century invention. She refers to the Victorian era's 'morass of revivalisms' and reveals how the nineteenth century shaped our entire modern perception of the archaic and the antique. As with sexual intercourse, or licentious behaviour in general, every generation throws up its expert commentators who like to postulate that the nostalgia of the present age is symptomatic of something that earlier revivalists have never experienced, some deeper condition or malaise denied to previous recipients. Nicolete Gray reveals that the Victorians invented that idea too.

The morass of typographical revivals that Gray documents were in abeyance by the end of the nineteenth century, as the idiosyncrasies of commercial type design gave way to the streamlined procedures of the giant American corporations. Those music-hall handbills of the 1840s, which John Lennon based an entire song on, presented a riot of clashing typefaces which, as Gray notes, were 'not visually related to each other or the words which they spell out'.[10] Such handbills had come to prominence precisely at the time when Pablo Fanque was advertising his amazing feats with trampoline leaps and hogsheads of real fire, and they accurately reflected the bizarre and diverse content of the shows they promoted. This blizzard of random, unrelated founts peaked in the 1850s and '60s, but like so many other aspects of Victorian social and cultural life, they had been successfully corralled into order and uniformity by the end of the century.

Equally damning was the extent to which commercial type designers fell foul of the high-art/low-art divide, another nineteenth-century invention. Mass-marketed design belonged to the world of 'popular magazine design, to chocolate box and Christmas-card decoration', says Gray.[11] The 'cleavage which was to become fundamental to English taste up till the second world war', as she puts it,[12] lumped commercial design in with Hollywood cinema, jazz and art deco, and pitted them against modernism in all its progressive forms: Vorticism, the stark, functional, unfussy look of the new typography, brutalist modern architecture, etc. 'Perhaps today the two streams meet again, at least superficially, in the avant-garde artists' espousal of pop art,' says Gray in the 1976, and final, edition of her book.[13] She died in 1997 and lived

long enough to witness the vindica-
tion and validation of everything she
believed in.

A Very British Happening

If the Great War of 1914–18 seared its
way into the psyche of the nation like so
much mustard gas, the Second World
War had a more visible effect on the
physical landscape. Abandoned pill-
boxes, unused gun turrets, disused air-
fields and Nissen huts, emergency rail
links, fenced-off Ministry of Defence
land – all of these things dotted the
small town where I grew up in the late
1950s and early '60s, enduring reminders of the invasion that never came.
Some are still there to this day, crumbling and rusting away, weeds growing through cracks, as nature reclaims
them. In time they will take on the
appearance of Neolithic sites, their
function to be pondered over by future
generations several millennia from
now. One of the great iconic reminders of the continuity between Britain
during wartime and the pop explosion
of the 1960s is the decaying remnants
of the old army and navy forts constructed at the outbreak of the Second World War and still visible from
the busy shipping lanes of the Thames
estuary. Between 1964 and 1967 these

imposing, long-abandoned structures
were briefly commandeered by several
of the offshore pirate radio stations,
as enterprising individuals like David
'Screaming Lord' Sutch and pop-group
manager Reg Calvert claimed squat-
ters' rights and broadcast non-stop pop
music from them.

Compared to the demoralised and
bereft aftermath of the Great War, a
sense of hope and reparation thrived
after the Second World War and there
was a massive demand for communal recreation. Bankrupt, and with its
collective arse hanging out of its torn
trousers, London still managed to
host the 1948 Olympic Games, and in
1951 it was the venue for the Festival
of Britain. The festival, conceived by
the Labour government, was intended
to serve both as a morale-booster during times of continued austerity – 'new
Britain springing from the battered
fabric of the old', as MP Herbert Morrison optimistically put it – and as an
opportunity for innovative collaboration between artists, architects and
designers.

What emerged was a very British
Happening, distinctly homespun in
the way that it went about exhibiting
the old and the new. Modernism and
tradition were presented side by side,
not as an either/or but as parallel paths

and interweaving threads. Futuristic architectural constructions like the Skylon and the Dome of Discovery and displays of the very latest radar and television technology happily rubbed alongside the quaint and the commonplace. The Lion and Unicorn Pavilion was so named because it was supposed to depict a nation of diehards and dreamers in harmonious coexistence. 'The British character' said Dylan Thomas in a BBC talk to commemorate the event, 'that stubborn, stupid, sea-bound, lyrical, paradoxical dark farrago of uppishness, derring do and midsummer moonshine, all fluting, snug and copper-bottomed.'[14] Given equal prominence under the same pavilion roof were traditional representations of British endeavour (everything from Shakespeare to the nation's nautical history) and an 'urban beach' installation that conveyed the English love of the seaside: 'The netted and capstaned, bollarded, buoyed, seashelled, pebbly beautiful seaside of summer childhood gone,' as Dylan Thomas inimitably put it.[15] A display entitled Eccentrics Corner self-consciously played up the British capacity for the quirky and the bonkers, complete with Dadaist contraptions such as an Egg Roundabout, a Smoke Grinding Machine and a tea set made of salmon bones. At the

entrance to the exhibition visitors were greeted by a life-size tableau of *Alice Through the Looking Glass*, with models based on Sir John Tenniel's original illustrations. A purpose-built Pleasure Garden at Battersea contained an American-style funfair, a miniature railway, an illuminated tree walk, a grotto and a dance pavilion that housed regular music-hall shows for those who wished the music hall had never gone away. Drum majorettes, orange girls, match girls and flower-sellers, resplendent in Victorian dress, paraded among the crowds. Nicolete Gray's revivalist lettering – Figgins, Thorne and Austin's original 1815 Roman and Italic – was the official festival typeface.

The Festival of Britain was part village fete, part futurescape. Contemporary design coexisted with Victoriana. Walls of brutalist avant-garde architecture were adorned with murals and mosaics both folksy and abstract. The kitsch and the defiantly outdated nestled happily in the shadow of space-age monuments (which themselves would look kitsch and outdated soon enough). Indeed the Skylon, a 250-foot-high cigar-shaped tensile-steel structure, clad in lacquered aluminium and suspended on hidden cables, served no other function than to look futuristic. It reflected light by day and looked even more impressive at night, when it was lit from within and gave the illusion that it was suspended in space. The popular joke at the time was that the Skylon was symbolic of Britain, as it had no visible means of support. (Displaying a similar sardonic wit a 1946 exhibition of British industrial design, 'Britain Can Make It', was variously dubbed 'Britain Can't Have It' or 'Britain Can't Afford It'.) The day before Skylon's official unveiling, a University of London student, Philip Gurdon, disguised himself as a workman, climbed to the top of the structure at midnight and attached a University of London Air Squadron scarf. The original plan had been to hang a pair of girl's knickers, but Gurdon's commanding officer forbade it. This typically British mixture of bravado and irreverence says as much about the spirit of the festival as the exhibits themselves.

The most significant event took place not at the main festival site on the south bank of the Thames but over in east London, at the Whitechapel Art Gallery. Barbara Jones and Tom Ingram's *Black Eyes and Lemonade* exhibition ran almost concurrently with the main festival, and if anything had a greater and more long-lasting impact. Its influence was particularly felt by a generation of budding young pop artists.

Jones was the first person to use the term 'pop art', writing it at the head of a checklist in her notebook of materials bought for the exhibition. In response to the question 'What Is Art?' Jones's answer was 'Everything'. What Nicolete Gray did for the retrieval and reinvention of typography Jones did for the everyday art object. In the same year that the Festival of Britain was held Jones's book *The Unsophisticated Arts* was also published. Its original title was *The Vernacular Arts* – the shift to the more confrontational '*Unsophisticated*' left the reader in no doubt as to the polemical implications of her work. Half a century earlier folklorists had set about preserving songs that had been passed down through oral transmission and were now in danger of being destroyed by industrialisation. By documenting the ephemera and artefacts of the machine age Jones provided a corollary to that mission. She visited fairgrounds, amusement arcades, tattoo parlours, funeral parlours, waxworks, taxidermists, high-street shops and seaside piers. She sought out canal-boat dwellers on the neglected and forgotten waterways of Britain, studied food decoration and funeral florists' armatures, and faithfully and non-judgementally documented both the way of life and the decorative art that went with it.

Jones's definition of what constituted art included household items that could be bought in the shops, bill posters from street hoardings, tinplate advertisements on barns, shop frontages and railway stations, comic postcards, pub signs, beer labels, agricultural trademarks and the decorative insignia found on farm machinery, costermongers' barrows and burlap sacks, Guy Fawkes effigies, greetings cards, Christmas decorations and party toys. Memorable exhibits at the Whitechapel Gallery included a talking lemon (which said, 'Lemonade is good for man, woman and child'), an edible model of St Paul's Cathedral made entirely from icing sugar, a paddle boat made of coloured glass beads, fire irons made of corn stalks, a fireplace in the shape of an Airedale dog, a 1910 milk float and Nora, a funfair horse. 'The museum eye must be abandoned before they can be enjoyed,' Jones commented waspishly in the exhibition catalogue. Items on display were arbitrarily arranged in order to resist what she called 'bogus sociological implications'. Defending the preponderance of dogs and cats in the exhibition, she noted dryly: 'Though English painters have been much influenced by the techniques of Picasso, they are slow to copy his interest in animals.'[16]

Jones discovered a naïf painter, Miss M. Willis, working in a small flat above a tattooist's shop that was about to be demolished to make way for the festival, and promptly offered her space in the exhibition. When she commended the painter's work to potential gallery sponsors, she was told that Miss Willis produced the wrong kind of primitivism. Not bright and pretty enough, was the verdict. Jones similarly defied categorisation: too playful for the intellectuals, too esoteric to be pigeon-holed, too restless to be tied to one particular style. Her idea of kinetic art was to advocate that the V&A should have a fairground roundabout on permanent display; her idea of an installation was to have pavement artist George McEarnean *in situ* in the Whitechapel Gallery. McEarnean, who normally worked a pitch outside the British Museum, demonstrated his skills beneath a huge Miss Willis canvas entitled *Lord Kitchener in His Coffin*. In truth, all of Jones's exhibits could be called installation art. The way she went about presenting her subject matter was in itself installation art. Her definition of the term was broad enough to include butchers and fishmongers, who, although handicapped by post-war rationing, could be observed decorating their 'almost empty shops into enchanting fantasies with white wrapping paper cut into patterns'. 'All through the exhibition the new and commonplace were seen near the old and safe,' she noted. 'And by the end most people felt able to accept a talking lemon extolling Idris Lemon Squash, and Bassett's Liquorice Allsorts isolated under a spotlight.'[17]

Jones was five years ahead of the game. Astutely anticipating the new pop-art sensibility she refused to make a distinction between hand-made and machine-made items. One of the most popular sections of the *Black Eyes and Lemonade* exhibition was an entire room devoted to Joseph Thorley's, a cattle-feed firm whose distinctive tin-plate advertising signs were seen widely on railway stations and shop hoardings. The idea for the section came about when Jones discovered that many people's memories were evoked by the advertising signs they had seen as children. One particular favourite was the iconic Start-Rite shoes poster showing a little boy and girl walking down a winding road lined with poplar trees. But it was the name Thorley's that kept cropping up, prompting Jones to phone the company's headquarters in King's Cross. Thorley's sent her to its run-down warehouse by the side of the Regent's Canal, where she found a treasure trove of ephemera, 'thickly black with London grime'.[18] 'More than a century's advertising,' as she put it, 'tin plates, glass plates, leaflets that unfolded to show chicks bursting from the egg, and portraits in oils of prize animals fed on Thorley's.' These items were lovingly restored and given pride of place in the Whitechapel Gallery. Seemingly unwittingly, Jones had tapped into a potent strain of nostalgia, one driven not by evocations of antiquity but by the fondly remembered familiarity of commonplace objects and their peculiar facility to trigger the most profound and intense recollections. It's an impulse that a decade later drove John Lennon and Paul McCartney to write 'Strawberry Fields Forever' and 'Penny Lane', Syd Barrett to write 'Matilda Mother', Pete Townshend to write 'Dogs', Ray Davies to write just about everything. It's an impulse that momentarily diverted an entire generation of songwriters and inspired them to start writing songs about Bonfire Night and autumn leaves, hats with 'Kiss me quick' on and deserted beaches. In *Black Eyes and Lemonade* Jones located the true source of the English penny Arcadia: the residual group memory of things, themes and places – fairgrounds and fairy tales, children's comics and Saturday-morning pictures, Ovaltine commercials and Radio London jingles, penny liquorish sticks, Bazooka Joe bubblegum cards and the corner shops that sold them. It is the same impulse that sent the Small Faces scurrying to Ogden's tobacco factory in search of an original nineteenth-century design for the cover of their *Ogdens' Nut Gone Flake* LP, an initiative that pays simultaneous homage to Nicolete Gray and Barbara Jones.

Futuristic structures like the Dome of Discovery and the Skylon dominated the Festival of Britain landscape with their sheer inventiveness and ingenuity, but no amount of public spending or morale boosting could quite conceal the sense that, as writer Brian Aldiss put it, the country was still convalescent after the war. Naysayers in the Tory press grumbled about the cost of the event during a time of austerity. Others criticised it for being parochial, inward-looking and nostalgic. Edward Lucie Smith remembered the 'air of enforced jollity . . . the fixed grin of a scoutmaster determined that one should enjoy oneself' ('within the limits of British decency', as Buster Bloodvessel would no doubt have put it). He castigated 'the hypocrisy of a second-class power still masquerading as a first-class one' and described the post-war pomp and pageantry as 'too obviously fancy dress, and rather scanty costume

at that – so diaphanous you could still see the bruises'.[19] Others remembered more mundane inconveniences like the queues for stale Swiss rolls and the reliably dismal weather. But eight million people still came, cavorted, diaphanous costumes, bruises and all, to dance bands in the pouring rain, marvelled at the fountains and coloured lights, and briefly forgot about ration-book Britain and the Blitz. 'The festival is London,' claimed Dylan Thomas. 'The arches of the bridges leap into light; the moon clocks glow; the river sings; the harmonious pavilions are happy. And this is what London should always be like, till St Paul's falls down and the sea slides over the Strand.'[20]

Speaking twenty-five years after the event even a modernist sceptic like Reyner Banham could begrudgingly acknowledge the galvanising effect the festival had on an entire generation of what he called 'impressionable but beady-eyed school children and teenagers . . . For them it was not an instruction in the appreciation of good design, not a new awareness of our great national inheritance of dotty humour and professional eccentricity. It was a turn on, man.'[21] Banham saw the seeds of the swinging sixties being sown right there and then in the futuristic vistas and Victorian pleasure gardens of bomb-strewn London. 'It was a pre-view of the human environment as a zone of enjoyment and its design as an occupation of pleasure,' he said. 'When the British became self-confident enough again to rejoice without having to be ordered to by Herbert Morrison, sophisticated enough to enjoy them-selves without needing instruction from kindly ex-officers and gentlemen, and affluent enough to do it without threatening national bankruptcy, then there was a generation at hand . . . to whom the Festival had shown the way if not the style.'[22]

Banham was only half right. The festival had not only shown the way, it had shown the style too. It was hybrid in nature, simultaneously forward-thinking and reflective, resistant to either/or dogma and easy categorisa-tion, and it impacted upon creativity at every level. In the light of the festival architectural historian Nikolaus Pevs-ner renounced his earlier unconditional support for modernism, re-evaluated Victorian design aesthetics, and subse-quently championed a uniquely British synthesis of what Nigel Whiteley called 'the intellectual rigour of modernism and the emotional appeal of Victori-ana'.[23] Artist John Piper, who provided *The Englishman's Home* mural for the festival's Homes and Gardens Pavilion,

had similarly aligned himself with European abstractionism in the 1930s, but in the post-war years made a simi-lar volte-face to Pevsner, which resulted in him returning to the English land-scape, to churches and country houses, for his inspiration and subject matter.

More than anything the Festival of Britain dispelled the idea that the 1950s were drab, grey and conform-ist. The decade is frequently depicted as culturally moribund, a time when, apart from the outpourings of a few angry playwrights, little of creative sig-nificance occurred. The fifties were, in fact, a time when many ideas that were more fully articulated in the sixties first took root. Perhaps the most insid-ious cliché about the 1950s is that it was a black-and-white decade. All this really means is that much of the era's news footage was shot and viewed in monochrome and there was still a lot of rubble about. Writers of lazy his-tories notice that the men were still predominantly dressed in national ser-vice khaki or demob-suit grey and that most women couldn't afford Dior's new look, and they tailor their superficial assumptions accordingly. In fact, the 1950s were a riot of colour – in cinema, in fashion, in painting and in interior and graphic design. The Teddy Boys, the first recognisably British youth cult, a group that predates rock-and-roll music by several years, wore fluorescent pink, green and purple socks and similarly shocking trim on their adapted Edwardian frock coats. These in turn had been appropriated from the clique of gay fashionistas who had first adopted the look. CinemaScope and Panavision dominated the cinema. Picture postcards and billboard ads were enhanced with hyper-real colouring. Dylan Thomas described the Telecinema at the Festival of Britain as 'spots with scarlet tadpole tails, and spottedly sinuous tintacks dancing with dissolving zebra heads, and blobs and nubbins and rubbery squirls receding to zig zag blasts of brass down nasty polychrome corridors, a St Vitus's gala of abstract shapes and shades in a St Swithin's day of torrential dazzling darning needles'.[24] Does any of this sound remotely colourless to you? It sounds like a light show and an acid trip without the acid to me.

The same post-war advances in polyurethane paints, dyes, soluble acrylics and primary-coloured plastics that inspired the light-show pioneers in the US made their presence felt on everything from home furnishings and wallpaper to fashion magazines. In recipe books and food advertising ubiquitous brown tints were replaced by lavish displays and garishly saturated colouring that amounted to culinary porn. This ubiquitous bombardment of gluttonous luminosity verged on the hallucinatory. In ration-book Britain its promise of plenty had a delirious effect. A dream vision of an Americanised consumerist future was being constructed, so tantalisingly aromatic you could practically taste it.

'A Place Painted Regardless and by Hand'

In 1951, while the Festival of Britain and the *Black Eyes and Lemonade* exhibition were offering an immersive environment that was part global village fete, part knick-knack emporium, the twenty-four-year-old Bruce Lacey was witnessing a light-show display at the Royal Academy of Arts by American John Hoppe. Hoppe's *Mobilux* utilised a refracted light source that was shone onto a chromium-plated surface overlaid by moveable stencilled figures, whose shape could be modified and manipulated at will. Hoppe saw the commercial potential of *Mobilux* and wanted to use it primarily as an advertising tool; indeed, it did eventually become a regular feature in advertising and TV credit sequences. By 1954 Hoppe was collaborating with the first generation of pop artists and his *Mobilux* spectaculars were getting a regular airing on the NBC television network. Bruce Lacey, however, saw how *Mobilux* could be used in a performance context and customised the technique accordingly. With the help of a few willing collaborators at the Royal College of Art he started to overlay musique concrète onto the pliable images and began exploring what would later become standard practice in light-show displays during the psychedelic era.

Britain may not have produced a convincing surrealist painter on a par with René Magritte, Max Ernst or Juan Miró, but it did produce Bruce Lacey. Lacey is the missing link between Marcel Duchamp and the *Magical Mystery Tour*. Indeed, had things been different there is no reason why he should not have been on the Beatles' bus in 1967. He had, after all, appeared as George Harrison's flute-playing gardener in *Help!*, and had worked with Ivor Cutler previous to that. Cutler as tour guide and Lacey as kinetic-machinery manipulator might just have been the double act that the *Magical Mystery Tour* needed.

During his time at the RCA Lacey developed a great hatred for his teachers. He thought many of them were little more than embittered drunkards and he despised the aggressively male culture in which they thrived. Nevertheless, he learned what he referred to as the double-talk of artspeak, chiefly so that he would be suitably equipped to fight aesthetic with counter-aesthetic. While at art school he set up a film society, where among other things he ran Laurel and Hardy flicks at high speed. He also developed a circus act consisting of incompetent magic tricks, and instigated art pranks such as sending up huge inflated balloons and then reporting them to the police as UFOs. He performed 'Flight of the Bumble Bee' with an exploding piano, 'Show Me the Way to Go Home' on the spokes of a penny-farthing bicycle and 'I'm Forever Blowing Bubbles' on a wind-up gramophone that blew bubbles from its speaker. Encouraged by surrealist painter Conroy Maddox he began exhibiting and selling his own assemblages (although, ever the autodidact, 'assemblage' was a term he'd never heard until this point).

Between 1956 and 1960 Lacey gave up painting and began making trick props and special effects for television. He worked briefly for Tommy Cooper, but Cooper's manager thought him too esoteric. 'I didn't fit into the art world and I didn't fit into the showbiz world,' he noted.[25] He worked with Spike Milligan on programmes such as *Idiots Weekly*, *Fred* and *Son of Fred*, and on former Goon Michael Bentine's flea circus. In 1960 Lacey formed the Gnits with Joe McGrath and animator Bob Godfrey, with whom he had worked on the Milligan shows. The trio made several short comedy films, which were shown on the ITV pop show *Cool for Cats*. Also in 1960 he made the props for – and appeared uncredited in – Peter Sellers's *The Running, Jumping and Standing Still Film*, where he provided the best visual gag in the movie. Playing the part of a poncey aesthete, his reverie is interrupted by Sellers as he stands gazing thoughtfully into a field. The two men circle each other warily for a moment before Sellers walks off, at which point Lacey takes a gramophone record from under his coat, places it on the flat base of a sawn-off tree trunk and, using his finger as a stylus, begins whirling dementedly around the tree.

In 1963 he began working with the Alberts, a crazed double act immersed in Victoriana. The Alberts were the inspiration for all the trad satirists who followed in the mid-sixties: the Temperance Seven, the Bonzo Dog Doo Dah Band et al. all owe a debt to their mould-breaking antics. That same year Lacey appeared with Ivor Cutler in the fondly remembered *An Evening of British Rubbish*. *Times* critic Bernard Levin laughed so hard he was physically sick. Peeping nervously through the curtain to see how the show was progressing, Lacey saw Levin writhing in his seat and assumed he was having a heart attack.

In 1965 Lacey was involved in two of the English underground's seminal events: the basement Happenings at Better Books with Jeff Nuttall and John Latham, and the International Poetry Incarnation at the Albert Hall. At the latter gathering Lacey unleashed the radio-controlled robot John Silent. Named after John the Silent, the fifth-century ascetic Christian saint, Lacey's robot was programmed to produce farting and belching noises. At the International Poetry Incarnation it provided some welcome kinetic counterpoint to some of the more unseemly farting and belching on the stage. In 1966 Lacey announced that John Silent had undergone a sex change and was now to be known as R.O.S.A. B.O.S.O.M (Radio. Operated. Simulated. Actress. Battery. Or. Standby. Operated. Mains). During this period Lacey also appeared in several feature films, including *It's Trad, Dad!*, *Casino Royale* and, most memorably, the 1967 swinging-sixties romp *Smashing Time*. With a sharp satirical script written by George Melley and shot mostly in the then unfashionable and run-down Camden Town, *Smashing Time* starred Lynn Redgrave and Rita Tushingham as two Liverpudlian girls trying their luck in a swinging London populated by predators, snake-oil salesmen and fly-by-night boutique owners. Lacey and his machines have a starring role in a party sequence filmed at the Roundhouse. His kinetic army machine-guns half the audience and molests the other half with huge extended arms fitted with boxing gloves. The robots explode balloons full of feathers and leave lipstick on the faces of everyone they assault. They rampage, like Lacey himself, uncontained and uncontrollable through the debris of the swinging sixties, leaving muddy robot footprints all over the furnishings.

Being an island race doesn't make you insular, it just makes things further away, and it's inevitable therefore that certain artefacts take on a cachet of exoticism. This occurred on numerous occasions in the two decades after the Second World War. It happened with New Orleans jazz and it happened with the Delta blues, which were both recast in the eyes (and ears) of the aficionado. Pop artists fetishised the American visual landscape and its consumer indurables. The mods did something similar with French films and Italian suits and scooters. Exoticism became part of the fabric. Because Britain never marched to the tune of fascism or totalitarianism one movement or one way of thinking has never simply swept away another. A certain displacement might have occurred periodically but what generally happened is that a multiplicity of cultural tendencies learned to coexist and coalesce. The schism between abstraction and figuration that dominated post-war thinking about art was never really perceived as a crisis in the UK. Here painters moved freely between idioms and happily incorporated a range of competing styles into their work. By the end of the 1950s such congregations of incongruities were everywhere. English art schools, as Bruce Lacey illustrates, fostered a unique interrelationship between jazz, humour, sculpture and design. Here again collaboration and diversity rather than demarcation and rigidity were the key elements in the cultural mix. Bebop and trad jazz, for example, had a simultaneous impact both on the subject matter of British painting and on the social life of British art students. Modernists and traddies are generally treated as irreconcilable opposites by those pop-cultural commentators who like their history served up factional and friction-ridden. In fact, there was considerable crossover between the two forms, both among the musicians who played jazz and those who listened to it. Barry Miles once told me that as an unabashed musical snob and fan of modern jazz he was initially so ignorant of the Beatles that he had to go and look at a record sleeve to see what instrument Paul McCartney played when he was first introduced to him. At the same time he remembers the social functions at Cheltenham art school, which he attended, all featured trad bands because even hipsters liked to dance and consort with the opposite sex when the occasion presented itself. The humour of radio shows like *The Goons* and, later, *Round the Horne* was satirical, surreal and subversive, but both programmes featured traditional-jazz or light-entertainment vocal groups as their musical guests. The juxtaposition is made more paradoxical when you consider that many of the members of those light-entertainment house bands were moonlighting bebop musicians.

In British humour that blurring of trad and modernist tendencies was integral to the comedy. The Goons took off on verbal flights of fancy that made full use of radio's capacity for providing better pictures, and for dismantling not just the fourth wall but all four walls, but the storylines and set-ups themselves were more often than not rooted in recognisable domestic scenarios and familiar comic tropes, which frequently involved the lampooning of stock military, political and bureaucratic figures.

The irreverent madcap nature of such escapades may be the very reason why Britain did not produce a Dalí, a Tanguy, a Rrose Sélavy, but produced a Bruce Lacey, a Tommy Cooper, a Peter Sellers, a Peter Cook instead. Even our surrealism is nostalgic – nostalgic for the pre-apocalyptic, nostalgic for the age of unreason, nostalgic for the unruly and the unruleable. European surrealism concerned itself with dream states and Freudianism; British surrealism adopts a less po-faced take on repression and the sublimated urge. We incorporate a certain kind of self-mocking humour into our surrealism in a way that few other countries do. I'm not talking about the visual conundrums of a Magritte (although with his emphasis on the domestic he really should be claimed as an honorary British surrealist); I'm talking about that implacable sense of British daftness that manifests itself with compulsive ingenuity whenever authority needs deflating. It's Peter Cook's police inspector floating helplessly in a hot-air balloon above the post-apocalyptic gathering in Richard Lester's 1969 film adaptation of Spike Milligan's *The Bed Sitting Room*, shouting, 'I didn't join the force just to float aimlessly into the void.' It's also Cook offering himself as a benign dictator at the end of that same film, reassuring the H-bombed congregation from the vantage point of his wicker balloon basket that 'At times of great national emergency you'll find that a new leader tends to emerge – here I am. So watch it.'

When I interviewed the artist Anthony Stern for my Syd Barrett biography, *A Very Irregular Head*, we talked at length about the light shows, which were a crucial feature of psychedelia. While giving due credit to Mark Boyle, Peter Wynne Wilson et al., Stern casually related that the first time he had encountered what he called 'light boxes' was through writer and portrait artist Reg Gadney. 'At that time he was at King's College when I came up to St John's, and he had built this ginormous lightbox in his room. It was like looking at something very contemporary, like an LED screen, this great big box with fairly complicated electrical equipment behind it, and very bright spotlights, shining on the diffuse screen. And it

had these extraordinarily interesting phases of change, things moving round each other in turn. And there was a cycle to it, so colours went round one way and shadows were cast on the diffusing screen at the front.' Stern didn't mention the obvious debt to Moholy-Nagy's Light Space Modulator in all this but he did cite the influence of Man Ray and the Russian constructivists. 'It was sculpting with light. That's what they were on about. It involved having electric motors turning things round and upside down and inside out, and then projecting that image without means of a spotlight onto a screen. It was abstract film-making in a way. They were all very much into architectural forms in space.' What was most intriguing about this recollection, more intriguing than the avant-garde lineage that Stern acknowledges, was the revelation that undergraduates were doing this as a matter of course in their halls of residence in Cambridge in the late 1950s and early 1960s. It evokes an enduring Heath Robinson spirit of garden-shed boffinry that has existed since amateur scientists made cat's whisker radios from kits or tried to invent perpetual-motion machines with little more than tin foil and sticky-back plastic. It's what Dylan Thomas defined at the Festival of Britain as 'the gay, absurd, irrelevant, delighting imagination that flies and booms and spurts and trickles out of the whole bright boiling'.[26] It's a form of nostalgia in itself: a nostalgia for invention, a reversion to DIY experimentation and a spirit that thrived in the days before ideas were patented and invention was commodified. Bruce Lacey and his kinetic robot army are a walking, talking, short-circuiting embodiment of those ideals.

Once you understand all this you begin to understand why we wouldn't necessarily want to draw a moustache on the *Mona Lisa* but why we might be inclined, given favourable circumstances, to drape a pair of knickers from the Skylon.

Camelot Boutique

In *Nineteenth Century Ornamented Typefaces* Nicolete Gray noted how architectural lettering survived in only a few select places at the start of the twentieth century. The examples she gave were the more lavishly illustrated children's books, terracotta, mosaic and glass. But even the eagle-eyed Cecil Sharp of typographica neglected to mention the one place where a stylistic jumble of anachronistic lettering remained visible, the one place where

it had never entirely been eradicated: the streets. It was there in signage and shop fronts, in decorative motifs and ornamented doorknobs – anywhere, in fact, where a tradesperson was unwilling or simply couldn't afford to update their nameplate or, more often than not, where the occupant simply liked things the way they were. The streets remained the one true amalgam of the old and the new, the site where enterprising young go-getter entrepreneurs resided side by side with those who were oblivious or indifferent to the whims of contemporary taste, those to whom keeping up with the Joneses wasn't an option because they didn't even know the Joneses existed. The street remained the ever-present hidden visible that everybody saw but nobody noticed.

There is a classic moment at the beginning of part two of Martin Scorsese's Bob Dylan documentary *No Direction Home* that shows Dylan, during his British tour of 1966, gazing at two adjacent advertising boards outside a pet shop in a side street in London's Knightsbridge. One sign reads, 'Animals and birds bought or sold on commission'; the other, 'We will collect, clip, bath and return your dog.' A phone number is rendered in the arcane metropolitan runes of the pre-SDT dialling code – KNI 7727 – and underneath that it says, 'Cigarettes and tobacco'. Dylan stares quizzically, reading the unfamiliar vernacular slowly, and sounding out each letter and digit of the phone number like it's some secret code. Behind him a huge red arrow on a cardboard sign points the way to Camelot Boutique.

Suddenly Dylan starts conjuring with the wording, jumbling the adjacent lettering into fragmented speed prose. Phrases spill out in ever more surreal incantations. 'I am looking for a place that is going to animal my soul, knit my return, bathe my foot and collect my dog.' And so on. Briefly we get to experience the living landscape of mid-sixties London as a cut-up seen through the eyes of a pop-art Rimbaud. It's the most potent image in the film. All our yesterdays meet some of our tomorrows. Camelot Boutique indeed. Here is Bob Dylan in 1966, the clown prince of beatitude, zeitgeist fizzing and sparking from every live-wire tentacle of his curly head. And he's riffing on antique signage.

A year later, at a time when psychedelia was in full flow, a forty-five-minute film documentary entitled *The London Nobody Knows*, presented by the actor James Mason, revealed the other side of the swinging city. The tall cranes and the wrecking balls of redevelopment are evident in much of the footage, but so too are frequent sightings of the typography that Nicolete Gray documented and the unsophisticated arts that Barbara Jones revered. The film was an adaptation of Geoffrey Fletcher's book of the same name. First published in 1962 and marginally updated in 1965, *The London Nobody Knows* documents a world where trendy fashion houses and dolly-bird emporia shared terrace blocks with sweatshops and pawnbrokers' balls; where one sweep of the eye would take in Mary Quant, Quorum, Take Six, the red and white striped pole of a barber's shop and flaking enamel tin-plate ads for St Bruno's Tobacco and Thorley's Cattle Feed.

Geoffrey Fletcher documents this world in the same way that Barbara Jones describes the interior of a canal-boat home or Nicolete Gray notes a revivalist fount. He lovingly lists the contents of junk shops that spill their wares out onto the pavement: 'feeble watercolours, vases of impossible shapes and sinister hues, fans, gramophones, olive green aspidistra pots (hallmarks of gentility) and books'.[27] He notes the ancient train carriages still in use on some of London's backwater branch lines 'travelling forward in space as it were but backwards in time'.[28] He laments the disappearance of gas-lamp lighters, 'a dying race – not quite gone, like the muffin men, but almost'.[29] Echoing Jones's waspish observations on Picasso and animals, Fletcher notes how 'the English steered clear of Cubism when offered in the form of easel paintings but promptly accepted it on cheap suburban wall-papers'.[30] He watches the buskers and one-man bands working Dept-ford High Street. Of the disappearing organ-grinders, 'whose instrument is properly termed "a street piano"', he notes that 'there is still one firm left hiring out the pianos in London, near Saffron Hill: look for the pictures of Edwardian beauties on the panel of the organ'.[31] Fletcher visits Victorian oyster rooms, Belgravia pharmacists, Mayfair gunsmiths and the ripped-out guts of former music halls. He spots the totters and the tarts, the horse troughs still in use on busy thoroughfares, and the narrow Spitalfield streets unchanged since the days of Jack the Ripper. Like Nicolete Gray he documents what he calls the 'nineteenth-century Middle Ages' of London gothic. Like Barbara Jones he greets delicately wrought iron-work and garish amusement arcades with equal impartiality. His depiction of the 'dreadfully badly drawn figures

supposed to resemble men' that stand outside barbers' shops makes them sound worthy of inclusion in the *Black Eyes and Lemonade* exhibition. 'Here are the plastic toys which the Eng-lish believe to be a source of amuse-ment to budgerigars,' he says of a pet store. 'There is something touching in the idea of a nation losing its Empire wholesale and at the same time devot-ing itself to budgerigars.'[32] Marvelling at the marble-clad bar and billiard room with horsehair seats of the Crown pub 'on the edge of St John's Wood and mistressy Maida Vale', he urges the reader to 'go there in a straw boater in summertime; smoke a Woodbine and think about Kitchener'.[33] He also notes, not entirely approvingly, the passing of the older generation of pavement artists in favour of 'the new generation – the long-haired youths who wear peaked caps in the style favoured by David Copperfield and Little Jack Horner'.[34] Nor does he care much for 'the youth-ful deadbeats of indeterminate sex, for example, long-haired, often barefooted, scruffy and displeasing, who spend long hours on the steps of the Eros fountain or hang about those of the National Gallery or drape themselves about the terrace overlooking Trafalgar Square, all with dirty beards, dirty hands and grubby, tight toggery and a general air of desiccation'.[35] If all this points to a reactionary streak, an air of 'You got a better class of down and out in the old days', it is partly because Fletcher senses what embourgeoisement and gentrification are doing to the spirit of the place.

The final page of *The London Nobody Knows* is an angry lament. 'Most of the things in this book are destined to go the same way in a London that has become the prey of bureaucrats, developers and destroyers,' he says. Indeed, several of the footnotes in the updated 1965 edition make reference to what has already disappeared in the three years since the book was first published. The film version ends on a less pessimistic note. 'There's no need to be too sad about it,' says James Mason as the bomb-site clearance that's taken twenty years to instigate rumbles all around him and wrecking balls take out slum terraces, allowing us to peer in at their gutted doll's house remains. 'After all, most of Victorian London was fairly hideous,' he says. Fletcher's conclusion is less equivocal: 'Of the new London, the London of take-over bids and soul-destroying office blocks, the less said, the better.'[36]

Both the book and film versions of *The London Nobody Knows* are full of reminders of what England's capital – what much of England, in fact – looked like when the Beatles were recording *Sgt Pepper* and the Carnabetian army was in full cry. Fletcher's book serves as another key reminder of where so much English nostalgia comes from. Longing and loss are embedded in the landscape, in its memory-scented dream life and its psychogeography. Melancholic reflection endures in actual physical sites, emotional residue is stirred up in the fust and dust of slum clearance and in the spectral imprint that remains long after the actual structures have gone. If memory echoes resonate in the disappeared and the disappearing, it shouldn't be surprising that they are there in the music too. One of the many songs that illustrates Oscar Wilde's maxim about Britain and America being two countries divided by a common language is Joni Mitchell's 'Big Yellow Taxi'. Mitchell sings about loss too: the loss of green spaces to concrete shopping malls, the loss of the eco-structure to insecticides, the loss of her father. In 'Big Yellow Taxi''s most quoted line she sings, 'You don't know what you've got till it's gone,' but I don't think that's true of Britain. It certainly wasn't true of Britain in the sixties. Most of the time people were only too aware of what they had and what was being taken away from them. That oft-derided stoicism of the British, that 'putting up with', masks passions both sentimental and embittered that find expression in all kinds of places, people and things. Remembrance of the dis-membered, deracinated past surfaces in all kinds of conspicuous and incon-spicuous displays, and it comes out in the music too. You don't always hear it, or may not think you hear it, but you do. It's inescapable, it's ingrained.

All those tendencies that had been quietly bubbling away in seemingly dis-parate and disconnected areas of Brit-ish cultural life – in the fine and not so fine arts, in architecture, invention, film, TV, radio, comedy and music – suddenly explode with renewed conver-gent energy in the mid-1960s. Echoing a legacy of revival and renewal that had periodically surfaced throughout the twentieth century, English psychedelia fused state-of-the-art sonics to nostal-gic sentiments. It applied cutting-edge technology to songs about penny-farthings and puppet shows. What are such juxtapositions if they are not vibrant manifestations of Nigel White-ley's 'rigour of modernism' married to the 'emotional appeal of Victoriana'? What else are the curlicues, cornices and gildings of late-sixties pop if they aren't a contemporary expression of the garish ornamentation first displayed in

the mock baroque of Victorian archi-tecture? What were those cluttered music-hall handbills if they weren't the typographical predecessors to the 'everything but the kitchen sink' pro-ductions that could be heard on many psychedelic records a century later? What, indeed, is English psychedelia if it isn't one long carnival procession comprising the raggle-taggle conscripts of Geoffrey Fletcher's ephemeral army, a dutiful ensemble of organ-grinders, one-man bands and other bloody but unbowed survivors from a bygone age, all decked out in discarded insignia and junk-shop spillage and pursued to the echo by a dream whirl of calliopes, melodions, player pianos and ice-cream chimes? And resplendently leading this tatty and frazzled procession is the 1910 handcart displayed at the *Black Eyes and Lemonade* exhibition, liberated from some dusty museum vault and paraded the length of Carnaby Street by one of Fletcher's fey young things in a Donovan cap. In his flowery evoca-tion of the joys of the Festival of Britain Dylan Thomas eulogised 'something very odd indeed, magical and paro-chial: a parish pump made out of flying glass and thistledown gauze-thin steel, a roly-poly pudding full of luminous, melodious bells, wheels, coils, engines and organs, alembics and jorums in a

palace of thunderland sizzling with scientific witches' brews, a place of trains,
bones, planes, ships, sheep, shapes,
snipe, mobiles, marbles, brass bands
and cheese, a place painted regardless
and by hand'.[37] He could have been
describing a good night down at UFO,
Middle Earth or the Roundhouse. He
could have been describing psychedelia
full stop.

Along the spine of the original
mock-up for her 1951 book *English
Vernacular Art* (as it was still called
then, the demo tape, if you like), Barbara Jones etched – in a riot of clashing founts, naturally – a list of intended
topics: Fairs, Taxidermy, Food, Birth,
Marriage, Death, Toys, Canals, Seaside, Riverside, Tattooing, Shops, Waxworks, Fire Works, Christmas, Sweets.
It reads like a prophecy of psychedelic
subject matter, Madame Zaza's end-of-
the-pier guide, swirling in her crystal
ball, ready to take shape, substance and
song form a decade later. There weren't
too many psychedelic songs about
canals, but pretty much everything else
in Jones's inventory got an airing.

The Go-Go. Gone

In 1962 the first episode was shown
on British TV of *Steptoe and Son*,
Ray Galton and Alan Simpson's sitcom
about two rag-and-bone merchants.
The father-and-son team of Albert and
Harold Steptoe was played by Wilfred
Brambell, who appeared in 1964 as
Paul McCartney's grandfather in the
first Beatles feature film, *A Hard Day's
Night*, and Harry H. Corbett, a student
of Stanislavski's Method school and a
product of Joan Littlewood's experimental East End Theatre Workshop.
The show was set in Oil Drum Lane
in Shepherd's Bush, a district of west
London where horse-drawn totters'
carts were still a daily sight on the
streets. Galton and Simpson made a
shrewd decision very early on to make
the two main protagonists a father-and-
son team rather than neighbours or
rival rag-and-bone merchants, both of
which had been considered at the planning stage. They reasoned that making the central characters kith and kin
would give the show its underpinning
dynamic. They were right beyond their
wildest expectations. *Steptoe and Son*
was Samuel Beckett set in a junkyard.
Most scenes were filmed either in the
yard itself or inside the Steptoes' ramshackle house, overflowing with items
from the daily haul. The widowed father,
Albert, is happy in his habitat, content
among his mess, with a ready sneer set
against the wider world in all its folly.
Son Harold perennially yearns for the

better life that he is sure exists somewhere outside of the drab confines of the daily rag-and-bone round. Already in his late thirties by the time he took the part, Harry H. Corbett (like Galton and Simpson's previous star turn, Tony Hancock) brought something of his own creative frustrations and misplaced grandeur to the role. As Harold he is the ageing swinger, doomed by demography to miss out on the full fruits of the permissive society. Whether trying to smuggle a 'bird' into his bedroom, better himself socially (also a Hancock staple) or simply free himself from the choking claustrophobia of Oil Drum Lane, Harold is constantly thwarted by the actions, and sometimes the mere presence, of his father. The die is cast in the very first episode, where after deciding to strike out on his own Harold is told he can take the cart but not the horse. In a bleak scene unparalleled in the annals of sitcom pathos, Harold tries to lift the heavy cart but cannot budge it an inch. 'I can't go,' he cries, crumbling into tears. 'I can't get away.' His father's defiant expression softens into pity. 'I'll go and put the kettle on and make a cup of tea, shall I?' he says. 'It's a bit late to start going anywhere now, isn't it?' Albert reasons, gesturing at the fading light that symbolises so much more. 'I'm still going. I'm not

staying,' sobs Harold. 'Of course you are,' says Albert. This moving scene sets the tone for what *Steptoe and Son* would play out comedically for the next ten years. 'Shall we go?' says Vladimir at the end of *Waiting for Godot*. 'Yes, let's go,' replies Estragon. 'They do not move,' reads Beckett's stage instruction. That's Harold Steptoe's life in a hundred weekly prime-time episodes.

That same interplay between stasis and desire is present in the early-1970s sitcom *Whatever Happened to the Likely Lads?* Starring childhood friends Bob Ferris (Rodney Bewes) and Terry Collier (James Bolam), and set in the north-east of England, the show, written by Dick Clement and Ian La Frenais, reprised its successful 1960s predecessor *The Likely Lads*. That earlier incarnation had featured two Jack the Lads in the prime of their youth, but the changes that have occurred in the intervening period give the follow-up series an added frisson. The embittered and culturally entrenched Terry has missed 'the swinging sixties' while serving in the army. Bob has a newly acquired petit-bourgeois taste for the good life. In the opening credits of *Whatever Happened to the Likely Lads?* the engaged and soon-to-be-married Bob stands proudly on the front step of his newly built property on the Elm Lodge housing estate, while Terry is shown desperately running for and missing a bus. The symbolism is unmistakable. In the very first episode of the return series the two men are reunited unexpectedly on a Newcastle-bound train, after visiting London seperately. Terry launches into his litany of lost opportunities. 'I missed it all. Swinging Britain was just hearsay to me,' he says. 'The death of censorship. The new morality, *Oh! Calcutta!* Topless waitresses in see-through knickers.' 'They didn't catch on,' says Bob mournfully. 'I'd like to have been here to have seen them not catching on,' fumes Terry.

In a memorable episode entitled 'Moving On', first shown in January 1973, the two men pay a visit to their old stamping grounds in the post-industrial heartland. The trip is initiated when Bob decides to show a disbelieving Terry how much has changed during the five years he's been away. They drive through a landscape in the throes of redevelopment and reminisce about former haunts against a backdrop of half-demolished slums, acres of wasteland cleared for new building plots and newly erected high-rise blocks. A multi-storey car park now stands on what used to be the Go-Go Rock Club. 'The North's premier music Mecca,'

muses Bob. 'The Go-Go? Gone?' says a stunned Terry. In a denouement worthy of Ray Davies a disenchanted Terry decides to hook up with an old army colleague who had grand plans when they were in the forces together, but when Bob tracks him down in Berwick-upon-Tweed Terry is working in a car wash and his old army pal is running a greasy-spoon cafe.

Between Harold Steptoe's inability to shift an unmoveable object in 1962 and Terry Collier's pained dislocation from the past in 1972 an entire pop culture pours in. Rodney Bewes even managed his own pop denouement by singing in a bleakly wistful voice the bleakly wistful theme tune to another early-seventies sitcom, *Dear Mother . . . Love Albert*, in which he stars as the central character. Like *Steptoe and Son* and *Whatever Happened to the Likely Lads?*, the show frequently slipped into lachrymose moods that would be unthinkable in a contemporary youth-orientated sitcom. Albert sends regular missives home to his mother from a London that only really exists in his dreams. 'I'll buy Buckingham Palace / you all can come and stay,' goes the theme song. 'I'll buy the Albert Hall / me dad can sit and play.'

Steptoe and Son and *Whatever Happened to the Likely Lads?* express themes that crop up frequently in the pop music of the mid- to late sixties: yearnings for the good life (usually a mythical good life based on assumptions about the one they think everyone else is living), tempered by a longing for security. Discontentment and frustration with life's lack of opportunities is frequently cancelled out by fear of change. Some move on, some remain rooted, wedded to familiar fixtures and fittings. Others, like Bob and Terry, revisit their youth, only to find it buried beneath the rubble. It's a perennial theme in the prematurely aged pop songs of the late 1960s.

That push and pull between leaving and staying plays a prominent role in many of the best lyrics of the period. 'A modern nostalgic can be homesick and sick of home at once,' says Svetlana Boym,[38] and that's Ray Davies to a tee. 'Where did my go go? / Where did the pleasure go?' he sings in 'Where Did the Spring Go?', a lamentation that would have done Bob Ferris and Terry Collier proud. Entrenchment is constantly doing battle with restlessness and the desire to get away in his songs. The suspicion that the other man's grass is always greener is constantly undermined by the fatal discovery that when he does arrive at his desired destination, there isn't actually any grass to be green about. Ray Davies creates Arcadias, but they are only ever temporary, and only ever as stable as his anxieties will allow. Penny Lane is in Paul McCartney's ears and eyes. Ray Davies's idylls are all in the mind. His Arcadia is only ever film-set scenery, flimsy theatrical partitioning, and about as robust. When he sings, 'But I don't feel afraid,' in 'Waterloo Sunset', he does actually sound a little bit afraid. In 'Days' he sings, 'I'm not frightened of this world, believe me,' and you don't quite believe him then either.

Up until the end of 1967 the dominant themes in Davies's writing were class, status, social conditions and societal expectations, all rendered masterfully in a prolific outpouring of witty, acerbic three-minute sketches. From 1968 onwards his muse seemed increasingly adrift in limbo land, expressing a mindset that was vaguely post-colonial and pre-welfare state. At times his writing seems almost Orwellian, not Orwell the *1984* dystopian, but Orwell the *Tribune* essayist, the chronicler of *Boy's Own* comic and the decline of the English murder story, Orwell the celebrator of the Moon and Sixpence, the fictitious pub he evokes in order to mourn a dying culture. Like Orwell, Davies developed an unsparing eye for detail, an economy of description and an inability to pen a dull or superfluous line. In other ways he seems reminiscent of a Bloomsbury essayist, Harold Nicolson wryly recollecting past colleagues and acquaintances while slyly blurring the line between biography and autobiography, as he does in his 1927 collection *Some People*. At other times Davies resembles an E. M. Forster of the pop age, perpetually worrying about the little man in the era of Big History, and faithfully documenting emotional anxiety and political impotence in the context of societal upheaval. He chronicles the lives of people who are permanently at the beck and call of social forces bigger than themselves, forever enslaved by the relentless grind of progress and the ruthless march of time.

These are the themes that dominate the 1968 album *The Kinks Are the Village Green Preservation Society*. Twelve months earlier, during the first full flowering of psychedelia, Eric Burdon offered a historical roll call of those who heralded the winds of change. He namechecked King Oliver, Duke Ellington, Jelly Roll Morton, Bessie Smith, Robert Johnson, Chick Webb, Charlie Christian, Billie Holiday, Alan Freed, Big Joe Turner, B. B. King, Charlie Parker, Louis Jordan, Ray Charles, Chuck Berry, Fats Domino, Elvis Presley, the Beatles, the Rolling Stones, Frank Zappa, the Mamas and the Papas, Ravi Shankar and Jimi Hendrix. A year later Ray Davies defiantly celebrated the winds of unchange. His lineage comprises Donald Duck, vaudeville and variety, Desperate Dan, strawberry jam ('and all the different varieties'), draught beer, Mrs Mopp, Old Mother Riley, custard pies, the George Cross, Sherlock Holmes, Fu Manchu, Moriarty, Dracula, little shops, china cups and virginity, Tudor houses, antique tables and billiards. As Davies put it in *X-Ray*, 'While everyone in the world was gravitating towards love, peace and San Francisco, the Kinks were in a London suburb making this strange little record about an imaginary village green . . . While everybody else thought that the hip thing to do was drop acid, do as many drugs as possible and listen to music in a coma, the Kinks were singing songs about lost friends, draught beer, motorbike riders, wicked witches and flying cats.'[39]

The Kinks Are the Village Green Preservation Society was no bland exercise in little England sentimentality or revivalism. The green is as much a metaphor as an actual physical place. It's a wilfully picturesque representation of the rural from an urbanite's perspective, a rurality that was in decline long before the Kinks celebrated it. *Village Green* is informed in the main not by cosy nostalgia but by fear and anomie and a plea for safe haven and sanctuary. Its central themes are change and resistance to change. The village green itself only ever seems a village-hall petition away from the bulldozers, the redevelopers and the road-widening scheme. It's the world that George Orwell chronicled in his 1939 novel *Coming Up for Air*, where on a whim the central protagonist, George Bowling, decides to revisit the rural haunts of his youth, only to find that the property speculators and the concrete spread of suburbia have got there first. Even the fondly remembered village pond where he once fished has been filled in with rubbish. The themes Orwell wrote about were just as prevalent in 1968 as they had been in the 1930s. Slum clearance may have erased some of the dead-end streets, but as the film version of *The London Nobody Knows* clearly illustrated, these were simply making way for the high-rise slums of the future. All people really wanted was indoor plumbing, but their communities (and the community consciousness that went with them) were demolished in the name of progress. This is the world that Ray Davies so meticulously chronicles. The *Village Green* album cherishes and celebrates English iconography, but it also mourns the ways of life that went with these now vanished mementos. The writer Jeremy Seabrook once said that English working-class people are only nostalgic because they are always having things taken away from them. Ray Davies recognised that too.

In 'Do You Remember Walter?', the narrator fondly remembers an old school friend, the good times they had together and their childhood dreams and ambitions. But even Walter is a metaphor, 'just an echo of a world I knew so long ago', and in the song's crushing denouement the narrator is left with little but lingering regret as he realises he and his old school pal would have little in common and nothing to talk about even if they did meet again. He rails against Walter, imagining that he's probably fat and married now, but readily acknowledges that he is the one stuck in the past and that he would bore Walter with his reminiscences. It's Walter who has moved on and he who has the rosy view of the past. By the time we get to the closing track, 'People Take Pictures of Each Other', the music-hall lilt of the melody is constantly being undermined by the pessimistic tone of the lyric. People take photos 'to prove that they really existed', sings Davies, offering a weary 'don't show me no more, please'.

The most splendidly Arcadian album of them all was the Zombies' famously misspelled 1968 masterpiece *Odessey and Oracle*. Recording began during the first week of June 1967, the very week that *Sgt Pepper* was released. 'Three-hour sessions,' remembers keyboard player Rod Argent of the Abbey Road studios' notoriously rigid work practices. 'Two till five. Tea break. Then seven till ten. Finish at ten on the dot.' 'And they all wore white coats when they came in and moved the pianos about,' says bass player Chris White. 'Lunchtime was strict hours too.' Despite the regimented procedures, the Zombies took full of advantage of Abbey Road's sumptuous facilities and the engineers' proactive approach to augmentation. 'The chaps with the long coats they had their own maintenance department, so not only was something fixed very quickly down in the basement by very efficient guys when it went wrong, but if you wanted something a bit different they were willing to rejig the studio to facilitate whatever you wanted to do,' remembers vocalist Colin Blunstone. This blend of discipline and indulgence, strict adherence to routine coupled with creative licence, produced some

of the most adventurous English LPs of the late 1960s. All of the Beatles' best work, the Pink Floyd EMI albums and the Zombies' *Odessey and Oracle* itself all bear testimony to this approach.

When I interviewed the surviving members of the Zombies in 2008 to commemorate the fortieth anniversary of the album's release, a more quintessentially English scene you could not have conjured. In the melancholic late-afternoon light of an autumn day we sat in the restaurant garden of Abbey Road studios, under a spreading horse chestnut tree. Bass player Chris White expertly threaded a conker with the help of his Swiss army penknife and time-honoured skills remembered from childhood. For the entirety of our chat my interview tape was periodically punctuated by the sound of horse chestnuts falling and splitting open on the stone flagging below. Occasionally a robin redbreast issued shrill territorial warnings from the bushes. This being London in the twenty-first century a police surveillance helicopter occasionally buzzed menacingly overhead, drowning out the voices on the tape. It was as befitting a scenario as you could have imagined for this most English of bands, and it seemed to sum up the *Odessey and Oracle* album perfectly. Idyllic English pastimes undermined by darker forces. Birdsong and spies in the sky vying for attention with the sound of autumn shedding its skin.

Odessey and Oracle was a thing of rare beauty, a delicate, softly spoken anachronism in the age of 'Street Fighting Man' and armchair revolution. It doesn't make grand statements about the human condition, just a series of gently reflective ones. Every jaunty, carefree sentiment has an unsettling or bittersweet counterpoint. For every song of celebration, friendship and conciliation there's one about absence, fear and loss. Unabashed optimism is tempered by melancholic reflection. Svetlana Boym's suggestive synecdoche of memory dominates the album.

'I think most of our songs even from the beginning had a bit of a melancholy thing, or a slightly darker thing,' says Rod Argent. 'Harmonically as well as lyrically.' When I interviewed the band I was determined to hang an entire treatise on such observations and I pressed them to elaborate, hoping that we might somehow alchemise the recipe for olde English pop melancholia out of thin October air. But after a few minutes of bemused reflection the formula remained as elusive and mercurial as Colin Blunstone's fragile and wistful enunciation and we went back to making small talk about exquisite things.

The album's vocal arrangements made full use of the increasing sophistication of studio technology, which at the time was in a period of transition between four- and eight-track. The multi-tracking of voices was clearly influenced by the Beach Boys' *Pet Sounds*: two- or three-part harmonies appear on almost every track. But on *Odessey and Oracle* Brian Wilson's 'Four Freshmen on acid' approach was anglophiled into soaring Home Counties bel canto and choral overlays that owed more to high church than high times. Inspired too by 'Strawberry Fields Forever', the Zombies added mellotron to their already rich sound world. Like everything else on the album, the mellotron presents itself unobtrusively and is weaved seamlessly into the rich textural tapestry of the songs. Musically the whole affair is characterised by an absence of indulgence. No idea is stretched too thin. No song outstays its welcome. There are no guitar pyrotechnics, no psychedelic longueurs. There is no jamming, no noodling, no surplus. And no drugs either.

'We all drank, but Hugh the drummer was the only one who even smoked cigarettes at that time,' remembers Chris White. 'We did believe in peace and love because that was that short period where it was a wonderful expansion of human existence, but the psychedelic thing in our minds wasn't necessarily linked with drugs. It was just an expansion of the mind.' This mild-mannered English attitude to excess was very Zombies: tolerant of others but not prone to indulgence themselves. 'We obviously knew people who took drugs, and I didn't mind that at all, but personally I wasn't attracted because it always seemed quite a crude way to expand your mind,' rationalises Argent. He describes drugs as 'a crude mechanism', likening their function to throwing a spanner in the works just for explosive effect. The band did, though, get into transcendental meditation. 'We never went to India. We never flew or levitated. Just used it for relaxation. Still do,' says White.

Odessey and Oracle's opening track, 'Care of Cell 44', sets the tone perfectly. On the surface it's a song about homecoming, until you discover that the girl he's serenading is in prison. 'A Rose for Emily' is a similarly sombre vignette. Like 'Eleanor Rigby', it's a song for the unloved and the lonely. Reflection and remembrance cast long shadows over the entire album. White's material in particular conveys a palpable air of longing. 'There was a harking back to halcyon times in a lot of our

songs,' he admits. 'But don't forget, it was the post-war period. We'd only just come out of rationing. My parents had a shop when they retired and I remember we took ration cards in the shop. It was a period of growth and a period of looking back, all at the same time.' 'Beechwood Park' was White's 'Penny Lane', his 'Itchycoo Park', his 'Blackberry Way', his Home Counties Arcadia. 'It was a girls' school in a village called Markyate, between St Albans and Dunstable,' he explains. The song took its title from the boarding school that stood in acres of beautiful countryside, bordered by woodland. 'We used to deliver groceries from the shop up there. They used the school as the army camp for the film *The Dirty Dozen* in 1967. I remember what it was like walking in the lanes around Beechwood Park, that lovely feeling on a hot summer's day when you've just had a rainstorm and the steam is rising up and everything smells fantastic.'

Odessey and Oracle was an out-of-kilter curio, unmistakably of its time and yet out of time, rare, precious and a little too ornate for its habitat. Shortly after its release the album slipped quietly out of public memory, a soon forgotten remnant of some other age. It had arrived without bombast or hype, and for a long time its unassuming nature looked to have sealed its fate. Slowly but surely, though, it snuck up on history's inside lane. Hip kids began to discover it, as hip kids are prone to do, and it is now regarded as one of the most accomplished works of its era. It's the musical equivalent of Geoffrey Fletcher casting his sights skywards above the grim featureless streets and spying some beautiful wrought-iron work on a balcony railing, or Barbara Jones spotting a carefully etched decorative motif on an overgrown mossy seat or abandoned canal barge. The album's misspelled title only adds to its charm, like the incorrectly inscribed shop-front sign that nobody can be bothered to paint over. Nicolete Gray, Barbara Jones and Geoffrey Fletcher, themselves relatively uncelebrated and unsung, taught us how to look afresh at the neglected, the ephemeral, the forgotten. It's somehow fitting that *Odessey and Oracle* should have been subject to those same processes of re-evaluation.

Don't Show Me No More, Please

'Is this a significance which *I* read into them? In other words, is there a mythology of the mythologists?' asks Roland Barthes in the introduction to his book *Mythologies*. 'No doubt, and the reader will easily see where I stand,' he replies, readily admitting to his own subjectivity.[40] I'm admitting to my subjectivity too. Nostalgic yearnings are subjective. Madeleine moments can be triggered by the most unlikely stimuli – a dunked biscuit here, a déjà vu there. They genuflect to the strains of long-forgotten chord sequences from long-forgotten tunes heard in long-forgotten circumstances, but they can just as easily be triggered by the smell of a freshly creosoted fence, the sight of a Thornley's Cattle Feed sign, a war memorial in the town square, much like the one you were walking past when you first heard that tune.

Which brings us finally to the Ian MacDonald quote at the beginning of this chapter. Although divided in age by six years – he would have been seventeen, I was only eleven – I have almost identical memories of the summer of 1966, right down to the sky-gazing epiphany. Offshore radio was at its peak and my listening habits were simple and uncomplicated. I tuned in to one pirate station and only tuned to another when they played a bad record, an extended ad break or donated half an hour to one of those sponsored religious programmes that helped pay the bills. Like MacDonald, I can remember entire uninterrupted passages of time when every record they played was great. There is much else I remember about that summer. The constant sunshine – not a case of false-memory syndrome, it was a long hot summer – made activity sporadic even to a sugar-fuelled eleven-year-old. The Lovin' Spoonful's 'Summer in the City' emanated from the sticky heat of urban LA, but its montage of traffic noise and road drills played just as well in my small town, as the tar melted in the roads and the thistle-down tumbled on wavy layers of heat. 'The long days seduce all thoughts away,' wrote Elizabeth Smart in *By Grand Central Station I Sat Down and Wept*. 'And we lie like the lizards in the sun, postponing our lives indef-initely.' That was my summer of '66 in a nutshell. Grime-ridden and rusting steam trains still occasionally chugged by and much of my six-week summer holiday was spent lounging with my mates on the luggage trolleys on plat-form four of our local railway station, taking down numbers, playing shove ha'penny into the perfectly shaped cylindrical holes in the barrows and flicking the dial from Radio Caroline to Radio London to Radio England to Radio City and back again. The railway station employed a gardener, as railway stations still did back then,

and the town's name was spelled out in the luscious flower beds. The toilets stank. The sun shone. Somewhere in the nearby faraway distance the drone of a woodyard buzz saw sounded. The chimes of competing ice-cream vans played on a forever loop. No one both-ered us and we bothered no one. The summer of 1966 is as freeze-framed for me as the Edwardian era must have been for many who survived the horrors of the Great War and lived to tell, or, more often than not, suppress, the tale. I'm not citing like for like. I'm not comparing the growing pains and rites of passage of a 1960s adolescence with the experiences of a boy not much older than I was then crouching scared witless in the rat-infested trenches of Ypres. But I am suggesting that they evoke the same impulses, and they both emanate from an identical desire that is wont to take remembrance and escape in its emotional grip, a hold that the passing of time can never loosen.

I suspect that something similar happens with all nostalgic impulses. Piece by piece a psychological barrier is built, until we can but peer through peepholes in the Wonderwall, through knot holes in a freshly creosoted fence, through wormholes in the fabric of time and marvel at what's on the other side, knowing that we can never go back there and suspecting that we wouldn't really want to anyway even if we could, but missing some aspect of its essence, and acknowledging its continued allure all the same. In the midst of fame, in retreat from the madness of Beatlemania, Lennon and McCartney cast their minds back to the certainties of childhood days. Wouldn't you?

16

INFANTASIA

Kinder Psych and Toytown Pop

At first glance nostalgia is a longing for a place, but actually it is a yearning for a different time – the time of our childhood, the slower rhythms of our dreams.

SVETLANA BOYM[1]

Somehow the sun does not seem to shine so brightly as it used; the trackless meadows of old time have shrunk and dwindled away to a few poor acres. A saddening doubt, a dull suspicion creeps over me. Et in Arcadia ego.

KENNETH GRAHAME, *The Golden Age*[2]

Et in Arcadia ego. Even in Arcady, there am I. Death is even in Arcady. And in Arcadia I am. Even in Arcadia I exist. Regardless of which translation you accept, Kenneth Grahame's Latin lamentation essentially means one thing: nothing lasts for ever and nothing disappears so rapidly (and yet retains its emotional hold so assiduously) as childhood. In 'The Olympians', the prologue to *The Golden Age*, which the above passage concludes, Grahame reminds himself, as so many other writers have done, that amid the idyllic splendour of temporary paradise death of a kind always lurks: the death of innocence, the death of unawareness or, as the mind grapples with its own biological inevitability, the death of childhood itself. Lewis Carroll mourns this too. *Alice in Wonderland* is about many things, but more than anything it is about a girl on the threshold of maturity, confronting the turbulence of growing up. It is through her eyes that we are invited to view the world in all its haphazard manifestations. Grahame's lament, written in 1895, ends: 'Can it be that I also have become an Olympian?'[3] – Olympian being the writer's synonym for the encroachment of adulthood. He acknowledges in *The Golden Age*, and in its companion volume *Dream Days*, published in 1898, that his entire perspective on life is filtered through the misty veil of reminiscence. These are not children's books. They are books that mourn the passing of childhood. The distinction is crucial.

At the end of 'Fall Out', the final episode of the 1967/8 TV series *The Prisoner*, Patrick McGoohan, as Number 6, having finally escaped the Village enacts a childlike mime to a bemused police officer as he tries to explain what he has been through. It's an apposite in-joke to end on. McGoohan's exaggerated gestures, shown in long shot on the busy streets of London, are as impenetrable to the police officer as much of the series was to the watching public. After seventeen episodes, during which he has been incarcerated for refusing to be 'pushed, filed, stamped, indexed, briefed, debriefed and numbered', the only way he feels he can explain his plight to the outside world is through the expression of child mime. *The Prisoner*, although ostensibly about espionage and betrayal, always had a distinctly prelapsarian feel to it. Evocations of childhood surface throughout the seventeen episodes. The servitude of the helpless occupants of the mysterious Village is little different to that experienced by the average child. The confined habitat is essentially Alice's dream world with added cold-war sensibilities, and is populated by similarly Carrollesque passive-aggressive character types. The Village seems to be one huge kindergarten for displaced adults, a place where the recalcitrant are made regressive and the conformists get to wear bright primary colours and ride around in toytown taxis. In episode fourteen, 'The Girl Who Was Death', first shown in January 1968, a child's

storybook is the method the authorities use to try and get inside the mind of No. 6. Adventure-book illustrations are shown fleetingly throughout the episode, but the nature of the mind-control technique is not made explicit until the final scene, when No. 6, having successfully resisted the interrogation, puts down the book and the contented children go to sleep. Turning to the surveillance cameras he says, 'Goodnight, children . . . everywhere,' echoing the wartime catchphrase of the BBC's *Children's Favourites* presenter Uncle Mac. 'Goodnight Children Everywhere' was also the title of a much-loved song by Vera Lynn that became something of an anthem during the Second World War for the parents of evacuees. When McGoohan turns to the camera and utters those same three words, he offers a powerful double-edged rejoinder, taunting to his captors, but poignant to those who recall the broken bonds of childhood. It's psychedelia in microcosm: the hopscotch steps back to infancy abetted or disrupted by the presence of adulthood.

William Empson, in his 1935 essay 'Alice in Wonderland: The Child as Swain', locates the origins of this yearning for childhood certainties in the work of the nineteenth-century Romantic poets, particularly Wordsworth and

Coleridge. 'It is the whole point of the "Ode to Intimations" and even of "We are Seven",' he says. 'The child has not yet been put wrong by civilization, and all grown ups have been.'[4] Empson claims that scientific rationalism is the source of this flight from reason. The child as embodiment of loss, he argued, arose with the age of utility, and it 'runs through all Victorian and Romantic literature; the world of the adult made it hard to be an artist, and they kept a sort of taproot going down to their experience as children'.[5] That same taproot plunges deep into the subterranean well of psychedelic pop. In its various ways psychedelia too sought out the trackless meadows of old time. On 'Bike', a song both charming and sinister, Syd Barrett invited us into 'the other room', a place that chimed to the sound of clockwork automata and nightmarish loops. Many followed Barrett into that 'other room' and inhaled the 'doll's house darkness / old perfume' that he refers to in another childhood evocation, 'Matilda Mother'. The Straw Headed Peter silhouettes of Barrett's best childhood songs cast shadows on the womb-like walls of all English nursery pop. The dominant image of Haight-Ashbury in its heyday was all those love children skipping and gambolling around Golden Gate Park, the air thick with unconfined joy as they also sought out the slow rhythms of their dreams. In England too, in London at least, participants in the great psychedelic masquerade gleefully dipped into the dressing-up box and pulled out the pixie dresses and the elf cloaks. There were times in the late 1960s when the English counter-culture seemed to resemble one huge kindergarten party. To a large extent it was a middle-class retreat from affluence and progress – for nineteenth-century rationalism read 1950s scientific management – but fear of the A-bomb, the H-bomb and all the other bombs to come had a lot to do with it too. It was the nuclear threat that caused the most pandemic retreat of all. Kurt Vonnegut once said that he grew up believing that science was truth and that he would live long enough to see a photograph of God on the front of *Time* magazine – and then, as he put it, 'they dropped truth on Hiroshima'. *Et in Arcadia ego*.

Add a microscopic droplet of LSD to these tender sensibilities and you have a recipe for playtime games without frontiers. Exultation at the altar of acid sometimes led to mystic communion with the godhead, but it could just as easily induce a state of childlike euphoria. Opening all those neocortex filters and saturating the body's inhibitory mechanisms with all that unprocessed sensory data prevents the adult mind from carrying out its normal blah blah blah. It can no longer modulate, moderate or instigate the necessary rationale that prevents us all from living in a permanent state of regressive grace. The nine-to-five mindset cannot function smoothly, distracted as it is by the universal 'wow' and the desire to fasten the brain to a pretty balloon. Ordinarily only two groups get to function like this on a regular basis: small children and the certifiably insane. LSD doesn't just cleanse the doors of perception, fathom hell and soar angelic, it also opens the Wendy house windows of the soul.

Edward Lear, Lewis Carroll, Kenneth Grahame, Hilaire Belloc, C. S. Lewis, Beatrix Potter, Charles Kingsley, J. M. Barrie and Enid Blyton were all consumed avidly by the baby-boomer generation born in the post-war years. This was the generation that hit its teens and twenties during the psychedelic sixties. Lewis Carroll's influence had been a constant in British fantasy life ever since the Great War revived the appeal of the *Alice* stories and sent readers fleeing to whatever womb-like Arcadia they could find. A model of John Tenniel's White Knight beckoned Festival of Britain visitors

into the Lion and Unicorn Pavilion in 1951, and an elaborate tableau of Alice going through the looking glass awaited them inside. With the miniature model railway, the funfair and the coloured fountains gushing 'indigo water waltzing to music', as Dylan Thomas put it, there was a strong childhood element to the entire festival. The psychedelic subtext of *Alice's Adventures in Wonderland* and *Alice Through the Looking Glass* became abundantly clear once LSD usage became widespread. *Alice*-inspired imagery found its way into an abundance of songs. Jefferson Airplane's 'White Rabbit', which namechecks Alice, the caterpillar, the White Knight, the Red Queen and the dormouse, was probably the most famous, but direct references or allusions to Lewis Carroll's best-known work can also be found in 'I Am the Walrus' (the Beatles), 'House for Everyone' (Traffic), 'Alice Is a Long Time Gone' and 'The Mad Hatter's Song' (the Incredible String Band), 'Little Girl Lost and Found' (Garden Club), 'Alice in Wonderland' (Central Nervous System), 'Jabberwock' and 'Which Dreamed It' (Boeing Duveen and the Beautiful Soup), 'Looking Glass Alice' (the Bunch), 'Who Planted Thorns in Miss Alice's Garden?' (Tom Northcott/ the Explosive), 'Alice Designs' (the

Sugarbeats), 'The Lion and the Unicorn' (Skip Bifferty) and 'Alice in Wonderland' (Berkeley Kites).

Even when songs didn't make direct reference to *Alice* the influence was there in the dreamtime ambience and the startling jump cuts and lurches in tempo. Reading the books afresh now it's not hard to see how they were so readily appropriated as psychedelic texts. In *Alice's Adventures in Wonderland* the main character experiences extreme size distortions; she grows and shrinks seemingly at will. These distortions usually occur after she has drunk an unnamed liquid from a bottle labelled 'Drink Me' or nibbled on a small cake found in a glass jar marked 'Eat Me'. When she is small Alice almost drowns in the pool of tears she had wept when she was nine feet tall. When she is nine feet tall Alice muses on what it would be like to send presents to her own feet ('*Alice's Right Foot, Esq., Hearthrug, near the Fender*').[6] In *Through the Looking Glass* she floats 'gently down without even touching the stairs with her feet, then she floated on through the hall, and would have gone straight out at the door in the same way if she hadn't caught hold of the door post'.[7] Schizophrenic-like inner voices are present in both books but are frequently more disturbing in *Through*

the Looking Glass. Sometimes they speak alone, at other times in a maddening chorus. 'I hope you understand what thinking in chorus means,' Carroll interjects, 'for I must confess that I don't.'[8]

Bad-trip scenarios loom up suddenly and unexpectedly in both books. In the *Wonderland* chapter 'Pig and Pepper' the cook throws fire irons, saucepans, plates and dishes at the Duchess and her baby, who eventually turns into a pig. In *Through the Looking Glass* the White Queen, who lives backwards, slowly forsakes human language, begins to bleat and gradually turns into a sheep. She screams 'so exactly like the whistle of a steam engine that Alice had to hold both her hands over her ears'.[9] The Red Queen screams at the top of her voice when she proposes a toast to Queen Alice. Humpty Dumpty also frequently raises his voice to a nightmarish scream.

As Queen Alice prepares to make her acceptance speech, the size distortions reappear just as she is rising to speak. 'And she really did rise as she spoke, several inches,' says Carroll, 'but she got hold of the edge of the table and managed to pull herself down again.'[10] The candles on the table spiral up to the ceiling, 'looking something like a bed of rushes with fireworks at the top'[11] – one of the most hallucinatory images that Carroll ever summoned. Meanwhile, back at the banquet table the bottles pick up plates and attach them as wings, and use the cutlery as legs. The White Queen disappears into the soup tureen, and by the end of the chapter 'several of the guests were lying down in the dishes and the soup ladle was walking up the table towards Alice's chair, and beckoning her impatiently to get out of the way'.[12] In the midst of this culinary turmoil it is comforting to note that Carroll slips in an impeccably English observation on good manners and that the ladle gives Alice fair warning of its intentions.

Over the years the *Alice* stories have lent themselves to all kinds of analysis: historical, theological, political, philosophical. Everyone from the Freudians to the Darwinians has claimed a piece of the landscape. It shouldn't, therefore, come as any surprise that in keeping with the tradition of treating the *Alice* stories as endlessly interpretable, acid users in the 1960s should claim them as their own and treat them as route maps to the unconscious, to be read alongside, and at times a great deal more instructively than, *The Doors of Perception* and *The Politics of Ecstasy*. For these readers LSD revealed in *Alice* not layers of obscurantism to be

academically pondered and pored over, but an all-too-familiar dream logic.

On Wednesday 28 December 1966, as English psychedelia was about to pass through the gates of dawn, the BBC showed Jonathan Miller's bold TV adaptation of *Alice in Wonderland*. Miller presented Lewis Carroll's tale as a disorientating Kafkaesque dreamscape, and the tempo of his small-screen adaptation remained faithful to the pace of the book: slow, contemplative and drowsy episodes punctuated by occasional hysteria. The milieu is the Victorian drawing room, the morning room, fussing nannies, decrepit octogenarians, walled gardens, derelict greenhouses, Escher-like staircases that lead to tiny rooms and endless elongated corridors. The Caucus-Race is reimagined as a St Vitus-charged chase of doddering idiots who stumble round the quadrants of what could be a university but could just as easily be an insane asylum; in Miller's knowingly analogous world the distinction is a thin one.

The production begins with a recitation from Wordsworth's 1807 'Ode: Intimations of Immortality from Recollections of Early Childhood'. This is followed by the opening bars of the hymn 'Immortal Invisible (God Only Wise)', struck slowly on a cimbalom. Informed as much by a close reading of

William Empson's 'The Child as Swain' as he was by Kafka, Miller draws on that familiar taproot that goes back to the Romantics. He prefaces his tale with Wordsworth's 'It is not now as it hath been of yore' rather than Carroll's equally serviceable and arguably more celestial 'where childhood dreams are twined / in memory's mystic band'. And he reprises Wordsworth's 'Ode' at the end, as Alice rouses herself from her dream sleep in the summer meadow, again in preference to Carroll's closing soliloquy about a 'dream of Wonderland of long ago', but the message remains the same. *Et in Arcadia ego.*

Miller wished his central character to look 'Rossetti-like, rather than Tenniel',[13] but his Alice still has something of the Tenniel illustration about her. She drifts through the story, looking perennially bent out of shape, as if all those bodily contortions have mildly disfigured her. When she runs she presents an elongated spectacle with her starchy triangular frizz of hair, egg-timer waist and billowing petticoats and skirt. Miller cast well-known names in many of the leading roles: his *Beyond the Fringe* colleagues Peter Cook and Alan Bennett played the March Hare and the Mouse; Wilfred Brambell was the White Rabbit; Gordon Gostelow, who also played Perks

in *The Railway Children*, was 1st Gardener; Leo McKern, who played one of the most memorable Number 2s in *The Prisoner*, dragged up to play the Duchess; John Gielgud and Malcolm Muggeridge, as the Mock Turtle and the Gryphon, pranced about on a pebbled Sussex beach like a couple of old hams as they recited 'The Lobster Quadrille'. The only unknown, Alice herself, was played by the thirteen-year-old Anne-Marie Mallik. After giving a memorable performance of one of the most iconic roles in children's literature Mallik never acted again in her life.

In one of the adaptation's most blatantly psychedelic scenes Michael Redgrave recites the lines of the Caterpillar, *sans* hookah. He is first seen seated at a table in a dimly lit morning room, where he absently dusts the disassembled wooden interior of a model Christopher Wren-style church. It's a clever visual joke, Venetian classical architecture ripped apart to reveal its innards, a knowing nod to the world of logic and proportion which Carroll similarly tears asunder. Agitated by the intrusion into his private domain the Caterpillar asks Alice the question she has just whispered to herself: 'Who are you?' In the book she answers haltingly, nervously, 'I–I hardly know, Sir, just at present – at least I know who

I *was* when I got up this morning, but I think I must have been changed several times since then.'[14] In Miller's adaptation she replies distractedly as she gazes around the room. There are other subtle changes too. 'Just at present' in the book is changed to 'Just at the moment'. 'Moment' conveys the vivid immediacy of sensations more than the more generalised blurry 'present' of her dream state. 'I must have been changed' becomes 'I've changed', making Alice the knowing and defiant mistress of her own destiny, rather than simply the subject of external forces. The constant inner dialogue that Alice has with herself is transposed to a lower key. The frenetic jabberings of the book are related in hushed whispers. Meanwhile, the action teeters constantly, as William Empson put it, 'between the luscious nonsense world of fantasy and the ironic nonsense world of fact'.[15] Miller's Alice exudes an air of inner calm and bemusement, expressing only occasional mild annoyance at the idiocy that surrounds her. The episodic hysteria of the original text is reduced to a muted irritability. In the face of adult regression the child Alice remains diffident, haughty, aloof.

The dreamlike quality of Carroll's narrative is visually illustrated with time-lapse cinematography and distorted lens. The Mad Tea Party seems to go on for a year and a day as thoughts ossify, conversation dribbles into inconsequentiality and food sits unattended on the long table. In her dream state Alice appears belladonna-eyed and uncomprehending, but knowing just enough to realise that most of what she encounters is nonsense. In other words, she confronts the world as any imaginative child would. The adaptation's soundtrack was provided by Ravi Shankar, whose sitar drones enhance the dreamlike quality of the action. Peals of raga notes accompany Alice as she skitters through the long grass in pursuit of fleeting glimpses and visitations. By eschewing the string quartet and drawing-room piano more commonly associated with Victorian adaptations Shankar's soundtrack serves a dual purpose: it adds a shimmering veer of psychedelic exotica to the story, but places the story in its colonial context too. 'Miller has argued that he wanted to bring the empire back in using the score to evoke the images of India that Alice Liddell would have been familiar with, no doubt from copies of the *Illustrated London News* left around the house,' says Rohan McWilliam. 'The film is a reminder that Britain in the 1960s was trying to come to terms with the loss of the empire that the Victorians had built up. It acknowledges the imperial content that is ostensibly invisible in so many Victorian texts.'[16]

Miller did not envisage his adaptation as an LSD trip. It just looks that way. It had, in fact, been three years in the planning before it was aired, so even allowing for the prescient use of Ravi Shankar, psychedelia was clearly not an influence. But its hazy replications of the logic twists and warped perceptions of the LSD trip were unmistakable. By the time it was shown a second time on 2 April 1967 psychedelia had moved on apace and the subtext was abundantly clear. *Alice* was by now ripe for appropriation and a whole new generation took fresh inspiration from its hallucinatory inversion of the ordered moral universe.

A preponderance of nursery-rhyme pop songs emerged at the height of the psychedelic era. As usual the Beatles started it, with their summer of 1966 single 'Yellow Submarine', and it should never be forgotten that at the height of their fame they lent their likeness (and some of their best psychedelic songs) to an animated feature film of the same name. They probably ended it too with 'Maxwell's Silver Hammer'. And in the space of three months at the end of 1967 three Top 10 hits in the UK charts featured children or childlike voices in a prominent role. On Keith West's 'Excerpt from a Teenage Opera' a chorus of children sang the main 'Grocer Jack' refrain. Traffic's 'Hole in My Shoe' featured a young girl reciting a fairy-tale evocation of climbing onto the back of a giant albatross and being transported to a land where happiness reigned all year round. 'Kites' by Simon Dupree and the Big Sound featured the actress Jacqui Chan reciting faux Orientalism in a little-girl voice over the instrumental break. In July 1968 another unlikely Top 30 hit, a radical adaptation of Leonard Bernstein's 'America' by the Nice, featured an altogether less innocent and awestruck eulogy as a child with a pronounced Home Counties accent hesitantly declared, 'America is pregnant with promise and antic-i-payshun, but is murdered by the hand of the inevitable,' over the track's explosive climax. Walt Disney it wasn't.

On 29 March 1967 Simon Dupree and the Big Sound were filmed at Stonehouse Church hall in Gloucestershire for a BBC *Man Alive* documentary, 'The Ravers'. The documentary shows them performing in front of an excitable, albeit camera-conscious crowd of young females, most of whom look like they would happily strip the group down to their eyelashes and carry home the spoils if the film crew wasn't there. The performance footage features the group's two most recent singles, 'I See the Light' and 'Day Time, Night Time', the former an organ-driven, hand-clapping stomper, the latter moody soul pop, both typical of their oeuvre and their era. By the end of the year Simon Dupree and the Big Sound would be in the Top 10 with 'Kites', a gentle psychedelic song complete with wind-machine effects, Chinese gong, mellotron and vibraphone. The nucleus of the group comprised Portsmouth-based siblings Derek, Phil and Ray Schulman, three blue-eyed soul brothers who started off life as the Howling Wolves and then the Roadrunners, performing R&B standards and more than holding their own against the Geno Washingtons of this world. 'Kites' changed everything. Like many a contemporary combo who had other ideas about where their interests lay, they hated the hit, performing it self-consciously, even mockingly on stage, and all they could do in its wake was search in vain for that elusive follow-up success. They made nifty novelty pop ('There's a Little Picture Playhouse'), irritating novelty pop ('Broken Hearted Pirates'), frantic floor scorchers ('Reservations') and yearning psych pop ('She Gave Me the Sun',

'Thinking about My Life', 'For Whom the Bell Tolls'), all of it played with the tight-assed, neatly coiffured proficiency of musicians who had honed their craft in provincial youth clubs and ballrooms. In 1968 they appeared incognito as the Moles on a single called 'We Are the Moles', a Parlophone publicity stunt that was briefly and unconvincingly passed off as the work of the Beatles. 'We Are the Moles' was, in fact, the most psychedelic thing they ever recorded and would have made a credible official follow-up to 'Kites', but the record was sunk by its hype and there never was a follow-up hit. Affronted by the drudge life of the cabaret circuit and the dawning realisation that life was turning into one endless frilly-shirted soft-pop B-side, Simon Dupree and the Big Sound reinvented themselves as the progressive rock group Gentle Giant, where they wore the mythological mantle as naturally as they had previously passed themselves off as Howling Wolves.

Mark Wirtz was a talented young German-born staff producer taken on by EMI in 1966. He had already made a name for himself with his Mood Mosaic series of CinemaScope-style instrumentals; one of these, 'A Touch of Velvet – A Sting of Brass', had been a massive club hit and was widely known as the theme tune to the Dave Lee Travis show on Radio Caroline. In partnership with engineer Geoff Emerick, Wirtz produced and arranged several psychedelic classics, including 'My White Bicycle' by Tomorrow, '10,000 Words in a Cardboard Box' by the Aquarian Age and 'Shy Boy' by Kippington Lodge. Early in 1967 Wirtz began to formulate ideas for his own ambitious project, which he called *A Teenage Opera*. He envisaged the *Opera* as 'a kaleidoscope of stories, a bouquet of allegorical, tragic comic tales about a variety of characters and their fate, all related to each other by the common thread of living in the same imaginary turn-of-the-century village'. Borrowing vocalist Keith West and future Yes guitarist Steve Howe from Tomorrow, he created what was intended to be the first part of the work, 'Excerpt from a Teenage Opera'. According to Wirtz, when he presented the completed single to EMI in April 1967 their first reaction was that no one would buy a four-minute classically inspired pop record with children on it. The single, released under the name of Keith West in July 1967, reached number two in the UK pop charts and was played extensively during the final weeks of offshore pirate radio. It was only prevented from reaching number

one by Engelbert Humperdinck's 'The Last Waltz'. The lyric, written by West, concerned an elderly grocer called Jack who struggled to keep up with his daily deliveries and whom everyone took for granted until the day he dropped down dead, at which point the townsfolk were consumed with guilt over their previous neglect. The record featured a chorus of children supplied by the Hammersmith-based Corona Stage School, who sang spectacularly out of tune when they performed it live on *Top of the Pops*. With its assembled cast of innocents singing 'Is it true what Mummy says / you won't come back?' in saccharine voices, 'Excerpt from a Teenage Opera' could have come straight out of a mawkish music-hall melodrama, but the epic sweep of the arrangement, the compelling storyline and the strong moral message ('Now they wish they'd given Jack / more attention and respect') clearly struck a nerve among a substantial section of the record-buying public.

As its title tantalisingly suggested, the story of Grocer Jack was supposed to be the first part of an actual pop opera. In fact, only two further singles were released. 'Sam', the five-and-a-half-minute follow-up, concerned another old man. This one spent his days lovingly preserving a railway engine called

Glory, until he was made redundant for working on an uneconomical route. The song featured the same chorus of children who had sung on 'Excerpt from a Teenage Opera', singing a remarkably similar refrain too – 'Dear old Sam, we miss you so / we wish you would come back.' One further single was released, a barnstorming everything-but-the-kitchen-sink production called '(He's Our) Dear Old Weatherman', arranged and sung by Wirtz himself. When it also failed to reach the Top 20, EMI pulled the plug on the entire venture.

Toytown pop took many forms, embracing everything from the cutesy and the sentimental to the unsettling and the macabre. If you were of a brittle disposition or discerning musical persuasion, this sudden outbreak constituted as unbearable a congregation of the winsome and the execrable as it was possible to contemplate in the late 1960s. Frequently the twee factor spiralled out of control like an eighteen-foot beanstalk knitted by elves in paisley waistcoats. To any diehard mod still reeling at the fact that their Ray Charles-influenced heroes of yore had gone all soppy and soft while prancing round the mulberry bush and worshipping at the feet of rainbows, the prospect of them mincing about with picnic baskets and trilling about fluffy bunnies

and ice lollies must have been beyond the pale. The Alan Bown Set were a classic example of what happened when soul boys reverted to little boys. A well-respected club act led by a trumpeter who had formerly played with the John Barry Seven, their line-up featured a young Jess Roden on vocals, as well as future members of King Crimson and Supertramp. Their early live material featured an impressive mixture of soul and jazz covers. By 1967 they had ventured into the sprightly psych-pop territory that ensnared many English beat groups of the time. TV footage exists of them performing some exuberant Dadaist piss-take mime on the French pop show *Dim Dam Dom* in May 1967, where they perform music from the Alain Jessua film *Jeu de massacre* (*The Killing Game*). Guitars and saxophones are wielded as guns; Jess Roden pretends to drill a hole in his head with his microphone; keyboard player Jeff Bannister plays with his elbows and then extracts a magic-trick hanky from his mouth; the guitarists wield their instruments sitar-style. Everyone acts indecorously, in a way that simply wouldn't have been permissible on a buttoned-up English pop show. In the autumn of 1967 the Alan Bown! jumped aboard the puff-puff train with an MGM single, 'Toyland', backed with

'Technicolour Dream'. The B-side was a wistful romp through the spectrum (of colours and emotions), with brassy backing, stretchy vowels and a fade-out refrain of 'It's a dream / it's a dream,' just in case anyone hadn't got the message yet. The A-side was set to a flute and acoustic-guitar arrangement and commenced with an unambiguous invitation to 'Let's go down and blow our minds / in Toyland.' Clearly, the nursery dreams of children was now where it was at, rather than sharing a Marquee bill with Jimmy James and the Vagabonds. Jess Roden sings about mice, bears, honey and buttercups, when only a matter of months earlier he had been belting out Edwin Starr and Little Anthony and the Imperials covers.

Groups who didn't want to skip the whole length of the yellow brick road would frequently get to record one side of a single, usually the B-side, in their chosen style, thus allowing them to show off their musical chops. The other side would normally be written by an established publishing-house writer with an eye on commercial success and a shrewd ear for what was currently in vogue. This often led to groups sounding like Cream on one side of a record and Bernard Cribbins on the other. On 'Little Man with a Stick'/'Model Village'

by the Penny Peeps the A-side was composed by Les Reed and Barry Mason, purveyors of classic balladry to the pop gentry (Engelbert Humperdinck, Tom Jones, etc.). It boasts a great shimmering orchestral arrangement by Reed and an enchanting lyric by Mason, who when he wasn't penning 'The Last Waltz' and 'Love Grows (Where My Rosemary Goes)' turned out idiosyncratic solo singles like 'Rowbotham Square', a homage to a nighterie in Wigan that played 'music to blow your mind'. 'Little Man with a Stick' was an arch little tale of an encounter in the park ('after dark', naturally, but only because it rhymes with 'park') with a fool-on-the-hill type who in successive verses claims to be conducting an orchestra and wielding a sword in battle, but really he's just picking up litter. 'Little Man with a Stick' is out of the same leaf mould as 'Autumn Almanac' and in its own sweetly sinister way it deserves to be spoken of in the same breath as 'Arnold Layne'. The song acknowledges a great undocumented tribe that not even Geoffrey Fletcher noticed in the late sixties: those welfare-state longhairs who shuffled between council jobs with the parks and gardens department and whatever commune or ashram would take them. The B-side, 'Model Village', bears the unmistakable stamp of the Who, the Move, Tomorrow and the Yardbirds. Naturally, the band hated the A-side, as bands often did when material was foisted upon them by the Denmark Street publishing houses. In fact, 'Model Village' is the more derivative song of the two, sounding like an amalgam of 'My White Bicycle', 'Real Life Permanent Dream', 'I Can Hear the Grass Grow' and 'I'm a Boy', any one of which can be sung over its main riff.

'Toffee Apple Sunday'/'Romeo and Juliet' by the Newcastle group Toby Twirl similarly captures the yin and yang of toytown pop. The A-side, an organ and brass-led number, celebrates the annual Spanish City Fun Fair in Whitley Bay. It mentions the ghost train, the strongman, the penny arcade and winning a goldfish, but being versed in late-sixties melancholia it still finds time to lament the day after the fair has packed up and gone ('nothing left but the dew on the grass'). The flip side, 'Romeo and Juliet', transposes Shakespeare's tale of doomed love into the teenage terrain of the 1960s, with the singer asking, 'Would things be so different today?' Phrases are lifted directly or minimally adapted from the original play ('what light by yonder window breaks', 'parting was such sweet sorrow', 'with this kiss I take my life') and transport Elizabethan angst into the turmoil-tossed landscape of modern adolescence. It's

a surprisingly effective conceit, aided immensely by the song's stately tempo and anthemic brass, although I'm pretty certain that Shakespeare never said, 'Hang about / hey, hey / whatever would your mother say?'

'Weatherman' by John Bromley is a whole other toybox full of broken marionettes. A typically jaunty late-sixties string arrangement accompanies a song (which Bromley performed live on the children's TV show *Rainbow* in 1969) about two figures in a weather clock doomed never to meet. He comes out, she goes in. When it's rainy for him, it's sunny for her. With the power invested in the singer by the willing suspension of disbelief, the two figures are allowed to meet in the final verse. This is, after all, toytown pop and not 'Cease to Exist' by Charlie Manson.

'Two Little Ladies (Azalea and Rhododendron)' by Crocheted Doughnut Ring is a lily of the valley-scented tale of two old dears – 'delicate and antique', like the song itself. It's all tinkling pianos, tinkling teacups and a sprinkling of phasing. Azalea and Rhododendron parade up and down the street like animated porcelain figurines, greeting passers-by ('their friends and relations and all the creations to be') before tottering off to the sanctuary of their tidy little home, where there is a place for everything and everything is in its place. Lacking a B-side, the A-side was vaporised into pure abstraction by producer Peter Eden, with the aid of some deft tape manipulation, echo and distortion. He called it 'Nice'.

At the height of the beat-group boom the language of puppy love took a series of twists and turns that perhaps not even Bobby Rydell and Bobby Vee could have contemplated. The subject of adolescent crushes, often dealt with in tracks sung by men well into their twenties or even thirties, crops up frequently in the second half of the 1960s. 'Pamela Pamela' by Wayne Fontana, 'Fire Brigade' by the Move and 'Carrie Anne' by the Hollies are just three of the chart hits in which love, or rather lust, manifests itself in hopeful gropes, classroom notes and playground games. In the same way that certain aspects of Victorian childhood portraiture now look creepy and inappropriate, adult pop no longer harks back to skipping-rope rhymes and would never entertain the pervy role play of 'Carrie Anne''s 'I played a janitor / you played a monitor,' but these were if not more innocent times, then certainly less wary ones, and songwriters thought nothing of referencing love's first gaze across the classroom or playing field, and then having

it sung by paisley-shirted lotharios with dubious intentions. 'Amelia Jane' by the Sheffields is a bus-shelter snog of a song, a piece of late Mersey-inspired pop that unfashionably extols the virtue of staying true to your first love. People ask the singer how he first met his girl, and he harks back to the playground days when he first saw her. In its own giddy way the 'even then I knew' refrain embodies as much emotional certainty as John Lennon's 'everything was right'. 'The Muffin Man' by World of Oz is more traditional boy-meets-girl fare, with the nursery rhyme about a man plying his trade in Drury Lane replaced by the tale of a woebegone boy who is all fingers and thumbs as he serves sweetmeats to the girl he adores. 'Gingerbread Man' by the Mirror has 'Lucy'-style lyrics about 'lemonade trees and chocolate cheese and houses made of sugar'. World of Oz and the Mirror can be seen performing these songs on the German TV show *Beat Club*, both in identical ruff shirts, the cabaret popster's apparel of choice in 1968. The Mirror display toothy grins and mime badly. Their lead guitarist wears a Hendrix perm and a look that says he'd rather be almost anywhere than under the unforgiving glare of the studio lights singing about 'lemon drops and candy clocks'.

Songs about ice-cream men, sweet shops and toy shops are so prevalent during this period they probably deserve a category of their own in the toytown-pop pantheon. 'Ice Cream Man' by Clover featured a Grocer Jack-style kiddie chorus and seaside seagull effects, as well as the splendidly sibilant 'spend their pocket money on some slushy grub'. 'Uncle Joe the Ice Cream Man' by the Mindbenders could also have been taken direct from *Teenage Opera*, and concerned a much-loved elderly shopkeeper. The jollity of the chorus, with its 'Lucy'-esque lemons, cherries and tangerines, can't quite disguise the song's underlying melancholy as the old man remembers a time when his parents worked in the shop, a time when all the mums and dads he serves now were children like him. 'Man in a Shop' by Marmalade is a darkly whimsical vignette about a shopkeeper who spends his days gazing out at the children who gaze in at his window display. He's lonely and the children are unfulfilled in their fantasies of things they will never possess. Even the window dummy eventually gets discarded like an unwanted toy, relegated to the cellar to make way for a younger model.

When R&B groups weren't singing about ice cream and gingerbread they were communing with the sprites and the goblins. 'Happy Castle' by Crocheted Doughnut Ring commences with a 'Kites'-style Chinese gong, before skipping merrily down la-la lane, spraying the hedgerows with oxidising shards of fuzz guitar as it goes. 'Dogs in Baskets' by the splendidly named Geranium Pond is barely two minutes long and is one of the true bib-dribbling masterpieces of English psychedelic pop. Set to a simple two-note keyboard figure on what sounds like a Fisher Price mellotron, interspersed with erratic string-quartet splashes of colour, the song's stuttering stop–start cadences of incomprehensibility are sung in the mock posh of someone who has sucked up far too much diethylamide. It might be about kitsch paintings of puppies, but the line about orbiting the Earth in caskets suggests that it might just as easily be about Laika, the unfortunate Russian mongrel who preceded Yuri Gagarin into outer space in 1957 in *Sputnik 2* and died within hours of take-off, a canine martyr to interplanetary exploration. 'Talking in a tongue of no man,' recites Mr Pond, before a swirling finale transports us back through the ionosphere into the more familiar realm of rave-up mod pop.

Of all the acts whose careers floundered in the post-Merseybeat era Billy

J. Kramer made perhaps the boldest attempt to adapt to the changing times. Rather than reinvent himself as a raucous rocker or bland balladeer he turned to songs with childhood themes and released two singles of exceptional quality: 'Town of Tuxley Toymaker', written by Maurice, Robin and Barry Gibb, and '1941', a Harry Nilsson composition about a boy who runs away to join the circus. The Gibb brothers' song takes a theme that is present in the fairy tales *Pinocchio* and *Petrushka*: the marionette that comes alive, or in the case of the Bee Gees' composition, the toy wished into everlasting life by its maker. Featuring the Gibb brothers on backing vocals, the song, with verses in 3/4 time and a 4/4 chorus, has a haunting Turkish/Arabic flavour. Kramer recalls in Bilyeu, Cook and Hughes's Bee Gees biography that he chose 'Town of Tuxley Toymaker' from a plethora of demos that the Gibb brothers presented to him.[17] The song was recorded in a Saturday-morning session (10 a.m. to 1 p.m.) in March 1967, with a lavish budget that provided for a full session orchestra, the first time that Kramer had worked with such a full complement of musicians.

Set to a nursery-rhyme beat and with trilling flutes and piccolos, 'Glasshouse Green, Splinter Red' by the Kinsmen tells the tale of a lonely gardener who buys a greenhouse when he retires, only to hurl himself from his balcony through the glass when he decides he can't take any more. All of this is set to the merrily inoffensive tra-la-la of late-sixties commercial pop. Death can be conveyed in many ways in pop song, from the mawkish to the existential. The song's writer, John Pantry, takes John Steed and Emma Peel as his role models and greets his hapless subject's tumble and untimely demise with a quizzical smile and pithy homily. Pantry, it should be mentioned, also wrote and sang the Factory's mod-supreme anthem 'Try a Little Sunshine', and was later ordained as an Anglican minister.

As 'Glasshouse Green, Splinter Red' amply illustrated, there was a thin line between some of the more idiosyncratic oddities of toytown pop and the quirkier end of the psychedelic music hall. Perhaps the greatest straight-faced ode to macabre misfortune was Thunderclap Newman's 'Accidents', the follow-up to their summer of '69 number one 'Something in the Air'. Like a sinister 1960s public-service information film about the dangers of larking about next to rivers, we encounter, albeit only briefly, Johnny playing in the middle of the roundabout with his paper aeroplane; Mary by the riverside, who thinks the queen is coming; Sammy on the railway bridge trainspotting; and Jimmy larking about on the milk float in his granddad's shoes. A terrible fate awaits them all. The bathos is beautifully weighted throughout and the song ends with a philosophical homily worthy of the group's mentor, Pete Townshend: 'Life is just a game / you fly a paper plane / there is no aim.' Curiously, this sentiment failed to resonate with a record-buying public who had been drawn to the plight of Grocer Jack in their thousands, and despite being played constantly by Kenny Everett on his Radio 1 show, 'Accidents' has to go down in history as possibly the greatest follow-up to an equally great number one that failed to make the charts. For aspiring hit-makers the message was clear: songs featuring cute children stood some chance of chart success. Child death by banal misfortune was not so profitable.

'Skeleton and the Roundabout' by the Idle Race was a bizarre tale about a fairground man who operates his roundabout by hand but laments his lack of customers. As a result he can't afford to buy food and soon becomes as thin as a skeleton. Enterprising and optimistic to the last, he realises that there might still be work for him as a scary apparition on the ghost train,

and he is promptly employed as a horror prop, in which role he spends his days contentedly flapping from a gate. Flushed with his new-found success he grows fat and as a result no longer looks convincing in his role. Consequently he finds himself back on the roundabout, and the song ends where it began ('And here I yam'). As in fairgrounds, as in the roundabout of life.

As might be expected, fairgrounds and circuses crop up frequently in toytown pop, and for many children the fairground was their first experience of the immersive environment. Barbara Jones devoted an entire chapter to fairground rides in *The Unsophisticated Arts*. Entitled 'The Demountable Baroque', the chapter draws attention both to the mechanical ingenuity of the fairground roundabout and the sheer grotesque beauty and bizarre zoological and mythological juxtapositions of the animals on the rides. Jones depicts mermaids and dragons' heads, weird hybrids of ostriches and turkeys, horses with wild, unruly manes and bared teeth, and sometimes with masks carved into their throats or breasts. All these wondrous beasts were glazed, as Jones puts it, 'with transparent colours in a limited range, such as carmine, yellow, viridian and Prussian blue, suggestive of the colours that can be used for tinting magic-lantern slides'.[18] She documents the rich visual iconography of the fairs, noting how hoardings and displays were garishly painted and elaborately decorated, with a cavalier approach to the exotic and the ornate: jungle animals, film-star caricatures, pre-pop-art signage, patriotic emblems, mysterious Green Man-like visages, coats of arms of no known lineage. Well into the post-war years, right up until record players and juke-boxes replaced them, in fact, the musical accompaniment on the fairground rides and exhibits was provided by huge art nouveau-adorned Bioscope organs. These had been purpose-built for the earliest mobile cinemas and were subsequently bought up by French and Belgian dance halls when the travelling cinema shows died out. Jones lovingly describes the unreality of these instruments, with their rococo carvings and their peculiarly inanimate automaton figures: 'anything up to half life size, with leather-jointed arms and sticks or flutes in their hands. They stare rigidly before them out of blue eyes set in dusty, porcelain-tinted faces, and beat their monotonous accompaniment to the organ on a little drum or cymbal'.[19]

Jones called it 'The Demountable Baroque' but 'Demountable Rococo' would have been just as accurate. The fixtures and figurines she depicted had previously been a hallmark of the follies designed for the royal households of eighteenth-century Europe at the height of the rococo movement. Augustus the Strong built a lavish Japanese palace on the banks of the Elbe in Dresden, in imitation of the great emperors of the east, but it bore only the faintest resemblance to the architecture of a country that neither Augustus nor his architect had visited. Frederick the Great of Prussia built a similar fantasy version of a Chinese pavilion in Potsdam. It featured supporting columns that were shaped like Middle Eastern palm trees and sculpted musicians who played inventions that looked vaguely luteish or violinish but adhered to no known instruments. Frederick's palace offered a similarly exoticised approximation of Chinoiserie, with its inauthentic wall murals and porcelain artifacts. Barbara Jones noted the same cavalier approach to historical accuracy in many fairground carvings. They might be medieval, Arcadian or English rustic shepherds, pantomime figures, occidental, oriental or hitherto unimagined combinations of any of these: 'But all the clothes have been seen through a fresh eye, have been a little distorted by someone unskilled in historic costume, and make a new period and place of their own, an unprecedented category.'[20] That 'unprecedented category' just as readily describes the stylistic hybrids, fish eye-lensed perceptions and peculiar phantasmagoria that manifest themselves in psychedelic pop in the late 1960s. It is no accident that so many psychedelic songs, from 'Being for the Benefit of Mr Kite' onwards, borrow their imagery and their atmosphere from the enchanted, impermanent spectacle that is (or at least was) the travelling English fairground.

Jones describes hoardings depicting Boar War scenes, tiger hunts and jungle battles between teeth-bared beasts, all done in an identical style borrowed from Rousseau and 'painted with so much innocent charm that they completely fail to alarm even the smallest child'.[21] I think she seriously underestimates the fevered imaginings of the overstimulated, sugar-coated, candy floss-fuelled child at this point, but she's right in one crucial respect:

those sideshow hoardings and their vivid apparitions displayed the familiar sinister we all grew up with, the vivid apparitions that loomed round every straw-pathed corner and blended in with all the other sights, sounds and smells of the five-day wonder that was, and perhaps still is, the English fairground. 'Even in Arcady there I am,' but it never comes like that again. Not like it did in childhood dream days, when the sheer auditory delight of it all assaults the malleable young brain, which is intuitively alive to all sensations. The montage mash-up of the merry-go-round, the dodgems, the ping and smash of the rifle range, the clunky jerks and tinkling small-change payouts from the one-armed bandits, the constant hum and diesel-scented air around the generators – they all converge in a starter-kit Happening, a junior media massage, a synaesthetic collide-oscope, a temporary pleasure garden of unearthly delights.

17

SITAR POP, RAGA ROCK
AND THE EXOTIC OTHERS

*At this particular stage I find myself
in, I seem to be going through a modal
phase . . . There's a lot of modal music
that is played every day throughout
the world. It's particularly evident
in Africa, but if you look in Spain
or Scotland, India or China, you'll
discover this again in each case. If you
want to look beyond the differences in
style, you will confirm that there is a
common base.*

    JOHN COLTRANE, 1963[1]

*The fiction of a purely indigenous
culture has been destroyed more
effectively today than at any time in
the past. As a student of history I have
never come across any culture which
was pure at any time in the world. In
our Indian language we have a term
called* kitchree. *This means a medley.
Culture must be* kitchree. *In fact it
has always been* kitchree, *but then the
purists came along and worked on it
to try and discover elements of purity
which do not exist.*

    HUMAYUN KABIR, 1964[2]

In April 1966 the Byrds turned up at the press conference to launch their new single 'Eight Miles High' with Roger McGuinn cradling a sitar. During the launch party McGuinn and Dave Crosby spoke enthusiastically, evangelically even, about their love of Indian music. McGuinn was photographed plucking gently at the sitar's strings, even though he couldn't actually play the instrument. A sitar doesn't actually appear on 'Eight Miles High', or indeed on any other Byrds record.

Later that same year a comment, variously attributed to Brian Jones, Donovan and George Harrison, has one of them responding to a journalist's question about their own recent adoption of the sitar with: 'I've been practising the instrument for nearly three months now and I'm really getting into it.' The story, possibly apocryphal, or a misquote at least, reflected a suspicion that the sitar was simply being used as exotic adornment and that pop musicians were adopting a Bert Weedon *Play in a Day* approach to the complexities of Indian music. The term applied to this short-lived enthusiasm was 'raga rock', and several sitar manuals were published to cash in on the trend. The best of these – *Introduction to the Sitar* by Harihar Rao (1967) and *The Sitar Book* by Allen Keesee (1968) – sold in their thousands and helped publicise the new-found interest in the instrument in the West. Rao, a California-based protégé of Ravi Shankar, also played in the Hindustani Jazz Sextet with trumpeter Don Ellis and did much to encourage the west-coast fusion between Indian music and jazz. He later played a pivotal role in the organisation of 1971's Concert for Bangla Desh.

For anybody other than the fully committed, learning to play the sitar presented considerable practical problems. When George and Pattie Harrison spent six weeks in India in 1966, at Ravi Shankar's invitation, Shankar made it clear that all he could do in that time was introduce the Beatles' guitarist to the correct sitting positions and some basic fingering exercises. Harrison later admitted that mastering the correct posture alone, while wielding a heavy and cumbersome instrument, took some getting used to. Many who eagerly purchased Rao's or Keesee's manuals with the same initial enthusiasm never got past the first few pages, once they discovered that without extensive yogic training they would merely develop cramp in their legs rather than musical expertise and spiritual insight.

Despite these obstacles the sitar was enthusiastically incorporated into pop music's expanding palette in the 1960s. The instrument's drone-like sound and its facility to create vibrating harmonics on its unplayed 'sympathetic strings' opened up a whole new world of possibilities, and it briefly took its place alongside a range of gadgetry – the fuzz box, the wah-wah pedal, the Binson Echorec, etc. – that offered similar opportunities for blurring texture and timbre. The sitar was capable of producing long, steady notes with extensive microtonal variations. It produced wider variations in sharps and flats than are normally heard in Western music, as well as slow continuous slides and slurs from one tone to another. It was capable of marked oscillation, as well as note-bending and delicate ornamentations that were beyond the capacity or range of the electric guitar. The sitar was, therefore, tailor-made for guitarists already versed in the slide and bottleneck techniques of the blues. The improvisational nature of raga music also appealed to their sense of showmanship and the rock culture's growing emphasis on virtuosity.

Initially, the sitar and other Indian instrumentation found their way into the sound palette of East–West fusion music on a number of groundbreaking jazz records by Yusef Lateef, Gábor Szabó and Alice Coltrane, among others. The sitar's exotic colouration was also a great favourite among those west-coast 'cool school' musicians who had emerged from Harihar Rao's Hindustani Jazz Sextet, such as Bill Plummer, Emil Richards and Tom Scott. These hybrid explorations enjoyed their most perfect realisation in Joe Harriott and John Mayer's 1966 recording *Indo-Jazz Suite* and its 1968 follow-up

Indo-Jazz Fusions. The sitar also added an exotic layer of otherness to the more experimental end of folk music and was used by a range of groups and artists, most prominently Donovan, Pentangle and the Incredible String Band. And, for a short period, the sitar had a direct influence on the sound of Anglo-American pop, appearing on numerous Top 10 records in both Britain and America. It was championed by the Beatles, the Rolling Stones, Traffic, the Pretty Things, the Moody Blues and many others. In the same way that mod groups mutated into psych groups by embellishing R&B beats with fuzz tones and frazzled lyrics, it became commonplace for sitar window dressing to be added to pop songs in order to give them an aura of mystery and enchantment. The instrument was, though, only ever briefly in vogue. Typecast by its novelty value, it had fallen out of favour again by the end of the decade, and by the early 1970s any rock group using a sitar on a record would have been considered passé.

The catch-all term 'raga rock' was, in fact, something of a misnomer, and was frequently misapplied to any record that used non-European instrumentation or musical styles to denote its exotic qualities. The two records chiefly credited with introducing raga motifs into Western pop are the Yardbirds' 'Heart Full of Soul' and the Kinks' 'See My Friends', both released in 1965, but equally radical tonal experiments were going on elsewhere at the time. In the folk world, Davey Graham's arrangement of the Irish ballad 'She Moved Through the Fair' as a guitar raga appeared on the Decca EP *From a London Hootenanny* in 1963, and was just one example of Graham's innovative fusion of blues, jazz, folk and ethnic styles, which he set to unorthodox guitar tunings. In America John Fahey had been blazing a trail for these kinds of unorthodox stylistic hybrids for some time. In fact, 'Heart Full of Soul' and 'See My Friends' weren't even the first records to put the drone into the pop charts. Although it carried significantly less cultural cachet, Rolf Harris's number-one hit 'Sun Arise', released in Australia in January 1961 and eighteen months later in the UK, featured the mesmerising didgeridoo sound of the indigenous Australian Aborigines. In 1961, though, Aborigines and their Dreamtime were not high on anyone's cultural agenda, and so 'Sun Arise' was regarded as a novelty, a one-off, rather than a trailblazer.

Given the vibrant state of the club scene in several of the UK's largest cities, and the fervent cross-pollinations of jazz, folk, blues and pop that were being explored by those who performed and socialised in those clubs, it was perhaps inevitable that someone would come up with a 'See My Friends' or 'Heart Full of Soul' sooner or later. Professional musicians are sociable beings and thieving magpies by nature. They trade anecdotes, influences, records and licks. They pass endless hours in rehearsal rooms and at soundchecks, noodling away on their instruments. They hang out at each other's gigs, watching, jamming and developing their repertoire. The first thing Jimi Hendrix did when he came to England was jam. D. A. Pennebaker's documentary film of Bob Dylan's 1965 UK concert tour, *Don't Look Back*, frequently shows Dylan in dressing rooms and hotel suites. He's either strumming his guitar or hammering away at his typewriter. In one revealing scene Alan Price hangs out backstage. He has just left the Animals, and Dylan casually enquires what he is going to do next. Price reacts with a grimace and a casual shrug. Apropos of nothing he begins to explain to Dylan the curiously beguiling stage act and snaky hand gestures of Dave Berry. He then breaks into an impromptu performance of Berry's current hit single 'Little Things' at the piano. The assembled backstage throng immediately pick up

the threads and join in. As a cameo of the workaday life of the average pop superstar in the mid-1960s it's as accurate as any scene in the film.

The Price/Dylan encounter was filmed in May 1965. One month earlier the Yardbirds had recorded 'Heart Full of Soul', which featured Jeff Beck replicating the sound of a sitar with the aid of a fuzz box. At an initial recording session producer Giorgio Gomelsky hired two Indian session musicians to play sitar and tabla, but even with the addition of reverb and echo it was found that the sitar notes decayed too quickly and didn't have the necessary impact or attack. At a second session Beck reworked the song's three-pitch riff on guitar and created a distinctive exotic sound. Equally noteworthy were the bursts of Gregorian plainchant that accompanied every second line in 'Heart Full of Soul''s verses and underpinned the concluding line to the chorus. Gregorian chant was another exotic motif that became fashionable in the mid-sixties. Like the raga it was the product of an oral culture passed down from generation to generation mnemonically. We have no real evidence of either the key or tempo it was originally sung in, only the liturgical context it arose from. There is no concrete evidence to suggest that it was invented by Pope Gregory, and it isn't strictly chanting either, but 'thirteenth-century solemn proclamation' doesn't trip off the tongue half as well, so 'Gregorian chant' was what the musicologists settled for. It became another of those convenient short-hand terms to describe a certain style of sonority, and in the sixties was applied in the same cavalier fashion as raga rock.

The Yardbirds' vocalist Keith Relf sounded singularly unconvincing when he tackled Chicago blues staples like 'Smokestack Lightning' or 'Good Morning Little Schoolgirl', but on the group's run of hit singles from 'For Your Love' in March 1965 to 'Happenings Ten Years Time Ago' in October 1966 the spooked and sinister inflections of that otherwise unremarkable baritone really came into their own. There was more than a touch of 'machismo gone wrong' in Ray Davies's singing too. On the Kinks' earliest hits, those raucous three-chord rewrites of 'Louie Louie' 'You Really Got Me' and 'All Day and All of the Night', he sounds like he's borrowing equally from the girl groups and Beatlemania, but there was always something a little too shrill and sibilant in his pronunciation to convince. In time Davies made that lisping and arch delivery his forte. On 'See My Friends' you can hear the transition. Written in January 1965 but not released until a month after 'Heart Full of Soul', 'See My Friends' had a sexually ambivalent lyric and used drone techniques both in its melody and in the drawled vocal. The song is lauded as a landmark but stylistically it's a continuation of the lazy tempo of two previous Kinks hits, 'Tired of Waiting' and 'Set Me Free', in which the drawl and the elongated vowels are already evident.

As influential as they were neither 'Heart Full of Soul' nor 'See My Friends' could strictly be called raga rock – both incorporate Middle Eastern and East European rhythms and melodies rather than Indian ones – but Keith Relf was clearly anticipating the changing times when he told Richard Green of *Record Mirror* in March 1965 that 'rhythm and blues is becoming what trad became'. The band was moving away from 'the old 12-bar bit', he said. Commenting on Jeff Beck's guitar experimentation, Relf likened it to 'musique concrète or musique electronique'. Such exploration sat well within the band's remit and on their singles in particular they illustrated a capacity to expand way beyond their original blues brief. Their first hit record, 'For Your Love', pioneered a distinctively English hybrid of garage baroque. 'Shapes of Things' and 'Over Under Sideways

Down' featured Turkish and Arabic folk melodies. 'Heart Full of Soul', 'Still I'm Sad' and 'Turn into Earth' made extensive use of Gregoriana. 'Happenings Ten Years Time Ago' made a feature of pick-up manipulation and atonality. And on 'Mister, You're a Better Man than I', recorded in September 1965, Jeff Beck unleashed the fifty seconds of noise that would serve as the prototype for all future psychedelic guitar solos.

Ray and Dave Davies grew up in north London, in the Golders Green/ Muswell Hill hinterland, and were exposed to a plethora of Russian-Jewish melodies. These were as much a part of their musical development as any of the more commonly cited influences. An unmistakable Jewish sonority runs through the title track of their 1968 LP *The Kinks Are the Village Green Preservation Society*, and on tracks like 'Phenomenal Cat' and 'People Take Pictures of Each Other' the band never sound more than half a beat away from a mazurka or a right old Russian Orthodox knees-up. In his autobiography *X-Ray* Davies was reluctant to make extravagant claims for 'See My Friends', merely citing a trip to Australia in 1964, when the Kinks made a stopover in India and saw fishermen chanting as they carried their nets.[3] In the same book he claims that his

nasal singing style on the song was an attempt to copy Hank Williams!

Exoticism was, in fact, abundant in Western music almost a couple of centuries before 'Heart Full of Soul' and 'See My Friends' graced the pop charts. In the post-Ottoman Empire years there was a vogue for Turkish music and for what became known as the 'Alla Turca' style. Mozart popularised it in 1778 with his 'Rondo Alla Turca'. Dave Brubeck revived the form in the 1950s with his 'Blue Rondo à la Turk', a version of the Mozart piece performed in 9/8 time. (In 1968 the Nice turned the same composition into a raucous and unrestrained Hammond-organ freak-out.) The Yardbirds' own version of 'Turkishness', then, was not so much five minutes ahead of its time, more like catching a wave that had been flowing in one form or another for the best part of two centuries. But with each successive appropriation came accusations of superficiality and decoration for its own sake, all of which resurfaced when sitar pop first appeared in the mid-sixties. American musicologist Joseph Kerman blamed Meyerbeer's *L'Africaine* and Verdi's *Aida* for creating the vogue for the 'careless application of local colour in opera', and noted that Puccini's final work, *Turandot*, had 'bogus orientalism lacquered over every page of the score'[4] Claude Debussy, no slouch himself when it came to exotic colouration, 'curtly dismissed Delibe's *Lakmé* (1883) as sham imitative Oriental bric-a-brac'.[5] One of Debussy's most famous gamelan-inspired pieces, 'Pagodas', was written after his second visit to the Javanese gamelan at the Paris World's Fair of 1900. But as music professor Mervyn Cooke points out, 'the title does not conjure up a specific image of Indonesia, where pagodas are not to be found'.[6] Benjamin Britten illustrated the same shaky sense of geography in his 1957 ballet *The Prince of the Pagodas*. Although he faithfully adhered to the architecture of the music by utilising direct transcriptions of Balinese music, he seemed less familiar with the architecture of Bali itself, which is singularly lacking in pagodas. Britten's gamelan for *The Prince of the Pagodas* was actually made up of conventional Western percussion and offered what Cooke called 'an accomplished pastiche of the Balinese kebyar style'. Similar renditions of 'accomplished pastiche' would serve sitar pop well in the 1960s.

What was also similar was the shared sense of epiphany. Ever since Claude Debussy witnessed a display of Javanese music and dancing during the Paris World's Fair in 1889 the gamelan had played a major part in revolutionising the compositional techniques of two successive generations of composers. In fact, the gamelan fulfilled the same exotic function in the first half of the twentieth century that the sitar did in the 1960s. In addition to those mentioned above, Francis Poulenc, Olivier Messiaen, Béla Bartók, Henry Cowell, Harry Partch, Lou Harrison, John Cage and Terry Riley were all seduced by the unfamiliar tunings and polyphonic textures of the Javanese and Balinese gamelan and the opportunities it afforded them to break away from conventional harmony and notation. Debussy's awestruck introduction to Javanese tonality was identical to the rapture experienced by Roger McGuinn, David Crosby, George Harrison and many others when they first heard the music of Ravi Shankar. Javanese music 'made our tonic and dominant seem like ghosts', claimed Debussy.[7] In his piano writing he began using the sustain pedal in the same way that rock musicians later utilised the fuzz pedal, blurring melody lines in order to create what Mervyn Cooke called 'a resonant wash of sound'. Cecil Taylor would later refer to the piano as eighty-eight tuned drums. Debussy wished to eliminate the instrument's percussive element completely and spoke of a need 'to make the piano appear as if it were an instrument "sans marteaux" i.e. without hammers'.[8]

In his desire to explore the acoustic possibilities of the piano, and with his emphasis on vibration and harmonics rather than tempo and Western tonality, there are direct historical parallels between Debussy's radical break with the past and the endeavours of a generation of post-war jazz musicians (and, later still, of the more adventurous rock musicians) who similarly wished to free themselves from traditional blues scales. John Coltrane, in his quest to find a 'common base' for all creativity, suggested that once the discerning listener disregarded the ethnic characteristics and folkloric aspects of music, they were left with what he called 'the presence of the same pentatonic sonority of comparable modal structures'.[9] Jazz music had developed an ear for the exotic very early on. In 1936 Duke Ellington offered a languid faux-Arabian adaptation of Juan Tizol and Irving Mills's 'Caravan'. Dizzy Gillespie's 'Nights in Tunisia' (1944) became one of the classics of the bebop era in the hands of the Charlie Parker Quintet. Miles Davis and Gil Evans's 1959 orchestration *Sketches of Spain* was an adaptation of Joaquín Rodrigo's 1940 work *Concierto de Aranjuez* – itself an evocation of nineteenth-century Spain,

written by Rodrigo when he was living in Paris. John Coltrane based the title track of his 1961 album *Olé Coltrane* on a Spanish folk song.

Given this preponderance of exoticism in Western music it's puzzling why sitar pop was ever seen as problematic. The dread hand of traditionalism was evident in much of the disapproval, as was the suspicion that pop was getting above itself and had no right to be meddling in more elevated forms. The *kitchree* quote at the head of this chapter was taken from a speech Humayun Kabir made at the Conference on the Music of East and West, held in Delhi in 1964. The author who uses the quote, playwright Gopal Sharman, disparages the *kitchree* theory and adds a footnoted disclaimer: 'Hash would be a more apt translation for this culinary metaphor,' he suggests disdainfully.[10] Sharman viewed non-indigenous hybridity as an abhorrent mish-mash of clashing, incompatible components. Caught in the crossfire of this argument was Ravi Shankar, the man who had done so much to bring Indian classical music to wider public attention in the West. In his autobiography *My Music, My Life* Shankar noted the contradictory nature of his position. 'I have been facing criticism from the very "traditional" people in India who say that I am commercializing and cheapening my music with the pop influence and lowering my standards of playing the sitar,' he said.[11] In fact, Shankar abhorred the culture of drug-taking that he witnessed in the West, particularly among the counter-cultural devotees who so adored his music. 'It was of course gratifying to see that many people loved India and all its culture; but their expression of this love was very superficial,' he said. 'Wearing beads and bells and flowers and carrying joss sticks came across as a mimickry and mockery of the real thing.'[12] When he first came to England he was shocked by the behaviour of younger concert-goers, and was highly critical of their behaviour and ignorance of basic concert etiquette. 'Often they sat there in front of me carrying on indecently with their girlfriends or boyfriends and many of them even lit cigarettes (if that in fact is what they were) whenever they pleased. Their conduct disgusted me.'[13] Initially, Shankar had similar misgivings about the sitar's role in Western pop. 'Except for a few groups who I think are musically creative and adventurous' – sadly he didn't give examples – 'pop musicians are using the sitar in an extremely shallow way, just a new sound or gimmick.' Despite this disapproval he remained philosophical.

'Those who sincerely love Indian music as classical music should not be upset by this,' he said. 'One instrument can serve many styles of music.'[14] As an example he cited the guitar, which had managed to become a mainstay of rock and pop without unduly affecting its standing as a classical instrument.

When George Harrison and Ravi Shankar first encountered each other in 1965, it was not so much a case of West meets East as West meets westernised. Often portrayed as the fortuitous collision of contrasting musical cultures, the two men actually had much in common. By the time he met Harrison, Shankar had already enjoyed three decades of success in Europe and America. Although he came from a Bengali Brahmin family and was steeped in Indian music and folklore, his father was an Oxford-educated barrister who practised in London and Calcutta. Unlike contemporaries such as Ustad Imrat Khan, who could trace his lineage through an unbroken line of master musicians back to the sixteenth century, Ravi did not come from a musical dynasty. His initial passion was dance and he spent his youth touring Europe and America as part of his older brother Uday's very successful troupe, Uday Shankar and His Hindu Ballet. Ravi was an enthusiastic dancer and only gave it up to study music in 1938, by which time he was eighteen. During his dance apprenticeship he enjoyed all the benefits of a privileged Western lifestyle, sitting on the knee of Andrés Segovia (who lived two doors away) in Paris as a child and seeing Toscanini conduct and Penderecki play the piano. On their first tour of America Uday's troupe played Broadway theatres, and the young Ravi attended Hollywood parties with Jean Harlow (whom he idolised), Clark Gable, Greta Garbo and Joan Crawford. At thirteen he wanted to be a Hollywood film star. He was still enjoying this life of glitz and glamour when he met his guru, the multi-instrumentalist Baba Allaudin Khan. A Muslim by birth, Khan had been a musician in the court of a maharaja and initially chastised the young Ravi for being 'a butterfly', for-ever flitting from one artistic form to another. He also criticised his dandyish taste in clothes. Shankar always cred-ited 'Baba' with putting him on the righteous path, comparing the great man to a 'Himalaya', and in 1938 he submitted himself to a strict seven-year musical apprenticeship under Baba's tutelage. Baba's daughter, and Ravi's fellow pupil, Annapurna played the surbahar (bass sitar) and in 1941 would become Shankar's first wife. The

marriage was a stormy one and they separated briefly in the 1940s, when Ravi had a well-publicised affair with dancer Kamala Shastri. Although they performed together frequently during the 1950s, Annapurna, said by many to be the more skilled musician, proved less willing to 'westernise' Indian clas-sical music than her husband. When they divorced in 1962, she retired from public performance completely, and to this day secretly taped recordings of concerts she gave in the 1950s are highly prized among collectors. Such background details cast fascinating light on the idea that Shankar's encoun-ter with George Harrison was simply one of devout unblemished master and impulsive secular pupil, although, to put things into cultural perspec-tive, it's instructive to observe what the two men were doing at eighteen, when they undertook their respective musical apprenticeships: Ravi Shankar had entered a strict regime of monastic dedication and austere discipline under the watchful eye of Baba Allaudin Khan; George Harrison was playing the Reeperbahn while John Lennon goose-stepped and *Sieg Heil*-ed around the stage with a piss pot on his head

In the same way that his older brother had popularised Indian dance, Ravi Shankar was the great populariser of Indian music. He became a cultural ambassador, liaising with diplomats and politicians and performing his music all over the world. This approach did not please everyone. Shankar combined Western and Indian instrumentation in his orchestrations, introduced westernised motifs into his playing and risked offending purists with his modifications of centuries-old traditions. He shortened the prelude section of the raga (the so-called alap) and condensed the length of the raga itself to suit the time limitations of LPs, the performance slots of All India Radio and the endurance of Western concert-goers. Shankar always maintained that such modifications were necessary if Indian music was to be enjoyed more widely. His own congregation of voices at this time was *kitchree* personified, comprising as it did styles drawn from both north and south Indian classical traditions, Persian music and Indian light orchestral music, as well as his own highly idiosyncratic stylistic innovations. By the 1960s his sitar-led performances had become synonymous in the West with Indian classical music.

Mervyn Cooke ends his appraisal of the gamelan's effect on Western music by suggesting that more often than not it 'acted as a catalyst by throwing up fortuitous musical parallels that focused [the composers'] attention on the more radical aspects of their own styles'.[15] That is also true of an entire generation of Western pop musicians in the 1960s who incorporated the sitar into their musical development. In a number of cases it was undoubtedly part of a sincere spiritual quest; in the majority, though, the impulse came from time-served inquisitiveness and a desire to get a good tune out of the thing.

Session guitarist Big Jim Sullivan fell into both camps. His day job saw him playing on some of the UK's biggest chart records of the 1960s. As a general rule of thumb, if it wasn't Big Jim playing session guitar on a record it was Jimmy Page – who for a time was known as 'Little Jim' in honour of his mentor – and more often than not it was both of them. In late 1964, while working on an EMI session, Sullivan heard Ustad Vilayat Khan playing sitar in Abbey Road studios, and subsequently took up the instrument himself. Under the tutelage of ethnomusicologist Nazir Jairazbhoy he quickly attained a degree of proficiency on the instrument while continuing to make his living playing on hits for the likes of Dusty Springfield, Dave Berry and P. J. Proby. In August 1967 he recorded an album called *Sitar Beat*, which was produced by Lou Reizner, released on the Mercury Label and marketed not at the rock audience but as part of its 'Super Stereo Sound' series, which also showcased albums by the likes of Quincy Jones, Xavier Cugat and Michel Legrand and His Orchestra. It wasn't the UK's first pop sitar album. That accolade goes to Chim Kothari's 1966 LP *Sound of Sitar*, an early release on the newly formed Deram label. Despite the excruciatingly toe-curling tone of its sleeve notes ('May we humbly suggest you dig his scene, Sahib?'), *Sitar Beat* contained imaginative arrangements of the Beatles' 'She's Leaving Home', Donovan's 'Sunshine Superman' and 'Fat Angel' and Jeff Beck's 'Tallyman', as well as Sullivan's own compositions 'LTTS', 'The Koan' and 'Flower Power'. One of the guitarists on the sessions was John McLaughlin, who had done his R&B apprenticeship with popular club outfits like the Graham Bond Organisation, Georgie Fame and the Blues Flames, the Brian Auger Trinity and Herbie Goins and the Nightimers. Within eighteen months of playing on Sullivan's *Sitar Beat* sessions, McLaughlin would be part of Miles Davis's group. From cover versions of 'Sunshine Superman' to *In a Silent Way* and *Bitches Brew* within a year and a half: all part of life's

rich pageant for many a jobbing sixties musician.

The sitar was used in various ways on pop records: sometimes embedded within the overall textures of the sound, sometimes as counterpoint to the vocal line, sometimes doubling up with the guitar or replacing it as lead instrument. John Renbourn utilised the instrument with great dexterity in his work with Pentangle. At their best Pentangle created an ensemble sound that did for folk music what *Rubber Soul*-era Beatles did for pop and John Coltrane's classic quartet did for jazz. Renbourn's sitar-playing on tracks like 'Once I Had a Sweetheart' and 'Cruel Sister' sat perfectly within the group sound, complementing Terry Cox's sensitive brushwork, Danny Thompson's liquid bass and Bert Jansch's subtle, unshowy guitar work. On his 1969 album *The Lady and the Unicorn* Renbourn seamlessly wove sitar textures into his arrangements of a series of melodies inspired by medieval music. Dave Mason's sitar played a similarly integral role in Traffic in their early days. It was a key element in the sound the group developed on the *Mr Fantasy* LP and on their hit singles. The sitar was equally prominent in the Incredible String Band's sound, which also drew upon a pan-global palette of bells, whistles, gongs, ouds, lutes, flutes and myriad other instruments they brought back from their travels or found in the post-colonial debris that was the British junk shop of the early 1960s.

Numerous other bands featured the sitar prominently on their psychedelic material. 'Love' by Virgin Sleep was lazy-tempo dream pop with a melody line similar to the Troggs' 'Love Is All Around', some voguish Gregorian chanting and a quick burst of 'Om Mani Padmi Hum' on the fade-out. More faux-monastic chanting introduces the wonderfully preposterous 'Wallpaper' by Pregnant Insomnia, an innuendo-laden tribute to the joys of interior decorating that can't make up its mind whether it wants to be the Spencer Davis Group's 'Somebody Help Me' or the Rolling Stones' 'Paint It Black'. Somewhat less ludicrously sitars were combined with R&B and folk stylings to excellent effect on a range of records. Among the best of them were 'Three Kingfishers' by Donovan, 'Mr Carpenter' by the Fox (with Dave Mason guesting on sitar), 'Real Life Permanent Dream' by Tomorrow, 'Defecting Grey' by the Pretty Things, Bob Grimm's 'It Never Stays the Same', 'Cave of Clear Light' by the Bystanders and 'Worn Red Carpet' by Idle Race. The last item was issued in 1969, just months before

lead singer and guitarist Jeff Lynne joined the Move, a band he had clearly been attempting to emulate for the previous two years. Lynne was arguably one of the last sixties musicians to hold a candle for psychedelic motifs, and he utilised its tricks and tropes well into the next decade, long after everyone else had jettisoned such stylistic trappings. Several ELO hits, including 'The Diary of Horace Wimp' and 'Mr Blue Sky', could easily have been late-1960s psych-pop singles. Lynne's subsequent co-writing partnership with George Harrison on Harrison's myth-busting 'When We Was Fab' and his integral production role in the 'Threetles'' 'Free as a Bird' and 'Real Love' should have surprised no one.

After George Harrison the most famous pop musician to explore the possibilities of Eastern music was the Rolling Stones' multi-instrumentalist Brian Jones. Jones was not a diligent devotee like Harrison; he was an inspired dabbler, and his wayward personal life and fragile psyche mitigated against him making a more lasting contribution to East–West fusions, but in June 1966 he did what no one else had done: he took the sitar to number one in the pop charts with 'Paint It Black'.

Jones had an intuitive musical talent and rapidly worked out how to

play blues harp and slide guitar profi-
ciently. At the height of the Stones' pop
fame he brought the same proficiency
to the dulcimer and the sitar, and his
exotic embellishments are all over the
group's records during what many
regard as their finest period. It was
Jones's slide-playing that toughened up
the Stones' debut hit, a cover version of
Lennon and McCartney's 'I Wanna Be
Your Man', and it was his equally deft
bottleneck work that took their version
of Howlin' Wolf's 'Little Red Rooster'
to number one in December 1964. As
a musical force Jones was at his peak
during the band's classic pop period
between 1965 to 1967, a period that
Marianne Faithfull accurately summarised as a 'blend of blues mythology and
King's Road noblesse oblige'. Jones's
marimba on 'Under My Thumb', 'Out
of Time' and 'Yesterday's Papers', his
sitar on 'Mother's Little Helper' and
'Paint It Black', dulcimer on 'Lady Jane'
and 'I Am Waiting' and sax and oboe
on 'Dandelion' are more than mere
musical embroidery. Sometimes the
contribution is simplicity itself – merely
repeating the vocal melody on 'Lady
Jane' or running up and down the scales
on 'Paint It Black' – but these elements
are integral, the making of those songs.
In one of the most telling episodes in
her autobiography Marianne Faithfull
describes the moment in the studio
when Jones first plays the beautiful lilting recorder melody that would eventually become 'Ruby Tuesday'. Keith
Richards picks up on it and starts shaping it on the piano. Jones tells him that
it's a cross between John Dowland's
'Air on the Late Lord Essex' and a
Skip James blues. The comment goes
unacknowledged.

Jones was the first Rolling Stone
to check out the west-coast music
scene. He knew Keith Anger and the
Expanded Cinema film-makers. Keith
Altham, who interviewed him for *NME*
in 1966, remembers him playing experimental free-form tapes that he was
working on. 'We just sort of laid back
and listened to what they were doing
in Frisco, whereas Brian was making
great tapes, overdubbing,' Keith Richards told *Rolling Stone* in 1971. 'He
was much more into it than we were.
We were digging what we were hearing
for what it was, but that other thing in
you is saying, "Yeah, but where's Chuck
Berry?"'

In late 1966 Jones composed the
soundtrack score for Volker Schlön-
dorff's film *A Degree of Murder*.
Jimmy Page plays guitar on the record,
Nicky Hopkins piano and Kenny Jones
drums. Brian Jones plays sitar, organ,
recorder, cello, bass guitar, dulcimer,

banjo, clarinet and harmonica, and also co-arranged the orchestration with Mike Leander. Jones's increasingly debilitated condition from 1967 onwards didn't stop him adding some inspired multilayered Moroccan brass at the end of 'We Love You' and some deft mellotron augmentation to *Their Satanic Majesties Request*. In January 1968 he sat in on the sessions for *Electric Ladyland* and contributed piano and sitar to early takes of 'All Along The Watchtower'. Later that year he went to Morocco and put together the *Pipes of Pan at Joujouka* album, a project he entered into with all the anthropological fervour of a Samuel Charters or Alan Lomax. Jones's doctoring of the primitive tapes, made on a simple four-track, is proto-dub in all but name.

Brian Jones was in the end fated to become the poster boy for sixties excess and became rock's first notable drug death. His musical trajectory through the decade – from blues purist to experimentalist to crushed spirit – mirrors wider changes that took place in the culture. His marginalisation within the Rolling Stones, the band he helped create, reflects something of the changing times, as experimentalism was reined in and rock returned to its roots. There wasn't much call for a dulcimer or a John Dowland air on 'Jumpin' Jack Flash'. By the end of the 1960s there wasn't really space for a dulcimer, or a sitar for that matter, in the rock repertoire at all, although with splendid irony Ananda Shankar, nephew of Ravi, recorded a supercharged version of 'Jumpin' Jack Flash' in 1970 that featured the sitar as its lead instrument. And so a cycle of appropriation had come full circle once again. It was Western rock and roll that was now the exoticised other.

AFTERGLOW (WHICH DREAMED IT?)

18

GAUCHE RIDERS IN THE SKY

Kitsch Psych, Part-Time Paradise People
and the Ersatz of Suchness

So it is that the in-scene of London is one big fancy dress ball. Men come as cowboys, Hussars and refugees from St Petersburg 1917. IT girls. If girls. Anyone for tennis girls. Odelisks from the harems of bygone Turkey mingle with kaftan slinkies from gay Arabia or boa-bedecked hoydens from the lids of ancient chocolate boxes. A super charade of happy Happenings, though it might be fun if some designer somewhere thought something up entirely new.

RANK ORGANISATION, *Look at Life*, 1967[1]

And obviously before long (and even now in fact) we will witness the anti-family kitsch, the kitsch of hippies and long-haired youths, the kitsch of addicts and beatniks. We cannot escape kitsch: as soon as something becomes conformist and traditional it can seldom be saved, and then only with great difficulty.

GILLO DORFLES, 1969[2]

Kitsch is a beautiful word.

BARRY RYAN, 1969

When you look back now at the early TV or film appearances by some of the most hip and happening pop stars of the 1960s, it's hard not to be struck by how gauche they all appear. Rockstar biopics in more recent times have relied on rebellious signifiers and mannerisms based on some mythical construct of how film producers assume 'Keef' Richards, say, or Iggy Pop acted in their 1970s junked-up prime; they certainly don't reflect the reality of the 1960s. Watch the way in which Jack Bruce and Ginger Baker submit to a teasing from 'the headmaster' in the risible 1965 pop flick *Gonks Go Beat*. After a barnstorming performance from the Graham Bond Organisation (at that time the tightest R&B act on the UK club circuit) the future Cream members are required to mug, contort and conform to beat type for the good of the plot. Bruce even endures a polite tap from the headmaster's cane. 'Dig?' the master threatens. 'Dig, sir. Dig,' replies the future rock god who could play Shostakovich by the time he was twelve. Ginger Baker's pursed-lipped look indicates that he might well be contemplating punching the guy out, but even he acquiesces to the facile dialogue. In the equally dire *The Ghost Goes Gear* from 1966 – a film that gives up on any pretence of plot development after about forty minutes – Steve Winwood of the Spencer Davis Group looks as uncomfortable as it's possible for a teenage prodigy to be in front of the camera, but he still submits himself to the imbecilic requirements of what might loosely be called 'the script'. These same painful displays of inept and awkward behaviour spill over into the earliest promo films made by

543

some of Britain's most famous groups. Cream gambol about in monks' habits in a promo for 'I Feel Free'. The Move enact a Mad Hatter's tea party in the woods for 'I Can Hear the Grass Grow', before a bevy of lurking dolly birds leap out from behind the trees and strip them of their Carnaby Street threads. Procol Harum trudge self-consciously across a park for their 'Whiter Shade of Pale' promo, while Pink Floyd try to look all art-school aloof and sinister for 'Arnold Layne' but ruin the effect when Roger Waters and Syd Barrett have a mock punch-up like the good grammar-school roister-doisters they really were underneath all that garb. The only time the Small Faces ever looked gormless or anything less than cool was in their promo films. In one of the most bizarre photo sequences of the period Jimi Hendrix tousles the hair of Liberal Party leader Jeremy Thorpe, while Thorpe throws unconvincing shapes with the guitarist's V-shaped Strat. In fact, it's rare to find photos of any group at the height of the beat era or the dawning of the psychedelic age in which they don't at some point feel obliged to goof around or hang legs akimbo from the back of a Mini Moke. Leap in the air, boys. Play the game, boys. Accentuate the zany. 'Suck your glasses,' says a photographer to a bemused, amphetamine-addled Bob Dylan in D. A. Pennebaker's 1966 film *Eat the Document*. The lensman clearly assumes that the singer will conform to the deep-thinking archetype, as many writers and musicians will have done before him. But Dylan is having none of it. 'Do you want to suck my glasses?' he replies, refusing to play the game. Dylan, though, was untypical in his refusal to don the appropriate mantle. Most pop stars did play the game, even if they looked painfully uncomfortable while doing so. Notice the shy smile that played across the face of Brian Jones whenever the TV camera lingered a second too long and he couldn't maintain that moody pout a moment longer. John Lennon covered his discomfort by chewing imaginary gum or running through his well-rehearsed repertoire of gurning goons. Different tics for different flicks but they all expressed the same endearing lack of media savvy. Audiences on TV pop shows were just the same, either shuffling awkwardly out of the way of the marauding cameras at the behest of an in-shot floor manager, or gawping up at the monitors, simultaneously thrilled and amazed to see their out-of-body selves as others might see them. In a 1961 episode of his BBC comedy show Benny Hill played all of the characters in a sketch which spoofed *Juke Box Jury*. He gets the haughty and gawky, smarmy and oily, facile and flirtatious, stiff and idiotic reactions of the panellists down to a pencil-sucking tee, but more importantly he gets the studio audience spot on too, perfectly capturing those moments when the camera lingered obtrusively on their unwitting features and they slowly stiffened into rictus grins and other mortified postures of embarrassment. It's one of the defining images of the TV sixties, the sixties that resolutely refused to swing, not while it was under surveillance anyway. Hill's devastatingly accurate pastiche captured an audience still relatively unaware of the intrusiveness of the medium and only slowly beginning to come to terms with the idea of how it might present itself. Things hadn't changed significantly by the end of the sixties. Society had, but pop TV hadn't. It's a 1960s I remember all too well: watching *Juke Box Jury*'s weekly re-enactments of social awkwardness and observing girls in horn-rimmed glasses and lacquered helmets of hair and thick-lipped spotty boys with Brylcreemed barnets melting into blushing puddles of shyness under the hot studio lights, or dissolving into mumbled politeness when they were presented with prizes on whatever pop TV show

was handing out its baubles and record tokens that week.

The light-entertainment sixties that actually existed, as opposed to the one that is sometimes presumed to have existed, was both more bizarre and more banal than is usually portrayed by most chroniclers of pop. It was a 1960s in which Scott Walker could appear on the *Billy Cotton Band Show* in August 1967 singing Jacques Brel's 'My Death' and no one think it even mildly incongruous. A sizeable proportion of that Saturday-evening prime-time audience had lived through six years of global conflict between 1939 and 1945, and would almost certainly have known someone who died in it. An equally significant proportion of that prime-time audience would have been Catholic, as was Jacques Brel. To them the ceremony of death was all part of the wine-and-wafers fabric of life, and Scott Walker's existentialist serenade would barely have raised a murmur from sofa to scullery. It's almost de rigueur to exoticise such circumstances now, but in the 1960s bookings like this were the norm. *Top of the Pops* was the most obvious light-entertainment neutral zone for this kind of encounter, but everywhere you looked the schedules reverberated with cross-genre pollinations. *The Ken Dodd Show* featured avant-garde mime acts and experimental puppetry. Visiting singer-songwriters like Leonard Cohen, Tim Hardin and Tim Buckley appeared in whatever light-entertainment slot was available. The Who performed 'Magic Bus' on the children's TV show *Cracker-jack*. The Kinks appeared on *The Basil Brush Show*. In three successive weeks in May 1968, while rioting French students were ripping up paving stones in search of the beach, Grapefruit, the Herd and Eric Burdon and the Animals (in their psychedelic incarnation, no less) appeared on the Sunday-evening ATV light-entertainment game show *The Golden Shot* with host Bob Monkhouse. The defining moment in this mash-up of cultural incongruities probably took place on *Juke Box Jury* in 1964, when Howlin' Wolf's 1956 recording of 'Smokestack Lightning' was reissued as a single. The record (which subsequently made the Top 30) was played to the duly unimpressed jury, who voted it a miss, at which point all six foot six and 300 pounds of Chester Burnett himself walked out from behind the partition and was revealed by host David Jacobs as the show's mystery guest. History does not record the shock or embarrassment on the faces of the panellists, or the degree of indifference or humiliation registered by the blues legend himself – the show, like so many others, has been wiped – but the episode illustrates just how common-place these occurrences were during the early days of pop TV.

It was in such hit-and-miss circum-stances that the majority of beat groups took their chances, as they submitted to the trial-and-error, suck-it-and-see, throw-enough-mud democracy of the showbiz sixties. In the late summer of 1966 the Moody Blues had just fin-ished another nightclub gig in a long line of routine nightclub gigs. It had been eighteen months since they had reached number one in the pop charts with their cover version of the Bessie Banks song 'Go Now', and they hadn't had a Top 10 hit since. At the very point when the Beatles had decided to give up live performance and pop was shift-ing up a gear, the Moody Blues were doing a cabaret turn for the chicken-in-a-basket crowd, the fate that awaited all beat groups once the hits, the pack-age tours and the prestige bookings dropped off. After this particular gig, at a Newcastle night spot, an aggrieved punter came backstage (some versions of this story say it was the club's pro-moter) to tell them they were the worst band he had ever seen. So abrupt and abrasive was this verdict that recent band recruit singer-guitarist Justin

Hayward burst into tears. During the long quiet journey back down the A1 the more pragmatic members of the Moodies conceded that the assailant may have had a point and that they should either call it a day or radically change their act. They settled on the latter course and ditched the blue suits and corny cabaret patter. As drummer Graeme Edge put it, 'Fuck it, we're miserable and unhappy and broke playing music we don't like, so let's be miserable, unhappy and broke playing music we do like.'[3] Expecting to be released by Decca Records, they relocated briefly to Belgium and played out the remainder of their contract happily broke but creatively fulfilled. The titles they recorded between the supper-club slap-down and their unlikely reinvention at the end of 1967 reveal a band in transition. Tracks like 'Fly Me High', 'Love and Beauty' and 'Long Summer Days' were mellifluous, folksy and slightly druggy, and they were a taste of what was to come. Fortuitously, Decca handed them a lifeline and asked them to record a demonstration album for the label's new Deramic Stereo Sound system. The Moody Blues' working brief was a pop version of Dvořák's New World Symphony and the album was to be called Days of Future Passed, a title suggested by the record company.

Instead the band, along with producer Tony Clarke, went into the studio and reinvented themselves as cosmic troubadours. Forsaking Dvořák, they recorded a lushly textured album of their own songs, with the help of the London Symphony Orchestra. Decca were mildly enthusiastic but thought it lacked a hit single. The album sold reasonably well, although not spectacularly, and the chosen single, 'Nights in White Satin', barely scraped into the Top 20, but the Moody Blues never played a cabaret club again.

The Moody Blues' story illustrates the slender thread that divides fame and failure. One minute you're top of the pops; the next you are leaving thirty-second inserts between songs so that you can have a bit of pre-rehearsed banter with the resident DJ at Wallflower's in Wolverhampton or the Go-Go club in Hartlepool. Rock critics rarely took the Moody Blues seriously during the psychedelic era. They were generally regarded as a bit laughable, a bit infra dig. They even warrant a mention in Gillo Dorfles' 1969 study Kitsch: The World of Bad Taste, albeit for their sleeve art rather than their records, but in this area too they generally received a bad critical rap. Like the Bee Gees, they didn't conform to hippie type. There was always assumed to be something a bit suspect about this physically mismatched bunch of straight-looking guys, with their Athena-poster version of pop psych and their songs full of alliterative doggerel about man's place in the bigger scheme of things. As the band themselves put it on one of their puzzled contemplations of the riddles of the universe, isn't life strange? And yet, when you examine the evidence, the Moody Blues' psych credentials were rock solid. They were directly implicated in the three-part *News of the World* exposé in February 1967 on drug-taking in pop, and the group were indeed enthusiastic converts to the lysergic cause. Keyboard player Mike Pinder's '(Thinking Is) The Best Way to Travel' on the Moodies' *In Search of the Lost Chord* is one of the great 'show me the universe and get me home for tea' acid songs. The use of 'thinking' in this context, of course, directly contravenes the unwritten Hays Code of pop euphemism. Anyone who mentioned 'thinking' in a 1967/8 pop song generally meant 'on drugs'. Similarly blatant and unambiguous were the mentions of Timothy Leary in flautist Ray Thomas's 'Legend of a Mind'. But as with everything else they did from 1967 onwards the Moody Blues' use of LSD was purposeful and productive. Justin Hayward's intake,

he later admitted, was minimal, just a dozen or so visits to planet otherplace.

In the late 1960s, at around the time they started their own record label, Threshold, the Moody Blues were photographed for the music mags, suited and sprawled on a Surrey lawn looking like slightly hip stockbrokers. They admitted in interviews that they held regular business meetings. Such disingenuous honesty merely confirmed the prejudices of that portion of the rock press who already thought them interlopers and bread-heads. Never mind that former LSE student Mick Jagger regularly attended record-company meetings to discuss percentage points, or that several of the people whom the rock press did revere at the time now appear regularly in rich lists with fortunes measured in the millions if not hundreds of millions, the Moodies were dressed in business suits in the pop papers. Prepare the ducking stool. Light the Wicker Man. Despite these critical disapprovals, the best of the Moody Blues' music between 1967 and 1970 possessed a grace and grandeur all of its own. Like the Beatles, they combined a sense of the epic with economy of style and execution, and they understood how pop songs worked as ensemble pieces. None of them were particularly virtuosic or showy musicians, and they all willingly subsumed their individual sensibilities within the group sound. They also explored the textural possibilities of the mellotron better than any other group in pop. And, unlike a lot of their peers, they could recreate their entire studio sound in live performance, sumptuous vocal harmonies, temperamental mellotronics and all. On a hot August weekend when everyone bemoaned Jimi Hendrix for being lacklustre and the Doors for being sluggish, the Moodies' set at the 1970 Isle of Wight festival, performed as the sun went down on the Saturday night, was the highlight of the entire event.

Days of Future Passed, the album that saved their career, was completed in just three weeks, with the orchestral and group components being recorded separately. Not surprisingly, the two elements sound rushed and never fully integrated. The Moodies' light-bulb moment came when they realised they could provide the orchestral textures themselves simply with the aid of a mellotron, and that's precisely what they did on subsequent albums. *In Search of the Lost Chord* (1968), *On the Threshold of a Dream* (1969), *To Our Children's Children's Children* (1969) and *A Question of Balance* (1970) are characterised by a unified sound: multilayered instrumentation overlaid with banks of luscious choral harmonies. The end result managed to sound both ethereal and full-bodied. In Justin Hayward the Moody Blues had one of the truly underrated singers of the 1960s. Hayward had a distinctive yearning quality to his voice, a high baritone with a choir-boy tremor. The point where he asks, 'Just what is happening to me?' on 'Voices in the Sky' is one of the great heart-rending moments in sixties pop. A stick-thin man-child from Swindon, he could easily have hidden behind Scott Walker, or passed himself off as his shadow. Possibly the least physically demonstrative vocalist in pop – 'When Justin gets worked up he taps his foot,' joked drummer Graeme Edge – Hayward was also one of the first to voice the opinion that middle-class boys from the shires shouldn't be pretending to be blues men, they should be pretending to be something else instead. And so the Moody Blues became psychedelic ambassadors and philosophical questers. Their lyrics spoke for everyone who, like Michael Caine's Alfie, had at some point turned to that little mongrel dog on the Waterloo Bridge of their mind and asked, 'So what's the answer? That's what I keep asking myself – what's it all about? Know what I mean?'

Yes, some of their lyrics were trite. It's hard to believe that the same man who wrote 'Legend of a Mind' and 'Dear Diary' could also write, 'Floating free as a bird / sixty-foot leaps / it's so absurd.' Then again, perhaps it isn't. And it's not always easy to keep a straight face during some of the more purple passages, or when Graeme Edge recites the poems that commence each album. But delivering lines like 'to burst up through tarmac' in a hysterical Birmingham brogue is no more absurd than well-bred boys from Shepperton or Chertsey singing about their wing-wang. The Moody Blues at their most florid were certainly no worse than Traffic or Eric Burdon's psychedelic Animals at their most jejune, or anyone else who sang about eternity's road or the fluttery flickery candle of life. And while it's true that the line 'face piles and piles of trials with smiles' should have been embroidered onto a range of tea towels, eiderdowns and antimacassars and sold in hippie emporia to anyone who lived in a little hobbity wizard world inside their heads, the Moody Blues also sang of real emotions like loneliness and love and trying to find one's place in this life. Furthermore they presented these existential tribulations with far less mordancy and infinitely more *joie de vivre* than Roger Waters, say, or ELP or King Crimson. Their lyrics may have been full of imponderables and prone to uncertainty, but their sound was as snug as an electric blanket. They were in some ways a curiously indefinable band, and it's easy to see in retrospect how they could have evaded the critics' grasp. They rarely displayed whimsicality but they weren't discernibly humourless either. They helped invent pop bombast, but even their grandiosity was delivered with a lightness of touch that eluded their more ponderous pomp-rock rivals. Their classical motifs are always reassuringly familiar. Everything is built on steady progressions; nothing ever jars or wanders off into atonality. There is dissonance but there is no abrasion in their music. It is these components – the ordinary-guy philosophising, the comforting rendering of uncomforting landscapes – that explain both their massive appeal and why a certain breed of pop writer bestowed shallowness and kitsch upon them. Critics who were scornful of their quest were generally scornful of commonplace aspirations as well.

And those accusations of kitsch were wildly off target anyway. In the end, perhaps even in the very beginning too, everything could be reduced to kitsch, and psychedelia embraced kitschness more readily than most, drawing willingly as it did from the deep well of the gaudy and the decorative. Its rococo roots (and routes) were apparent from the very start, as were its borrowings from the Pre-Raphaelites and art nouveau. Many a floaty nocturnal apparition down at UFO or the Roundhouse looked like Millais' doomed Ophelia risen up from the watery shallows to take her rightful place among the beautiful people, all diaphanous display and belladonna eyeballs. Psychedelic posters borrowed their florid lines from Alphonse Mucha and their swirly lettering from the French Metro. 'One moment it is not there and then suddenly, from about 1899, the pastel shades and seductive contours of this false dawn are visible everywhere,' said Cyril Connolly of art nouveau,[4] and the same is true of psychedelia, with the emphasis firmly on the false dawn. Connolly argued that art noveau was not the precursor that paved the way for modernism. He thought it 'more correct to see the style as complete in itself, an unattainable end, no doubt, but one having very little to do with modern art as we now know it'. And that is true of psychedelia too, again with the emphasis on unattainable end. As a visual and audible style psychedelia came and went very quickly. It emerged from the noonday underground in 1966, peaked in 1967 and was all but gone by the end of 1969. One minute everyone was adorning their record sleeves and their lyrics with rainbow arcs; the next no one was. For a short while sound engineers reversed everything that formerly ran clockwise. They phased cymbal hiss and vocals to within an inch of their lives, but by 1970 such strategies had disappeared from the manual. As a bunch of stylistic options psychedelia seemed to swell up all at once, before deflating as quickly as a balloon once the party moved on. Walter Crane described art nouveau as 'that strange decorative disease'.[5] It's a description that applied equally to psychedelia.

In the end psychedelia was a style like any other and a lot of unlikely people fell for its seductive charms. And how rapidly its allure was assimilated. Clearly, if Des O'Connor could have his *I Pretend* album sleeve adorned with bubble graphics and yellow swirls, and Cilla Black could record a song called 'Abyssinian Secret' that coyly invited you to sample exotic wares recently smuggled back from the Near East, then psychedelia's entry into the mainstream, if not the bloodstream, was all but complete. In the summer of 1967 cabaret crooner Vince Hill followed up his number-one hit version of 'Edelweiss', from *The Sound of Music*, with a portentous release called 'When the World Is Ready'. Penned by John Scott and Don Black, and taken from the movie *The Long Duel*, starring Yul Brynner and Trevor Howard, 'When the World Is Ready' was an unlikely peacenik anthem. Embellished with a mournful sitar line played by Big Jim Sullivan, the song was transplanted into an action movie set during the days of the Raj in which blacked-up actors played Indian police officers and Yul Brynner once again proved that he was the go-to guy for stage and screen exotica. 'When the world is ready / all wars may cease,' intones Vince as B-52s continue to carpet-bomb Vietnamese villages on the other side of the world. A similar sitar accompaniment can be heard on Paul and Barry Ryan's 'Pictures of Today', the last song the duo recorded together before Barry went solo and elevated his brother's compositions to a whole new level of rococo overload. 'Pictures of Today' was written by Peter Morris, a library-music writer and jack of many trades. It was perfect off-the-peg psychedelia, full of storybook reveries and lines like 'ever glowing / never showing signs of latent fears at all', which like a lot of psych-pop lyrics is both achingly suggestive of

meaning and splendidly meaningless. For years I misheard the chorus phrase 'touch my heart' as 'Taj Mahal'. The point is, it doesn't make the slightest bit of difference to the song if you substitute one for the other.

Taking his cue from that song's lovelorn landscape, Barry Ryan embarked upon a series of late-sixties singles that were kitsch classicism in extremis. His 1968 Top 10 hit 'Eloise' was a silk-blousey romp of a song, with bridal choruses that crescendoed and climaxed like a host of Tin Pan Alley valkyries. The orchestra, conducted by session supremo Johnny Arthey, crashes through the score with all the scale-rate abandon and panache you would expect from musicians who had seen it all, done it all and were off to Shepherd's Bush Green to fulfil a BBC light-entertainment booking the minute that studio clock struck six. 'Eloise' was five and a half minutes of pop bombast, ever glowing, never showing signs of latent fear at all. It set the tempo for everything Barry Ryan (and, indeed, a distinctively British form of pop baroque) did for the next two years. After 'Eloise' Ryan carried on making the same record with different words, till the wave broke, the tide subsided and nobody wanted their bombast to sound like that any more. When 'Eloise' entered the UK pop charts in November 1968 its grandiloquence didn't sound out of place at all. It was released just months after Jim Webb's seven-and-a-half-minute epic 'MacArthur Park', and there is something of that song's ambition and intent about 'Eloise', and indeed in all of Paul Ryan's subsequent compositions for his brother. The confident young Ryan reputedly went up to Webb at a London showbiz party and brazenly announced, 'I'm writing songs like that.' And he was. 'Eloise' and its follow-ups 'Love Is Love', 'The Hunt' and 'Magical Spiel' had lyrics that were camp, predatory and Oedipal all at the same time. 'The Hunt' was the sound of Oliver Tobias chasing an off-duty bunny girl round Annabel's while Peter Wyngarde looked disdainfully on and discreetly slipped a suspiciously fizzy something into an unattended drink. 'Magical Spiel' was a veritable cornucopia of kitschness, with Ryan spelling out the title's bewitched and bewildering acrostic 'M is for Magdalene / A is for Alchemist / G is for the Grecian god of light', etc. Merlin, Aphrodite, Lucifer, Incest, Ouija boards – they're all in there. And then, during the long hot summer of 1970, came the love that finally dared speak its name. 'Kitsch' was possibly the best of Barry Ryan's singles. Had it been the first it would be the one that everyone would remember now and the one that the Damned would have felt compelled to give a goth-punk makeover to. 'Kitsch' begins with a dream apparition. 'I saw the shape of things to come / then I awoke / it was no joke / I'd seen the shape of things to come,' and who dared doubt him as the session cats turned those sheet-music pages with mounting incredulity, the bridal choruses were screeched even more dementedly and Ryan burst ever more primally out of his blouse. '"Kitsch" is a beautiful word / it's a beautiful lullaby,' he screamed. He even rhymes 'moon' with 'June' without making it sound jejune.

The other great purveyors of late-sixties pop baroque were Ken Howard and Alan Blaikley, a writing team whose psychedelic-era credits included the Herd hits 'From the Underworld' and 'Paradise Lost', and 'Last Night in Soho' and 'The Wreck of the Antoinette' for Dave Dee, Dozy, Beaky, Mick and Tich. 'From the Underworld' rewrote the Orpheus myth for pop consumption and it worked a treat. The mini-opus opens with funereal bells, fuzz guitars and Yardbirds harmonies, and picks up a steady galloping pace. The lyric flows like the River Styx from verse to verse, pausing only for 'Penny Lane' trumpet interludes. No chorus, no bridge, no middle eight, just that remorseless lovers' march towards a doomed finale, when Orpheus forgets his promise and turns to look at Eurydice. Howard and Blaikley had another stab at the formula with the follow-up single 'Paradise Lost', but although the song made the Top 20, the writers lost their nerve second time around and succumbed to the first law of camp by introducing the song with a pastiche of David Rose's 'The Stripper' theme. After that nipple-tassled intro any attempt at building the doomed momentum that characterised 'From the Underworld' went out of the window. 'Experience has dulled my eyes / With repetition wonder dies,' sings Peter Frampton in the final verse, altogether too clever by half and seemingly in on the joke as they cue that stripper music once more for the burlesque outro. By the time they scored a third successive hit with 'I Don't Want Our Loving to Die' Howard and Blaikley had dropped the classical references entirely and returned to the more familiar realm of everyday pop love. The sound is scaled down too. Busy orchestration is replaced by those chunky trebly organ stabs that became ubiquitous in 1968 as keyboard players stopped bowing down to the holy trinity of Smith, McGriff and McDuff and traded in their blue notes for a little

Reginald Dixon Wurlitzer action. Like a lot of half-decent musicians from that era, the Herd badly wanted to show they had chops. Their final single, a group composition called 'Sunshine Cottage', was perfect psych-pop euphemystica, with clanging Beatley guitars, ba-ba-ba-ba vocals and time-served metaphorical eulogising to a domicile made out of drugs. 'Sunshine Cottage' boasted 'excellent price / reasonable view' (when seen through 'magic spectacles' no doubt), but when the song failed to match the success of its predecessors, Pete Frampton was off to join Steve Marriott in Humble Pie as quick as you could say 'Face of '68'.

Howard and Blaikley's compositions for Dave Dee, Dozy, Beaky, Mick and Tich matched the melodramatic sweep of their work with the Herd. Like that other great Wiltshire combo the Troggs, Dave Dee and Co. never took themselves seriously enough to garner serious critical attention. By rights their early hits – 'Hideaway', 'Hold Tight' and 'Save Me' – should have been garage-band staples and inspired cover versions in the same way that the Troggs' 'I Can Only Give You Everything' did, but no one took the bait. Even though the opening riff of 'Hold Tight' will be pounded out at football grounds for the rest of time, it never ended up in the hands of the Shadows of Knight or the Standells, where it really belonged. Like the Troggs, Dave Dee and Co. had their bamboo-butterfly moments. On 'The Sun Goes Down', the B-side to 'Zabadak', they gave full vent to their nasal Gregoriana and fuzz-wah tendencies. It's a magnificent slab of noise that could easily be mistaken for late-period Yardbirds, but they are forever fated to be best known for novelty fare like 'Bend It' and 'Zabadak'. The group's final Top 20 flourish was with a brace of Howard and Blaikley compositions: 'Last Night in Soho' and 'The Wreck of the Antoinette'. The former was a psycho-drama set in gangland. With a middle eight straight out of Lionel Bart and Joan Littlewood, it told the tale of the little guy who tries to go straight but succumbs to temptation and strongarm persuasion, and in the pay-off finds himself heading for a prison sentence and a tearful farewell to his trusting gal. Its follow-up, 'The Wreck of the Antoinette', released in September 1968, was emblematic of a style of kitsch melodrama that Howard and Blaikley championed and others dared to follow. This was the last great age of orchestration on pop records before Marshall stacks, heavy rockers and sensitive singer-songwriters rewrote the rule book and the budgetary requirements of the music industry. It was also the last gasp of the character songs as bands began to reject bespoke vignettes about Grecian myths and dodgy dealings in gangland and settled for solipsism and songs about the bulging contents of their loon pants instead.

Trace the evolution of UK pop (as opposed to rock) to the end of the decade and you can hear the trace elements of psychedelia slowly evaporating, as Status Quo put it, like ice in the sun. 'Ice in the Sun' was written by Marty Wilde, who had been one of the most promising acts in Larry Parnes's home-grown stable of UK rockers in the late 1950s. Wilde's own version of the song appeared on his 1969 solo album *Diversions*, along with a clutch of pop ballads arranged in that particularly English style of pop orchestration that was enjoying its last hurrah at the end of the decade. The album's cover showed a photo of Wilde in John Lennon granny glasses and was adorned with the kind of flowery pencil doodles that fifth-form girls used to decorate their art folders with. *Diversions* is the sound of someone going mildly psychedelic. It's full of radio-friendly flourishes and frills, all gussied up by the A-list of British arrangers: Peter Knight (Dusty Springfield, Scott Walker, the Moody Blues), Johnny Arthey (Barry

Ryan, Mary Hopkin, every Trojan reggae record that had a string arrangement) and Cy Payne (a man whose CV includes assistant music director on Jack Good's *Oh Boy!*, as well as writer of children's TV themes and the official regimental music for Trooping the Colour). *Diversions* reverberates not with paisley-coloured skies and hissy phasing but clattering percussion and parping brass. The occasional arbitrary sound effect is thrown in for good measure and the studio controls are set to chirpy, no matter how moody and reflective the balladry is trying to be. There was a lot of it about in the late 1960s; it's that peculiarly parochial version of Vegas via Club Tito's in Stockton-on-Tees, the kind of place where Scott Walker fetched up during his sabbatical years. For Walker it was a kind of gap life, and one which conveniently fulfils that most necessary of critical contrivances, the bridge between fame and third act, but for many it was the norm, just another career opportunity, one door opening as another closed.

The closing track on *Diversions*, 'Abergavenny', was a hit for Wilde in America, where it was released under the pseudonym of Shannon, reaching the *Billboard* Top 50 in August 1969. Set to a pounding beat with trilling piccolo and oompah brass, 'Abergavenny' paid a bracing and carefree homage to unfashionable British seaside resorts, with just enough archly enunciated innuendo in 'taking a trip up to Abergavenny' to give it some analogous cachet. The song also contained the winning couplet 'passing some time with paradise people / paradise people are fine by me', and essentially that's what all these latter-day psychsploitation contenders were doing as they pursued with varying degrees of conviction and pizzazz what Aldous Huxley, in a splendidly apposite phrase, called 'the ersatz of suchness'. Huxley was making a point about art's inability to convey the splendour and totality of the religious experience, its inadequacy (or at least the inadequacy of bad art) in the grander scheme of things. In one of the most contentious and yet throwaway comments in *The Doors of Perception* he seems to be suggesting that almost all creativity is ersatz. 'Art, I suppose, is only for beginners,' he says. It's for those who are content with 'symbols rather than what they actually signify, with the elegantly composed recipe in lieu of actual dinner'.[6]

Some would argue that that's ultimately what psychedelia was too – the elegantly composed recipe rather than the sustenance of the meal itself. There is certainly something deeply symbolic about the way that LSD heightened awareness of the ungraspable. Pop records, in attempting to convey that elusiveness, added a further layer of distortion, while those who didn't take psychedelics at all added a final layer of illusion by simulating what they presumed the drug experience to be like, until in the end bamboo butterflies swell to twice their normal size and everyone stares, mesmerised by multiples of their own fleeting image in an ever-receding hall of mirrors, never knowing which is facsimile and which is real.

Marty Wilde was certainly no stranger to ersatz, having penned 'Elizabeth Dreams' and 'Paradise Flat', two of Status Quo's best LP tracks, but in the end, if Huxley's dictum is adhered to, ersatz is what everyone was offering. It was the only rainbow-chasing game in town. From the four stately kings of EMI to those who romped in the mud at Max Yasgur's farm during the very month that 'Abergavenny' was in the US chart. All those Aquarian-age aspirants, bandwagon jumpers and bums. All those one-hit or no-hit wonders who briefly donned butterfly wings and looking-glass ties, who fastened the buttons on their multicoloured dreamcoats and went in search of sunshine cottages, satellite jockeys and a skilful

enough song plugger to propel their effort to number 42 in the chart. They were all wallowing in the ersatz splendour of LSD's suchness.

In the same way that a significant number of pop releases in 1965 and 1966 anticipated psychedelia with their decentred subject matter, their disembodied longings, their melancholic moods and their disruptive tempo shifts, many of the outpourings of the late 1960s, although not psychedelic in anything other than the loosest terms, were records that would not have been made, or at least would not have sounded the way they did, had the musical climate not been so full of 'drink me' elixir and hallucinogenic sparkle. The Flowerpot Men was an alias for the John Carter–Ken Lewis writing team, who as members of the Ivy League sang back-up on the Who's 'I Can't Explain' and enjoyed several Top 20 hits of their own. The Sagittarius cover version of the Ivy League's 'My World Fell Down' and Music Explosion's 'Little Bit O' Soul', which appeared on the *Nuggets* compilation, were both Carter–Lewis compositions. In the grand tradition of pan-Atlantic cultural ricochet, Carter and Lewis took Gary Usher and Terry Melcher's Sagittarius reworking of 'My World Fell Down' as the template for their own homespun refinement of the

Californian sound. The most successful realisation of this was the hit single 'Let's Go to San Francisco', an invitation that few if any of the record's UK listeners were in a position to take up. 'Let's Go to San Francisco' was six minutes twenty seconds long and had to be spread over two sides of a single when it was released in August 1967. That running time hinted at more grandiose intent, and Carter and Lewis subsequently embarked upon two further ambitious full-length works, *The Peace Album* and *Past Imperfect*. Both projects, unreleased at the time, were testimony to the vainglorious dreams that British pop frequently threw up in the late 1960s: Mark Wirtz's *Teenage Opera* springs to mind, as do several mad-brained song suites that Robin Gibb claimed to be working on at the time. Only a few pieces of Carter and Lewis's mosaic emerged in the late 1960s, but both albums were pieced together in a CD reconstruction in 2000. Like *Teenage Opera*, the reconstructions gathered together the ad hoc elements of a grander plan and presented them as they might have been had the world not moved on. 'The Cooks of Cake and Kindness' on *The Peace Album* had previously been released by a pop harmony group called the Californians, who hailed not from the west coast but the West Midlands. 'Mythological Sunday', one of the great ersatz of suchness song titles, was a six-minute B-side released in the summer of 1968. 'Blow Away' was a ringing twelve-string endorsement of a Byrds who had stopped sounding like that three years earlier. Both *The Peace Album* and *Past Imperfect* sounded like an extended coda to a sixties that had long since been and gone. In 1969 Carter and Lewis even recorded a reprise of 'Let's Go to San Francisco' called 'Let's Go Back to San Francisco', by which time the Haight-Ashbury they were eulogising was full of boarded-up shop fronts. As Charles Perry put it, 'House cats did not dare walk on the streets that year; they hid behind bushes because needle freaks – speeders and junkies – were hunting them for food.'[7] When 'Let's Go Back to San Francisco' was finally released in 1971, it could have qualified for heritage funding as a form of restoration pop. By this time love, peace and universal brotherhood were far more likely to be illustrated by swaying in 'perfect harmony' to 'I'd Like to Teach the World to Sing' while endorsing Coca-Cola. What had sounded like a pop epiphany in 1967 now sounded like cabaret fodder. 'Let's Go Back to San Francisco' would have slotted seamlessly into a nightclub set, introduced with a ready quip and a bit of banter with the DJ and sung by whichever group of individuals was touring as the Flowerpot Men by 1971. This was the past imperfect the Moody Blues had left behind a lifetime ago but one which more pragmatic souls returned to when their own mythological Sunday never arrived. It was here, on the scampi-and-chips, Mateus Rosé-in-a-wicker-basket club circuit, that UK pop psych came home to die. All that had once melted into air solidified into well-rehearsed stagecraft in the smoke-filled rooms of the club circuit: the Caesar's Palaces, Cinderellas', Rafters, Tiffanys' and Locarnos, the dress-code, two-drink minimum, eight till late (but not that late) go-go emporia where patter calcified into cliché and hits-of-the-day medleys were compulsory. Collars grew wider, jackets more velveteen, long hair more layered, lacquered and groomed. Year on year the flock wallpaper was kippered with another coating of nicotine, the compère continued to do that Norman Collier thing with the mic and week by week the resident house band seemed to grow a little more glam and glittery. Oh, and the stories that dressing-room mirror could reveal. 'Did I tell you we had the Moody Blues here once? Back in '66 it was. Worst bloody band I ever booked.'

The Avant-Garde Rearguard

In one of those barely believable instances of historical happenstance C. S. Lewis, Aldous Huxley and John F. Kennedy all died within a few hours of each other on 22 November 1963. Seismically epochal portents could be contrived out of such synchronicity, and some would argue that the psychic energy released by that unlikely congruence of fatalities contained the nebulous gases that formed the psychedelic sixties. On the one hand you have the author of the *Narnia* books, whose wardrobe portal into a netherworld of wickedness and redemption unleashed the dreams of those who believed Turkish Delight to be the one true gateway drug. In close mortal conjunction, receiving lysergic sacrament on his deathbed, you have the polymath who gave intellectual and spiritual justification to a generation's romantic proclivities and their chemical transformation. Finally, and most conspiratorially, you have the murder of the dreams and hope that sprang if not eternal, then certainly youthful from the body politic of Kennedy's Camelot. These three deaths conjoined thesis, antithesis and synthesis in a multiplicity of unconscious and uncoordinated desires.

To others, though, the really significant event took place the following day, Saturday 23 November, when at teatime the BBC unveiled its new children's sci-fi drama, *Doctor Who*. While many were intrigued by the strange tale of a strange man who lived in a phone box that was bigger on the inside than the outside, even more were spellbound by the opening credits: a warped and wavy white-haired apparition, accompanied by some of the strangest oscillations ever heard on TV, a theme tune that more than half a century on still fanfares a future we haven't quite acclimatised ourselves to yet. Delia Derbyshire's 1963 treatment of Ron Grainer's melody for the *Doctor Who* theme signified a far-off world at a time when the charts were full of Merseybeat and Trini López. As the sixties wore on Time Lords and their adversaries came and went, but that theme tune never stopped sounding eerie. The disconnect between clunky action sequences, ham acting and cardboard sets on the one hand and the radiophonic bleeps and squalls of the *Doctor Who* theme and the programme's incidental music grew ever larger as the years went by; yet another manifestation of that peculiarly British juxtaposition of avant-garde noise and trad narrative. Dr Who may have been teleported from another dimension but he frequently teamed up with stiff-upper-lipped, khaki-wearing military men in order to have showdowns with makeshift papier mâché monsters in disused quarries. And all of this glorious kitsch nonsense was choreographed to the tape-treated, time-warped, analogue-looped world of Delia Derbyshire, Desmond Briscoe, Dick Mills, Daphne Oram, Brian Hodgson, Paddy Kingsland and all the other make-do-and-mend Heath Robinson heroes and heroines of the BBC Radiophonic Workshop.

This was the avant-garde's rearguard, the experimentalist's revenge, the lab boys and girls who innovated to order and produced atonal noise on commission that could be bought by the yard. The BBC Radiophonic Workshop maintained a constant high-profile presence throughout the 1960s and '70s. It could be heard in school programmes, local-radio themes and jingles, in incidentals and subliminals everywhere, the true tomorrow's world that fanfared the banality of today. This is where psychedelia settled once it stopped hailing newspaper taxis and sliding down rainbows. Its legacy does not lie in periodic pop press-hyped revivals of a 'sound'. It sits deeply embedded within the subversive functionality of library music. A world of ranked and filed options where the accompanying client-orientated track descriptions form a haiku poetry of their very own:

> Slow relaxed rhythm
> With mysterious build-up
> Romantic restrained

> Driving dramatic
> Pulsating hard and lively
> Frantic up-tempo

> Eerie atmosphere
> Swirling strings persistent beat
> Repetitive riff

Julie Burchill once claimed in a typically withering *NME* singles column that because most of that week's new releases were so dispiritingly alike, they should have been graded by the same criteria as wallpaper samples or paint manufacturers' colour codings. She clearly meant it as an insult but in the world of library music this is the standard Dewey-eyed approach to pop classification. The splendidly cosmic paradox is that many of the endeavours created in the name of client-orientated creativity now sound far more out there than most of the efforts that were really trying to be out there. 'Soon these things will acquire period charm; the cycle of taste, revolving ever

faster, will quickly bring them, with cinema posters and jazz lino, within our range of aesthetic appreciation,' said Barbara Jones of the vernacular arts she championed in 1951. Shrewd to the last she even predicted the pattern of their route to respectability and canonisation. 'Their steady ritual progress will follow clearly ordained lines: via the appreciation of common man into almost total oblivion, out again to the intellectual home, onwards to the antique shop and finally to permanent deification in wealthy drawing rooms and museums.'[8] The avant-garde's rearguard follows a similar process. For the intellectual home read irony, camp and post-modern commodification; for antique shops, drawing rooms and museums read record shops, collectors and cult appeal. Kitsch psych, session psych, soundtrack psych, library psych and all their attendant made-to-measure noise codes didn't bear any of these names at the time. Nor did they constitute a movement of any kind. They were assimilated not by sales figures or prestige but by osmosis. Lacking any semblance of cultural capital they became a non-genre genre virtually by default, and with the minimum of fuss and seemingly with zero publicity and promotion. They slid imperceptibly into our daily lives, where they ingratiated themselves by stealth, as adverts and jingle stings, theme tunes, film scores, elevator drones, restaurant ambience. They became the residual psychedelic musak of our souls, anonymous, everywhere.

There were hundreds of these albums. They were released through all kinds of unlikely outlets and performed by the cream of a session generation. As with kitsch portraits of dogs playing cards and dolls' houses made out of sequins and seashells, ask not who bought these records or even who they were aimed at, ask what they can still do for you now that everything is endlessly retrievable and shelf life is measured in samples and bytes. They have a timeless yet time-bound beauty of their own, and in their more outré moments they are as much a part of psychedelia's legacy as light shows and sugar cubes.

Footprints on the Moon

In May 1967 Andrew Loog Oldham's Immediate label released a single called 'The Changing of the Guard'. Credited to the group Marquis of Kensington, the song was penned by arranger Mike Leander, performed by session musicians and sung by former Kinks manager Robert Wace, who adopted the tones of a louche young Scottish laird as he delivered his droll tale of an empire on its uppers. It's a world in which aristocrats can no longer afford a butler or maid, Lady Londonderry has flogged the family silver, and Lord Windermere has raised a mortgage on the mansion and shows visitors round 'for a half a dollar fee', and if the song's loyal and stoical subjects ever get invited to the palace, 'then we'll all go there by bus'. The song, like so many others of the period, is indebted to Wace's former charge Ray Davies, although Davies in his prime would never have penned that final verse's dreadful pun about a rich girl down on her luck who is now a belly dancer, 'and not because she comes from a naval family'. When he performed 'The Changing of the Guard' on the German pop show *Beat Club* Wace was accompanied by two panda-eyed models who clapped along in a disinterested manner, missed their miming cues by at least half a bar and generally treated the whole affair with perfectly judged insouciance. Peter Whitehead gave prominence to 'The Changing of the Guard' at the start of his 1967 documentary *Tonite Let's All Make Love in London*. Here the song accompanies the annual Trooping the Colour ceremony on Horse Guards Parade. The sight of all that pageantry and procession throws the lyrics into sharp relief. It anchors the song to the time of its origins and a world that doesn't look like that any more. We see chinless gin-flushed men in bowler hats, and ladies in twin sets and Ascot hats who regard the camera with expressions that range from wary distrust to haughty disgust. These impeccably groomed onlookers serve as iconic reminders of the swinging sixties' other fashion parade, of empire-bonded loyalties and unbreakable allegiances. This portion of White-head's film freeze-frames a square mile of Belgravia and Knightsbridge that remained impervious to the march of the Carnebetian army. It's also a telling reminder that in the UK the beneficiaries of wealth and privilege, young and old alike, could coexist and not remotely threaten each other. Indeed, that's probably Lady Annabelle Barley, the belly dancer's mother, scowling at the camera.

'The Changing of the Guard' was achingly arch and mildly satirical, and its tone was not so different from those Pathé newsreels and Rank Organisation cine features that filmed swinging England in all its Technicolor glory. These were then overdubbed with the kind of witheringly amused commentary that made it perfectly clear that the swinging sixties could tolerate all but its most dangerous eccentricities to death. The tone of those Pathé pieces has the practised sanguinity and 'Oh well, if you must' world-weary acceptance that permeated every media angle on youth culture. It became the default lingua franca that informed everything from the BBC's pop programming and satire sketches to all those rip-and-read news-agency items wired around the Western world in breathless show-biz patois. It's a world where, if you believe the glib official pitch, everyone did everything for 'the fun of it', in a 'Look, no strings, no Daddy's trust fund' meritocracy of fab boutiques and even fabber accessories. That carefree and breezy view of the era covers up a multiplicity of contradictions, of course, but it has endured surprisingly well and has hardened into a kind of official orthodoxy. In an age when everything can be reduced to its iconography, and when post-modernism commandeers irony, kitsch and camp and coats them in a depoliticised surface sheen, those newsreels take on a freshly replenished life of their own. The same archive clips of the same people trying on the same clothes in those same cramped boutiques play on a forever loop until it's the only sixties we know. It would be easy to say that irony, kitsch and camp killed the swinging sixties – killed the sixties full stop, in fact – but that would mean disregarding the fact that there was always an ironic, kitsch and camp element to it all. Was anybody ever more arch, blasé and knowing than the Chelsea set? When Peter Cook and Dudley Moore urged *Private Eye* readers, via the medium of flexi-disc, 'If you want a kinky caper / then suck a blotting paper,' on a song called 'Psychedelic Baby' in December 1966, it was clear that consciousness-raising was as ripe for satire as any other aspect of popular culture. On Boxing Day 1966, a year to the day before *Magical Mystery Tour* caused such a furore, Cook and Moore slipped an equally brazen song called 'LS Bumble Bee' into their *Not Only . . . But Also* Christmas special. The song was included in a sequence that also featured a guest appearance from John Lennon as the doorman of London's fashionable Ad-Lav club. Cook, playing the visiting American reporter Hiram J. Pipesucker in 'The Pipesucker Report', goes to visit brash young record producer Simon Accrington, played by Moore and obviously based on Mickie Most and Andrew Loog Oldham ('he's young, adventurous and horrible'). Accrington takes Pipesucker to see his new young charges – the Mothers, who perform an exquisite pastiche of a musical form that barely exists yet. It has

pitch-perfect synaesthetic lyrics ('I hear with my knees / run with my nose'), seagull sound effects and the same mispronunciation of 'psychedeelic' that features on the *Private Eye* flexi-disc. Cook and Moore perform 'LS Bumble Bee' clad à la mode in Nehru jackets. Cook wields a faux-Indian instrument fashioned from a cricket bat. During the middle eight Moore strokes miked-up water in a goldfish bowl. It's the Alberts, Bruce Lacey, knickers hung from the Skylon and the great spirit of UK Dada all over again. And it precedes *Sgt Pepper* by five months.

A few months later, when Vivian Stanshall slipped a far from subliminal 'take a trip' into the Bonzos' 'Cool Britannia', no one raised an eyebrow. Benign tolerance and a modicum of ridicule – it's the British way. Those waspish cinema-reel voice-overs captured that blithe spirit in all its glory. The man responsible for the dry, acerbic *Look at Life* quote which commences this chapter was Michael Ingrams, appropriately enough, the step-brother of *Private Eye* founder Richard Ingrams. In his commentary Ingrams was sufficiently astute to recognise that for those who were lucky enough to be at the centre of things, it was all one big fancy-dress ball, and that identity was malleable, interchangeable and up for grabs. He might also have mentioned that one of the most distinctive things about pop fashion in 1967 was that there was a big 1920s revival going on. It would make icons of Bonnie and Clyde and build the cathedral of Biba. Those *Look at Life* features were beamed into a thousand provincial Gaumonts and Odeons. They were sharp, witty and pithily scripted, and they offered a window on another world. They were how most people saw the swinging sixties – the media-patented swinging sixties, that is. They saw it from the outside looking in, sandwiched between the Pearl and Dean ads and the main feature.

One of the more simple truths lurking among all the complex ones is that once fashion moved on, the music moved on with it. By the turn of the decade disposability was shunned and suddenly whole aspects of the sixties that had previously been revered, or at least indulged, looked shallow, materialistic and pointlessly frivolous. Nobody wanted irritatingly zany movies, dolly-rocker dresses, newspaper dresses (or newspaper taxies), enamel-disc belts, PVC boots and macs, plastic visors and all the other accoutrements of mid-sixties space chic. Nobody wanted plastic anything. Faux-ethnicity was the new thing. Laura Ashley, oatmeal and dungarees. What also killed

mid-sixties space chic – what finally killed the psychedelic sixties full stop – was the moon landing. On 21 July 1969, almost eight years after John F. Kennedy had pledged to outdo Russia's colonial expansionism into the astronomical final frontier by putting a man on the moon, America finally did just that, and what we saw shattered any lingering illusion that outer space could provide better pictures than inner space. The news bulletins showed grey grainy footage. We all heard Neil Armstrong's halting and hesitant delivery as he misquoted Richard Nixon's Pentagon-approved soliloquy about small steps and giant leaps. Armstrong and Buzz Aldrin played space golf and goofed around on a piece of illuminated cold rock that, despite the monumental historical significance of the occasion, continued to look far more beautiful from down here than it did from up there. The BBC's coverage of that same momentous occasion (subsequently wiped, naturally) was accompanied by a specially commissioned composition by Pink Floyd. Variously known as 'Moonhead', 'Trip on Mars' and 'Corrosion', the piece captures Pink Floyd in their own gravity-free limbo – post-Syd Barrett, pre-*Dark Side of the Moon* – where they sound magnificently exploratory and abstract.

'Moonhead' reclaimed inner space for those who didn't want their visions contaminated by facile commentary or homilies written by crooked presidents. It was the purest moment in the BBC's entire coverage.

The one Apollo mission that did truly resonate with the jaded and the reverential alike was unlucky 13 in April 1970, when that great epochal (and frequently misquoted) understatement 'Houston, we've had a problem here' was uttered, and James Lovell, John Swigert and Fred Haise almost slipped the surly bonds and nearly re-entered the Earth's orbit not as All-American heroes but as spam in a can. Drifting up there alone for four long days, with only their frozen piss and their prayers for company, they captured hearts and minds in a way that no gravity-free bounce on the moon's tideless beaches ever could. By the time Apollo 15 got to the moon in July 1971 the whole billion-dollar spectacle had started to seem like a long-haul commute. The Netherlands-based offshore pirate radio station Radio Northsea International used to commence its nightly mission updates with the eerie flute intro to arranger Johnny Harris's composition 'Footprints on the Moon'. The echo-chambered woodwind, the sparse, yearning piano melody and its Sea of Tranquillity chorale presented a more ghostly, melancholic evocation of deepest darkest space than all the Apollo missions put together. 'Footprints on the Moon' soundtracked a far stranger domicile: our inner dream homes and heartaches, rendered in uneasy listening and beamed to lonely souls, uninhabited satellites and barren planets alike – all of them so far away and yet so near.

19

PAINT AMERICA LOVE

Feeling then, not that I was drugged,
but that I was in an unusual degree
open to reality I tried to discern the
meaning, the inner character of the
dancing pattern which constituted
both myself and the garden, and
the whole dome of the night with its
coloured stars. All at once it became
obvious that the whole thing was love
play, where love means everything
that the word can mean.
ALAN WATTS, 1960[1]

Imagine a parallel world where you might be watching some dumb sitcom, and it's suddenly interrupted without too much rhyme or reason by one of your favourite garage-rock bands. You could call the show, I dunno, something like *The Mother-in-Law*. It would feature a typical all-American extended family and the action could take place in a typical all-American sitting room. The set-up would be that the son has this band he wants to promote and he's running the contract past his sceptical father-in-law in an attempt to secure some up-front funding. The resident pragmatists are converting 10 per cent of $100,000 into soft furnishings and luxury goods. 'That's $10,000,' says Mom approvingly. 'Or six million, two hundred and fifty thousand, one hundred and forty-seven lire,' says the daughter of immigrant stock. The band could be called the Warts just to maximise the hilarity factor.

Cut to the next scene. The audition. There are amplifiers and instruments set up in the living room. The son-in-law gestures towards the back door. 'Ladies and gentlemen, loveable backers. Here they are, the Warts.' And, get this, in walk Sly Saxon and the Seeds, fully decked out in pop-star threads: kaftans, capes, loud flowery shirts, the works. The assembled family gathering go through the whole gamut of wriggling discomfort and confusion as the Warts set up to play. There's the usual misunderstandings of generational argot, endless riffing on terms like 'heavy', 'bread', 'bag', 'do your thing', etc. 'When Jerry told us what you were going to do for us, it really blew our minds,' says Sly Saxon. 'Oh, that's too bad,' says Mom, looking concerned.

'You people are really heavy,' says Sly. 'Now don't get personal,' says pipe-smoking Pa, getting up from the sofa and looking good and ready to slug these scuzzy drop-outs who have invaded his living space. 'Just give us a couple of minutes and we'll get into our bag,' says Sly. 'They sing in a bag?' asks Mom. With the older family members shouting clueless encouragement ('Go ahead and jump into your bag'; 'Yeah, blow your brains out'), the Warts who are really the Seeds launch into the garage classic 'Pushin' Too Hard', hamming it up something rotten for the prime-time audience. Wouldn't that be a gas? 'If only life were like this,' as Woody Allen says as he brings on Marshall McLuhan to correct a know-nothing critic in *Annie Hall*. Except that on this occasion life really was like this. The above scenario happened. Of course it happened. Half of you have seen it on YouTube, and the other half of you were probably far enough ahead of the conceit to know that 1960s media America was wild enough and strange enough and large enough to accommodate almost anything. Performers of every showbiz persuasion appeared in front of the prime-time lenses of Ed Sullivan, the Smothers Brothers, Dick Cavett, Dick Clark, Andy Williams et al. What's

more, the TV networks and production companies who made these shows kept the footage to prove it. Maybe that's why such occurrences seem less anachronistic to American audiences than to us tape-wiped/memory-bereft/ mythed-up Brits. John Cage appeared on the TV game show *I've Got a Secret* in 1960. Frank Zappa played a bicycle wheel on *The Steve Allen Show* in 1963. Lesley Gore appeared in *Batman*. The Beau Brummels appeared in *The Flintstones*. We probably need to get over the idea that there is anything game-changing or idiosyncratic about any of this.

The twenty-sixth of October 1967 was the fiftieth anniversary of the Bolshevik Revolution in Russia. Meanwhile, Gotham City was under threat from an assailant every bit as menacing as the Red Peril. In season three, episode seven of *Batman*, arch criminal Louie the Lilac, played by comedian Milton Berle, plans to capture the entire 'flower generation' by kidnapping Princess Primrose, the organiser of a forthcoming 'flower-in' to be held in Gotham City Park. Louie brainwashes Princess Primrose with his Stupefying Aromatic Spray, as a prelude to taking control of the rest of the young generation with his giant man-eating lilacs. Hearing of Louie's fiendish plot, Batman and the

Boy Wonder apply a flower decal to the Batmobile and into action they go. After a little judicious zap, splaaaat and thwaaaarp the Dynamic Duo, dependable as always, restore order in the final reel. As Louie and his henchmen are carted off to jail Batman delivers a touching homily to the spirit of '67. 'The flower children think we're cool, man. Like we turn them on, you know?' says Robin. 'Yes, please be gentle with your visitors,' Batman urges the police chief, Commissioner Gordon, who is clearly no Mayor Daley. 'Although it may not be understood by more literal minds, in their own way they're doing what they can to correct the world's woes with love and flowers.'

Meanwhile, over in Palo Alto even the Merry Pranksters found their acid escapades incorporated into the network combine when an episode of the popular TV cop show *Dragnet* featured a juvenile drug dealer called Blue Boy. *Dragnet*'s tag line – 'The story you are about to see is true. The names have been changed to protect the innocent' – was more prescient than usual on this occasion, as Blue Boy was based on Prankster Paul Foster, who at the Watts Acid Test in February 1966 painted his face half blue and half silver. Foster, who had wandered around at a previous Acid Test in a Second World War

gas mask and with a sign round his neck reading 'I'M IN THE PEPSI GENERATION AND YOU'RE A PIMPLY FREAK', could never have known that a year later his lysergic-inspired antics would be immortalised in a prime-time cop show, or that the Magic Bus and the Acid Tests would also get a namecheck.

The episode in question – the first to be aired in colour, appropriately enough – went out in January 1967 and its plot was broadly faithful to the timeline of LSD's evolution from thrill-seekers' new discovery to criminal felony. There is even a brief scene where a scientist accurately describes the drug's history to date. Dialogue and plot development, however, were another matter. We are first alerted to Blue Boy's existence with reports that a youth dressed as an Indian is down in the park 'chewing the bark off of a tree'. When Joe Friday and his dependable sidekick Bill Gannon arrive, they find the blue-faced youth head down in a pile of bark, claiming that he's peering down into the centre of the Earth, where he can apparently see 'purple flame and a pilot light'. When they read him his constitutional rights, he replies: 'There I am. I'm over there now. I'm not here any more. My hair's green. I'm a tree.' From here on in the plot is as implausible as the dialogue. 'You stay in that chair,' they tell Blue Boy at his interrogation. 'I am the chair,' yells Blue Boy as he upends office furniture. The drug, we are reliably informed, has its own street slang and is variously known as 'the ticket, the ghost, the beast, the chief, the hawk or simply 25'. Two girls aged fourteen and fifteen are picked up on Sunset Strip, high on said 25. 'I saw all these weird colours and then I saw an eye. You know what I mean? A human eye,' one of them tells the concerned cops. 'It kept coming closer and closer. Then all of a sudden everything started to melt. Just melting on down. The sidewalk melted. The street melted. Just everything.'

'LSD?' asks Bill Gannon.

'Both of them,' confirms the arresting officer. 'Dropped a cap apiece. Paid three bucks for them.'

'Three bucks a tab?' says Gannon. 'When it drops to 50 cents, the grammar-school kids will have a big time in recess, won't they?'

'It's really getting popular,' says the arresting officer. 'Have you seen that bus up on the strip on a Friday, Saturday night? Big sign on it says can you pass the Acid Test? Pay a dollar and find out. For a buck they drive you up to the Hollywood Hills to an acid party.'

'Before we're through they'll be listing it in the Yellow Pages,' says Gannon, who, as you'll have guessed by now, gets all the best lines.

Cut to the chase. 'What do you fellows figure he's going to put in all those capsules?' says the man from the Apex pharmacy, who has just exercised his constitutional right to legally sell 3,000 empty ampules to a man with his face painted half blue. 'A lot of misery,' intones Joe Friday. Blue Boy is eventually located at an apartment a couple of blocks away, but the cops are too late. He has died from an overdose of LSD. As you do.

Inasmuch as it was possible to get your drug education from a network TV show that featured a character called Sgt Eugene Zappey, *Dragnet* was typical of the media portrayal of the growing acid peril, maintaining a moral tone that managed to be simultaneously titillating, exploitative and disapproving. That same tone is evident in countless psychsploitation movies. It's there in the soundtrack to *Mondo Hollywood* and *Teenage Rebellion*, two 1967 movies with incidental scores by Mike Curb. In the latter (billed as 'The truth about the "Now" generation') Curb casts a worried eye on teenage pregnancy, narcotic addiction, prostitution and homosexuality. There is a great moment on a track called 'Pot Party' where the spoken narration outlines the perils that await the unsuspecting young teenager. 'Come over to a similar apartment in the village. Smoke a joint. Burn a little grass. Pop party. Roach party. Mainliner. Skin pop. Shoot some crystal. The language of the narcotic and marijuana user. The language of a large and ever-increasing number of teenagers,' the narrator intones as he recites from his copy of *How to Speak Hip*. And then comes the moment of magic. 'Starting in high school on Benzedrine and pep pills,' he says, and at that precise moment the soundtrack that up to now has been content to lay down a burlesque backbeat suddenly spirals into an approximation of the speed buzz, 'it is not long before many soon graduate to marijuana, the teething biscuits to a whole adolescent generation . . . And if marijuana is the appetiser, the advent of the space-age technology has provided the main course: LSD, the crazy acid.' By this point the electronic bleeps and squawks of the soundtrack are making the whole experience sound so damned seductive that an entire generation reared on John Glenn and the Cape Canaveral Right Stuff would have been queuing up for their teething biscuits, or asking the nearest blue boy where they might procure some ticket, ghost, beast, chief or hawk.

There were countless variations on *Mondo Hollywood* and *Teenage Rebellion*. They featured groovy 'in the style of' incidental music and played in fleapits and drive-ins from coast to coast. The soundtracks were usually churned out by session combos on a commission. They are the unsung heroes of American psychedelia, the musicians for whom no job was ever too ersatz. Session musicians played on some of the most pivotal rock albums of the late sixties. Frank Zappa was shrewd enough to use LA's finest on the Mothers' debut LP *Freak Out!* They also provided the orchestral flourishes on Love's *Da Capo* and *Forever Changes*. Roger McGuinn was the only Byrd who played on 'Mr Tambourine Man'. The crowning glory of LA plasticity was, of course, the Monkees. Here was a manufactured band, put together from an ad placed by TV execs Bert Schneider and Bob Rafelson in *Variety* and the *Hollywood Reporter* in September 1965 that asked for 'spirited Ben Franks types', i.e. the sort of people who frequented the famously hip all-night diner on Sunset Strip where the scenesters hung out. And types was what they got. They got the cute English type. The droll southern type. The cool dreamy folkie type (who was required to act the ditzy misunderstood talentless type) and the

zany hellzapoppin' showbiz type. And
in the period between the placing of
that ad and the moment in December 1968 when the Ben Franks types
committed hara-kiri with the movie
Head, they made fifty-eight half-hour
TV shows, five albums (the first two
of which didn't contain a single note
played by the band themselves) and
sold approximately twenty-three million records before embarking upon in
a spirited attempt to storm the reality
temple and wrest control of their own
creativity. Despite the insipid promise
of a theme tune that claimed 'We're
too busy singing to put anybody down,'
the Monkees tore up their showbiz
brief, renegotiated their life script and
were more than happy to put themselves down. By episode 57 they were
introducing Frank Zappa to discerning twelve-year-olds on network TV.
Zappa also had a walk-on part in *Head*,
leading a cow across the Screen Gems
parking lot and informing Davy Jones
that he should spend more time on his
music 'because the youth of America
depends on you to show the way'.

The final episode of *The Monkees*
concluded with minimal fanfare. Micky
Dolenz quietly announced, 'This is
Tim Buckley,' and Buckley sang 'Song
of the Siren'. It seems a remarkably
magnanimous gesture now, and it was

unprecedented on pop TV at the time,
but it typified the efforts the Monkees
made during the final series of their
TV show to destabilise the very notion
of a manufactured act. Despite this
they remained the butt of every music
snob's derision. At the Monterey pop
festival Micky Dolenz, resplendent in
Native American headgear, spectacularly misread the fancy-dress code
and, like Laura Nyro, chose the wrong
outfit. He spent the entire weekend
strutting around in his halo of feathers,
oblivious to the ridicule he was leaving
in his wake. Brian Jones, in his capacity (or incapacity) as benighted MC,
made similarly snide comments about
fellow attendee Peter Tork to reporters. Even after the Monkees had split
up and Mike Nesmith was attempting
to establish a solo career he had to
endure members of the Flying Burrito
Brothers sneering from the wings and
cat-calling for the Monkees.

The way in which the Monkees
came to personify hype and insincerity
reeks not just of a certain west-coast
snobbery but jealousy too. In rock-
and-roll terms the group never had
to pay their dues. They could call on
the best of the Brill Building writers
to pen their hit singles and they were
showbiz from Micky Dolenz's grin to
Davy Jones's stacked heels, but then,

as Bill Graham reminded the Jefferson Airplane, what other business was there? Just when they seemed beyond redemption the Monkees vindicated their entire existence with the self-lacerating, demythologising celluloid suicide note that was *Head*, a movie which begins and ends with the drummer jumping off Golden Gate Bridge into the ocean below. The slow symbolic death of Micky Dolenz is bathed in multicoloured tints. Every writhe, twist and turn is choreographed to the dreamy drift of Goffin and King's 'The Porpoise Song', a 'Walrus'-tinged anthem to disavowal and escape. One line leaps out more than any other as Dolenz sinks into the inky blue depths: 'An overdub has no choice / an image cannot rejoice.'

The Monkees were merely the most famous and blatant example of the manufactured outfit, but their experience was not untypical. Several prominent garage bands underwent line-up transformation and changes in musical direction at the whim of a record producer. The Chocolate Watch Band was one of the most distinctive groups to emerge from the Bay Area savant-garde. Singer Dave Aguilar could do a more than passable Mick Jagger, and his band had all the growling, scowling prerequisites of the era. None of this

prevented producer Ed Cobb from filling their albums with hired hands and his own ideas. On their 1967 debut *No Way Out* the instrumental cuts 'Expo 2000' and 'Dark Side of the Mushroom' were performed by a session group led by recording engineers Richie Podolor and Bill Cooper. The title track, which evolved from a group jam in the studio, had further instrumentation and tape trickery added by Podolor and Cooper, as well as a completely new vocal from session singer Don Bennett. The first three cuts on the band's follow-up album – 'Voyage of the Trieste', 'In the Past' and the title track 'Inner Mystique' – featured no members of the group at all. On 'Medication' and 'Let's Go, Let's Go' Aguilar's vocals were once again replaced by those of Don Bennett. On a slowed-down cover version of We the People's 'In the Past', the original's balalaika sound is replaced by Richie Podolor's sitar. Podolor can also be heard playing the instrument on Steppenwolf's 'Snowblind Friend'. Previously he had played guitar on Sandy Nelson's 'Teen Beat' and 'Let There Be Drums', as well as the Hondells' surf hits. He issued his own surf albums under the name Richie Allen and the Pacific Surfers, and played on the Castaways' 'Liar, Liar'. Before going on to produce and engineer for the Grateful

Dead, Three Dog Night, Steppenwolf and Iron Butterfly, he and Bill Cooper played on records by the Turtles and were heavily involved with the first two Electric Prunes albums. The latter outfit, like the Chocolate Watch Band, also found themselves the victims of an identity heist when producer David Axelrod, charged with producing the band's third and fourth albums, was instructed by the Electric Prunes' own manager to dismiss the members who had previously made two great psychedelic LPs and use session musicians instead. *Mass in F Minor* and *Release of an Oath*, both released in 1968, were magnificent kitsch artifacts, full of opulent, tightly scored orchestral arrangements and cod religiosity. The former album took the Latin Mass as its starting point; the latter utilised Christian and Jewish liturgy to forge an unlikely hybrid of psychsploitation incidental music and multidenominational requiem.

Ed Cobb's cavalier attitude towards his charges – replacing their endeavours without notifying them, recycling backing tracks and sharing composition credits on their album cuts – was not untypical. It was done shamelessly and was seen as a perfectly legitimate way of boosting publishing revenue. Perhaps the most blatant of all the session

recyclists was guitarist Jerry Cole. Cole was one of the leading lights in the Wrecking Crew. Like Hal Blaine, Carol Kaye and the rest of the gang, he's all over half the hit records made in the 1960s. He led the pit bands in TV shows like *Shindig!* and *Hullabaloo* and knew every lick, trick and beat in the book. When commissioned to produce 'in the style of' albums for budget labels like Crown, Custom, Command and Contessa, he and his LA session colleagues would churn out an LP a day, making Hawaiian, Latin, country, R&B, rock, easy-listening and surf albums to order. By 1967 they were hacking out session psychedelia to order too. Cole's various ensembles put out material under a number of names, including T. Swift and the Electric Bag, the Projection Company, the Animated Egg, the Id, the Generation Gap, the Haircuts and the Impossibles. This material would be endlessly tweaked and rehashed, and then leased under different band names to a variety of labels, most of which seemed to share the same South Normandie Avenue address in Los Angeles. Two of Cole's recycled efforts – *Dance Party Time* by the Electric Firebirds, issued on the Crown label, and *Top Hits of Today* by the Associated Soul Group, issued on Contessa – even shared a recycled sleeve: an identical image of a suede-clad female sprawled among a collection of randomly strewn LPs. The Electric Firebirds' disc boasted track titles that sounded as if they had been run through a hip-jargon generator set to random: 'Woodstock Hour', 'Let's Make It', 'Moon Right On', etc. The typography of the cover (i.e. slapdash and bearing little resemblance to the order of the tracks on the LP) makes it look as if the closing cut is called 'Heavy Doors Time'. In fact, there are two separate tracks, 'Heavy' and 'Doors Time', but the point is it wouldn't have mattered if there had been a track called 'Heavy Doors Time', any more than if 'Moon Right On' had been two separate tracks called 'Moon' and 'Right On'. The titles were free-floating signifiers and could be used in any order and affixed to any track. Titles were tweaked from album to album to give them that necessary 'Heavy Doors Time' vibe when the era called for it. This was generically codified underground music in its most blatant form, and there was something wonderfully utilitarian about its barefaced cheek. What is striking about Cole's output from this period is the stylistic continuity. Tracks custom-made for surf cash-ins in 1964 could be readily adapted to the psychedelic freak-outs of 1967

without having to change a single note.

Cole and his Wrecking Crew buddies played on some of the greatest and some of the most abysmal pop hits of the day – and they treated those imposters the same, signing for their fee and splitting for the next gig. It might be Brian Wilson's *Smile*. It might be a Coke commercial. It might be a Top 40 radio station jingle package. On *Hot Hits of Today* by the Associated Soul Group, Cole's combo play a stripped-down version of 'Are You Experienced' that gives an indication of what Hendrix might have sounded like if he hadn't left the bar-band circuit or discovered LSD. It's followed by a winsome version of Jim Webb's 'Up, Up and Away', and that's exactly as it should be. The Cole albums and countless others like them were true pop-art statements. They are the pop-music equivalent of Warhol's silkscreen prints, multiple reproductions of the same basic template: this one tinted blue, that one bleached white, some filtered, some overexposed. And they say as much about a culture's sense of disposability as pop art ever did.

Every nuance, every time-warped, echo-chambered riff that psychedelia could emit was emulated, imitated, even occasionally innovated by the session gang. In 1966 another Wrecking Crew combo working under the name the Folkswingers recorded *Raga Rock*, a selection of Eastern-tinged cover versions, which was released on the World Pacific label. In 1966 the trend for Indian classical cash-ins had barely begun, but there was Hal Blaine, Larry Knechtel, Herb Ellis and the rest of the Crew, along with sitar tutor Harihar Rao, soon to be a member of Ravi Shankar's LA set-up, all giving the generic exotica treatment to instrumental versions of 'Eight Miles High', 'Paint It Black', 'Norwegian Wood', 'Along Comes Mary' and 'Homeward Bound'. This was the sound of session musicians laying down homogenised versions of Eastern beats that had been borrowed by Western pop groups, inspired as often as not by the illusory magic of LSD. How many more simulated layers could you add? How much more inauthentic could music get? The answer was: by devising an instrument that electronically replicated the sound of the sitar. Various companies manufactured customised versions of the sitar and several individuals claim they invented the device, claims that Ravi Shankar refuted. 'It is supposed to be a new invention,' he wrote in 1969, 'but I have been listening to people play electric sitars for the past 25 years in India, and I was presented with several of them by various manufacturers

in Delhi and Bombay quite a few years ago . . . The instrument has been widely used for several years now in film music and different forms of popular music in India.'[2] The version most widely adopted in the 1960s was developed by the Danelectro Corporation in Neptune City, New Jersey. The Coral Electric Sitar still allowed the guitarist to play full chords; additionally, it had a four-octave range and strings that could provide a sitar-like drone tone simply by being stroked in open tuning. That distinctive open-tuned strum can be heard at the beginning of Eric Burdon and the Animals' 'Monterey', and between 1967 and 1969 the vast majority of sitar sounds on pop records were provided by the ubiquitous electric version of the instrument. Most of these were played by just one man, Vincent 'Vinnie' Bell. It's Bell's Coral Electric Sitar that you hear on an abundance of late-sixties hits: 'Colour My World' by Petula Clark, 'Good Morning Starshine' by Oliver, 'Green Tambourine' by the Lemon Pipers, 'The Rain, the Park and Other Things' by the Cowsills, 'Games People Play' by Joe South, 'Cry Like a Baby' by the Box Tops and many more besides. Bell also played the instrument on 'No Matter What Sign You Are' by the Supremes, 'Band of Gold' by Freda Payne and countless other soul hits from the late 1960s and early '70s. A customised 'buzz bridge' developed by Bell, plus the incorporation of sympathetic strings similar to those found on a traditional sitar, gave exotic resonance to all the above records. To the trained ear it doesn't sound at all like an actual sitar, but its artificial exotic sheen added a flourish of textural colour to an abundance of pop records in the late 1960s.

The Lemon Pipers used the Coral Electric Sitar on all three of their UK and US hits – 'Green Tambourine', 'Rice Is Nice' and 'Jelly Jungle (of Orange Marmalade)' – and on several album tracks too. Due to a somewhat reluctant association with the Kasenetz–Katz stable of Buddha-label bands (1910 Fruitgum Company, Ohio Express, Crazy Elephant, etc.), the Lemon Pipers were transformed from a band with underground credibility who had played the Fillmore and Avalon ballroom into one of the main purveyors of what retrospectively became known as bubblegum music. Top 40 radio pioneer Bill Stewart maintains that the term was entirely a music-industry invention, used primarily by record-company execs as a marketing tool. 'I think that most programme directors fall into the "trick bag" – feeling that they are playing their music

for the record promoters, or the people who live in the same apartment building or for the people they meet in places where you don't run into average people,' he said. 'I keep reading everywhere about "bubblegum" music. Well, you ask the average person what bubblegum music is and he won't know. Try it sometime. Stand on a street corner and ask the first ten people who pass, "What do you think about bubblegum music?" They won't know what the hell you are talking about. And yet this is one of the most accepted terms in our industry.'[3]

'Bubblegum' rapidly entered into common critical parlance as a put-down, a catch-all term used to pour scorn on a whole range of catchy late-1960s commercial AM radio-friendly pop songs that otherwise had little or nothing in common. Suddenly everything from Tommy James and the Shondells and the Monkees to the Banana Splits, the Archies and the Brady Bunch was 'bubblegum'. People who had no trouble embracing the bubblegum equivalent of the immersive environment or the soothing *kinder*-comforts of Buckie Fuller's geodesic wombs sneered at the shimmering pop magnificence of a 'Crimson and Clover' or a 'Crystal Blue Persuasion'. Al Kooper, the man who laid down the distinctive root-chord organ sound on Bob Dylan's 'Like a Rolling Stone' and participated in numerous super-sessions with the cream of his genera-tion, also played in the Banana Splits' house band and contributed some of the best tracks to the show's soundtrack LPs. If this book required any further evidence at this late stage of just how paper thin and precarious those ten-uous categorisations of pop and rock really were, the whole high art/low art demarcation surely collapses when faced with the knowledge that there is an unbroken line of development between Bob Dylan and the Banana Splits; not even six degrees of separa-tion, but one simple diary-entered leap from session booking to session book-ing. In the greater trickle-down scheme of things children were acid pop's last, although possibly its most grateful and unquestioning, recipients. By the late 1960s techniques of visual display that had once been the sole preserve of avant-garde art movements were now staples of kids' TV. It didn't matter if it was *Rowan and Martin's Laugh-In, The Smothers Brothers Show* or some regional opt-out featuring an annoy-ing clown and a talking bird, the wow graphics and cartoon bubbles all spelled out the same welcoming mes-sage in a candy-coloured fount.

The lexicography of the love gen-eration eventually permeated every available channel of mass communica-tion and was promoted with ruthless efficiency by the large media cor-porations. What happened with TV occurred simultaneously in radio too. During 1967 several Top 40 stations, mostly in the San Francisco Bay area, but in New York and Chicago as well, began to run streamlined versions of the free-form radio format that had been pioneered by Tom Donahue's KMPX and KRLA. Not only did they extend their playlists and broaden their formats to incorporate psychedelic rock and pop (a great deal of which was beginning to appear in the Top 40 anyway), they also began to appro-priate psychedelic style and jargon in order to sell in these huge urban mar-kets. Pretty soon it was not uncommon to hear beer or hairspray ads accom-panied by sitar music, or news promos set to a throbbing psychedelic-rock backing. Ad copy was set to suitably hippiefied terminology:

Rush to your local Lester Burgers.
Lester's regular deluxe burgers
are only 19 cents. Outtasight. Man
that's a love in!
  (KYNO Fresno advert, 10
  February 1968)

In June 1967 a promotion for the annual KRLA Arts Festival paraphrased the lyrics of the Beatles' 'All You Need Is Love' as 'Nothing you make that can't be displayed,' to which a station announcer breathlessly added: 'So manifest your vibrations in art and send us your love.' He concluded, without discernible irony: 'All entries become the property of KRLA.' During the same month a promotion aired on KFRC for Revlon lipsticks began with a laid-back husky male voice intoning, 'Have you ever heard the sound of colour? In a world of TOO MUCH, Revlon slices colour to a pale juicy minimum. Only Revlon could make it happen.' An advert for knitting patterns aired on KYA Los Angeles in November 1969 similarly illustrated the extent to which sales speak on mainstream radio had become fully psychedelicised:

Carol's a dancer. She makes jumpsuits and low, hip, long, leggy, flared pants. Rebecca's kinda moody. Into a lot of heavy things. I guess that's why she wears earth colours. And there's Ginger, who could buy anything but makes it instead. Ginger could wear anything and does. Did I tell you what they all have in common? Sewing. The word's out about Penny's. Because Penny's is fashion patterns and far-out fabrics and everything that makes sewing come together.

By the end of the decade the pop and rock airwaves from coast to coast were utilising mind-blowing imagery, and blatant punning on words like 'trip' and 'experience' filled the ether in an attempt to get the youth demographic to part with its money. Although confined to urban markets at first, the psychedelicising of music radio soon spread to smaller outlets as stations continued to expand the frontiers of hippie consumerism. One station in DeKalb, Illinois, began promoting itself with the tagline 'With a flower in its tower and love on its lips this is your friendly psychedelic pussy cat, WLBK.' The hip argot sat somewhat inappropriately with the pro-Pentagon news items that continued to be broadcast by stations owned by Westinghouse, General Electric and all the other representatives of the military-industrial complex who had vested interests in South-East Asia. Only in the amoral montage of American pop radio in the late 1960s could an anti-Vietnam war song be followed by a government-sponsored public-service announcement urging listeners to register for the draft. In the midst of such wilful incongruity the love shuck didn't stand a chance. In July 1969 the ABC chain introduced its Love Network, a new service based in New York and beamed to twelve ABC FM affiliates, including WABC New York, WXYZ Detroit, WLS Chicago, KGO San Francisco, KQV Pittsburgh and KXYZ Houston. As part of its marketing campaign for the new network ABC ran full-page ads in the underground press. One of them read: 'JOHN LENNON. BOB DYLAN. PETER FONDA. If they mean anything to you try LOVE.' The promotional material that ABC sent to potential advertisers was equally shameless:

> *Like any business we invest in new products too. One of our latest is called LOVE. It communicates to a new kind of audience. The audience that feels and buys the same way. A group with whom the buying power of the country rests. And LOVE is the only concept on radio that is effectively reaching them. As marketing and business men, we anticipate the needs of the changing market. That's why it took almost a year of research and development to launch the LOVE format. A process similar to the way you market your new products.*

> *And though you won't find our new product on supermarket shelves, at least we can help you move yours off them.*

In the end everything could be reduced to hard sell and sales speak. Even love. Pop art, of course, had got there first. It got everywhere first. Robert Indiana had come a long way since the early 1960s, when he trawled the abandoned wharfs of Coenties Slip with Steve Durkee, hunting for discarded timber and signage. Indiana was one of the most iconoclastic and emotionally engaged painters in the pop-art movement and his distinctive one-word (mostly single-syllable) artworks – *EAT*, *YIELD*, *GOD*, *SOUL* – along with his mandala motifs and his playful sense of semantics vibrate throughout the 1960s with a shimmering optical energy all of their own.

In December 1964 Indiana sent his friends a series of pencil-and-crayon rubbings in the form of personalised Christmas cards. They all contained the word 'Love'. These frottaged Yuletide greetings with their grainy surfaces 'full of the shadow and highlights of the emergent image', as art critic Rosalind Kraus put it, were in marked contrast to Indiana's more typical hard-edged signage. 'The adjacent letters

LO and VE appear to touch almost erotically,' said Susan Elizabeth Ryan. 'The bottom serif of the L seems to stroke the lower part of the O, which leans towards it in response; while the E's rigidly extended top serif continues into the opening of the V.'[4] When the New York Museum of Modern Art commissioned Indiana to provide a design for its own Christmas cards in 1965, he reverted to his familiar hard-edged style but reprised the motif from the previous year. 'Indiana submitted several twelve-inch, hard-edged colour variations in oil on canvas,' said Ryan. 'The museum chose the most intense, rendered in high-saturation equal-value hues: red letters against a background of green and blue.'[5] The cards went on to become one of the museum's best-sellers. And in the years that followed Indiana's distinctive *LOVE* design went on to become the most plagiarised image in the history of American painting. By the time his own *Love Show* opened at New York's Stable Gallery in the spring of 1966 Indiana's original image had been reproduced commercially on thousands of Christmas cards, with the museum's copyright notice displayed discreetly on the back. The *LOVE* motif was also emblazoned on commercially available posters to publicise the Stable Gallery exhibition.

Unfortunately, no one thought to claim copyright on the image. This oversight proved to have considerable ramifications. Because he didn't want a copyright notice to cheapen the front of his design Indiana effectively surrendered all legal protection. When he put in a retrospective claim for copyright registration, it was rejected on the grounds that the law did not provide protection for a single word. 'Indiana realized only later that he should have disputed the ruling on grounds of creative enhancement,' said Susan Elizabeth Ryan. 'At the time he was advised to patent the image as a trademark, an unsatisfactory solution that the artist rejected.'[6]

There was recent precedence for this in the fine-art world. Bridget Riley, upon arrival in the US for MoMA's *The Responsive Eye* exhibition in 1965, was horrified to find that collector Larry Aldrich had transformed several of her op-art paintings into fabrics and dress prints. Within a year Riley's original designs were plastered all over everything from handbags to billboard ads. In the autumn of 1965 Yves Saint Laurent based his 'Go-Go' look on Mondrian's geometric style. *Vogue* magazine, as Ryan pointed out, had anticipated this trend in the 1950s, when it used Jackson Pollock's action paintings as the backdrop for a fashion shoot for its spring collection. For Indiana the experience was a salutary one. The wordage he utilised in his paintings had always been carefully chosen and carried great emotional resonance, much of it directly autobiographical. He was not a neutralist. He was not attempting to transform the word 'love' into a slogan or logo, but that's what happened anyway, and the effect it had on his reputation as an artist was considerable. Because of the commercial proliferation of the *LOVE* image many critics assumed, erroneously as it turned out, that Indiana was getting rich off the profits. John Canaday in the *New York Times* suggested that Indiana should do *MONEY* next, a put-down redolent of André Breton's infamous anagram of Salvador Dalí, Avida Dollars. Indiana didn't help matters any by allowing the motif to be used on everything from jewellery to album covers, although he did draw the line at *LOVE* paperweights. By the time he created a *LOVE* hologram for the University of Michigan in 1972 the image had long since passed into common currency. Naked cast members of the original Broadway production of *Hair* posed behind one of Indiana's original *LOVE* prints. The book jacket and promotional design for Erich Segal's 1970 novel *Love Story* featured a near as dammit

approximation of *LOVE*'s lettering and colour scheme, while being careful not to plagiarise the original design. Meanwhile, galleries stopped purchasing or commissioning Indiana's work. When John Perreault interviewed the artist for the *Village Voice* in 1972, he could make the following observation without fear of contradiction:

> Although Indiana's 'love' predates
> the flower-power hoax, because
> his design came to permeate
> the ambience, still present, of
> meaningless sentiment, it is
> impossible now to divorce the
> design, even in massive three-
> dimensional, two-color form,
> from the conditioned response of
> nostalgia for a media daydream.[7]

Indiana readily concurred with this indictment. 'It's like committing murder,' he told *Art News* in February 1973. 'Something done for the most personal reasons suddenly becomes notorious.' In an age when you can buy Cézanne fridge magnets and Monet tea towels this may not seem like much to get worked up about, but it mattered a great deal at the time. The *LOVE* paintings came to define a moment when the currency of commerce overwhelmed and then completely obliterated the idea of artistic integrity and intent. In finding against Indiana the legislature effectively argued that no individual artist owned words, or even the symbolic shaping of those words. In his reluctance to claim copyright for a logo Indiana revealed the paradox that lies at the heart of pop art and its aestheticisation of popular images and everyday objects, and it's no coincidence perhaps that pop art was eventually superseded by conceptual art: the pop artists, despite their celebration of surface, despite their reaction against the macho intensity and rugged romanticism of abstract expressionism, were in the end romantics themselves. They had dream desires too. They were nostalgic for now.

Pop music had no such crises to deal with. By the late sixties it too had developed its own distinctive signage, and it had long since become obvious that the machinations of mass production could be best read and most instantaneously assimilated via the creative outpourings of the pop-music world rather than the art world. Here the word 'love' had always been emblematic, analogous, logocentric. Love, as sentimental utterance, as loyalty pledge, as slogan, as word to rhyme with 'dove' or 'above', remained robust and durable regardless of

commercial imperatives. 'Message of Our Love'. 'Words of Love'. 'Love Is All Around'. 'Love Years Coming'. 'All You Need Is Love'. Psychedelia tie-dyed the word into the very fabric of pop music. And at the tail end of that era, at the twilight's last gleaming, as the light shows began to lose their lustre and the dream began to fade, all kinds of unlikely people dipped into the colour box, got busy with the brushes and began writing eulogies to love in translucent letters eight miles high.

Brian Wilson's legacy could be heard in virtually every note of what came to be known as sunshine pop. As retrospectively created genres go, sunshine pop is one of the better ones. The term speaks with iridescent, unbridled optimism of a music born out of affluence. It makes the unrelenting glare of Californian daylight a metaphor, as the Beach Boys, the Mamas and the Papas and so many others made California itself a metaphor. Sunshine pop spoke of inclusivity, not exclusivity. It countered rock's initiation rites with pop's unimpeachable democracy, replaced entropy with empathy, isolation with embrace, rebellion with reconciliation. Groups who would have been sneered at by the self-appointed canonisers of rock made music that welcomed you in unconditionally. From the subversively ambiguous connotations of their name to the sitars that adorned their records the Poppy Family were as psychedelic as the Ultimate Spinach or the Blues Magoos, but Susan Jacks delivered their songs about injustice, intolerance and wanderlust in a yearning Karen Carpenter stifled sob of a voice rather than a bourbon-soaked snarl. Those who took their drinks neat, their hunter-gatherer roles seriously and their old ladies for granted significantly underestimated the potency of unashamedly commercial pop to deliver messages every bit as raw-edged and radicalised as those that might be found on an MC5 album. There was a preponderance of this kind of surreptitious sunshine pop in the late sixties, music that was both disarmingly pleasant and potently message-driven. People still sang about candy bars and Cupid's arrow, but the grace notes of pop's angelic chorus gained added glister as acid's transformative influence continued to trickle down like so much heavenly rain. Most of it still came in the unabashed form of AM-friendly three-minute singles, but the more adventurous exponents threaded their visions like love beads and made works of conceptual unity to rival the very best of the rock crowd.

'Time for Hope. Time for Peace. Paint It Love'

In dulcet streams, in flutes' and
  cornets' notes,
electric, pensive, turbulent,
  artificial,
(Yet strangely fitting even here,
  meanings unknown before,
Subtler than ever, more harmony,
  as if born here, related here,
Not to the city's fresco'd rooms,
  not to the audience of the
  opera house
Sounds, echoes, wandering strains,
  as really here at home . . .)
WALT WHITMAN, 'Italian Music in Dakota'[8]

Frankie Castelluccio and the Varietones came up through the New Jersey club circuit in the 1950s, before changing their name to Frankie Valli and the Four Lovers and then to the Four Seasons. Joined by Bob Gaudio of the Four Teens (as in 'Who Wears Short Shorts?') and aided by the powerhouse production techniques of Bob Crewe, they enjoyed a consistent run of hit records between 1962 and 1966 that made no concession to the British invasion and promoted an unbroken line of harmonising that went back to the earliest days of doo-wop. Like a lot of Italian kids of diminutive stature, Frankie Valli grew up street tough beyond his years, with a voice that was street tough too: a three-octave register that ranged from a shrill altar-boy falsetto to the empty husk of a broken man. He always sounded pent-up, taut and troubled, even when he was serenading a sweetheart. Valli sang with the wary wavering tones of a man who had one eye on the comely silhouette in a first-floor tenement window and the other on the look-out for love rivals from the next block. 'Walk Like a Man', 'Big Man in Town', 'Let's Hang On', 'Working My Way Back to You', 'Opus 17' – these were pop operettas about pride, emptiness and regret. But by the late sixties that particular East Side story had run out of plot and the hits had dried up. So the Four Seasons teamed up with singer-songwriter Jake Holmes, who penned all the songs on their 1968 album *Genuine Imitation Life Gazette*, one of the great forgotten classics of its era. The album came wrapped in pop-art packaging, with a spoof daily newspaper, the *Genuine Imitation Life Gazette*, which contained cornball humour and insight in equal measure. There were mini-mart food offers for Moby Grapes, US Government-inspected Electric Prunes, and Country Joe's Fish. There were cut-out '15c off' coupons for 1910 Fruit Chewing Gum, Silver Apples and Four Seasons Salad Dressing. There were horoscopes by Constella ('Scorpio: Make a pal of your dad, he may be good for some bread later in the week. Start a rock group and call it "Scorpio". Don't practise'), suburban-cinema ads for Andy Warhol's fifty-seven-hour epic *Dandruff!*, juvenile teen flicks (*Born to Throw a Tantrum* and *Draft Dodgers in Paradise*), exploitation pics (*Hell's Angels' White House Weekend* and *While Wives Wait*) and mainstream Hollywood offerings such as *Guess Who's Coming to Pick Up the Garbage* and *Please Don't Darken My Doorstoop* ('positively no one admitted'). There were Robert Crumb-style cartoon funnies, and a defiantly anti-hip 'don't be a drop-out' message that read: 'Four Seasons Handy Hints – "don't fergit ta finish high school kids."' The sleeve also contained a Rauschenberg-style Stars and Stripes inlay of tinted band photos and song lyrics dressed up as news stories. The tone of the spoof news magazine veered between satire and sincerity. Jake Holmes's lyrics trod a similarly ambivalent line that addressed middle America's neuroses and the follies of the freak parade with equal scrutiny.

In the grand psychedelic tradition everything on the album is presented as a masquerade. High-society mores and small-minded tittle-tattle are taken to task in 'Mrs Stately's Garden', just one of several songs on the LP that depict a world where America seems to be forever taking tea on the lawn, oblivious to the ghettos that might be burning a few blocks away. 'Wall Street Village Day' contrasts activities in the financial sector – 'some are pinstripe, some are grey' – with those in the West Village – 'some are paisley, some are grey' – and concludes there isn't a great deal to choose between the two. The uptown department stores and the Greenwich Village boutiques are both filled with 'stylish trash and trinkets'. Love beads or luxuries, 'Wall Street Village Day' makes it clear that it's all consumerism in the end.

A yearning sense of broken morality surfaces throughout the album. On 'Saturday's Father' the kids of estranged parents get to dress in party clothes and go to a weekend puppet show, but Dad is the last one to leave and it's the adults who have to work hardest at faking their parts. After a few listens the song begins to sound like an analogy for an America separated from its young. The title track, 'Genuine Imitation Life', also presents reality as an illusion and suggests that everyone is just playing a part. With its false ending and mocking 'Hey Jude' refrain ('Hey, play it cool') 'Genuine Imitation Life' might just be the most accurate statement about the death of the American dream to appear on an album in the late 1960s. Like the *commedia dell'arte*, the Mime Troupe radicals and the Diggers, it takes wealth acquisition and love pageantry to task. 'Taking off their masks / revealing still another guise,' sings Valli in those empty aching tones. Reality is 'a lovely place to visit but I wouldn't want to stay'. Myriad layers of falsehood and illusion are heaped up then stripped way, until all that's left is a hollow sham.

From its opening bars to its finale the LP reeks magnificently of overambition and epic intent. Bob Gaudio's symphonic sweeps and Frankie Valli's raw-nerved ability to sing the body electric make *Genuine Imitation Life Gazette* one of the uncelebrated triumphs of psychedelic classicism. Another Italian-American, Lou Christie – Lugee Giovanni Alfredo Sacco to his mother – made another of the great unsung Italianate curios of the era. *Paint America Love*, released on Buddha in 1971, is by no means a masterpiece but it is Christie's crowning glory, a neglected gem of a song cycle in which columnated ruins domino in every chorus and salvation springs eternal from the debris. Christie started out back in the days of the girl groups and the puppy-love balladeers – the Brians, the Bobbys and the Fabians – but even then his songs seemed a little overwrought and out of step. Christie's immoderate falsetto could swing from the rhapsodic to the parodic in a fluttering heartbeat, while the chattering chants of his backing vocalists, often disconcertingly unconnected to the texture or subject matter of the song, provided a deranged siren choir. Twyla Herbert, Christie's arranger, co-composer and mystic muse, was a classically trained concert pianist twenty-two years his senior. The compositions they wrote together always seemed at odds with current trends, informed by the contemporary scene but defiantly not of it. Everything was writ a little too large and loud, even by the expansionist production values of the early sixties. Individual lines sounded like they should be blown up big and rendered in Roy Lichtenstein Ben-Day dots, with caption to match. 'Watch your heart after dark.' 'Don't trust anyone but me.' 'Make up or cover up.' 'Green for my envy. Red for my anger. Silver for my tears.' Between them Christie and Herbert painted a world where the night had a thousand spies and the streets were a Roman

wilderness of pain. Amazingly, they managed to maintain the style well into the beat-group era without remotely compromising its other-worldly nature and its over-magnified dynamics. Songs like 'Cryin' (in the Streets)' and 'Jungle' were augmented by stuttering coughs, yelps and hiccups seemingly assembled out of Hugo Ball phonetics and exotica concrète. Between 1966 and 1968 Christie embarked upon a run of extraordinary records for MGM that are unparalleled in content and scope. 'If My Car Could Only Talk' and 'Wild Life's in Season' were Jack Nitzsche-produced three-minute psychodramas of jealousy and untamed impulses. They are girl-group songs born out of their time, and they sound all the more remarkable for it. 'Wild Life's in Season' is a Sunset Strip sleaze-escape of cop cars, drug habits and unredeemable degradation. 'If My Car Could Only Talk' transports male suspicion into new realms of paranoia as Christie, adopting the role of a GI on leave, finds his photos ripped up in the ashtray of the car his girlfriend has borrowed and someone else's cigarette lighter, personally engraved to his Sarah Jane, under the driver's seat. Even by the standards of girl-group hyper-realism Christie presents a startling scenario as he implores his car to yield up its secrets. It's the ultimate machismo-in-peril oratorio, full of silver-teared Ben-Day dot lyrics that reek of neurosis ('a flash of suspicion') and flick-knife threats ('watch your step / you'll get yours yet').

A quartet of MGM cuts that Christie recorded in 1968 are even more remarkable. 'Genesis and the Third Verse', 'Rake Up the Leaves', 'The Johnstown Kite' and 'Canterbury Road' cast Catholic redemption through psychedelia's stained-glass prism and offer benediction to a bold new dawn. 'Genesis and the Third Verse' opens with a pop catechism ('Seems the earth can't see the children / and the children can't see the earth') and combines early stirrings of an eco-consciousness ('In this green cathedral / God put these people') with longings for post-Vietnam stability. It's *What's Going On* in microcosm, three years before Marvin Gaye's album appeared. Of the other songs 'Rake Up the Leaves' implores the listener to 'turn on the spirit', while 'Johnstown Kite' features Vinnie Bell's Coral Electric Sitar and suggests that fate makes its own momentum. The best of these recordings, 'Canterbury Road', was a rewrite of Curt Boetcher's 'There Is Nothing More to Say', which was first recorded by Boetcher's group Millennium and featured on

the group's *Begin* album. Bob Goldstein rewrote the lyric for Christie but retained the day-of-reckoning imagery of the original, combining Chaucerian pilgrimage ('in the early dust of morning on a shimmering day') with Martin Luther King's long march towards the promised land. The song envisages a new spirituality where rich man, poor man, church man, layman and journeyman will greet the stations of the cross with consciousness renewed. It's a Walt Whitmanesque epistle full of first-day-of-Creation stirrings ('the sun's a diamond dancing through the leaves') and prophetic intent, but it's all rounded off abruptly with a sudden irreverent poke at religious conformity. 'And the language won't be Latin la-la-la-la-la-la,' spits Christie, rhapsodic and parodic to the last.

That clutch of forgotten 1968 songs gave a hint of what would follow on *Paint America Love*. Had they been included on the album at the expense of a handful of weaker songs that are saddled with early-1970s chirpy pop arrangements, *Paint America Love* might now be regarded in the same light as Brian Wilson's *Smile* rather than as a flawed but fascinating curio. Like *Smile*, *Paint America Love* is a Steinbeckian journey across the great plains of an unsettled continent, an epic travelogue written up in small details. The album personifies America as a hippie drifter writing letters home to himself as he searches for security and yearns to return to his own personal Kansas. It documents a nation's troubled heart ripped apart by the war in Vietnam, attempts to summarise the long, strange trip of the previous ten years (Christie's and America's) and distils it all down in the end to that one word, love.

> *I could see that the intricate organization both of the plants and of my own nervous system, alike symphonies of branching complexity, were not just manifestations of intelligence – as if things like intelligence and love were in themselves substances or formless forces. It was rather that the pattern itself is intelligence and is love, and this somehow in spite of all its outwardly stupid and cruel distortions.*
>
> ALAN WATTS[9]

In *Paint America Love*'s valedictory trilogy of songs – 'Lighthouse', 'Look Out the Window' and the title track itself – Christie revisits themes laid down in 'Genesis and the Third Verse' and 'Canterbury Road' and imagines

Eden restored from a faded dream. Lapsed ideals are given one last try. 'Let us take the peace from the meadow / let it ring as far as the ghetto,' sings Christie as 'Lighthouse' fashions a new non-denominational faith, free of sanctimony and cant. 'Look Out the Window' catches the turning tide of public opinion as middle America increasingly begins to voice its opposition to the Vietnam war. The song arrangements are still as big and epic as they ever were but the quest is more humble now. By 1971 it needed to be, as a nation, unprepared for reckoning without recompense and peace with dishonour, attempted to piece together its own emotional reconciliation. 'Time to honour the best in ourselves,' sings Christie on the title track. 'Time for hope. Time for peace. Paint it love.'

'The carousel has stopped us here / It twirled a time or two and then it dropped us here,' sang Glen Campbell in 'Where's the Playground, Susie?', Jim Webb's sublime 1969 evocation of separation and regret. And if the multi-coloured carousel of karma has to drop us anywhere, it might as well be here, with Lou Christie's Italianate illuminations blinding us and his choir of angels ringing in our ears. *Paint America Love* asks us to endorse a dream, even as the dream light is fading. 'Where's the Playground, Susie?' is a song made entirely out of analogy and metaphor. The scattered toys, the sandbox, the unanswered puzzles and unfinished games, the carousel, the merry-go-round, the playground itself, they all stand for something else: lost innocence, lost opportunity, lost paradise, lost love.

It seems an appropriate place to end our journey through the word maze, a maze fashioned from analogy and metaphor and things not being what they seem and leading to who knows where. LSD was in the end a metaphor too, a metaphor for what we might at any one time choose to, or choose not to, define as reality, a simulacrum for all seasons. Acid sugar-cubed and blotter-soaked and tidal-waved its way across the universe in ways unparalleled before or since. Once upon a time in a land far away where they did things differently, although not that differently, LSD rampaged through innocence and experience alike, submitting the gracious and the ungracious to the same tricks and treats. It trickled into minds willing to be opened and tore apart some that weren't, irretrievably in some cases. It favoured those who lived in the precious moment, held them spellbound and made cherished seconds seem like a lifetime. Acid was every lost playground paradise, every lawn-swing vision of every child that soared high and peered over the picket fence into their neighbour's yard. It gave young hearts permission to run free and unencumbered 'through the recess, the chalk and numbers'. Free to shake off logic and skip down country lanes and yellow brick roads towards unreachable horizons. Free to build cathedrals of unimaginable splendour out of dreams that touched the sky. And still be home in time for tea.

NOTES

FRONTPIECE AND INTRODUCTION

1 *London Review of Books*, 26.4.2012

2 Barthes, Roland, *The Grain of the Voice: Interviews 1962–1980* (Oakland, University of California Press, 1992)

3 Benjamin, Walter, 'Protocol I: Highlights of the First Hashish Impression' (1927), from *Protocols to the Experiments on Hashish, Opium and Mescaline 1927–1934*, trans. Scott J. Thompson. http://www.wbenjamin.org/walterbenjamin.html

4 http://thequietus.com/articles/10502-jonathan-meades-interview

CHAPTER 1

1 Huxley, Aldous, *The Doors of Perception* (London, Chatto & Windus, 1954), p. 50

2 This and following quotes *Current Affairs – 24 Hours*, TX 66/07/01, 66/07/31, T58/512/1 (BBC)

3 Bedford, Sybille, *Aldous Huxley: A Biography. Vol. 2: 1939–1963* (London, Collins and Chatto & Windus, 1974), p. 223

4 Bedford, p. 163

5 Huxley, p. 26

6 Ibid.

7 Huxley, p. 38

8 Ibid.

9 Jordan Jnr, G. Ray, 'LSD and Mystical Experiences', *Journal of Bible and Religion*, vol. 31, no. 2 (1963), p. 119

10 Huxley, p. 46

11 Novak, Steven J., 'LSD before Leary: Sidney Cohen's Critique of 1950s Psychedelic Drug Research', *Isis*, vol. 88, no. 1 (1997), p. 93

12 Ibid.

13 Bedford, pp. 332–3

14 Durr, R. A., *Poetic Vision and the Psychedelic Experience* (New York, Syracuse University Press, 1970), p. ix

15 Koestler, Arthur, 'Return Trip to Nirvana'. In *Drinkers of Infinity: Essays 1955–1967* (London, Hutchinson, 1968), pp. 201–12

16 Watts, Alan, *In My Own Way: An Autobiography* (London, Jonathan Cape, 1973), p. 343

17 Novak, p. 89

18 Cohen, Sidney, *The Beyond Within* (Atheneum, New York, 1964), p. 107

19 Novak, p. 101

20 Eisner, Betty Grover, *Remembrances of*

LSD Therapy Past (2002), http://www.
maps.org/books/remembrances.pdf, p. 129
21 Jacobs, Adam, 'Acid Redux: Revisiting
LSD Use in Therapy', Contemporary
Justice Review, vol. 11, no. 4 (2008), p.
434
22 Eisner, pp. 71–2
23 Ibid.
24 Novak, p. 103
25 Bedford, p. 255
26 Eisner, p. 7
27 Carroll, Lewis, Alices Adventures in
Wonderland (London, Penguin Puffin
edition, 1972), pp. 65–7
28 Lee, Martin A. and Shlain, Bruce, The
Complete Social History of LSD: The
CIA, the Sixties, and Beyond (New York,
Grove Press, 1992), p. 152
29 Stafford, Peter and Golightly, Bonnie,
LSD – The Problem-Solving Psychedelic
(New York, Award Books, 1967)
30 Watts, p. 356
31 Ibid.
32 Eisner, pp. 98–9
33 Eisner, p. 127
34 Watts, p. 351
35 Watts, p. 356
36 Bedford, pp. 222–3
37 Novak, p. 100
38 Bedford, p. 335
39 Grof, Stanislav, LSD: Doorway to the
Numinous (Rochester, Park Street Press,
2009), p. xix
40 Watts, p. 346
41 Watts, Alan, This Is It: And Other
Essays (New York, Collier, 1958), p. 133
42 Bedford, p. 216
43 Huxley, p. 29
44 Nin, Anaïs, The Journals of Anaïs Nin.
Volume 6: 1955–1966 (London, Quartet,
1979), p. 332
45 Bedford, p. 271

46 Grof, Stanislav, LSD Psychotherapy
(preface) (Alameda, CA, Hunter House,
1994), cited at http://www.druglibrary.
org/schaffer/
47 Durr, p. xiii
48 Durr, p. xi

CHAPTER 2
1 Perry, Charles, The Haight-Ashbury:
A History (New York, Wenner Books,
2005), p. 199
2 Attali, Jacques, Noise: The Political
Economy of Music (Minneapolis, University of Minnesota Press, 1985), p. 11
3 Kostelanetz, Richard (Ed.), Moholy-Nagy: Documentary Monographs in
Modern Art (New York, Praeger Publishing, 1970), p. 151
4 Moholy-Nagy, Lázló, Vision in Motion
(Chicago, Paul Theobald and Company,
1965), p. 163
5 Salter, Chris, Entangled: Technology
and the Transformation of Performance
(Cambridge, MA, MIT Press, 2010), p. 90
6 Salter, p. 22
7 Salter, p. 43
8 Lee and Shlain, p. 81
9 Chtcheglov, Ivan. 'Formulary for a New
Urbanism' (1953), http://www.bopse-
crets.org/
10 All of the information in this paragraph
is distilled from Peacock, Kevin, 'Instruments to Perform Colour Music: Two
Centuries of Technological Experimentation', Leonardo, vol. 21, no. 4 (1988),
pp. 397–406
11 Zurbrugg, Nicholas, Installation Art –
Essence and Existence (Australian Perspecta, Art Gallery of New South Wales,
1991), p. 17
12 Moholy-Nagy, p. 268
13 Most of the information about Thomas

Wilfred is taken from Eskilson, Stephen, 'Thomas Wilfred and Intermedia: Seeking a Framework for Lumia', *Leonardo*, vol. 36, no. 1 (2003)

14 Bernstein, David W. (Ed.), *The San Francisco Tape Music Center: 1960s Counterculture and the Avant-Garde* (Berkeley and Los Angeles, University of California Press, 2008), p. 21

15 Moholy-Nagy, p. 163

16 Most of the biographical information about Tony Martin is taken from Bernstein, pp. 136–62

17 Youngblood, Gene, *Expanded Cinema* (1970), p. 371; http://www.vasulka.org/ Kitchen/PDF_ExpandedCinema/book. pdf

18 Most of the information about the Space Theater is taken from Holms, Thom, *Electronic and Experimental Music: Technology, Music and Culture* (London, Routledge, 2008)

19 Polt, Harriett R. and Sandall, Roger, 'Outside the Frame', *Film Quarterly*, vol. 14, no. 3 (University of California Press, spring 1961), p. 35

20 Youngblood, p. 389

21 Polt, p. 36

22 Youngblood, p. 161

23 Youngblood, p. 174

24 Youngblood, p. 159

25 Kostelanetz, Richard, *The Theatre of Mixed Means* (London, Pitman Publishing, 1970), p. 244

26 Kostelanetz, p. 252

27 Bernstein, pp. 184–5

28 Interview with Michelle Kuo, *Artforum*, May 2008

29 Youngblood, p. 349

30 http://www.nypl.org/blog/2012/06/04/ transmissions-timothy-leary-papers-psychedelic-show

31 http://www.billhamlights.com/

32 Ibid.

33 Huxley, p. 7

34 Kostalenatz, p. 74

35 Bernstein, p. 150

36 Rainer, Yvonne, 'Interview with Anna Halprin', *Tulane Drama Review*, vol. 10, no. 2 (winter 1965), p. 143

37 Ibid.

38 Doyle, in Braunstein, Peter and Doyle, Michael William (Eds), *Imagine Nation: The American Counterculture of the 1960s and '70s* (London, Routledge, 2002), p. 73

39 Cuncliffe, John W., 'Italian Prototypes of the Masque and Dumb Show', *PMLA*, vol. 22, no. 1 (1907), p. 146

40 Bernstein, p. 64

41 Bernstein, p. 43

42 Bernstein, p. 238

43 Perry, Paul, *On the Bus: The Complete Guide to the Legendary Trip of Ken Kesey and the Merry Pranksters and the Birth of the Counterculture* (New York, Thunder's Mouth Press, 1990), p. xv

44 Perry, p. 37

45 http://www.phinnweb.org/retro/garage/ lightshows.html

46 Lesh, Phil, *Searching for the Sound. My Life with the Grateful Dead* (New York, Back Bay Books, 2005), p. 61

47 Lesh, p. 38

48 Bernstein, p. 74

49 *Rolling Stone*, 20.1.72

50 http://www.postertrip.com

51 Suvin, Darko, 'Reflections on Happenings', in *The Drama Review*, vol. 14, no. 3 (1970), p. 135

52 Suvin, p. 137

53 Suvin, p. 134

54 Perry, p. 151

55 Johnson, Kim, *The Funniest One in the*

Room. The Lives and Legends of Del Close (Chicago, Chicago Review Press, 2008), p. 64

56 Bernstein, p. 243

57 Sculatti, Gene and Seay, Davin, *San Francisco Nights: The Psychedelic Music Trip 1965–1968* (London, Sidgwick & Jackson, 1985), p. 63

58 Wolfe, Tom, *The Electric Kool-Aid Acid Test* (London, Weidenfield and Nicolson, 1969), p. 271

59 Digger archives at http://www.diggers.org/

CHAPTER 3

1 Coyote, pp. 80–1

2 Diggers pamphlet, 'Time to Forget', 1967

3 Graham, Bill and Greenfield, Robert, *Bill Graham Presents. My Life Inside Rock and Roll* (Cambridge, MA, Da Capo, 2004), p. 168

4 Perry, p. 54

5 Bockris, Victor, *Warhol* (London, Penguin, 1990), p. 225

6 Perry, p. 68

7 Sculatti and Seay, pp. 89–90

8 Goldstein, Richard, *Reporting the Counter Culture* (London, Unwin Hyman, 1990), pp. 53–8

9 Dalton, David, *Janis* (London, Calder & Boyars, 1971), p. 6

10 Graham, p. 172

11 Oliver, Michael (Ed.), *Settling the Score: A Journey Through the Music of the 20th Century* (London, Faber and Faber, 1990), p. 280

12 Cavallo, Dominick, *A Fiction of the Past: The Sixties in American History* (New York, Palgrave, 1990), p. 141

13 Braunstein, Peter and Doyle, Michael William, p. 83

14 Grogan, Emmett, *Ringolevio: A Life Played for Keeps* (New York, New York Review of Books, 1990), p. 266

15 Grogan, p. 251

16 Coyote, Peter, *Sleeping Where I Fall* (Washington DC, Counterpoint, 1990), p. 80

17 Grogan, p. 238

18 Grogan, p. 274

19 Grogan, p. 269

20 Grogan, p. 274

21 Grogan, p. 276

22 Grogan, p. 277

23 Graham, p. 186

24 Peck, Abe, *Uncovering the Sixties: The Life and Times of the Underground Press* (New York, Citadel Underground, 1991), p. 45

25 Coyote, p. 80

26 Gourmetbather on www.hipforums.com, posted January 2009

27 http://globalia.net/donlope/fz/videography/You_Are_What_You_Eat.html

28 Coyote, pp. 117–18

29 Coyote, p. 73

30 Johnson, p. 116

CHAPTER 4

1 Unterberger, Richie, *Unknown Legends of Rock 'n' Roll* (San Francisco, Miller Freeman Books, 1998), p. 48

2 *Dancing in the Street*, episode 1: 'Whole Lotta Shakin'' (BBC Worldwide, 1998)

3 richieunterberger.com

4 Strausbaugh, John, *Rock Till You Drop* (London, Verso, 2001), p. 231

5 Hicks, Michael, *Sixties Rock: Garage, Psychedelic and Other Satisfactions* (Chicago, University of Illinois Press, 1999), p. 32

6 Hicks, p. 34

CHAPTER 5

1 Derek Taylor, *World Countdown News*, July 1967.
2 Lesh, p. 105
3 Selvin, Joel, *Summer of Love: The Inside Story of LSD, Rock & Roll, Free Love and High Times in the Wild West* (New York, Dutton, 2004), p. 124
4 Paul Grein's sleeve notes for *The Mamas and Papas Complete Anthology* (MCA, 2004)
5 Nelson, in Miller, Jim (Ed.), *The Rolling Stone Illustrated History of Rock & Roll* (London, Picador, 1981), p. 234
6 Taylor, *World Countdown News*, July 1967
7 Ibid.
8 Ibid.
9 Porter, Lewis, *John Coltrane: His Life and Music* (Ann Arbor, University of Michigan Press, 1999), p. 209
10 Rogan, Johnny, *Byrds: Requiem for a Timeless Flight* (Bury St Edmunds, Rogan House, 2012), pp. 28–9
11 Rogan, p. 94
12 Lesh, p. 130
13 Ibid.
14 Lesh, p. 136
15 Greenfield, Robert, *Dark Star: An Oral Biography of Jerry Garcia* (New York, Morrow, 1996), p. 128

CHAPTER 6

1 Mekas, Jonas, *Film Culture*, issue 43, winter 1966
2 Miller, Leta E. and Lieberman, Fredric, *Lou Harrison: Composing a World* (Oxford, Oxford University Press, 1998), p. 45
3 Gropius, Walter (Ed.), *The Theater of the Bauhaus* (Middletown, CN, Wesleyan University Press, 1961), pp. 29–30

4 Scott, Felicity D., *Architecture or Techno-utopia: Politics after Modernism* (Cambridge, MA, MIT Press, 2007), p. 192
5 Scott, p. 194
6 Scott, p. 191
7 Miller and Lieberman, p. 45
8 Perry, p. 64
9 Perry, p. 172
10 Interview with Michelle Kuo, *Artforum*, May 2008
11 Bernstein, p. 43
12 Kostelanetz, p. 74
13 Ibid.
14 Bernstein, p. 238
15 Kostelanetz, p. 74
16 Graham, p. 202
17 *Artforum*, May 2008
18 Greenfield, p. 89
19 Bockris, p. 295
20 Bockris, p. 293
21 *Artforum*, May 2008
22 Scott, p. 189
23 Scott, p. 315
24 Lyric to the Fantastic Zoo's 'Light Show'
25 Scott, p. 189
26 Gropius, p. 88
27 Graham, p. 277
28 Ibid.
29 Grunenberg, Christoph and Harris, Jonathan, *Summer of Love: Psychedelic Art, Social Crisis and Counterculture in the 1960s* (Liverpool, Liverpool University Press, 2005), p. 291
30 *International Times*, issue 9, p. 2
31 Huxley, p. 19
32 http://theboweryboys.blogspot.co.uk, 4 December 2009
33 Scott, p. 198

CHAPTER 7

1 Eisen, Jonathan (Ed.), *The Age of Rock: Sounds of the American Cultural Revolution* (Vintage Books, New York, 1969), p. 67
2 Marks, J. (Ed.), *Rock and Other Four Letter Words: Music of the Electric Generation* (New York, Bantam Books, 1968), p. 19
3 Wolfe, p. 238
4 Wolfe, p. 239
5 Wolfe, p. 240
6 Perry, p. 122
7 http://www.diggers.org
8 Grogan, p. 288
9 Grogan, p. 323
10 Goldstein, pp. 120–1
11 Goldstein, p. 121
12 Grogan, p. 324
13 Ibid.
14 Perry, p. 174
15 Lesh, p. 97
16 Selvin, p. 343
17 Dalton, p. 132
18 Dalton, p. 149
19 Dougan, John, 'Objects of Desire: Canon Formation and Blues Record Collecting', *Journal of Popular Music Studies*, vol. 18, issue 1 (2006), p. 58
20 *International Times*, issue 161, p. 17
21 Gilroy, Paul, *The Black Atlantic: Modernity and Double Consciousness* (London, Verso, 1993), p. 49
22 Porter, p. 211
23 Kofsky, Frank, *Black Nationalism and the Revolution in Music* (New York, Pathfinder Press, 1970), p. 56
24 http://www.soul-patrol.com/funk/chambers.htm
25 Ibid.
26 Bangs, Lester, *Phonograph Record*, June 1973
27 Ibid.
28 Ibid.
29 Kofsky, p. 125

CHAPTER 8

1 Peck, p. 51
2 Didion, Joan, *The White Album* (London, Flamingo, 1993), p. 42
3 Sleeve notes to the Fugs' *Don't Stop! Don't Stop!* (Fugs Records/Ace, 2008)
4 Bangs, Lester, *Mainlines, Blood Feasts and Bad Taste* (Ed. John Morthland) (London, Serpent's Tail, 2003), p. 218
5 Ibid.
6 Quoted in Turner, Fred, *From Counterculture to Cyberculture: Stewart Brand, the Whole Earth Network, and the Rise of Digital Utopianism* (Chicago, University of Chicago Press, 2006), p. 78
7 Gordon, Alistair, *Spaced Out: Radical Environments of the Psychedelic Sixties* (New York, Rizzoli International, 2008), p. 285
8 Stevens, Jay, *Storming Heaven: LSD and the American Dream* (London, Paladin, 1989), p. 352
9 Stevens, p. 353
10 Stevens, pp. 352–3
11 Watts, p. 352
12 *Billboard*, 30.8.69
13 Peck, p. 180
14 Didion, p. 101
15 Bangs, p. 139

CHAPTER 9

1 *Wire* magazine, April 2003
2 MacDonald, Ian, *Revolution in the Head* (London, Pimlico, 1995), p. 77
3 Hicks, p. 110
4 Thomson, Elizabeth and Gutman, David, *The Lennon Companion* (London, Macmillan Press, 1987), p. 97

5 *The Times*, 27.12.1963

6 Thomson and Gutman, p. 99

7 Leary, Timothy, Metzner, Ralph and
  Alpert, Richard, *The Psychedelic Experience: A Manual Based on the Tibetan
  Book of the Dead*, p. 12 (http://www.
  erowid.org/)

8 Bernstein, p. 54

9 Wenner, Jann, *Lennon Remembers*
  (London, Penguin, 1972), p. 76

10 Jordan, p. 116

11 Wenner, p. 77

12 Miles, Barry, *Ginsberg: A Biography*
   (London, Viking, 1989), p. 304

13 *Rolling Stone*, issue 512, November–
   December 1987

14 Watts, p. 347

15 Ibid.

16 Mellers, Wilfred, *Twilight of the Gods:
   The Beatles in Retrospect* (London,
   Faber and Faber, 1973), p. 86

17 MacDonald, p. 204

18 Eisner, p. 23

19 Beatles, *The Beatles Anthology* (London,
   Cassell and Co., 2000), p. 179

20 Rose, Barbara, quoted in Branden,
   W. Joseph, 'White on White', *Critical
   Enquiry*, vol. 27, no. 1 (autumn 2000), p.
   92, footnote 7

21 Thomson and Gutman, p. 247

CHAPTER 10

1 Green, Jonathon, *Days in the Life:
  Voices from the English Underground
  1961–1971* (Heinemann, London, 1988),
  p. 140

CHAPTER 11

1 Cavanagh, John, *The Piper at the Gates
  of Dawn* (New York, Continuum, 2003),
  p. 52

2 Huxley, p. 30

3 www.sydbarrett.com/news/Irregular-
  Head_June10.pdf

CHAPTER 12

1 Whiteley, Nigel, *Pop Design: From Modernism to Mod* (London, Design Council, 1987), p. 104

2 Dalton, David, *Rolling Stone*, 3.5.69

3 Huxley, p. 21

CHAPTER 13

1 'Banned Records – 1967', R44/670/1
  (BBC)

2 Ibid.

3 Ibid.

4 Ibid.

5 Ibid.

6 'Censorship of Programmes: Songs,
  Records and Music 1960–70', R34/1249
  (BBC)

7 Ibid.

8 Ibid.

9 Ibid.

10 Ibid.

11 Ibid.

12 'Pop Music Policy – 1964–69',
   R19/1530/2 (BBC)

13 R34/1249 (BBC)

14 Ibid.

15 Bilyeu, Cook and Hughes, p. 143

CHAPTER 14

1 Huxley, p. 38

2 Russell, Dave, *Popular Music in England, 1840–1914* (Manchester, MUP,
  1997), p. 108

3 http://www.angelfire.com/home/tell-
  everyone/RONNIELANEINTERVIEW-
  byAlanVorda.html

4 Kift, Dagmar, *The Victorian Music Hall:
  Culture, Class and Conflict* (Cambridge,
  Cambridge University Press, 1996), p. 49

5 Russell, p. 126
6 Kift, p. 37
7 Kift, p. 38
8 Fletcher, Geoffrey, *London's Pavement Pounders* (London, Hutchinson, 1967), p. 11
9 Fletcher, p. 68
10 Fletcher, p. 94
11 Munthe, Axel, *Memories and Vagaries* (London, John Murray, 1898), p. 12
12 Kift, p. 37
13 Ibid.
14 Kift, p. 47
15 Kift, p. 50
16 Connolly, Cyril, *The Evening Colonnade* (New York, Harcourt Brace Jovanovich, 1975), p. 134
17 Kift, p. 42
18 Kift, p. 43
19 Ibid.
20 Priestley, J. B., *Essays of Five Decades* (London, Heinemann, 1969), p. 293
21 Kift, p. 61
22 Ibid.

CHAPTER 15

1 Gorman, Paul (Ed.), *In Their Own Write: Adventures in the Music Press* (London, Sanctuary Publishing, 2001), pp. 41–2
2 Boym, Svetlana, *The Future of Nostalgia* (New York, Basic Books, 2001), p. 54
3 Ibid.
4 Blunden, Edmund, *Cricket Country* (London, The Imprint Society, 1945), p. 48
5 Owen, Wilfred, 'The Send-Off', in *The Works of Wilfred Owen* (Ware, Hertfordshire, the Wordsworth Poetry Library, 1994), p. 19
6 Gray, Nicolete, *Nineteenth Century Ornamented Typefaces* (London, Faber and Faber, 1976), p. 8

7 Gray, p. 9
8 Gray, p. 93
9 Gray, p. 108
10 Gray, p. 138
11 Gray, p. 109
12 Ibid.
13 Ibid.
14 Thomas, Dylan, 'The Festival Exhibition 1951', in *Quite Early One Morning* (London, J. M. Dent, 1968), p. 55
15 Thomas, p. 51
16 Banham, Mary and Hillier, Bevis, *A Tonic to the Nation: The Festival of Britain 1951* (London, Thames & Hudson, 1976), p. 131
17 Ibid.
18 Banham and Hillier, p. 132
19 Banham and Hillier, p. 189
20 Thomas, p. 57
21 Banham and Hillier, p. 196
22 Ibid.
23 Whiteley, p. 35
24 Thomas, p. 56
25 Bruce Lacey interviewed by Gillian Whiteley, C466/99 ('National Life Stories: Artists' Lives' at http://sounds.bl.uk/), p. 73
26 Thomas, p. 52
27 Fletcher, Geoffrey, *The London Nobody Knows* (London, Penguin, 1965), p. 20
28 Fletcher, p. 36
29 Fletcher, p. 64
30 Ibid.
31 Fletcher, p. 98
32 Fletcher, pp. 69–70
33 Fletcher, p. 118
34 Fletcher, *London's Pavement Pounders*, p. 58
35 Fletcher, *London's Pavement Pounders*, p. 11
36 Fletcher, *The London Nobody Knows*, p. 132
37 Thomas, p. 52

38 Boym, p. 50
39 Davies, Ray, *X Ray: The Unauthorised Autobiography* (New York, Overlook Press, 1996), p. 361
40 Barthes, Roland, *Mythologies* (London, Paladin, 1986), p. 12

CHAPTER 16
1 Boym, p. xv
2 Grahame, Kenneth, *The Golden Age* (New York, Signet, 1964), p. 22
3 Ibid.
4 Phillips, Robert (Ed.), *Aspects of Alice: Lewis Carroll's Dreamchild as Seen Through the Critics' Looking Glasses, 1865–1971* (London, Penguin, 1971), p. 406
5 Ibid.
6 Carroll, p. 34
7 Carroll, p. 204
8 Carroll, p. 221
9 Carroll, p. 255
10 Carroll, pp. 336–7
11 Carroll, p. 337
12 Ibid.
13 McWilliam, Rohan, 'Jonathan Miller's *Alice in Wonderland* (1966): A Suitable Case for Treatment', *Historical Journal of Film, Radio and Television*, 31.2.2011, p. 232
14 Carroll, pp. 65–6
15 Phillips, p. 414
16 McWilliam, p. 235
17 Bilyeu, Melinda, Cook, Hector and Hughes, Andrew Mon, *The Ultimate Biography of the Bee Gees: Tales of the Brothers Gibb* (London, Omnibus Press, 2000), pp. 189–90
18 Jones, p. 40
19 Jones, p. 42
20 Ibid.
21 Jones, p. 43

CHAPTER 17
1 Porter, p. 211
2 Sharman, Gopal, *Filigree in Sound: Form and Content in Indian Music* (London, Andre Deutsch, 1970), p. 118
3 Davies, pp. 275–6
4 Locke, Ralph P., in Bellman, Jonathan (Ed.), *The Exotic in Western Music* (Boston, MA, Northeastern University Press, 1998), p. 127
5 Cooke, Mervyn, '"The East in the West": Evocations of the Gamelan in Western Music', in Bellman, p. 258
6 Cooke, p. 260
7 Cooke, p. 259
8 Cooke, p. 262
9 Porter, p. 211
10 Sharman, p. 118
11 Shankar, p. 93
12 Shankar, p. 94
13 Shankar, p. 96
14 Shankar, p. 93
15 Cooke, p. 280

CHAPTER 18
1 Rank Organisation, *Look at Life: In Gear*, 12.3.67
2 Dorfles, Gillo, *Kitsch: The World of Bad Taste* (London, Studio Vista, 1969)
3 *NME*, interview with Keith Altham, 20.10.73
4 Connolly, p. 392
5 Connolly, p. 393
6 Huxley, p. 15
7 Perry, p. 276
8 Jones, p. 15

CHAPTER 19
1 Watts, p. 145
2 Shankar, p. 93
3 Hall, Claude and Hall, Barbara, *This Business of Radio Programming* (New

York, Billboard Publications, 1977), p. 169

4 Ryan, Susan Elizabeth, *Robert Indiana: Figures of Speech* (New Haven, Yale University Press, 2000), p. 205

5 Ryan, pp. 205–6

6 Ryan, p. 212

7 Ryan, p. 224

8 Whitman, Walt, *Leaves of Grass* (New York, Signet, 1955), p. 315

9 Watts, p. 146

BIBLIOGRAPHY

Aaronson, Bernard and Osmond, Humphry (Eds), *Psychedelics: The Uses and Implications of Hallucinogenic Drugs* (Cambridge, MA, Schenkman Publishing Company, 1970)

Bangs, Lester, *Mainlines, Blood Feasts and Bad Taste* (Ed. John Morthland) (London, Serpent's Tail, 2003)

Banham, Mary and Hillier, Bevis, *A Tonic to the Nation: The Festival of Britain 1951* (London, Thames & Hudson, 1976)

Barthes, Roland, *Mythologies* (London, Paladin, 1986)

Beatles, *The Beatles Anthology* (London, Cassell & Co., 2000)

Bedford, Sybille, *Aldous Huxley: A Biography. Vol. 2: 1939–1963* (London, Collins and Chatto & Windus, 1974)

Bellman, Jonathan (Ed.), *The Exotic in Western Music* (Boston, MA, Northeastern University Press, 1998)

Bernstein, David W. (Ed.), *The San Francisco Tape Music Center: 1960s Counterculture and the Avant-Garde* (Berkeley and Los Angeles, University of California Press, 2008)

Bilyeu, Melinda, Cook, Hector and Hughes, Andrew Mon, *The Ultimate Biography of the Bee Gees: Tales of the Brothers Gibb* (London, Omnibus Press, 2000)

Bockris, Victor, *Warhol* (London, Penguin, 1990)

Boym, Svetlana, *The Future of Nostalgia* (New York, Basic Books, 2001)

Braunstein, Peter and Doyle, Michael William (Eds), *Imagine Nation: The American Counterculture of the 1960s and '70s* (London, Routledge, 2002)

Carroll, Lewis, *Alice's Adventures in Wonderland and Through the Looking Glass* (London, Puffin Books, 1972)

Cavallo, Dominick, *A Fiction of the Past: The Sixties in American History* (New York, Palgrave, 1999)

Cavanagh, John, *The Piper at the Gates of Dawn* (New York, Continuum, 2003)

Chapman, Rob, *Syd Barrett. A Very Irregular Head* (Faber and Faber, 2010)

Cohen, Sidney, *The Beyond Within* (Atheneum, New York, 1964)

Connolly, Cyril, *The Evening Colonnade* (New York, Harcourt Brace Jovanovich, 1975)

Coyote, Peter, *Sleeping Where I Fall* (Washington DC, Counterpoint, 1999)

Dalton, David, *Janis* (London, Calder & Boyars, 1971)

Davies, Ray, *X Ray: The Unauthorised Autobiography* (New York, Overlook Press, 1996)

Didion, Joan, *The White Album* (London, Flamingo, 1993)

Durr, R. A., *Poetic Vision and the Psychedelic Experience* (New York, Syracuse University Press, 1970)

Eisen, Jonathan (Ed.), *The Age of Rock: Sounds of the American Cultural Revolution* (Vintage Books, New York, 1969)

Eisner, Betty Grover, *Remembrances of LSD Therapy Past* (2002); http://www.maps.org/images/pdf/books/remembrances.pdf

Fletcher, Geoffrey, *London's Pavement Pounders* (London, Hutchinson, 1967)

Fletcher, Geoffrey, *The London Nobody Knows* (London, Penguin, 1965)

Gardner, Hugh, *The Children of Prosperity: Thirteen Modern American Communes* (New York, St Martin's Press, 1978)

Gilroy, Paul, *The Black Atlantic: Modernity and Double Consciousness* (London, Verso, 1993)

Goldstein, Richard, *Reporting the Counter Culture* (London, Unwin Hyman, 1989)

Gordon, Alistair, *Spaced Out: Radical Environments of the Psychedelic Sixties* (New York, Rizzoli International, 2008)

Gorman, Paul (Ed.), *In Their Own Write: Adventures in the Music Press* (London, Sanctuary Publishing, 2001)

Graham, Bill and Greenfield, Robert, *Bill Graham Presents: My Life Inside Rock and Roll* (Cambridge, MA, Da Capo, 2004)

Grahame, Kenneth, *The Golden Age* (New York, Signet, 1964)

Gray, Nicolete, *Nineteenth Century Ornamented Typefaces* (Berkeley, CA, University of California Press, 1976)

Gray, Nicolette, *XIXth Century Ornamented Types and Title Pages* (London, Faber and Faber Limited, 1938)

Green, Jonathon, *Days in the Life: Voices from the English Underground 1961–1971* (London, Heinemann, 1988)

Greenfield, Robert, *Dark Star: An Oral Biography of Jerry Garcia* (New York, Morrow, 1996)

Grof, Stanislav, *LSD: Doorway to the Numinous* (Rochester, Park Street Press, 2009)

Grogan, Emmett, *Ringolevio: A Life Played for Keeps* (New York, New York Review of Books, 1990)

Gropius, Walter (Ed.), *The Theater of the Bauhaus* (Middletown, CN, Wesleyan University Press, 1961)

Grunenberg, Christoph and Harris, Jonathan, *Summer of Love: Psychedelic Art, Social Crisis and Counterculture in the 1960s* (Liverpool, Liverpool University Press, 2005)

Hall, Claude and Hall, Barbara, *This Business of Radio Programming* (New York, Billboard Publications, 1977)

Hicks, Michael, *Sixties Rock: Garage, Psychedelic and Other Satisfactions* (Chicago, University of Illinois Press, 1999)

Holms, Thom, *Electronic and Experimental Music: Technology, Music and Culture* (London, Routledge, 2008)

Johnson, Kim, *The Funniest One in the Room: The Lives and Legends of Del Close* (Chicago, Chicago Review Press, 2008)

Jones, Barbara, *The Unsophisticated Arts* (London, Architectural Press, 1951)

Kaprow, Allan, *Assemblages, Environments, and Happenings* (New York, Abrams, 1966)

Kift, Dagmar, *The Victorian Music Hall: Culture, Class and Conflict* (Cambridge, Cambridge University Press, 1996)

Koestler, Arthur, 'Return Trip to Nirvana'. In *Drinkers of Infinity: Essays 1955–1967* (London, Hutchinson, 1968)

Kofsky, Frank, *Black Nationalism and the Revolution in Music* (New York, Pathfinder Press, 1970)

Kostelanetz, Richard (Ed.), *Moholy-Nagy: Documentary Monographs in Modern Art* (New York, Praeger Publishing, 1970)

Kostelanetz, Richard, *The Theatre of Mixed Means* (London, Pitman Publishing, 1970)

Leary, Timothy, Metzner, Ralph and Alpert, Richard, *The Psychedelic Experience: A Manual Based on the Tibetan Book of the Dead* (New York, Citadel Press, 1992)

Lee, Martin A. and Shlain, Bruce, *The Complete Social History of LSD: The CIA, the Sixties, and Beyond* (New York, Grove Press, 1992)

Lesh, Phil, *Searching for the Sound: My Life with the Grateful Dead* (New York, Back Bay Books, 2005)

MacDonald, Ian, *Revolution in the Head* (London, Pimlico, 1995)

Mellers, Wilfred, *Twilight of the Gods: The Beatles in Retrospect* (London, Faber and Faber, 1973)

Miles, Barry, *Ginsberg: A Biography* (London, Viking, 1989)

Miller, Jim (Ed.), *The Rolling Stone Illustrated History of Rock and Roll* (London, Picador, 1981)

Miller, Leta E. and Lieberman, Fredric, *Lou Harrison. Composing a New World* (Oxford, Oxford University Press, 1998)

Moholy-Nagy, Lázló, *Vision in Motion* (Chicago, Paul Theobald and Company, 1965)

Munthe, Axel, *Memories and Vagaries* (London, John Murray, 1898)

Nin, Anaïs, *The Journals of Anaïs Nin. Volume 6: 1955–1966* (London, Quartet, 1979)

Oldham, Andrew Loog, *2Stoned* (London, Seeker and Warburg, 2002)

Oliver, Michael (Ed.), *Settling the Score: A Journey Through yhe Music of the 20th Century* (London, Faber and Faber, 1990)

Peck, Abe, *Uncovering the Sixties: The Life and Times of the Underground Press* (New York, Citadel Underground, 1991)

Perry, Charles, *The Haight-Ashbury: A History* (New York, Wenner Books, 2005)

Perry, Paul, *On the Bus: The Complete Guide to the Legendary Trip of Ken Kesey and the Merry Pranksters and the Birth of the Counterculture* (New York, Thunder's Mouth Press, 1990)

Phillips, Robert (Ed.), *Aspects of Alice: Lewis Carroll's Dreamchild as Seen Through the Critics' Looking Glasses, 1865–1971* (London, Penguin, 1971)

Porter, Lewis, *John Coltrane: His Life and Music* (Ann Arbor, University of Michigan Press, 1999)

Priestley, J. B., *Essays of Five Decades* (London, Heinemann, 1969)

Rogan, Johnny, *Byrds: Requiem for a Timeless Flight* (Bury St Edmunds, Rogan House, 2012)

Russell, Dave, *Popular Music in England: 1840–1914* (2nd edn) (Manchester, MUP, 1997)

Ryan, Susan Elizabeth, *Robert Indiana.*

Figures of Speech (New Haven, Yale University Press, 2000)

Salter, Chris, *Entangled: Technology and the Transformation of Performance* (Cambridge, MA, MIT Press, 2010)

Scott, Felicity D., *Architecture or Techno-utopia: Politics after Modernism* (Cambridge, MA, MIT Press, 2007)

Sculatti, Gene and Seay, Davin, *San Francisco: Psychedelic Music Trip 1965–1968* (London, Sidgwick and Jackson, 1985)

Selvin, Joel, *Summer of Love: The Inside Story of LSD, Rock and Roll, Free Love and High Times in the Wild West* (New York, Dutton, 1994)

Shankar, Ravi, *My Music, My Life* (London, Jonathan Cape, 1970)

Sharman, Gopal, *Filigree in Sound: Form and Content in Indian Music* (London, André Deutsch, 1970)

Stafford, Peter and Golightly, Bonnie, *LSD – The Problem-Solving Psychedelic* (New York, Award Books, 1967)

Stevens, Jay, *Storming Heaven: LSD and the American Dream* (London, Paladin, 1989)

Strausbaugh, John, *Rock Till You Drop* (London, Verso, 2001)

Thomas, Dylan, *Quite Early One Morning* (London, J. M. Dent, 1968)

Thomson, Elizabeth and Gutman, David, *The Lennon Companion* (London, Macmillan Press, 1987)

Turner, Fred, *From Counter Culture to CyberCulture: Stewart Brand, the Whole Earth Network, and the rise of Digital Utopianism* (Chicago, University of Chicago Press, 2006)

Unterberger, Richie, *Unknown Legends of Rock 'n' Roll* (San Francisco, Miller Freeman Books, 1998)

Watts, Alan, *In My Own Way: An Autobiography* (London, Jonathan Cape, 1973)

Watts, Alan, *This Is It: And Other Essays* (New York, Collier, 1958)

Wenner, Jann, *Lennon Remembers* (London, Penguin, 1972)

Whiteley, Nigel, *Pop Design: From Modernism to Mod* (London, Design Council, 1987)

Wolfe, Tom, *The Electric Kool-Aid Acid Test* (London, Weidenfield and Nicolson, 1969)

Youngblood, Gene, *Expanded Cinema* (1970); http://www.vasulka.org/Kitchen/PDF_ExpandedCinema/book.pdf

JOURNAL ARTICLES

Branden, W. Joseph, 'White on White', *Critical Enquiry*, vol. 27, no. 1 (autumn 2000), pp. 90–121

Cuncliffe, John W., 'Italian Prototypes of the Masque and Dumb Show', *PMLA*, vol. 22, no. 1 (1907), pp. 140–56

Dougan, John, 'Objects of Desire: Canon Formation and Blues Record Collecting', *Journal of Popular Music Studies*, vol. 18, issue 1 (2006), pp. 40–65

Eskilson, Stephen, 'Thomas Wilfred and Intermedia: Seeking a Framework for Lumia', *Leonardo*, vol. 36, no. 1 (2003), pp. 65–8

Jacobs, Adam, 'Acid Redux: Revisiting LSD Use in Therapy', *Contemporary Justice Review*, vol. 11, no. 4 (2008), pp. 427–39

Jordan Jnr, G. Ray, 'LSD and Mystical Experiences', *Journal of Bible and Religion*, vol. 31, no. 2 (1963), pp. 114–23

McWilliam, Rohan, 'Jonathan Miller's *Alice in Wonderland* (1966): A Suitable Case for Treatment', *Historical Journal of*

Film, Radio and Television, 31.2.2011, pp. 229–46

Monod, David, '"Ev'rybody's Crazy 'Bout the Doggone Blues": Creating the Country Blues in the Early Twentieth Century', *Journal of Popular Music Studies*, vol. 19, issue 2 (2006), pp. 179–214

Novak, Steven J., 'LSD before Leary: Sidney Cohen's Critique of 1950s Psychedelic Drug Research', *Isis*, vol. 88, no. 1 (1997), pp. 87–110

Peacock, Kevin, 'Instruments to Perform Colour Music: Two Centuries of Technological Experimentation', *Leonardo*, vol. 21, no. 4 (1988), pp. 397–406

Polt, Harriett R. and Sandall, Roger, 'Outside the Frame', *Film Quarterly*, vol. 14, no. 3 (University of California Press, spring 1961)

Rainer, Yvonne, 'Interview with Anna Halprin', *Tulane Drama Review*, vol. 10, no. 2 (winter 1965), pp. 142–67

Reck, David R., *Asian Music*, vol. 16, no. 1, pp. 83–149 (University of Texas Press, 1985)

Sessa, B., 'Is It Time to Revisit the Role of Psychedelic Drugs in Enhancing Human Creativity?' *Journal of Psychopharmacology*, vol. 22, no. 8 (2008), pp. 821–7

Suvin, Darko, 'Reflection of Happenings', *The Drama Review*, vol. 14, no. 3 (1970), pp. 125–44

Zurbrugg, Nicholas, *Installation Art – Essence and Existence* (Australian Perspecta, Art Gallery of New South Wales, 1991)

INDEX

Abdabs, the, 334
Accent, the: 'Red Sky at Night', 382
Ace of Cups, 132–3
acid, *see* LSD
Acid Tests: aftermath, 83, 178, 252; audiences, 72–4, 78–9; first events, 68–9, 71–2, 193; Graduation Ceremony, 69, 77; Grateful Dead, 70, 72, 74, 78–9, 168, 184; masque play, 73, 292; origins, 272; participants, 69–71, 75–7, 299, 571; prototype, 71; Trips Festival, 74–5, 77–8; venues, 69
Action, the: 'Shadows and Reflections', 397
action painting, 50, 60, 583
Addrisi, Dick and Don: 'Time for Living', 144
Adler, Lou, 142, 143
A440: 'Torture', 125
Aguilar, Dave, 575
Alan Bown Set, 512–13; 'Toyland'/'Technicolour Dreams', 512–13
Alberts, the, 477, 564
Aldcroft, Richard, 58, 184
Alder, Twink: '10,000 Words in a Cardboard Box', 396
Alexander, Gary, 145
Alice in Wonderland: bad-trip scenarios, 505–6; 'Beautiful Soop' lyrics, 179; childhood theme, 501–2; 'I Am the Walrus' allusions, 302; 'Lucy in the Sky with Diamonds' lyrics, 294; 'Magic Potion' lyrics, 400; psychedelic subtext, 504, 506; songs inspired by, 504–5; teatime, 288; testing herself, 26; 'White Rabbit' lyrics, 90–1
Alice in Wonderland (BBC TV), 506–9
Alice Through the Looking Glass: bad-trip scenarios, 505–6; Festival of Britain tableau, 469, 504; 'Lucy in the Sky with Diamonds' lyrics, 295; psychedelic subtext, 504, 506; songs inspired by, 504–5
Alk, Howard, 107–8
Allen, Daevid: career, 313–16; deported, 320; Gong, 209, 324; LSD experience, 313; Mr Head, 317; Soft Machine, 313, 317–20, 328; *Live*, 315; 'Why Are We Sleeping?', 321
Allen Pound's Get Rich: 'Searching for My Love', 382
Alpert, Richard, 28–9, 41, 105–6, 145; *The Psychedelic Experience*, 272; *Psychedelic Review*, 32
Altamont, 128, 160, 249–54
American Breed, the: 'Bend Me, Shape

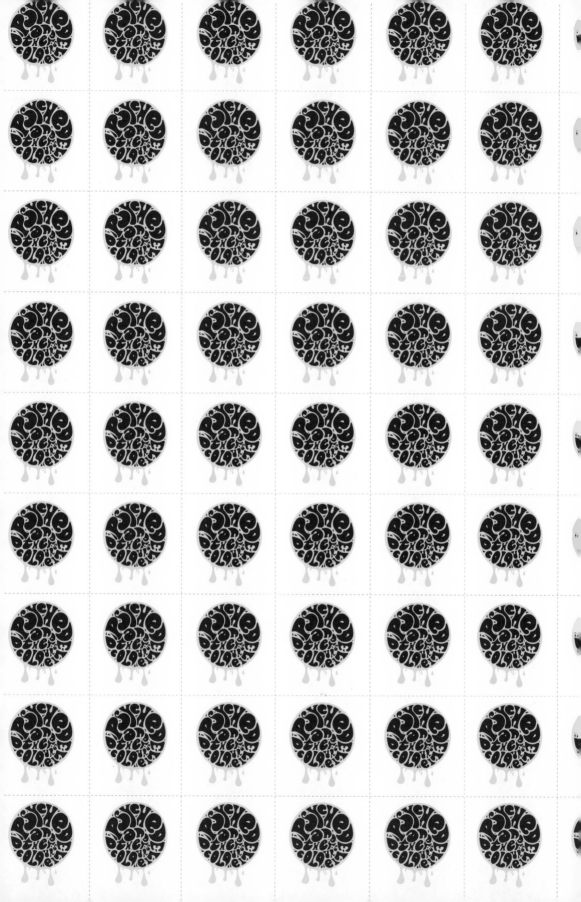